Gut and the Liver

Gut and the Liver

EDITED BY

H. E. Blum

Abteilung Innere Medizin II
Medizinische Klinik und Poliklinik
Universitätsklinikum Freiburg
Hugstetter Str. 55
D-79106 Freiburg
Germany

J. Ch. Bode

Abteilung Innere Medizin I
Zentrum für Innere Medizin
Robert-Bosch-Krankenhaus
Auerbachstr. 110
D-70376 Stuttgart
Germany

Ch. Bode

Abteilung für Ernährungsphysiologie
Institut 140
Universität Hohenheim
Garbenstr. 28
D-70593 Stuttgart
Germany

R. B. Sartor

Department of Medicine
Division of Digestive Diseases
CB#7080
Burnett Womack Building
Chapel Hill, NC 72599-7080
USA

Proceedings of the Falk Symposium 100 (Part III of the Intestinal Week in the Black Forest 1997) held in Freiburg, Germany, May 29–30, 1997

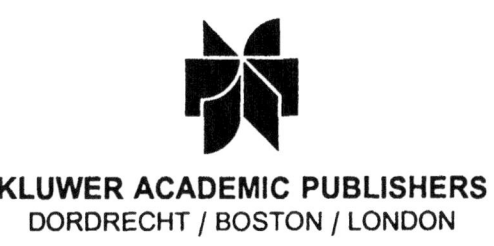

KLUWER ACADEMIC PUBLISHERS
DORDRECHT / BOSTON / LONDON

Distributors

for the United States and Canada: Kluwer Academic Publishers, PO Box 358, Accord Station, Hingham, MA 02018-0358, USA

for all other countries: Kluwer Academic Publishers Group, Distribution Center, PO Box 322, 3300 AH Dordrecht, The Netherlands

A catalogue record for this book is available from the British Library

ISBN 0–7923–8736–8

Contents

List of Principal Authors   ix

Preface   xiii

**SECTION I: THE 'MILIEU EXTERIEUR' AND
            'MILIEU INTERIEUR' IN THE GUT:
            CONFRONTATION AND COOPERATION**

1   Intestinal microflora: control and overgrowth
    Onderdonk AB   3

2   The intestinal immune system
    Marth T, Zeitz M   12

**SECTION II: GASTROINTESTINAL PERMEABILITY AND
             TRANSLOCATION**

3   The intestinal permeability barrier – what is measured,
    what does it mean?
    Gabe S, Jacob M, Bjarnason I   31

4   Bacterial translocation
    Berg RD   47

5   Intestinal permeability in inflammatory bowel disease
    Gardiner KR   61

6   Intestinal absorption of small particles
    Seifert J   75

SECTION III: BILE ACID, AMINO ACID AND DRUG METABOLISM – IT'S NOT ONLY THE LIVER, IT MAY BE THE GUT

7   State of the Art Lecture: Bile acids and intestinal bacteria: peaceful coexistence versus deadly warfare
AF Hofmann, Hagey LR   85

8   Gastric first-pass metabolism of alcohol: interaction with ammonia and associated gastritis
Lieber CS   104

9   Ethanol oxidation and acetaldehyde production by colonic microbes
Salaspuro M, Jokelainen K, Nosova T   124

10   Adaptation of liver cell function to enteral resorption: role of liver cell hydration
Häussinger D, Schliess F, Kurz A-K, Warskulat U, Heinrich S, Wettstein M, vom Dahl S   134

11   Amino acid metabolism in the gut
Plauth M, Roske A-E   153

12   Drug metabolism in the intestinal wall
Klotz U   163

13   The role of gut bacteria in drug metabolism
Bauer TM   177

SECTION IV: GUT-DERIVED BACTERIAL TOXINS AND LIVER INJURY

14   How bacterial toxins affect the intestinal mucosa: molecular mechanism of the action of *Clostridium difficile* toxins
Aktories K   185

15   Acute and chronic endotoxaemia: effects on hepatic neutrophil influx and respiratory burst
Spitzer JA   195

16   Experimental liver injury: the role of lipopolysaccharides and cytokines
Wendel A, Leist M, Gantner F, Künstle G   203

17   Endotoxin, Kupffer cells and alcoholic liver injury
      Thurman RG, Bradford BU, Knecht KT, Iimuro Y,
      Arteel GE, Yin M, Connor HD, Wall C, Raleigh JA,
      v. Frankenberg M, Adachi Y, Forman DT, Brenner D,
      Kadiiska M, Mason RP   222

18   Hepatic injury and biliary tract diseases associated with
      small intestinal bacterial overgrowth
      Sartor RB, Lichtman SN   241

19   Endotoxaemia in chronic hepatitis and cirrhosis:
      epiphenomenon or of pathological relevance?
      Fukui H, Tsujita S, Matsumoto M, Kitano H, Hoppou K,
      Morimura M, Takaya A, Okamoto S, Tsujii T, Bode Ch,
      Bode JCh   251

20   Endotoxaemia and disseminated intravascular
      coagulation in cirrhosis
      Violi F, Basili S, Ferro D   263

21   The role of gut-derived bacterial toxins (endotoxin) for
      the development of alcoholic liver disease in man
      Bode Ch, Schäfer C, Bode JCh   281

22   Endotoxaemia and cholestasis
      Walter E   299

      **SECTION V: GASTROINTESTINAL DYSFUNCTION IN
                  LIVER DISEASE**

23   Altered gastrointestinal motility in chronic liver disease
      Zetterman RK   307

24   Portal hypertensive intestinal vasculopathy
      Viggiano TR   316

25   Role of lipopolysaccharide and inducible nitric oxide
      synthase in gastrointestinal and hepatic disease: actions
      of selective inhibition of iNOS on microvascular integrity
      in the gut and liver
      Whittle BJR, Evans SM, László F   324

26   Bacterial overgrowth in the small intestine in chronic liver
      disease
      Casafont F, Martin L, Pons-Romero F   332

SECTION VI: SPONTANEOUS BACTERIAL PERITONITIS IN CIRRHOTICS

27   Spontaneous bacterial peritonitis: incidence, diagnosis
     and clinical course
     Ochs A   341

28   Treatment and prophylaxis of spontaneous bacterial
     peritonitis
     Rimola A, Navasa M, Rodés J   354

SECTION VII: LIVER INJURY IN PATIENTS WITH DISEASES OF THE GASTROINTESTINAL TRACT

29   Haemochromatosis: a defect in gut transport leads to
     liver injury
     Stremmel W, Smolarek C, Gehrke S   365

30   Liver and biliary abnormalities in ulcerative colitis and
     Crohn's disease
     Wiesner RH   381

31   Liver abnormalities in coeliac disease
     Jacobsen MB   398

32   Primary sclerosing cholangitis: new therapeutic strategies
     Stiehl A, Benz C, Sauer P, Theilmann L   401

33   Jejunoileal bypass: an unintended model of steatohepatitis
     (NASH syndrome) in humans
     Kaminski DL   406

     Index   417

List of Principal Authors

K Aktories
Institut für Pharmakologie und
  Toxikologie
Albert-Ludwigs-Universität Freiburg i.
  Br.
Hermann-Herder-Str. 5
D-79104 Freiburg
Germany

TM Bauer
Abteilung Innere Medizin II
Medizinische Klinik und Poliklinik
Universitätsklinikum Freiburg
Hugstetter Str. 55
D-79106 Freiburg
Germany

RD Berg
Department of Microbiology and
  Immunology
Louisiana State University Medical
  School
Louisiana State University Medical
  Center–Shreveport
Shreveport LA 71130
USA

I Bjarnason
Department of Medicine
King's College School of Medicine &
  Dentistry
Bessemer Road
London SE5 9PJ
UK

HE Blum
Abteilung Innere Medizin II
Medizinische Klinik und Poliklinik
Universitätsklinikum Freiburg
Hugstetter Str. 55
D-79106 Freiburg
Germany

Ch Bode
Abteilung für Ernährungsphysiologie
Institut 140
Universität Hohenheim
Garbenstr. 28
D-70593 Stuttgart
Germany

J Ch Bode
Abteilung Innere Medizin I
Zentrum für Innere Medizin
Robert-Bosch-Krankenhaus
Auerbachstr. 110
D-70376 Stuttgart
Germany

F Casafont
Hepatogastroenterology Unit
University Hospital Marques de
  Valdecilla
E-39008 Santander
Spain

H Fukui
Third Department of Internal Medicine
Nara Medical University
840 Shijo-cho Kashihara-shi
Nara 634
Japan

KR Gardiner
Department of Surgery
The Queen's University of Belfast
Institute of Clinical Science
Grosvenor Road
Belfast BT12 6BJ
UK

D Häussinger
Medizinische Universitätsklinik
Klinik für Gastroenterologie,
  Hepatologie und Infektiologie
Heinrich Heine Universität Düsseldorf
Moorenstrasse 5
D-40225 Düsseldorf
Germany

AF Hofmann
Division of Gastroenterology
Department of Medicine 0813
University of California, San Diego
9500 Gilman Drive
La Jolla, CA 92093-0813
USA

MB Jacobsen
Department of Gastroenterology
Østfold Sentralsykehus
N-1601 Fredrikstad
Norway

DL Kaminski
Department of Surgery
St Louis University
3635 Vista Ave at Grand Blvd
PO Box 15250
St Louis, MO 63110-0250
USA

U Klotz
Dr Margarete Fischer-Bosch Institut
  für Klinische Pharmakologie
Auerbachstr. 112
D-70376 Stuttgart
Germany

CS Lieber
VA Medical Center (151-2)
130 W Kingsbridge Road
Bronx, NY 10468
USA

T Marth
Innere Medizin II
Medizinische Klinik und Poliklinik
Universität des Saarlandes
D-66421 Homburg/Saar
Germany

A Ochs
Abteilung Innere Medizin II
Medizinische Klinik und Poliklinik
Universitätsklinikum Freiburg
Hugstetter Str. 55
D-79106 Freiburg
Germany

AB Onderdonk
Departments of Pathology and
  Medicine
Channing Laboratory
Brigham and Women's Hospital
Harvard Medical School
75 Francis Street
Boston, MA 02115
USA

M Plauth
IV Medizinische Klinik und Poliklinik
Klinikum Charité
Schumannstr. 20/21
D-10098 Berlin
Germany

J Rodés
Liver Unit
Hospital Clinic University of Barcelona
Villarroel 170
E-08036 Barcelona
Spain

M Salaspuro
Research Unit of Alcohol Diseases
University Central Hospital of
  Helsinki
Tukholmankatu 8F
SF-00290 Helsinki
Finland

RB Sartor
Department of Medicine
Division of Digestive Diseases
CB#7080
Burnett Womack Building
Chapel Hill, NC 72599-7080
USA

J Seifert
Chirurgie Forschung der Klinik für
  Allgemeine Chirurgie und
  Thoraxchirurgie der Universität Kiel
Michaelisstr. 5
D-24105 Kiel
Germany

JA Spitzer
Department of Physiology
Louisiana State University Medical
  Center
1901 Perdido Street
New Orleans, LA 70112
USA

A Stiehl
Department of Medicine GJ Unit
Bergheimer Str. 58
D-69115 Heidelberg
Germany

RW Stremmel
Department of Internal Medicine
University of Heidelberg
Bergheimer Str. 58
D-69115 Heidelberg
Germany

RG Thurman
Department of Pharmacology
CB# 7365 Mary Ellen Jones Building
The University of North Carolina at
   Chapel Hill
Chapel Hill, NC 27599-7365
USA

TR Viggiano
Gastroenterology and Internal
   Medicine
Mayo Clinic
200 First Street SW
Rochester, MN 55905
USA

F Violi
Policlinico Umberto I
Instituto di I Clinica Medica
Universita 'La Sapienza'
Viale del Policlinico
Roma
Italy

E Walter
Abteilung Innere Medizin II
Medizinische Klinik und Poliklinik
Universitätsklinikum Freiburg
Hugstetter Str. 55
D-79106 Freiburg
Germany

A Wendel
Fakultät für Biologie
Universität Konstanz
Postfach 5560-M 447
D-78467 Konstanz
Germany

BJR Whittle
The William Harvey Research
   Institute
Charterhouse Square
London, EC1M 6BQ
UK

RH Wiesner
Liver Transplantation
Mayo Clinic and Medical
   School
200 First Street SW
Rochester, MN 55905-0001
USA

M Zeitz
Innere Medizin II
Medizinische Klinik und Poliklinik
Universität des Saarlandes
D-66421 Homburg/Saar
Germany

RK Zetterman
University of Nebraska
Medical Center
600 42nd Street
Omaha, NE 68198-3332
USA

Preface

The Falk Symposium 100 was a milestone in the longstanding tradition of national and international scientific and clinical symposia organized by the Falk Foundation. The topics of these symposia traditionally encompass the whole spectrum of gastrointestinal as well as hepatobiliary diseases. For these diseases, the clinical as well as scientific aspects are presented by international authorities in the respective fields.

The Falk Symposium 100 comprehensively reviewed the physiological and pathophysiological interactions between the intestine and the liver as well as between intestinal and hepatic diseases. The book is divided into seven major sections:

(I)   The 'Milieu Exterieur' and 'Milieu Interieur' in the Gut: Confrontation and Cooperation;
(II)   Gastrointestinal Permeability and Translocation;
(III)   Bile Acid, Amino Acid and Drug Metabolism:
        It's not only the Liver, it may be the Gut;
(IV)   Gut Derived Bacterial Toxins and Liver Injury;
(V)   Gastrointestinal Dysfunction in Liver Disease;
(VI)   Spontaneous Bacterial Peritonitis in Cirrhotics;
(VII)   Liver Injury in Patients with Diseases of the Gastrointestinal Tract.

Apart from basic and experimental aspects of the interaction between the gut and the liver, novel clinical data demonstrating the significance of gut-derived bacterial toxins for the development of liver diseases and the effect of liver diseases on gastrointestinal functions are comprehensively discussed. Through state-of-the-art contributions of the speakers, the book summarizes in a unique way the highlights of the interactions between gut and liver at the molecular level as well as in clinical disease.

The Editors

Section I
The 'milieu exterieur' and 'milieu interieur' in the gut: confrontation and cooperation

1
Intestinal microflora: control and overgrowth

A. B. ONDERDONK

INTRODUCTION

The microbiota of the human intestine is one of the most complex ecosystems in nature. The terminal ileum and large intestine of humans harbours between 10^{10} and 10^{11} viable organisms per gram of lumen contents. Using classic taxonomic criteria it has been reported that over 300 separate phenotypes are present as part of the microbiological milieu[1-3]. These two facts define only the quantitative and qualitative dimensions of the intestinal ecosystem, however, and do not address the control mechanisms so important to determining which organisms are present and numerically dominant. One of the unfortunate aspects of modern microbiology is that little effort has been directed at understanding the complex ecosystem represented by the human large intestine in recent years. The best taxonomic studies were completed in the early 1970s, and little effort has been made to update the available data using the newer molecular biological techniques available today. With the exception of inflammatory bowel diseases, few studies characterizing the intestinal microbiota have been performed in the past decade. In order to discuss the control of normal microbiota, and the factors responsible for overgrowth of components of the microbiota, it is first important to consider the various elements normally associated with microbial growth within the gastrointestinal (GI) tract.

There are essentially three sets of factors responsible for determining the types and numbers of organisms present within the large intestine. These include: (1) host factors such as anatomy, secretions into the GI tract, peristalsis and local immune response; (2) dietary factors including both exogenous and endogenous components; and (3) bacterial-related factors including adhesins, bacteriocins, cofactors, synergistic relationships, antagonistic relationships and commensal relationships. Current research has revealed the influence of only a few of these factors on selected microbial species found within the lumen of the large intestine. A review of some of the described control mechanisms, and factors known to regulate the intestinal microbiota, are discussed below.

NORMAL MICROBIOTA OF THE LARGE INTESTINE

As stated above, the total number of viable organisms present within the large intestine approaches the physical limitations of the intestine (approximately 10^{11-12} colony-forming units (CFU)/g dry weight). Culture methods are thought to be able to account for 50–90% of the total bacterial population. For humans, the major genera present, and approximate numbers, are shown in Table 1. The major genera and species are all obligate anaerobes, with obligately anaerobic Gram-negative rods being numerically dominant. Facultative species including enterococci and members of the Enterobacteriaceae are present at a considerably lower concentration, often comprising less than 0.1% of the total viable bacterial population. At birth the GI tract is sterile; however, passage through the birth canal, followed by subsequent exposure to the environment, results in acquisition of a variety of species within a few hours after birth. During the first few weeks of life the oxidation–reduction potential (Eh) is relatively high (–50 mV), a diet consisting of protein and simple carbohydrates is most often consumed and facultative species such as lactobacilli, streptococci and various members of the Enterobacteriaceae dominate the microflora[1,3–5]. While there are clear differences between the intestinal microflora of breast-fed and formula-fed infants with respect to lactobacilli and bifidobacteria, the next major change in the intestinal microflora occurs when solid foods, including complex carbohydrates and fibre, become a regular part of the diet. The Eh decreases (–200 mV) and

Table 1   Major genera present in human large intestine

Genus/species	Log_{10} CFU/g[a]	Gram reaction and morphology

Bacteroides sp.
  vulgatus
  thetaiotaomicron
  ovatus
	10^{10-11}	Anaerobic Gram-negative rods

Fusobacterium sp.	10^9	Anaerobic Gram-negative rods

Eubacterium sp.
  contortum
  cylindroides
  lentum
	10^{10-11}	Anaerobic Gram-positive rods

Bifidobacterium sp.	10^{10}	Anaerobic Gram-positive rods
Lactobacillus sp.	10^9	Anaerobic Gram-positive rods
Peptostreptococcus sp.	10^{10}	Gram-positive coccus
Ruminococcus sp.	10^{10}	Gram-positive coccus

Clostridium sp.
  bifermentans
  perfringens
  ramosum
	10^{7-10}	Spore-forming Gram-positive rods

Enterococcus sp.	10^8	Gram-positive coccus

Enterobacteriaceae
  Escherichia coli
  Klebsiella
  Proteus
  Enterobacter
	10^8	Facultative Gram-negative rods

[a] Data from ref. 1.

Table 2 Factors influencing normal intestinal microflora

Factor	Population(s) affected
Eh	Obligate anaerobes
pH	All bacteria
Short-chain fatty acids	Enterobacteriaceae
Bile acids	Many species, particularly *Clostridium*
Nutrients	All bacteria
Competition for binding sites	????
Competition for nutrients	????
Host immune factors	????

short-chain fatty acids, such as butyrate, increase in concentration. Obligate anaerobes, particularly members of the genera *Bacteroides*, *Eubacterium* and *Fusobacterium*, become the dominant organisms, often referred to as the autochthonous microbiota. As the numbers of Gram-negative anaerobes increase, the concentration of the short-chain fatty acids increases and the numbers of coliforms decrease[1]. Once established, this microbial ecosystem is extremely stable over a broad range of conditions[6].

The normal intestinal microbiota can be visualized as a sphere containing many smaller spheres with the overall tendency to continuously increase in size. The large sphere, representing the total size of the viable bacterial population, is limited in size by external pressures such as available nutrients, pH, Eh, short-chain fatty acid concentrations, bile acids and host factors (see Table 2). Within this large sphere are many smaller spheres each representing a different bacterial phenotype. The size of each of the smaller spheres is controlled by the factors controlling the overall size of the total population, as well as phenotype-specific factors. These phenotype-specific factors are not well defined, but are thought to include competition for nutrients, competition for binding sites, production of bacteriocins and other toxic molecules, and use of cofactors produced by other bacterial species.

BASIC MICROBIAL CONTROL MECHANISMS

One of the major challenges for microbial ecologists is to define the mechanism(s) by which specific bacterial populations are controlled. This becomes even more difficult when multiple populations are growing within the same physical environment. The *in-vitro* growth system that best models the human large intestine microbiologically is a continuous-culture fermentation system. In such a system microorganisms grow at a rate determined by the rate at which new nutrients are added to the system and dead cells and spent growth medium are removed from the system. Traditional theory suggests that the total number of bacterial cells within a particular environment is determined by a specific limiting factor, such as a nutrient. This theory has been tested *in vitro* with a variety of microbial populations. However, the same factor cannot be growth-limiting for two bacterial populations within the same environment. The difficulty in defining such a system for multiple organisms growing simultaneously is determining what the limiting factors are for the various bacterial phenotypes[7,8], since this is often an important part of a basic control mechanism for a specific bacterial population.

Previous work indicates that among the major control mechanisms of microbial growth within the large intestine are Eh, pH, deconjugated bile acids, short chain fatty acids and hydrogen sulphide. The Eh is a measure of a liquid medium's propensity to take up or give up electrons versus a hydrogen half-cell. In general, the more dissolved oxygen in the environment, the higher (more positive potential) the Eh. Within the large intestine, obligate anaerobes usually do not grow well at Eh values of greater than –50 mV. The measured Eh for the large intestine of a variety of animal species is approximately –200 mV or lower. The tolerance for acidic or basic growth conditions is somewhat unique to the various bacterial phenotypes present within the GI tract. Certain organisms, such as lactobacilli and streptococci, grow well at pH values of 5.5 or lower. Other organisms, including many *Bacteroides* species, do not grow well at pH values of less than 6.0. When measured, the pH of the lumen contents of the GI tract is usually between 6.0 and 7.0. In addition to helping lower the pH of the large intestine, short-chain fatty acids, primary metabolites of obligate anaerobes, have been shown to be inhibitory to the growth of a variety of Enterobacteriaceae. Hydrogen sulphide is produced by several bacterial phenotypes and has been shown, *in vitro*, to inhibit the growth of other organisms apparently by inhibiting nutrient transport systems. Deconjugated bile acids are also potent antibacterial agents, even in relatively low concentrations[1]. While it is appealing to believe that growth inhibitors are responsible for control of microbial populations within the GI tract, the variable concentrations of such substances present over time suggest otherwise. It is likely that multiple factors are responsible for control of microbial populations, and that changes in one factor may be compensated for by co-dependent changes in other factors.

Our knowledge of other possible explanations for the types and numbers of bacteria present within the GI tract is often based on *in-vitro* studies or animal test systems. The relevance of such systems to the human condition is unknown in most instances. Among the most commonly cited factors explaining the presence or absence of a particular bacterial species or strain within a complex ecosystem is bacterial adherence. Experimental work using both gnotobiotic mice and continuous-culture methods has led to a mathematical model with which to test various assumptions[1]. Such models have led to the notion that strains with a superior ability to adhere within an environment are capable of replacing less adherent strains competing for the same adherence sites. Within the GI tract, however, the complexity of the physical environment provides an almost limitless number of adherence sites, ranging from the crypt epithelial cells, and surface mucopolysaccharides, to adhesion to other organisms attached to the underlying epithelial tissues. Although little information about the adherence characteristics of the normal microbiota has been generated since the 1980s, the importance of adherence for a number of intestinal pathogens, including *Vibrio cholerae*, *Salmonella* and *Shigella*, are well documented. Perhaps the best information available regarding control mechanisms within the human intestine comes from studies of the effect of dramatic alterations of the normal microbiota.

ALTERATIONS OF THE NORMAL MICROBIOTA

The intestinal microbiota is an important part of the health of the host. When the large intestinal microbiota is within the limits described as 'normal' it serves as a barrier to colonization by enteric pathogens and helps to recycle compounds such as bile acids via deconjugation and reabsorption. Presumably there is balance between the microbiota and the host immune system. However, when the microbiota becomes 'abnormal' a variety of clinical symptoms may occur. Although we cannot define 'normal' with precision, we do know that certain things will vastly alter the microbiota and lead to serious consequences for the host. In certain instances, such as *Clostridium difficile*-associated colitis or diarrhoea (CDAD), the sequence of events leading to disease has been well characterized. In other cases, such as ulcerative colitis or ileal pouchitis, the sequence of events is less clear.

Antibiotic-associated colitis

In the early 1970s the association between the use of broad-spectrum antibiotics and the development of severe pseudomembranous colitis was made. Subsequent research revealed that the cause of the disease was *Clostridium difficile*[9–13]. CDAD is now recognized as one of the major nosocomial infection problems within the hospital environment. Early research suggested that broad-spectrum antibiotics suppressed the normal intestinal microbiota, allowing the overgrowth of *C. difficile* and subsequent production of toxin(s) responsible for the clinical and pathological features of the disease. The data appeared to support microbial overgrowth as the mechanism by which disease occurred, and the causal association with antibiotic use was clearly established. However, a critical examination of the data revealed that antibiotics, such as ampicillin, which are rarely excreted via the large intestine in an active form, were most commonly associated with CDAD. Additional research in animals showed that metabolites of clindamycin (one of the antibiotics commonly associated with CDAD in early studies) lacking demonstrable antibacterial activity, were more active in provoking disease than the parent compound[14]. Moreover, quantitative culture of stool for *C. difficile*, from stool samples from patients with CDAD, rarely revealed this organism to be numerically dominant. The question that arises from these observations is whether the biological effect of antibiotics is directly on the microbiota or is an indirect effect of antibiotics on another control mechanism within the GI tract. It is also of interest to note that children and infant hamsters are both able to carry toxin-producing strains of *C. difficile* without apparent ill-effect[15]. It is possible that the effect of antibiotics is on bile acids, or other host factors, excreted into the GI tract which serve as important control mechanisms for clostridia[13,16,17].

Irrespective of the actual mechanism by which antibiotics contribute to the disease process in CDAD, it is clear that suppression of the normal intestinal microbiota provides a biological 'vacuum' that is often filled by undesirable organisms. An excellent example of this is the overgrowth of yeast in transplant and chemotherapy patients on long-term antibiotic prophylaxis.

7

Ileal pouch disease

An inflammatory condition associated with the surgical construction of an ileal reservoir for patients with ulcerative colitis, Crohn's disease and rarely for other purposes, has been described. Inflammation of the ileal pouch is commonly termed 'pouchitis' and refers to a constellation of symptoms and histopathological criteria[18] which can occur in up to 20% of patients following surgery. Because the characteristics lesions of this disease are similar to those noted for other inflammatory bowel diseases, a microbial involvement in the development of ileal pouch disease has been sought. Studies in our laboratory have been directed at assessing the potential microbiological involvement based on preliminary findings of bacteria within tissue biopsy specimens of patients with ileal pouchitis by electron microscopy. Tissue biopsy samples from patients with and without ileal pouches have been examined by both electron microscopic and quantitative microbiological culture techniques to determine the numbers and types of microorganisms closely associated with or within the tissue biopsy specimens[19]. Collaborative studies using the same biopsy materials have been performed in a blinded manner to determine whether patient specimens should be classified as pouchitis or non-pouchitis on the basis of both endoscopic and histopathological criteria[18]. Patient groups also included two patient control groups of non-pouch patients. The results of these studies indicated that microbiological and electron microscopic observations of microorganisms associated with pouch biopsy specimens were closely correlated. In addition, electron microscopic findings revealed certain unique features of ileal pouch patient tissues[20]. Microbiologically, it was noted that 82% of specimens yielded bacteria in detectable numbers. The total counts for facultatively anaerobic bacteria for samples from patients with pouchitis were significantly greater than for samples from patients in control groups. In addition, the number of samples from patients with normal pouches that did not contain obligate anaerobes was significantly less than from patients with pouchitis. The data suggested that no specific bacterial species was consistently associated with ileal pouchitis, but rather that ileal pouch disease might represent a significant imbalance of the intestinal microbiota which resulted in invasion of colonic tissues by a variety of bacteria capable of causing localized irritation.

The results of a study in which tissue biopsy specimens from the ileal pouches of patients were obtained in a longitudinal manner following surgery suggested that only a small percentage of patients have detectable numbers of bacteria closely associated with, or within, intestinal tissues at the time of surgery; however, most patient biopsy specimens had closely associated microorganisms within 6 weeks following surgery. The numbers of organisms present were generally less than 6.0 $\log_{10}$ CFU/g, which, according to our previous study, would be undetected by electron microscopy[21]. Little difference was noted in either the total aerobic or total anaerobic counts at the various sample times, irrespective of patient group. The qualitative data suggest that there are minor differences in the frequency with which specific bacterial species are isolated, with no apparent trend with respect to patient group. The one notable exception was the frequency of isolation for streptococci in pouchitis patients at the time of surgery.

The most unusual finding was the occurrence of *Escherichia coli* in a substantial number of specimens. Characterization of the *E. coli* strains from both pouchitis and non-pouchitis patients failed to reveal the presence of either eae or EAF elements commonly associated with enteropathogenic strains of *E. coli*.

The data, taken as an aggregate with previous studies, suggests that colonization of the mucosal epithelium with a variety of bacterial species is a common occurrence following ileal pouch construction. The finding of low levels of organisms within the tissues of these patients also appears to be normal both for patients who develop pouchitis and patients who remain symptom-free. The events which allow organisms to either grow within the tissues of pouchitis patients or enter the tissue in higher numbers remain to be elucidated. It may be that some perturbation of the normal colonization precedes the events leading to pouch inflammation. The absence of an essential control mechanism may be responsible for the changes in the microbiota in these patients.

Inflammatory bowel diseases

A variety of clinical conditions in which the primary tissue affected is the terminal ileum or large bowel, are classified as inflammatory bowel diseases (IBD). These include both Crohn's disease and ulcerative colitis. A great deal of effort has been directed at defining the aetiological mechanisms by which this inflammation occurs. Similar efforts have been directed at finding the actual initiators of the inflammatory process. Because the inflammatory process occurs within proximity to one of the largest naturally occurring microbial ecosystems[21,22], extensive inquiries into a microbiological aetiology have been made. Previous studies of an experimental model in guinea pigs simulating ulcerative colitis have clearly indicated that bacteria are causally involved in the initiating events[21-27], and have also identified a possible species, *Bacteroides vulgatus*, of interest for further study. These earlier studies also identified the important role of the host immune response to the development of IBD. Investigations with a variety of other animal model systems have implicated other bacteria or bacterial components, such as the peptidoglycan polysaccharides of Gram-positive organisms in the inflammatory process[28]. Current theory suggests that bacterial mediators of inflammation gain access to the underlying mucosal tissues via a variety of perturbations to the normal colonic microbiota. Once within the tissues, long-lived bacterial mediators provoke an inflammatory process. This process may include additional damage to the intestinal microbiota, thereby intensifying the disease state.

SUMMARY

The intestinal microbiota of the human large intestine is a complex ecological system governed by a multiplicity of environmental and host factors. The intact microbiota provides many benefits to the host, including colonization resistance, nutrient degradation and production of essential vitamins and cofactors. Alterations of the normal microbiota can be induced either by naturally occurring diarrhoeal diseases of known aetiology, surgical manipulations or by the use of broad-spectrum antibiotic agents. Once the microbial components of the GI tract have been altered, the possibility for more serious consequences such as the development of IBD become more likely. Current research using transgenic and knockout animals that spontaneously develop IBD clearly supports the role of bacteria in the development of the disease. Moreover, these experimental animals point to the importance of the host immune system in the development and continuation of the inflammatory process. Additional research into the growth and control mechanisms for the GI microbiota needs to be performed using the technological tools available today.

References

1. Hentges DJ. Human intestinal microflora in health and disease. New York: Academic Press; 1983.
2. Tannock GW. Normal microflora. London: Chapman & Hall; 1995.
3. Hill BS, Draser MJH. Human intestinal microflora. London: Academic Press; 1974.
4. Akhmed M [Microflora of the birth canal in normal labor and in the uncomplicated puerperium]. Pediatr Akush Ginekol 1978:53–4.
5. Evaldson G, Heimdahl A, Kager L, Nord CE. The normal human anaerobic microflora. Scand J Infect Dis Suppl. 1982;35:9–15.
6. Brunel A, Gouet P. Kinetics of the establishment of gastrointestinal microflora in the conventional new-born rat. Ann Microbiol (Paris). 1982;133:325–34.
7. Ross RA, Lee M-L, Delaney M, Onderdonk A. Use of continuous culture growth systems for modeling vaginal microflora behavior. Microecol Ther. 1995;23:16–17.
8. Onderdonk AB, Johnston J, Mayhew JW, Gorbach SL. Effect of dissolved oxygen and Eh on *Bacteroides fragilis* during continuous culture. Appl Environ Microbiol. 1976;31:168–72.
9. Bartlett JG, Onderdonk AB, Cisneros RL. Clindamycin-associated colitis in hamsters: protection with vancomycin. Gastroenterology. 1977;73:772–6.
10. Bartlett JG, Onderdonk AB, Cisneros RL, Kasper DL. Clindamycin-associated colitis due to a toxin-producing species of *Clostridium* in hamsters. J Infect Dis. 1977;136:701–5.
11. Bartlett JG, Moon N, Chang TW, Taylor N, Onderdonk AB. Role of *Clostridium difficile* in antibiotic-associated pseudomembranous colitis. Gastroenterology. 1978;75:778–82.
12. Bartlett JG, Chang TW, Gurwith M, Gorbach SL, Onderdonk AB. Antibiotic-associated pseudomembranous colitis due to toxin-producing clostridia. N Engl J Med. 1978;298:531–4.
13. Bartlett JG, Chang T, Taylor NS, Onderdonk AB. Colitis induced by *Clostridium difficile*. Rev Infect Dis. 1979;1:370–8.
14. Onderdonk AB, Brodasky TF, Bannister B. Comparative effects of clindamycin and clindamycin metabolites in the hamster model of antibiotic-associated colitis. J Antimicrob Chemother 1981;8:383–93.
15. Onderdonk AB, Bartlett JG. The biological and clinical significance of *Clostridium difficile*. Crit Rev Clin Lab Sci. 1981;13:161–72.
16. Cooperstock M, Riegle L, Woodruff CW, Onderdonk A. Influence of age, sex, and diet on asymptomatic colonization of infants with *Clostridium difficile*. J. Clin Microbiol. 1983;17:830–3.
17. Hirschhorn LR, Trnka Y, Onderdonk A, Lee ML, Platt R. Epidemiology of community-acquired *Clostridium difficile*-associated diarrhoea. J Infect Dis. 1994;169:127–33.
18. McLeod RS, Antonioli D, Cullen J *et al.* Histologic and microbiologic features of biopsy samples from patients with normal and inflamed pouches. Dis Colon Rectum. 1994;37:26–31.
19. Onderdonk AB, Dvorak AM, Cisneros RL *et al.* Microbiologic assessment of tissue biopsy samples from ileal pouch patients. J Clin Microbiol. 1992;30:312–17.
20. Dvorak AM, Onderdonk AB, McLeod RS *et al.* Axonal necrosis of enteric autonomic nerves in continent ileal pouches. Possible implications for pathogenesis of Crohn's disease [see comments]. Ann Surg. 1993;217:260–71.
21. Onderdonk AB, Bartlett JG. Bacteriological studies of experimental ulcerative colitis. Am J Clin Nutr. 1979;32:258–65.
22. Onderdonk AB, Hermos JA, Bartlett JG. The role of the intestinal microflora in experimental colitis. Am J Clin Nutr. 1977;30:1819–25.

23. Onderdonk AB. The carrageenan model for experimental ulcerative colitis. Prog Clin Biol Res. 1985;186:237–45.
24. Onderdonk AB, Cisneros RL, Bronson RT. Enhancement of experimental ulcerative colitis by immunization with *Bacteroides vulgatus*. Infect Immun. 1983;42:783–8.
25. Onderdonk AB, Bronson R, Cisneros R. Comparison of *Bacteroides vulgatus* strains in the enhancement of experimental ulcerative colitis. Infect Immun. 1987;55:835–6.
26. Onderdonk AB, Franklin ML, Cisneros RL. Production of experimental ulcerative colitis in gnotobiotic guinea pigs with simplified microflora. Infect Immun. 1981;32:225–31.
27. Onderdonk AB, Hermos JA, Dzink JL, Bartlett JG. Protective effect of metronidazole in experimental ulcerative colitis. Gastroenterology. 1978;74:521–6.
28. Onderdonk AB. Experimental models for ulcerative colitis. Dig Dis Sci. 1985;30:40–4S.

2
The intestinal immune system

T. MARTH and M. ZEITZ

INTRODUCTION

The mucosal immune system is exposed to a high and constant evolutionary pressure due to the influence of a complex antigenic array present at the surface of the gastrointestinal tract. The immune system of the gastrointestinal mucosa has therefore, not surprisingly, distinct structural and functional features as compared to the systemic immune system, and represents in many ways a separate immunological entity.

The mucosal immune system has a central role in dealing with potential pathogenic substances such as bacteria, viruses, parasites, dietary proteins and others. One major function of the intestinal immune system is to distinguish potentially pathogenic antigens from non-pathogenic antigens and physiological gut flora. Moreover, the gastrointestinal immune system differentiates between self and non-self. Thus, both mechanisms serve to recognize and protect against foreign antigens and ensure the integrity of the mucosal barrier[1].

Since most of the dietary antigens do not present a danger for the immune system, immunoregulatory mechanisms have evolved which prevent reactivity against most of the ingested dietary antigens. Accordingly, systemic T and B cell immune responses to an orally ingested antigen may be suppressed, a phenomenon known as 'oral tolerance'[2].

Although the majority of human pathogens enter the body across mucosal surfaces of the gastrointestinal, pulmonary, and genitourinary organs, relatively little is known about the induction, regulation, or importance of humoral immunity and cell-mediated immune responses at these mucosal sites. The importance of the best studied mucosal defence mechanism, the ability of secretory immunoglobulin A (sIgA) to prevent the attachment of microorganisms and toxins to the intestinal epithelium, has been demonstrated primarily by showing that levels of specific sIgA correlate better than systemic responses with protection against infection[3]. The contribution of sIgA secretion relative to systemic humoral immunity, or to mucosal or systemic cell-mediated responses in protection against a mucosal pathogen, however, is not known. It has been shown in prior work that more sIgA is produced than any other immunoglobulin isotype in the body, and that the number of lymphocytes present in the intestine is greater than that in all the systemic lymphoid organs combined, suggesting that the mucosal immune system is of major importance in protection against invading pathogens[3,4].

Taken together, oral antigens are capable of either stimulating or suppressing both mucosal immunity and systemic immune responses. The delicate balance of these functions is brought over by specifically evolved structures and functions of the mucosal immune system. The involved regulatory processes of antigen processing and presentation mainly occur at mucosal lymphoid sites specialized for the sampling and transport of luminal antigens, also defined by the acronyms MALT and GALT (mucosa-associated lymphoid tissues and gut-associated lymphoid tissues, respectively).

STRUCTURE OF THE GASTROINTESTINAL IMMUNE SYSTEM

Antigens can be taken up by different cells and structures of the inductive (or 'afferent') compartment of the mucosal lymphoid system. This part of the intestinal immune system encompasses the organized lymphoid tissues, i.e. the mucosal follicles. Stimulation of immunocompetent cells with orally administered antigens in the inductive immune compartment of the small intestine leads to the dissemination of these cells to other lymphoid sites and to intestinal effector tissues, the latter of which can also be described as diffuse lymphoid tissues. These structures consist, for example, of the lamina propria of the gastrointestinal mucosa and upper respiratory tract, and are the sites of the subsequent 'effector' antigen-specific sIgA antibody responses (Fig. 1).

Organized lymphoid tissues

Peyer's patches are lymphoepithelial structures in the small bowel which underlie the dome epithelium of the mucosa[5,6]. Peyer's patches present the primary areas of antigen uptake and antigen processing as well as the site of the generation of specific IgA immune responses. Many of the ingested antigens being taken up to the Peyer's patches are transported via the specialized M cells in the dome epithelium. The M cells (membranous cells) are flattened epithelial cells with abundant pinocytic vesicles but poorly developed brush borders, and a virtual lack of proteolytic structures, i.e. absence of antigen-processing machinery. The antigen is being taken up pinocytically into the M cells, vesically transported through the cell and released into the subepithelial 'dome' area[7]. In regard to non-protein antigens, it is noteworthy that only a part of the infectious organisms are transported through the M cells, probably depending on their surface virulence factors. In the dome area underlying the M cells, many cells expressing MHC class II molecules are located, such as macrophages, dendritic cells and B cells, all of which are capable of processing and subsequently presenting the antigen to T cells. The structure of the Peyer's patches is similar to peripheral lymphoid follicles: a follicular zone containing predominantly B cells surrounds the germinal centre in which differentiated B cells and activated T cells can be found. This is the initiation site of many of the immune responses[4,8].

Antigens may be taken up alternatively by intestinal epithelial cells which are found throughout in the epithelium of the small and large bowel. Newer studies

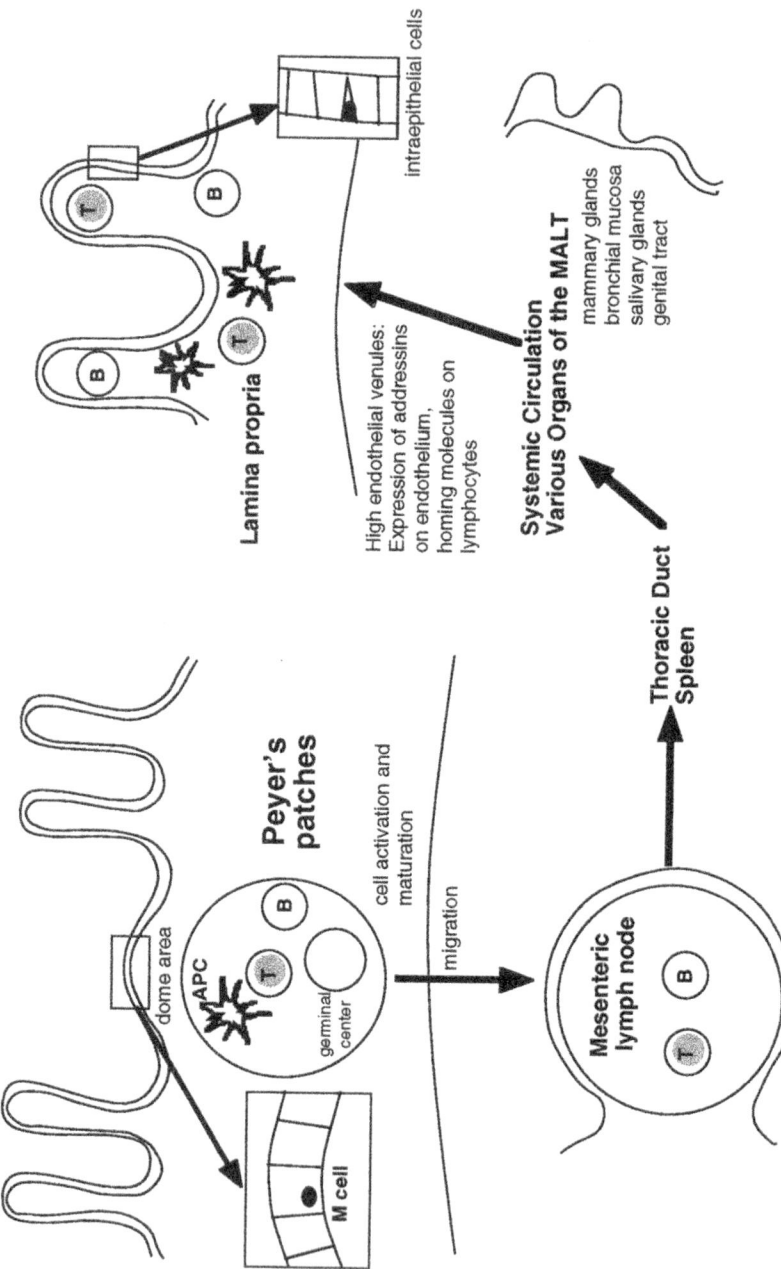

Figure 1 Structure of inductive and effector sites of the mucosal immune system

Labels within the figure:

intraepithelial cells

Lamina propria

High endothelial venules:
Expression of addressins
on endothelium,
homing molecules on
lymphocytes

**Systemic Circulation
Various Organs of the MALT**

mammary glands
bronchial mucosa
salivary glands
genital tract

**Peyer's
patches**

cell activation and
maturation

migration

dome area

APC

germinal
center

M cell

**Mesenteric
lymph node**

**Thoracic Duct
Spleen**

have shown that antigen processing and presentation is a function of intestinal epithelial cells; however, unlike antigen presentation by 'conventional' antigen-presenting cells such as MHC class II bearing macrophages, the presentation is mediated via 'atypical' MHC class I (MHC class I-like) molecules, CD1d, in conjunction with an accessory molecule designated as gp 180. In this model it is proposed that the antigen could be presented to $\gamma/\delta+$ CD8+ cells, e.g. to CD8 cells in the intra-epithelial compartment, although that remains to be formally proven. This process may be associated with an altered costimulatory signal to the T cells, and thus more likely result in a state of T cell unresponsiveness as referred to in detail in the following paragraphs[9-11].

Following the uptake of antigens in those lymphoid structures, there is typically a distribution and migration of activated B and T lymphocytes to other areas of the lymphoid tissues. After stimulation of T helper (Th) cells and IgA precursor B cells in the Peyer's patches by orally administered antigens, these cells exit the Peyer's patches, migrate to the mesenteric lymph nodes and then to the thoracic lymph duct. The cells subsequently enter the systemic circulation and some of them migrate back to mucosal effector sites, e.g. to the diffuse mucosal lymphoid tissue of the gastrointestinal tract, to salivary glands, to the bronchus-associated lymphoid tissue, to the mammary glands and to the female genital tract (Fig. 1). This migrational pattern is referred to as 'common mucosal immune system'. The mechanisms involved in regulating the so-called 'mucosal homing' are discussed below[12-14].

Diffuse mucosal lymphoid tissue

The diffuse mucosal lymphoid tissue in the intestine consists of two compartments, the intraepithelial cells (IEL) and the lamina propria lymphocytes (LPL).

The IEL population consists mainly of lymphocytes that are located above the basement membrane and between epithelial cells, and therefore could be capable of interacting with antigens that cross the epithelial barrier. IEL are mostly of the T cell lineage, i.e. are CD3-positive. Similar to peripheral T cells, the majority of the IEL T cells express the α/β and not the γ/δ T cell receptor; however, in contrast to peripheral T cells, more than 90% of the IEL T cells are CD8-positive. The IEL T cells are also characterized by specific phenotypic markers, such as the HML-1 activation antigen ($\beta7$ integrin, expressed on mucosal T cells) and express higher levels of memory T cell markers (e.g. CD45RO)[15-17]. In recent years evidence has accumulated suggesting that the α/β T cell receptor positive IEL T cell population is derived from the thymus, whereas another IEL T cell subset, the γ/δ positive and the α/β positive subset lacking the CD8 β chain, probably undergoes a thymus-independent development. Although the function of IEL T cells has not yet been clearly elucidated, recent work suggests that α/β T cell receptor positive IEL T cells have capabilities similar to cytotoxic and cytokine-secreting α/β T cells in the periphery. The γ/δ IEL T cells could be important in presenting heat-shock proteins or bacterial components[18].

While the majority of the lymphoid cells in the lamina propria compartment consists of lymphocytes, a considerable amount of non-lymphocytic cells is present in the lamina propria[19,20]. These cells include macrophages, dendritic cells, mast cells and eosinophils, some of which exhibit functions distinct from those of peripheral cells. In addition, the lamina propria contains natural killer cells which may exhibit cytotoxic functions in an antigen-unspecific fashion, since they are able to lyse their antibody-loaded targets after binding of the Fc portion. The lymphocyte population in the lamina propria consists mainly of B cells, which represent more activated B lymphocytes than the B cells in the peripheral blood. In contrast to the situation in the periphery, more than 80% of the B cells and plasma cells in the lamina propria produce IgA, around 15% produce IgM but only few B cells are capable of secreting IgG. While a greater proportion of the B and T cells in the lamina propria is derived from recirculated Peyer's patches cells, recent work suggests that some IgA-producing B cells may stem from the peritoneal cavity. About one-third of the lymphocytes in the lamina propria are T cells, most of which are CD4-positive and express the α/β T cell receptor. Moreover, many of the LPL T cells are characterized by higher expression of activation markers such as CD45RO, CD25 (IL-2 receptor α-chain), CD71 (transferrin receptor), and others. A smaller proportion of the LPL CD8 cells express, like the CD4 cells, the mucosal HML-1 antigen. Functionally, the LPL cells are capable of secreting cytokines in a fashion similar to peripheral memory cells, although their cytotoxic function *in vivo* has not yet been well documented[19].

FUNCTIONAL FEATURES OF THE MUCOSAL IMMUNE SYSTEM

Events following the uptake of antigen

The uptake of antigen can result in a secretory IgA response on the gastrointestinal mucosa, which then may prevent the absorption of further antigen. Alternatively, there may be a stimulation of systemic immune responses including the humoral and the cellular immune system following the uptake of the antigen, a situation required for a successful vaccination. In most cases, however, and for most antigens being taken up, oral antigen will induce a systemic tolerance encompassing the level of humoral and cellular immune responses[4].

Schematically, many of the orally administered antigens are taken up, as mentioned above, via the Peyer's patches. The antigens are ingested by antigen-presenting cells, processed intracellularly, and finally presented on the surface. This antigen is recognized in the context with the MHC class II complex by a specific antigen receptor on a T cell, the T cell receptor. Following the antigen recognition, and under the influence of associated cell surface molecules and costimulatory structures, an intracellular signalling cascade is activated in the T cell. In particular, it has become clear in recent years that the activation of a T cell may not only require the high-affinity binding of an antigen to the T cell receptor, but also a stimulation via costimulatory molecules such as CD40 (ligand CD40L), CD80/86 (ligand CD28), and CD2 (ligand CD58). The T cell activation is associated with phenotypical changes on the T cell surface (e.g. expression of CD25) and the initiation of T cell proliferation and cytokine secretion, as well as a T cell differentiation[21,22]. The concept of functional distinction of two helper subsets in the course of the CD4+ T cell differentiation is now well established. CD4+ T helper cells type 1 (Th1) are characterized functionally by the secretion of IL-2 and interferon-γ, and are mainly generated in the course of cellular immune responses. Their generation is influenced positively by IL-12 and interferon-γ, and inhibited by IL-4. In contrast, CD4+ Th2 cells secrete cytokines such as IL-4, IL-5, IL-10, and IL-13, and can be found mostly following allergic immune reactions and in parasitic diseases. The generation of Th2 cytokines is favoured by IL-4 and inhibited by interferon-γ[23,24]. The generation and differentiation of suppressor T cells and CD8+ T cells is currently much less well understood.

The primary T cell cytokine milieu in the intestine following conventional antigen feeding is not well defined. It has been shown that repeated intestinal feeding of the same antigen, for example in the model of experimental auto-immune encephalitis, is associated with a mucosal Th2 cytokine response as well as an immune tolerance[25,26]. Recent studies from our laboratory have demonstrated that feeding high doses of protein antigens (ovalbumin) up to three times leads to a generation of Th1 responses in the Peyer's patches which is similar to the Th pattern following systemic antigen exposure[27]. Many previous studies have also elucidated the generation of T helper classes following antigen feeding and the simultaneous use of adjuvants (for example cholera toxin). In those studies it was found that both Th1 and Th2 type cells may be induced by antigen feeding[28,29].

Finally, those T cell cytokines will have a wide array of influences on B cell function and differentiation, as well as on antigen-presenting cells (Fig. 2). In the course of the aforementioned activation processes and the complex interplay of regulatory events, cell activation may result in either local immunity, systemic immunity, or immunological tolerance.

B cell differentiation

In the course of the above activation events, B cells are stimulated and their differentiation to plasma cells is initiated. Like T cells, B cells carry antigen-specific molecules on their surface which are represented by membrane-bound immunoglobulins of a distinct subtype. Following the binding of an antigen the B cell may produce immunoglobulins with the same specificity as the membrane-bound form. It has become apparent that there are two types of antigens stimulating B cells: the first group may stimulate B cells directly (T cell-independent antigens), other antigens require a prior processing by other antigen-presenting cells and are presented to the B cells in the context with T cells (T cell-dependent antigens)[3,20].

The structure of antibody, the product of the plasma cells, is characterized by assembly of two heavy (H) chains and two light (L) chains, each of which contain constant (C) and variable (V) genetic regions. The structure of the constant regions of the heavy chains determines the specificity of antibody subtype. Thus, γ, μ, δ, ϵ, and α chains define the immunoglobulin subtypes IgG, IgM, IgD, IgE, and IgA, respectively. Functionally, the antibody can be divided into a Fab region which mediates the binding of antigen, and the Fc region which is involved in effector function such as opsonization and complement fixation[3].

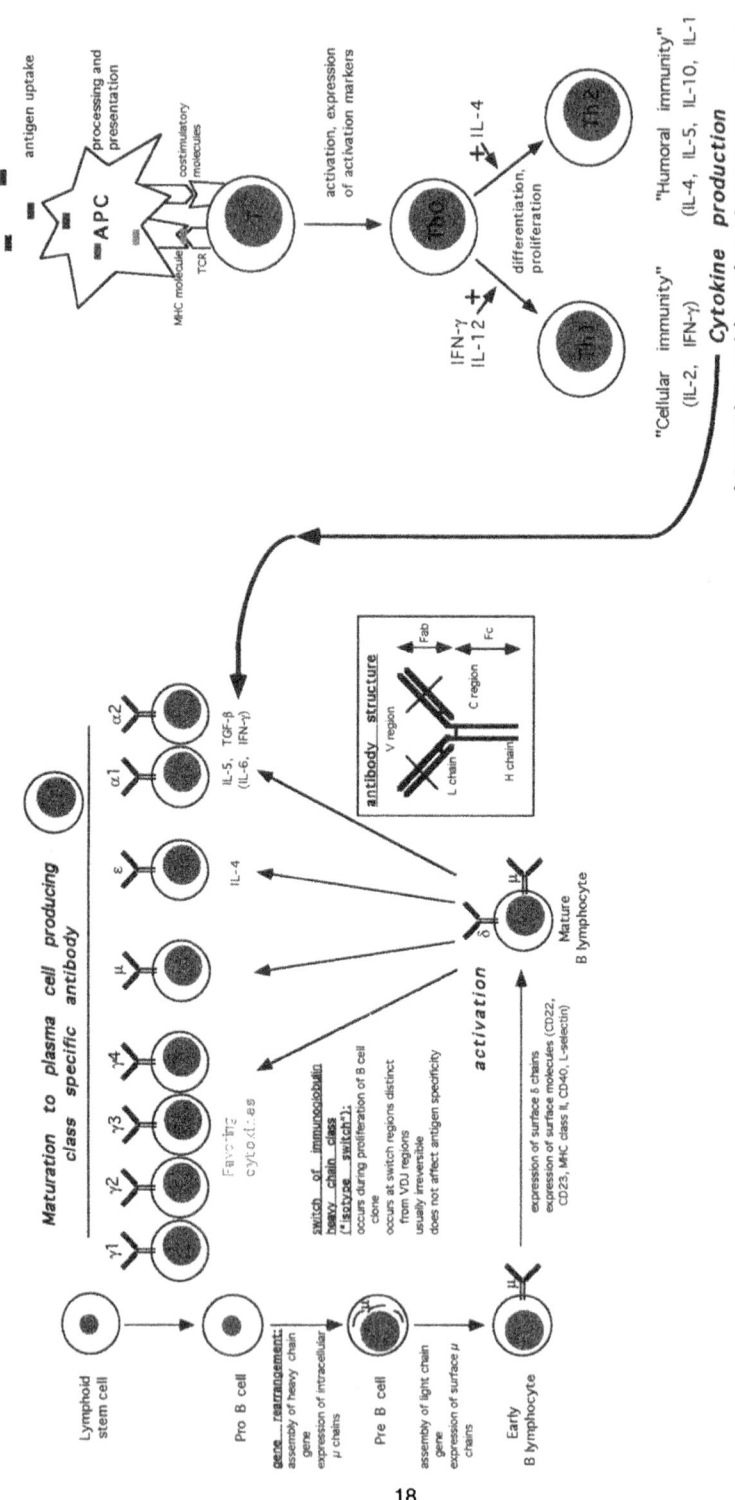

Figure 2 Development and function of B cells and T cells

18

B cells undergo a maturation from stem cells via pro-B cells, pre-B cells and immature B cells to mature B cells. The differentiation step from pro-B cells to pre-B cells is characterized by a gene arrangement of antibody subtype encoding molecules, which ultimately results in the intracytoplasmic expression of the μ-chain in the pre-B cells. In the stage of immature B cells the lymphocytes express the μ molecule on the surface (they are μ+), and mature B cells express both μ and δ. These double-positive mature B cells further differentiate under the influence of T cell cytokines to γ, μ, ϵ, or α expressing subtypes (see Fig. 2), a process called isotype switch. From this stage the final differentiation of the B cells to antibody-producing plasma cells may occur[30]. The activation processes for B cells mainly occur in the Peyer's patches where, under the influence of T cell cytokines, antibody-producing plasma cells (especially IgA plasma cells) are generated. The latter cells then undergo a migration to effector sites as discussed below.

Homing

A characteristic feature of the mucosal immune system is the property of mucosally derived cells to migrate back into effector sites of the MALT. As mentioned above, evidence has emerged that B cells and T cells derived from and activated at intestinal sites may migrate to other mucosal tissues such as the salivary glands, the bronchus-associated lymphoid tissue, the mammary glands and the female genital tract. The reason for the existence of this 'common mucosal immune system' may lie – in regard to B cell trafficking – in the antigenic specificities of IgA-producing B cells. Thus, the antigenic specificity of colostral IgA derived from B cells which migrated from the intestine to the breast, may reflect the antigenic exposure that these B cells experienced previously in the intestine. However, mucosal homing is not an antigen-trapping mechanism, since antigen-reactive cells migrate to both antigen-exposed and non-exposed areas, indicating that cell migration is not directed by antigen[12,14,31].

Following activation in the Peyer's patches, B and T cells migrate to mesenteric lymph nodes and then to the thoracic duct, before systemic distribution and remigration to mucosal sites occurs. This process usually takes 4–6 days. The majority of the homing B cells produce IgA. In comparison with B cells, fewer T cells have the capability to migrate back to intestinal sites (T cells migrate to the IEL and LPL compartment). Once located back in the lamina propria, T and B cells become sessile and exert specific functions according to their differential pattern (see below)[19,31].

The mechanisms involved in regulating the mucosal homing have become understood more completely in recent years. Lymphocyte migration is determined by adhering to and migrating between specialized endothelial cells (i.e. high endothelial venule cells) in postcapillary venules. There are receptors on lymphocytes and reciprocal ligands in tissues (for the endothelial cells called addressins) which regulate specific migration. For the mucosally derived lymphocytes, more or less specific markers such as LPAM-1 (in humans α_E or α_4 $\beta7$ integrin, i.e. the HML-1 antigen), PgP-1 (CD44), and others on lymphocytes may interact with their ligands on the endothelial cell and thus determine their migration to Peyer's patches or other mucosal sites[31,32].

Lamina propria T cells

T cells in the lamina propria represent a specific class of end-stage differentiated effector lymphocytes. As mentioned above, CD4+ and CD8+ T cells are found in the lamina propria in a similar ratio as in the peripheral blood; these T cells may either act as helper/inducer cells (CD4) or suppressor/cytotoxic cells (CD8). A further functional distinction of CD4 cells is possible by their surface expression of the CD45RA (inducer of suppressor cells) or the CD45RO molecule (memory cells mainly inducing Ig production). Recent work has elucidated that most of the lamina propria T cels are differentiated T cells expressing CD45RO, and thus providing helper function for Ig synthesis by plasma cells upon antigen challenge; in addition, they are characterized by higher expression of activation markers such as CD25 (IL-2 receptor α-chain), CD71 (transferrin receptor), and others. The helper function is brought over by production of specific T cell cytokines. In contrast to naive T cells, the differentiated T lymphocytes in the lamina propria do not proliferate, but produce larger amounts of cytokines following antigen stimulation (Table 1)[19,33-35].

IgA

Following the migration to the lamina propria, B lymphocytes and plasma cells may exert their specific Ig-producing function which is regulated by the interaction with T lymphocytes and other immunocompetent cells within the lamina propria. For the mucosal immune system, IgA has a special importance. IgA is the predominantly Ig subtype produced in the gastrointestinal mucosa, and has low complement-activating functions. In contrast to the periphery, it exists in two forms in the mucosa: the minority of the total mucosal IgA is regular, monomeric IgA structurally identical to the peripheral form, whereas most of the IgA in the intestine is the so-called secretory IgA (sIgA) which is produced as a dimer. The sIgA contains additional polypeptide chains, the secretory component, and the J chain which confers distinct functional features for the sIgA. The J chain mediates the polymerization of IgA molecules, and the membrane-bound secretory component which is expressed on intestinal epithelial cell and is involved in transporting dimeric IgA from the gut (e.g. from the lamina propria) to the intestinal lumen (therefore also called poly-Ig receptor). The function of

Table 1 Characteristics of LP T cells

	Naive T cells	Memory T cells	LP T cells
Phenotype			
CD45RA	↑↑	↓↓	↓↓
CD45RO	↓↓	↑↑	↑↑
Leu-8	↑↑	↓↓	↓↓
HML-1	↔	↔	↑↑
CD25	↓	↑	↑↑
Functional features			
Proliferation	↓↓	↑↑	↔
Cytokine production	↔	↑↑	↑↑

IgA and sIgA at mucosal surfaces consists mainly in the resorption of antigen within the gut, thereby preventing mucosal damage by microorganisms and other antigens. This function is ensured by its specific structure preventing rapid lysis by proteolytic enzymes[1,36,37]. In addition, newer studies show that IgA can also bind antigen in the lamina propria or within the intestinal epithelial cell, and is then transported via the poly-lg receptor to the lumen, thus contributing to the host defence[38].

ORAL TOLERANCE

Background

The term 'oral tolerance' describes the antigen-specific suppression of an immune response following administration of oral antigen. Both cellular and humoral immune responses are suppressed by such orally induced tolerance, and this tolerance is often associated with the generation of cytokine-producing suppressor T cells. The method of inducing oral tolerance is a well-known phenomenon and has been analysed in a variety of animal models, but just recently oral tolerance has begun to be tested in clinical medicine. Currently, there are several trials in humans, testing the potential of orally induced tolerance as a possible therapy for autoimmune diseases[2,39].

Characteristics of oral tolerance

Oral tolerance has been studied for a variety of applied antigens such as thymic-dependent antigens, heterologous cells (e.g. erythrocytes), killed bacteria and viruses, as well as soluble non-adjuvanted dietary proteins. The latter antigens probably present the dietary antigens of the highest immunological relevance. It has been shown that specific systemic immunoglobulin responses (IgM, IgG and IgE) can be suppressed by oral antigen feeding. The suppression of IgE responses can be achieved with relatively low amounts of fed antigens, and lasts usually for a long time, whereas reduction of other immunoglobulins may either be short term or may require higher doses of fed antigen[40,41]. The application of oral antigen also leads to the suppression of cellular immune responses. Thus, it has been shown that *in-vitro* parameters of cell-mediated immunity (proliferation and cytokine production), as well as *in-vivo* functions of cell-mediated immunity such as DTH reactions and contact hypersensitivity, can be suppressed by oral antigen feeding (Table 2). Similar to the IgE response, cellular immune functions can be suppressed relatively easily with low amounts of fed antigens, and the suppression of CMI persists over a longer time period.[27,40,42].

Mechanisms of oral tolerance

While there are considerable overlaps with the mechanisms explaining the occurrence of systemically induced tolerance, orally induced tolerance also has distinct characteristics. One major difference between systemic and orally induced tolerance seems to be based on antigen processing in the mucosal immune system. In this regard the generation of suppressor T cells at mucosal sites, as well as the intestinal proteolysis and the role of mucosal barrier, seems

Table 2 Features of oral tolerance

Definition	Systemic immunological unresponsiveness following oral administration of a soluble protein antigen.
Characteristics	Humoral and cellular immune responses are suppressed. Relative sparing of the mucosal IgA response. Inducible by a wide array of protein antigens.
Mechanisms	Processes involved in intestinal antigen processing. Induction of suppressive T cell cytokines ('active suppression'). Clonal anergy. Clonal deletion.
Clinical significance	Treatment of antigen-specific autoimmune diseases. Defects in oral tolerance may be important for the pathogenesis of food intolerance, gluten-sensitive enteropathy, inflammatory bowel diseases, and others.

to be important[43,44]. A growing body of recent work also implies that tolerance versus immunization following an antigen feeding may be influenced by the strength of activation of antigen-presenting cells. In this model the intestinal antigen proteolysis and antigen processing usually will not lead to a highly activated APC; thus the development of tolerance, rather than an active immune response, can occur[45,46]. While more work in this field is necessary, it is interesting to note that the costimulatory activity could be dependent on factors such as the cytokine milieu at intestinal sites, as well as strength and duration of T cell antigen receptor binding by the antigen.

As mentioned above, immunoregulatory mechanisms of orally induced tolerance have some common features with systemically induced tolerance. Thus, the well-studied phenomena of suppression, clonal anergy and clonal deletion of systemic tolerance can be also found in oral tolerance[22,39]. Suppression seems to be a significant mechanism of oral tolerance. It has been shown that adoptively transferred lymphoid cells from pre-fed animals can induce tolerance (mostly on the level of cell-mediated immunity) in the hosts[47]. It has become clear that the main mediators of suppression are cytokines, and subsequently the term 'active suppression', meaning a cytokine-mediated suppression of immune reactions, has been designated[39]. The cytokines associated with active suppression are Th2 cytokines such as IL-4 as well as IL-10 and transforming growth factor beta (TGF-β). The latter cytokine, TGF-β, seems to have a central role, since in a number of animal models (including the experimental autoimmune encephalitis (EAE) model), it was demonstrated that TGF-β mainly mediates the immunosuppressive and therapeutic effects. It has been suggested that TGF-β-producing cells may be a Th1- and Th2-independent population (i.e. Th3 cells)[26,39,48,49]. The current concept is that the TGF-β-producing cells generated in the intestinal mucosa, following antigen feeding, migrate to systemic lymphoid tissue and target organs (such as the central nervous system by the EAE model), and then upon activation specifically suppress immune responses of nearby T cells. This phenomenon has been termed 'bystander suppression'[50], and based on this principle therapy of autoimmune diseases should be possible even though the exact nature of the causative antigen may not be known.

Recent work from our laboratory has shown that the generation of TGF-β-producing cells can be regulated by IL-12 and Th1 cytokines. We observed in OVA-T cell receptor transgenic mice, fed high doses of OVA and simultaneously systemically treated with antibodies to IL-12, an augmentation of peripheral tolerance associated with a significant increase in the production of TGF-β (also by cells from mucosal lymphoid tissue, i.e. the Peyer's patches) and elevated levels of antigen-specific T cell apoptosis. These results therefore, together with others obtained in the trinitrobenzene sulphonic acid (TNBS) colitis model (see below), show the importance of the intestinal cytokine milieu and the interplay of TGF-β and Th1 cytokine responses for the occurence of oral tolerance[27,51].

The second mechanism observed in oral tolerance, clonal anergy, is defined as a state of tolerance of clonal T cells which can be reversed by IL-2, and was found in studies of oral tolerance mainly after one-time feeding of protein antigens[52]. Finally, it has been shown, by us and others, that feeding of high doses of antigen can lead to clonal deletion of T cells in the periphery by apoptosis is a significant regulatory mechanism for the limitation of immune responses[27,53].

Taken together, it has become clear that the occurrence of antigen-induced oral tolerance is dependent on a complex interplay of different immunoregulatory mechanisms. Most of the presented observations have in common that oral tolerance is more likely to occur when a Th1 cytokine response is being reduced and when, simultaneously, suppressor cytokines such as TGF-β and IL-4 occur[39,51].

Suppression of disease in animal models by orally induced tolerance

Much has been learned about immunological mechanisms of oral tolerance with the use of animals and animal models. Most of the animal models discussed here represent models of chronic relapsing autoimmune diseases which are in many cases similar to human diseases. Among others, the model of experimental autoimmune encephalomyelitis (EAE), collagen arthritis, diabetes in the non-obese diabetes (NOD) mouse, experimental autoimmune uveitis (EAU), and TNBS colitis have been used[39].

The induction of TNBS into Balb/c or SJL mice induces a chronic inflammatory colitis clinically and histologically resembling Crohn's disease in humans (i.e. transmural inflammation, generation of granulomas, massive infiltration of microphages and lymphocytes; severe weight loss, diarrhoea and rectal prolapse). Recent studies have shown that the disease is mediated by Th1-like cytokines such as interferon-γ, and that the colitis can be effectively suppressed by systemic administration of antibodies to IL-12. Interestingly, it has also been shown that the feeding of haptenized colonic proteins will suppress the Th1-type reactions from mucosal surfaces, and will lead to an increase of Th2 cytokines and TGF-β at those sites[54]. In studies by Elson *et al.* it has also been shown that the antigen-specific IgG2a and IgG2b responses were suppressible by prefeeding TNBS, and that this also prevented the clinical disease[55].

Oral tolerance in humans

There are a number of observations supporting the notion that orally induced tolerance can also occur in humans. One study has thus shown that antigen-specific suppression of delayed-type hypersensitivity reactions following oral administration of keyhole-limpet haemocyanin can be achieved in normal individuals[56]. Furthermore, it has been demonstrated that feeding sensitizing antigens can prevent induced cutaneous hypersensitivity[57]; this observation would agree with the historical phenomenon of prevention of hypersensitivity against poison ivy in South American Indians[58]. It should be noted, however, that a suppression of specific antibody response in humans has not yet been demonstrated, and that the results from the animal studies may be extrapolated to the human system only with caution.

Previous studies have speculated on the possible role of dysregulated oral tolerance in the pathogenesis of food allergies and gluten-sensitive enteropathies[40,59]. Several observations support this notion. First, in persons with intact mucosal barrier there is a low incidence of food allergies against ubiquitous dietary antigens. Second, in patients with disturbed mucosal barrier functions, such as patients with Crohn's disease, increased antibody titres against food dietary antigens can frequently be found. Third, allergies to dietary antigens in young calves can be prevented if the causative antigens are fed after weaning instead of feeding them before the weaning; that may be due to the lack of immunoregulatory mechanisms in the young animals. Clearly, more work is necessary to clarify the pathogenic relevance of oral tolerance in the occurrence of food allergies and gluten-sensitive enteropathies.

The detailed investigations in animal models, and the dissection of immunological mechanisms underlying the occurrence of oral tolerance, have led in recent years to the setting up of clinical trials in humans, which are designed to test the effect of oral antigen feeding on the cause of autoimmune diseases. An initial study in multiple sclerosis in 1993 revealed in 15 patients that oral antigen feeding of bovine myelin resulted in a lower frequency of severe relapses in the antigen group than in the placebo-treated group. The hypothesis that HLA DR2-negative men may have profited most from the oral antigen feeding is currently being tested in a phase III study. A study on 30 patients with rheumatoid arthritis has revealed that oral collagen application over a period of 3 months led to a reduction of joint swelling and disease index as compared to the placebo group. Based on these promising results further studies of oral tolerance in these and other human diseases (uveitis, diabetes) have been initiated[39].

References

1. Strober W, James SP. The mucosal immune system. In: Stites DP, Terr AI, Parslow TG, editors. Basic and clinical immunology. Norwalk, CT: Appleton & Lange; 1994:541–51.
2. Mowat AMcl. Oral tolerance and regulation of immunity to dietary antigens. In: Ogra PL, Lamm ME, McGhee JR, Mestecky J, Strober W, Bienenstock J, editors. Handbook of mucosal immunology. San Diego, CA: Academic Press; 1994:185–201.
3. Mestecky J, McGhee JR. Immunoglobulin A (IgA): molecular and cellular interactions involved in IgA biosysthesis and immune responses. Adv Immunol. 1987;40:153–245.
4. Kelsall BL, Strober W. Host defenses at mucosal surfaces. In: Rich RR, Fleisher TA, Schwartz BD, Shearer WT, Strober W, editors. Clinical immunology: principles and practice. St Louis, MO: Mosby, 1996:299–331.

5. Spencer J, Finn T, Isaacson PG. Human Peyer's patches: an immunohistochemical study. Gut. 1986;27:405–10.
6. Ermak TH, Owen RL. Differential distribution of lymphocytes and accessory cells in mouse Peyer's patches. Anat Rec. 1986;215:144–52.
7. Wolf JL, Rubin DH, Finberg R et al. Intestinal M cells: a pathway for entry of reovirus into the host. Science. 1981;212:471–2.
8. Kelsall BL, Strober W. Distinct populations of dendritic cells are present in the subepithelial dome and T cell regions of the murine peyers patch. J Exp Med. 1995;183:237–47.
9. Blumberg RS, Terhorst C, Bleicher P et al. Expression of a nonpolymorphic MHC class I-like molecule CD1d, by human intestinal epithelial cells. J Immunol. 1991;147:2518–24.
10. Panja A, Mayer L. Diversity and function of antigen-presenting cells in mucosal tissues. In: Ogra PL, Lamm ME, McGhee JR, Mestecky J, Strober W, Bienenstock J, editors. Handbook of mucosal immunology. San Diego, CA: Academic Press; 1994:177–83.
11. Panja A, Blumberg RS, Balk SP, Mayer L. Cd1d is involved in T cell : epithelial cell interactions. J Exp Med. 1993;178:1115–20.
12. McDermott MR, Bienenstock J. Evidence for a common mucosal immunologic system. I. Migration of B immunoblasts into intestinal, respiratory, and genital tissues. J Immunol. 1979;122:1892–8.
13. Asherson GL, Zembala M, Perera MACC, Mayhew B, Thomas WR. Production of immunity and unresponsiveness in the mouse by feeding contact sensitizing agents, and the role of suppressor cells in the Peyer's patches, mesenteric lymph nodes and other lymphoid tissues. Cell Immunol. 1977;33:145–55.
14. Mestecky J. The common mucosal immune system and current strategies for induction of immune responses in external secretions. J Clin Immunol. 1987;7:265–76.
15. Dobbins WO. Human intestinal intraepithelial lymphocytes. Gut. 1986;27:972–85.
16. Cerf-Bensussan N, Guy-Grand D. Intestinal intraepithelial lymphocytes. Mucosal Immunol. 1991;20:549–76.
17. Schieferdecker HL, Ullrich R, Weiss-Breckwoldt AN et al. The HML-1 antigen of intestinal lymphocytes is an activation antigen. J Immunol. 1990;144:2541–9.
18. Guy-Grand D, Cerf-Bensussan N, Malissen B, Malassis-Seris M, Briottet C, Vassalli P. Two gut intraepithelial CD8+ lymphocyte populations with different T cell receptors: a role for the gut epithelium in T cell differentiation. J Exp Med. 1991;173:471–81.
19. Zeitz M, Schieferdecker HL, Ullrich R, Jahn HU, James SP, Riecken EO. Phenotype and function of lamina propria T lymphocytes. Immunol Res. 1991;10:199–206.
20. Kagnoff MF. Immunology and inflammation of the gastrointestinal tract. In: Sleisenger MH, Fordtran JS, editors. Gastrointestinal diseases. 1993:45–86.
21. Schwartz RH. Immunological tolerance. In: Paul WE, editor. Fundamental immunology. New York: Raven Press; 1993;677–731.
22. Miller JFAP, Moraham G. Peripheral T cell tolerance. Annu Rev Immunol. 1992;10:51–70.
23. Mosmann TR, Coffman RL. TH1 and TH2 cells: different patterns of lymphokine secretion lead to different functional properties. Annu Rev Immunol. 1989;7:145–73.
24. Seder RA, Paul WE. Acquisition of lymphokine-producing phenotype by CD4+ T cells. Annu Rev Immunol. 1994;12:635–73.
25. Santos LMB, Al-Sabbagh A, Londono A, Weiner HL. Oral tolerance to myelin basic protein induces regulatory TGF-β secreting cells in Peyer's patches of SJL mice. Cell Immunol. 1993;157:439–47.
26. Khoury SJ, Hancock WW, Weiner HL. Oral tolerance to myelin basic protein and natural recovery from experimental autoimmune encephalomyelitis are associated with downregulation of inflammatory cytokines and differential upregulation of transforming growth factor b, interleukin 4, and prostaglandin E expression in the brain. J Exp Med. 1992;176:1355–64.
27. Marth T, Strober W, Kelsall BL. High dose oral tolerance in ovalbumin TCR transgenic mice: systemic neutralization of interleukin-12 augments TGF-β secretion and T cell apoptosis. J Immunol. 1996;157:2348–57.
28. Xu-Amano J, Kiyono H, Jackson RJ et al. Helper T cell subsets for immunoglobulin A responses: oral immunization with tetanus toxoid and cholera toxin as adjuvant selectively induces Th2 cells in mucosa associated tissues. J Exp Med. 1993;178:1309–20.
29. Taguchi T, McGhee JR, Coffman RL et al. Analysis of Th1 and Th2 cells in murine gut-associated tissues. Frequencies of CD4+ and CD8+ T cells that secrete IFN-γ and IL-5. J Immunol. 1990;145:68–75.

30. Kawanishi H, Saltzman L, Strober W. Mechanisms regulating IgA class-specific immunoglobulin production in murine gut-associated lymphoid tissues. II. Terminal differentiation of postswitch sIgA-bearing Peyer's patch B cells. J Exp Med. 1983;158:649–69.
31. Phillips-Quagliata JM, Lamm ME. Lymphocyte homing to mucosal effector sites. In: Ogra PL, Lamm ME, McGhee JR, Mestecky J, Strober W, Bienenstock J, editors. Handbook of mucosal immunology. San Diego, CA: Academic Press; 1994:225–39.
32. Stoolman LM. Adhesion molecules controlling lymphocyte migration. Cell. 1989;56:907–10.
33. Quiao L, Schuermann G, Betzler M, Meuer SC. Activation and signaling status of human lamina propria T lymphocytes. Gastroenterology. 1991;101:1529–36.
34. Zeitz M, Quinn TC, Graeff AS, James SP. Mucosal T cells provide helper function but do not proliferate when stimulated by specific antigen in lymphogranuloma venereum proctitis in non-human primates. Gastroenterology. 1988;94:353–66.
35. Zeitz M, Greene WC, Peffer NJ, James SP. Lymphocytes isolated from the intestinal lamina propria of normal nonhuman primates have increased expression of genes associated with T-cell activation. Gastroenterology. 1988;94:647–55.
36. Koshland ME. Structure and function of the J chain. Adv Immunol. 1975;20:41–69.
37. Mostov KE, Friedlander M, Blobel G. The receptor for transepithelial transport of IgA and IgM contains multiple immunoglobulin-like domains. Nature. 1984;308:37–43.
38. Mostov KE. Transepithelial transport of immunoglobulins. Annu Rev Immunol. 1994;12:63–84.
39. Weiner HL, Friedman A, Miller A *et al*. Oral tolerance: Immunologic mechanisms and treatment of animal and human organ-specific autoimmune diseases by oral administration of autoantigens. Annu Rev Immunol. 1994;12:809–37.
40. Mowat AMcl. The regulation of immune responses to dietary protein antigens. Immunol Today. 1987;8:93–8.
41. Challacombe SJ, Tomasi JB. Systemic tolerance and secretory immunity after oral immunisation. J Exp Med. 1980;152:1459–72.
42. Kay R, Ferguson A. The immunological consequences of feeding cholera toxin. I. Feeding cholera toxin suppresses the induction of systemic delayed-type hypersensitivity but not humoral immunity. Immunology. 1989;66:410–15.
43. Strobel S, Mowat AMcl, Drummond HE, Pickering MG, Ferguson A. Immunological responses to fed protein antigens in mice. II. Oral tolerance for CMI is due to activation of cyclophosphamide sensitive cells by gut processed antigen. Immunology. 1983;49:451–6.
44. Bruce MG, Ferguson A. The influence of intestinal processing on the immunogenicity and molecular size of absorbed, circulating ovalbumin in mice. Immunology. 1986;59:295–300.
45. Mowat AMcl, Parrott DMV. Immunological responses to fed protein antigens in mice. IV. Effects of stimulating the reticuloendothelial system on oral tolerance and intestinal immunity to ovalbumin. Immunology. 1983;50:547–54.
46. Strobel S, Mowat AMcl, Ferguson A. Prevention of oral tolerance induction to ovalbumin and enhanced antigen presentation during graft-versus-host reaction in mice. Immunology. 1985;56:57–64.
47. Thomas HC, Parrott DMV. Induction of tolerance to a soluble protein antigen by oral administration. Immunology. 1974;27:631–9.
48. Miller A, Lider O, Roberts AB, Sporn MB, Weiner HL. Suppressor T cells generated by oral tolerization to myelin basic protein suppress both *in vitro* and and *in vivo* immune responses by the release of transforming growth factor after antigen-specific triggering. Proc Natl Acad Sci USA. 1992;89:421–5.
49. Fukaura H, Kent SC, Pietrusewic MJ, Khoury SJ, Weiner HL, Hafler DA. Induction of circulating myelin basic protein and proteolipid protein-specific transforming growth factor-b1-secreting Th3 T cells by oral administration of myelin in multiple sclerosis patients. J Clin Invest. 1996;98:70–7.
50. Miller A, Lider O, Weiner HL. Antigen-driven bystander suppression after oral administration of antigen. J Exp Med. 1991;174:791–8.
51. Strober W, Kelsall BL, Fuss I *et al*. Reciprocal IFN-gamma and TGF-beta responses regulate the occurrence of mucosal inflammation. Immunol Today. 1997;18:61–4.
52. Whitacre CC, Gienapp IE, Orosz CG, Bitar DM. Oral tolerance in experimental autoimmune encephalitis. III. Evidence for clonal anergy. J Immunol. 1991;147:2155–63.
53. Chen Y, Inobe JI, Marks R, Gonella P, Kuchroo VK, Weiner HL. Peripheral deletion of antigen-reactive T cells in oral tolerance. Nature. 1995;376:177–80.

54. Neurath MF, Fuss I, Kelsall BL, Presky DH, Waegell W, Strober W. Experimental granuloma-tous colitis in mice is abrogated by induction of TGF-β-mediated oral tolerance. J Exp Med. 1996;183:2605–16.
55. Elson CO, Beagley KW, Sharmanov AT *et al.* Hapten-induced model of inflammatory bowel disease: mucosa immune responses and protection by tolerance. J Immunol. 1996;157:2174–85.
56. Husby SJ, Mestecky J, Moldoveanu S, Holland S, Elson CO. Oral tolerance in humans. T cell but not B cell tolerance after antigen feeding. J Immunol. 1994;152:4663–70.
57. Lowney ED. Immunologic unresponsiveness to a contact sensitizer in man. J Invest Dermatol. 1968;51:411–17.
58. Dakin R. Remarks on a cutaneous affection produced by certain poisonous vegetables. Am J Med Sci. 1827;4:98–100.
59. Ferguson A, Gillett H, Mahony SO. Active immunity or tolerance to foods in patients with celiac disease or inflammatory bowel disease. Ann NY Acad Sci. 1996;778:202–16.

Section II
Gastrointestinal permeability and translocation

3
The intestinal permeability barrier – what is measured, what does it mean?

S. GABE, M. JACOB and I. BJARNASON

INTRODUCTION

The non-invasive assessment of intestinal permeability has a short history, only becoming practically possible with the introduction of lactulose as a permeability probe and a reliable, sensitive and quantitative method for its detection in 1974 by Menzies[1,2]. The original idea was to assess the intestinal barrier function, as opposed to intestinal absorptive capacity, as impairments of the former would seem to have different pathophysiological connotations to the latter[3–5]. Hence increased intestinal permeability has been thought to play a possible role in both local inflammatory reactions and systemic disease[6–13], while impaired absorption clearly has nutritional implications. There has been rapid development in respect of technical refinements of the test procedure, although there are plenty of pitfalls for the uninitiated[3,14].

Tests of intestinal permeability have been accepted in the research laboratory for the study of the pathogenesis of disease. However, there is still some uncertainty about their precise place in the routine assessment of patients with abdominal symptoms and various diseases. Nevertheless, while the clinical implications of increased intestinal permeability are now becoming clear (i.e. the development of a uniformly severe inflammatory enteropathy which is associated with bleeding, protein loss, etc.) these are not widely known to clinicians. The wider use of these tests will undoubtedly benefit patients, as diseases not identifiable by other methods will be found and treated accordingly. Acceptance depends on a number of factors; not least the availability of the tests in routine laboratories and, perhaps more importantly, the level of care that the gastroenterologist is willing to provide.

PROCEDURE

Small intestinal permeability

The precise test procedure employed depends on the problem at hand, and the desired sensitivity and specificity of the procedure. Serious consideration of test dose composition and osmolarity is of paramount importance, as is the method of analysis of the markers[14–18]. In general there are three major options of assessing small intestinal permeability[3,17]. In all cases the tests are performed after an overnight fast (poor compliance with this requirement affects the sensitivity of the procedure) with a further 2–3 h fast after ingestion of the test dose. A 5–6-h or 24-h urine collection is made for marker analyses. The recommended tests are:

1. 24-h urinary excretion measurement of ^{51}Cr-EDTA (or somewhat less satisfactorily ^{99m}Tc-DTPA) following neat ingestion of the marker in water.
2. 5-h urinary excretion and calculation of a ^{51}Cr-EDTA/L-rhamnose ratio following their ingestion.
3. As in (2) but substituting lactulose for ^{51}Cr-EDTA.

The straightforward 24-h urinary excretion of ^{51}Cr-EDTA appears to be the most sensitive of the tests[15,16]. However, it is also associated with more frequent and apparent false-positive results when used as a screening procedure. The incorporation of L-rhamnose into the test increases the specificity of the test as a small intestinal disease marker, as opposed to the whole of the gastrointestinal tract, and it conforms to the principle of the differential urinary excretion of ingested test substances, with minor reductions in sensitivity. Substituting lactulose for ^{51}Cr-EDTA has the effect of reducing the sensitivity of the test[15,16], probably because of the luminal osmotic retention (withholds water and causes intestinal hurry) effect of the poorly permeating lactulose[18]. This is not particularly important when the test is used as screening for major gastrointestinal disease, such as coeliac and Crohn's disease, but more subtle changes, such as those seen with non-steroidal anti-inflammatory drugs (NSAID), may be missed. Provided that certain precautions are taken mannitol (mannitol is excreted in small quantities in man) can be substituted for L-rhamnose and the sugars quantified by high-performance liquid chromatography (HPLC)[19,20]. If mono or disaccharides are used in (2) or (3) it is possible to include 3-O-methyl-D-glucose and D-xylose into the test, allowing a much more complete assessment of intestinal absorptive capacity without affecting the sensitivity of the permeability procedure.

A brief note about the use of polyethylene glycol (PEG 400). PEG 400 comes as a range of polymers with a molecular mass of 194–502. The molecular cross-sectional diameter of the PEG polymers is similar in the 200–600 molecular weight range[21]. Analysis of PEG in urine is time-consuming, requiring extraction and quantitation by gas chromatography or HPLC[16,22–28]. PEG 400 fulfils many of the theoretical requirements of an 'ideal' test substance[22,23].

The drawback of the use of PEG 400 is that the completeness of urine excretion after intravenous administration is variable and unsatisfactory. Following intravenous instillation in pigs the 3-h urine recoveries were 74% for polymers 722–1206, but only 34–57% for polymer 282–678[25]. In humans, urinary recoveries increase from 26% for PEG 194 to 69% for PEG 502 in a 7.5-h urine collection following intravenous administration[16]. More importantly, normal subjects excrete between 20% and 50% of an orally ingested test dose of PEG 400 in urine, which is similar to that of monosaccharides whose permeation across the small intestinal mucosa is facilitated by specific carriers. This has suggested to a number of workers that PEG 400 may partition across the lipophil domains of the brush-border membrane[17,29,30], rather than across the tight junctions of adjacent enterocytes. This is, however, fiercely disputed by other workers[31]. The high permeation rates in normals, which by itself cast doubt on its use as a 'permeability' probe, and the fact that the permeation of PEG 400 in disease almost invariably increases as differential urinary excretion of di-/monosaccharides decreases and vice versa makes interpretation of the test very difficult, if not challenging.

Gastric permeability

It has been suggested that it may be possible to assess gastric permeability by the co-administration of sucrose with the permeability test solution[32]. The idea is that ingested sucrose is completely and rapidly hydrolysed by small intestinal sucrase so that all sucrose in urine following oral administration represents gastric permeation and can therefore serve as an index of gastric permeability[32,33]. While some authors have endorsed the test[34,35] others have voiced caution about the interpretation of the results[36]. Furthermore, if proof was required, administration of α-glucosidase inhibitors increases significantly, and at times spectacularly, the permeation of sucrose[37], and sucrose permeation is greatly enhanced in primary sucrasia[38]. Hence the method is not at all specific for the stomach, and its clinical use is still under investigation.

Colonic permeability

Consideration of the principle of the urinary excretion of test substances enables one to expand and devise new non-invasive tests of intestinal function. One such modification is to administer ^{51}Cr-EDTA with lactulose and L-rhamnose followed by a 0–5-h and a 5–24-h urine collection for marker analyses[39,40]. The underlying idea is that lactulose and L-rhamnose are both rapidly degraded by colonic bacteria, while ^{51}Cr-EDTA is not. Any difference in the total 24-h urine excretion of ^{51}Cr-EDTA and lactulose is due to colonic permeation, because the two behave identically in all other respects. Recent abstracts advocate sucralose as a substitute marker for ^{51}Cr-EDTA, but it is not at all clear what advantage it has over ^{51}Cr-EDTA. The reinvention of the wheel takes peculiar forms!

Small intestinal and colonic permeability

Perhaps the most demanding of all the tests is the technique designed by Teahon *et al.* to localize the site of intestinal permeability[41]. The principle of the technique is that a range of test substances, whose absorptive site is well defined to a particular region of the intestine, are given orally, with subsequent serum analyses[41]. The absorption profile of ^{51}Cr-EDTA in studies of intestinal permeability is then compared with that of the other markers, which allows the site of increased intestinal permeability to be assessed. The test substances are:

1. 3-O-methyl-D-glucose, absorbed predominantly from the jejunum by the glucose carrier (active mediated transport).
2. ^{57}Co-vitamin B_{12}, absorbed from the terminal ileum by specific carriers.
3. Sulphasalazine, which passes unchanged into the caecum where it is cleaved into 5-aminosalicylic acid and sulphapyridine by azo-reductase-containing bacteria. Sulphapyridine is rapidly absorbed and its appearance in serum indicates when the test solution enters the caecum.

Representative results are shown in Fig. 1. The absorption profile from patients with untreated coeliac disease shows increased serum levels of ^{51}Cr-EDTA which correspond to the 3-O-methyl-D-glucose absorption curve. Similarly the peak serum levels of ^{51}CrEDTA in patients with ileal Crohn's disease correspond to the appearance of the ileal and colonic marker, while patients with severe total colitis have increased serum levels of ^{51}Cr-EDTA some time following the appearances of vitamin B_{12} and sulphapyridine. This is the first *in-vivo* evidence showing that the site of increased intestinal permeability in patients with coeliac and inflammatory bowel disease is indeed the diseased intestinal mucosa itself. This test it too demanding (on patient and investigator alike) to be used, except for research purposes. It nevertheless holds particular promise for the assessment of the efficacy of drug-delivery systems which can be exploited in collaboration with the pharmaceutical industry.

USES OF INTESTINAL PERMEABILITY TESTS

There are many situations in which tests of intestinal permeability can be useful. The following is a brief description, but for comprehensive coverage the reader is referred to other reviews[3,14,42].

Intestinal permeability for diagnostic screening and monitoring of therapeutic responses

Tests of intestinal permeability may be used as non-invasive screening procedures to anticipate or even replace the need for more invasive investigations of the small intestine. In major diseases such as coeliac disease the tests are almost invariably abnormal[43–49], can be used to confirm the diagnosis of coeliac disease[46,50] and assess responses to treatment by gluten withdrawal[48–55].

Similarly most patients with Crohn's disease have increased intestinal permeability[56–62]. Again the tests are useful in assessing responses to treatment[63–65]. It has been suggested that the finding of normal intestinal permeability in patients with Crohn's disease may have a predictive value for their well-being[65,66]. Along with other observations, this has led to the hypothesis that disruption of the intestinal barrier is the central mechanism leading to relapse in inflammatory bowel disease[4,5].

Other common intestinal disorders such as giardiasis, Rotavirus infection, etc. are also consistently associated with increased intestinal permeability[67–69]. In geographical areas with a high prevalence of tropical sprue, which is associated

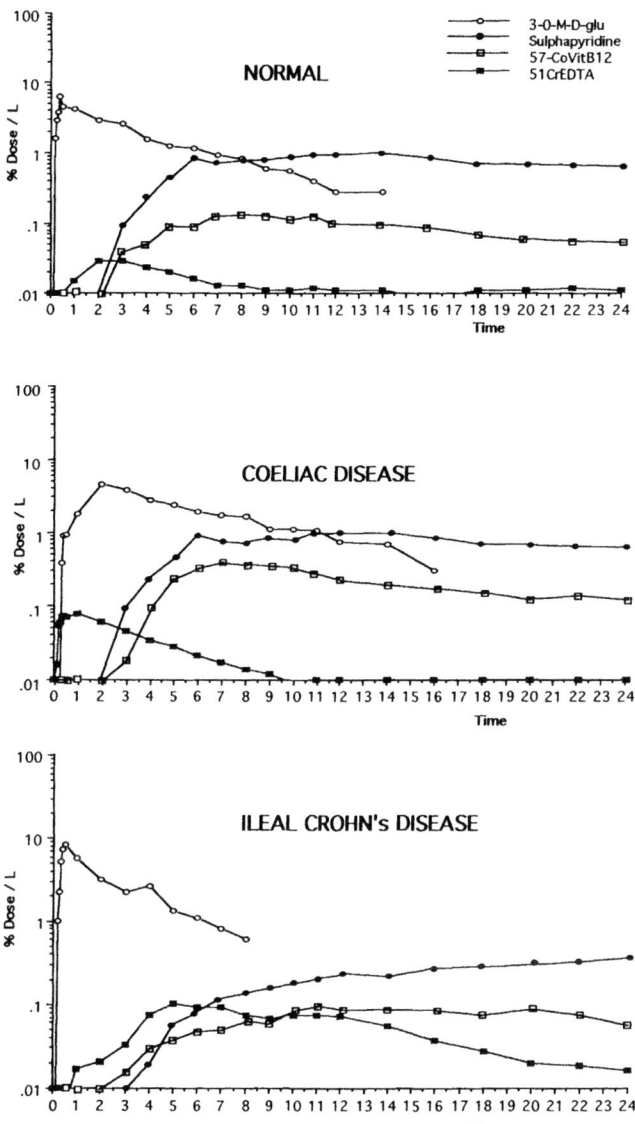

Figure 1 Localization of intestinal permeability changes. The site of increased intestinal permeability can be assessed by a technique described by Teahon *et al.*[41]. This involves an overnight fast followed by ingestion of a test solution containing: 3-O-methyl-D-glucose (absorbed from the jejunum), ^{57}Co-vitamin B_{12} (absorbed from terminal ileum), sulphasalazine (appearance of sulphapyridine in serum indicates that the test solution has entered the caecum), and ^{51}Cr-EDTA, the permeability marker. Blood is taken frequently over 24 h for marker analysis. In normals there is a rapid rise in the jejunal marker followed by low levels of ^{51}Cr-EDTA. The oro-ileal/caecal transit is 3 h in the representative result from a healthy volunteer shown above. In a patient with coeliac disease there is a marked rise (note that the scale is logarithmic) in the levels of ^{51}Cr-EDTA, which coincides with the jejunal marker. In a patient with ileal Crohn's disease the increased permeation of ^{51}Cr-EDTA occurs much later, at a time when the ileal/caecal markers are measured

with increased intestinal permeability, it may be difficult to define an effective normal range of intestinal permeability[70-72]. While tests of intestinal permeability clearly lack diagnostic specificity, they may be useful as a non-invasive marker to assess therapeutic response in a given individual[3].

Intestinal permeability and pathogenesis of disease

The interest in the role of increased intestinal permeability in the aetiology and pathogenesis of various diseases is substantial, ranging from Crohn's and coeliac disease, systemic autoimmune diseases, spondylarthropathies, rheumatoid arthritis to schizophrenia[6,8-11,13,73,74]. An intriguing question is whether altered intestinal permeability plays an aetiological role in Crohn's disease[8,9,75]. Hollander et al.[9,75] demonstrated that PEG 400 permeation was increased in a substantial proportion of first-degree relatives of patients with Crohn's disease. This suggested that a genetically determined abnormality of the intestine might underlie the disease, or that the families were exposed to a common environmental toxin. However, these findings have been challenged[76-78]. Intestinal permeability is usually normal in relatives when tested with the differential urinary excretion of sugars or ^{51}Cr-EDTA[76,79]. However, a proportion of relatives have an increased intestinal permeability (around 10% in most studies)[76,79-82]. A most impressive study[83] suggested that half of the first-degree relatives of patients with Crohn's disease had increased intestinal permeability, and this was associated with immunological markers of antigen presentation. This issue is likely to continue to be disputed.

The effects of drugs and toxins on intestinal integrity

Tests of intestinal permeability have shown that NSAID disrupt small intestinal integrity[84] within hours of ingestion. The mechanism is likely to involve mitochondrial damage[85-89], followed by reduced adenosine triphosphate (ATP) production and loss of control over the intercellular junctions between adjacent enterocytes[40,90-102]. Consequentially up to 65% of patients develop small intestinal inflammation with bleeding, protein loss and ileal dysfunction; the occasional patient may develop intestinal strictures termed 'diaphragm disease'[84,103-107].

Chemotherapeutic agents increase intestinal permeability[108-113], as do alcohol[114-116] and detergents[16,117].

Intestinal physiology

As alluded to above, the test dose osmolarity of the test solution, and how this is made up, profoundly affects small intestinal function[1,16,118-120]. The pioneering work of Menzies showed that the permeation of lactulose, in particular, is influenced by test dose osmolarity. In normal subjects this effect is most marked when the osmolarity is increased beyond 1500 mOsm/L[1,16,119,120] with absorbable osmotic fillers. The hyperosmotic effect is also evident when lactose, sucrose, melibiose, raffinose, stachyose and dextrans (mean molecular weight 3000) are used as test substances, but the permeation of monosaccharides (L-rhamnose, mannitol) is not affected, even when the solution is made up to

3600 mOsm/L[1,115,120,121]. The hyperosmolar effect of absorbed solutes contrasts with that of poorly permeable solutes, which retain fluid within the intestinal lumen and thus accelerate intestinal transit, reduce the contact time between the test probes and the area under interest[122,123]. As little as 5 g of lactulose is sufficient to reduce the permeation of L-rhamnose by 30%[18]. The principle of osmotic fluid retention of poorly absorbed substances is easily explained by diffusion principles[124–127] and does not require the more elaborate explanation of 'solvent drag'[128–134].

CONSEQUENCES OF INCREASED INTESTINAL PERMEABILITY

It is sometimes suggested that increased small intestinal permeability is synonymous with the enhanced permeation of macromolecules. Ingested food and luminal toxins might then permeate across the mucosa, upsetting the fine balance between the luminal aggressors and luminal defence. The consequences could be systemic and/or local. For this to be plausible it needs to be shown that increased intestinal permeability, as assessed with the low molecular weight markers, does indeed reflect increased macromolecular permeability.

Systemic consequences

There is circumstantial evidence to suggest that this is the case. Davin *et al.* found a significant correlation between intestinal permeability to ^{51}Cr-EDTA and IgA immune complex-plasma levels in patients with IgA-associated nephropathies[135]. Ramage *et al.* showed significant correlation between ^{51}Cr-EDTA permeation rates and increased permeation of ovalbumin in rats infected with *Nippostrongylus brasiliensis*[136]. Similarly the permeation of N-formyl-methionyl-leucyl-[125]L-tyrosine, a synthetic analogue of the bacterial chemotactic peptide N-formyl-methonyl-leucyl-phenylalanine, correlated significantly with intestinal permeability to ^{51}Cr-EDTA following dithiothreitol[137]. However, the permeation of PEG 4000, which otherwise behaves much like ^{51}Cr-EDTA and lactulose, does not appear to conform to the above[138,139]. However the permeation of a very large marker, polysucrose 15 000, appears to conform to data obtained with the low molecular weight (340–360 kDa) markers ^{51}Cr-EDTA and lactulose[140–142]. Collectively the data at present suggest that increased intestinal permeability to inert markers increases the possibility of significant macromolecular permeation. However, an increase in the permeation of macromolecules across the intestinal mucosa is not necessarily synonymous with an increase in its systemic effects. The overall effect of the permeating macromolecule will be dependent on the degradative processes and the effectiveness of local and systemic immunological factors.

Local consequences

The local consequences of increased intestinal permeability has come from integrated studies assessing and quantitating small intestinal inflammation in many diseases in which intestinal permeability is known to be increased. The result is the emergence and characterization of a number of 'new' inflammatory gut diseases in humans which are simply caused by an imbalance and interaction between intestinal mucosal integrity, luminal aggressors and mucosal defence. Here it is suggested that the inflammation in all these small bowel diseases is driven by mucosal exposure of luminal antigens, irrespective of the primary cause; the central mechanism of damage occurring because of a breach in mucosal permeability. Indeed all the above diseases are associated with similar changes of intestinal permeability and a nearly uniformly severe (low grade) inflammatory reaction, as shown in Table 1.

By comparison, patients with inflammatory bowel disease have similar changes in intestinal permeability. The inflammatory reaction, however, is an order of magnitude greater (10–70% of labelled white cells) than that shown for the low-grade enteropathies. The case for the importance of increased intestinal permeability in the relapse of inflammatory bowel disease has been made[4,14], but the intensity of the inflammatory response is the central issue that distinguishes classical inflammatory bowel disease from the above 'non-specific' inflammatory diseases.

INTESTINAL PERMEABILITY IN LIVER DISEASE

Blood leaving the intestine goes directly to the liver. The possible interaction between increased intestinal permeability and liver disease is therefore of considerable interest. Increased intestinal permeability occurs during acute hepatitis A infection, suggesting that the enterocytes may be affected[143]. Similarly intestinal permeability is increased in chronic alcohol misuse in humans[114] and such consumption has a number of effects on the small bowel[144–148] in experimental animals. Menzies found that when a test solution was made markedly hyperosmolar with alcohol it had no effect on the permeation of lactulose[1], which is unlike the effect of any other absorbed osmotic filler. Presumably this is due to

Table 1 Interaction between intestinal permeability and inflammation

	Intestinal permeability	Inflammation
Permeability breakers		
NSAIDs	×2–5	3.0%
Alcohol	×2–5	2.6%
Chronic renal failure	×2–3	5.2%
Radiation	×2–3	Mild*
Cytotoxic drugs	×2–5	Unknown
Impaired mucosal defence		
Hypogammaglobulinaemia	×2–7	6.9%
HIV–AIDS	×2–10	2.0%
Luminal aggressors		
Infections	×2–5	7.2%
Salmonella		
Shigella		
Yersinia		
Cystic fibrosis	×2–10	Unknown

* Based on the faecal excretion calprotectin.

the rapid absorption of alcohol from the stomach and duodenum. Similarly the permeation of ^{51}Cr-EDTA was unaffected by alcohol, given at a final osmolarity of 3600 mOsm/L, while an identical hyperosmolar stress induced by urea increased the permeation 10-fold[115]. However, a modest dose of alcohol (0.5 g/kg) 15 h before the test caused a modest but significant increase in the permeation of ^{51}Cr-EDTA[149]. It has been suggested that increased permeation of macromolecules may play a role in the system pathology of alcoholism, but this would be but one factor among many to bring about this damage, as the vast majority of patients with chronic end-stage liver disease (cirrhosis with portal hypertension) have normal intestinal permeability[150–152].

It is often postulated that in spontaneous bacterial peritonitis the infecting bacteria translocate from the gut lumen either directly through the serosa or indirectly via the blood. This remains unproved to date. The question of the pathophysiological role of increased intestinal permeability in bacterial translocation is also frequently raised in the critically ill. Damage to the small intestine, as assessed by an increase in intestinal permeability, has been shown to be present in critical illness[153], following cardiopulmonary bypass[154,155], major vascular surgery[156], liver transplants[157], multiple trauma[158] and severe burns[159]. These conditions are all associated with endotoxaemia, sepsis and multiorgan failure.

In burn patients Ziegler et al.[159] demonstrated that an increase in intestinal permeability correlated with the severity of sepsis, and that non-infected burn patients had normal intestinal permeability. In addition, patients with particularly high permeability values are at significant risk of sepsis[160]. The suggestion is that loss of intestinal barrier function contributed to the infection. This relationship is difficult to characterize, as a number of factors will influence both intestinal barrier function and infection rates in any given group. For example, endotoxin may permeate across a damaged mucosal surface and systemically administered endotoxin will increase intestinal permeability[161]. An additional factor to consider in severely ill patients is the effect of uraemia on intestinal permeability[162,163]. Clearly further studies are required in this very complicated field. A commonly overlooked factor in these studies is that while small intestinal permeability is being assessed it is the colon which is the main bacterial reservoir, and potentially a much more important site of bacterial translocation than the small intestine.

SUMMARY

Following the pioneering work of Menzies the non-invasive assessment of intestinal permeability is now within the capability of any decent chemical pathology laboratory. There are a number of potential pitfalls which are easily avoided by tailoring the test to the problem at hand, and by attention to analytical details of the markers. The clinically relevant consequence of increased intestinal permeability is the development of a uniformly severe, low-grade enteropathy, regardless of whether the permeability changes are primarily due to barrier breakers, increased luminal aggressiveness or reduced mucosal defence. The systemic consequences of increased mucosal permeability, in particular on the liver, are of questionable importance and require further study.

References

1. Menzies IS. Absorption of intact oligosaccharide in health and disease. Biochem Soc Trans. 1974;2:1040–6.
2. Menzies IS. Quantitative estimation of sugars in blood and urine by paper chromatography using direct densitometry. J Chromatogr. 1983;81:109–27.
3. Bjarnason I, Macpherson A, Hollander D. Intestinal permeability: an overview. Gastroenterology. 1995;108:1566–81.
4. Bjarnason I, Macpherson AJS, Somasundaram S, Teahon K. Non-steroidal anti-inflammatory drugs and Crohn's disease. In: Scholmeric J, Kruis W, Goebbel H, Hohenberger W, Gross V, editors. Inflammatory bowel diseases: pathophysiology as basis of treatment. Falk Symposium Lancaster: 67. Kluwer ;1993:208–22.
5. Bjarnason I, Macpherson AJ, Somasundaram S, Teahon K. Nonsteroidal anti-inflammatory drugs and inflammatory bowel disease. Can J Gastroenterol. 1993;7:160–9.
6. Walker AW, Isselbacher KJ. Uptake and transport of macromolecules by the intestine. Possible role in clinical disorders. Gastroenterology. 1974;67:531–50.
7. Warren S, Sommers SC. Pathology of regional ileitis and ulcerative colitis. J Am Med Assoc. 1954;154:189–93.
8. Shorter RG, Huizenga GA, Spencer RJ. A working hypothesis for the etiology and pathogenesis of nonspecific inflammatory bowel disease. Dig Dis Sci. 1972;17:1024–31.
9. Hollander D. Crohn's disease – a permeability disorder of the tight junctions? Gut. 1988;26:1621–4.
10. Dohan FC. Coeliac disease and schizophrenia. Lancet. 1970;1:897–8.
11. Mielants H, Veys EM, Cuvelier C, de Vos M. Ileocolonoscopic findings in seronegative spondyloarthropathies. Br J Rheumatol. 1988;27(Suppl. II):95–105.
12. Bywaters EGL. Historical aspects of the etiology of rheumatoid arthritis. Br J Rheumatol. 1988;27(Suppl. II):110–15.
13. Hong R, Amman AJ. Selective absence of IgA: autoimmune phenomena and autoimmune diseases. Human Pathol. 1972;69:451–96.
14. Bjarnason I, Macpherson A, Menzies IS. Intestinal permeability: the basics. In: Sutherland LR, Collins SM, Martin F, McLeod RS, Targan SR, Wallace JL, Williams CN, (editors). Inflammatory bowel disease: basic research, clinical implications and trends in therapy. Lancaster, UK: Kluwer Academic Publishers; 1994:53–70.
15. Bjarnason I, Maxton D, Reynolds AP, Catt S, Peters TJ, Menzies IS. A comparison of 4 markers of intestinal permeability in control subjects and patients with coeliac disease. Scand J Gastroenterol. 1994;26:630–9.
16. Maxton DG, Bjarnason I, Reynolds AP, Catt SD, Peters TJ, Menzies IS. Lactulose, [51]CrEDTA, L-rhamnose and polyethylene glycol 400 as probe markers for 'in vivo' assessment of human intestinal permeability. Clin Sci. 1986;71:71–80.
17. Menzies IS. Transmucosal passage of inert molecules in health and disease. In: Skadhauge E, Heintze K, editors. Intestinal absorption and secretion. Falk Symposium 36. Lancaster: MTP Press; 1984:527–43.
18. Menzies IS, Jenkins AP, Heduan E, Catt SD, Segal MB, Creamer B. The effect of poorly absorbed solute on intestinal absorption. Scand J Gastroenterol. 1990;25:1257–64.
19. Laker MF, Mount JN. Mannitol estimation in biological fluids by gas liquid chromatography of trimethylsilyl derivatives. Clin Chem. 1980;26:441–3.
20. Laker MF, Bull HJ, Menzies IS. Evaluation of mannitol for use as a probe marker of gastrointestinal permeability in man. Eur J Clin Invest. 1982;12:485–91.
21. Hollander D, Rickets D, Boyd CAR. Importance of 'probe' molecular geometry in determining intestinal permeability. Can J Gastroenterol. 1988;2(Suppl. A):35–8A.
22. Chadwick VS, Phillips SF, Hofman AF. Measurements of intestinal permeability using low molecular weight polyethylene glycols (PEG 400). II. Application to study of normal and abnormal permeability states in man and animals. Gastroenterology. 1977;73:247–51.
23. Chadwick VS, Phillips SF, Hofman AF. Measurements of intestinal permeability using low molecular weight polyethylene glycols (PEG 400). I. Chemical analysis and biological properties of PEG 400. Gastroenterology. 1977;73:241–6.
24. Blatzinger JG, Rommel K, Ecknauer R. Elimination of low molecular weight polyethylene glycol 400 in the urine following oral load, as a measure of intestinal permeability. J Clin Chem Clin Biochem. 1981;19:265–6.

25. Tageson C, Anderson PA, Anderson J, Bolin T, Kallberg M, Sjodahl R. Passage of molecules through the wall of the gastrointestinal tract. Measurement of intestinal permeability to polyethylene glycols in the 634–1338 dalton range (PEG 1000). Scand J Gastroenterol. 1983;18:481–6.
26. Irving CS, Lifschitz CH, Marks LM, Nichols BC, Klein PD. Polyethylene glycol polymers of low molecular weight as probes of intestinal permeability. I. Innovations in analyses and quantitation. J Lab Clin Med. 1986;107:290–8.
27. McClung HJ, Powers D, Sloan H, Kerzner B. A new micromethod for the quantitation of low molecular weight polymers of polyethylene glycol. Clin Chim Acta. 1983;134:245–54.
28. Delahunty T, Hollander D. New liquid-chromatographic method for measuring polyethylene glycol. Clin Chem. 1986;32:351–3.
29. Cooper BT. Tests of intestinal permeability in clinical practice. J Clin Gastroenterol. 1984;6:499–501.
30. Cox MA, Iqbal TH, Lewis KO, BT C. Viewpoints in intestinal permeability. Gastroenterology. 1997;112:669–70.
31. Ma TY, Krugilak P. Viewpoints in intestinal permeability. Gastroenterology. 1996;110:967–8.
32. Sutherland LR, Verhoef M, Wallace JL, Rosendaahl GV, Crutcher R, Meddings JB. A simple, non-invasive marker of gastric damage: sucrose permeability. Lancet. 1994;343:998–1000.
33. Meddings JB, Sutherland LR, Byles NI, Wallace JL. Sucrose: a novel permeability marker for gastroduodenal disease. Gastroenterology. 1993;104:1619–26.
34. Rabassa AA, Goodgame R, Sutton FM, Nou CN, Rognerud C, Graham DY. Effects of aspirin and *Helicobacter pylori* on the gastroduodenal mucosal permeability to sucrose. Gut. 1996;39:159–63.
35. Vogelsang H, Oberhuber G, Wyatt J. Lymphocytic gastritis and gastric permeability in patients with coeliac disease. Gastroenterology. 1996;111:73–7.
36. Cox MA, Iqbal TH, Lewis KO, Cooper BT. Gastric permeability in coeliac disease. Gastroenterology. 1997;112:314–15.
37. Bjarnason I, Batt R, Catt S, Macpherson A, Maxton D, Menzies IS. Evaluation of differential disaccharide excretion in urine for non-invasive assessment of intestinal disaccharidase activity caused by α-glucosidase inhibition, primary hypolactasia and coeliac disease. Gut. 1996;39:374–81.
38. Maxton DG, Catt SD, Menzies IS. Combined assessment of intestinal disaccharidases in congenital asucrasia by differential urinary disaccharide excretion. J Clin Pathol. 1990;43:406–9.
39. Jenkins AP, Nukajam WS, Menzies IS, Creamer B. Simultaneous administration of lactulose and ^{51}Cr-ethylenediaminetetraacetic acid. A test to distinguish colonic from small-intestinal permeability change. Scand J Gastroenterol. 1992;27:769–73.
40. Jenkins AP, Trew DR, Crump BJ, Menzies IS, Creamer B. Do nonsteroidal anti-inflammatory drugs increase colonic permeability? Gut. 1991;32:66–9.
41. Teahon T, Somasundaram S, Smith T, Menzies IS, Bjarnason I. Assessing the site of increased intestinal permeability in coliac and inflammatory bowel disease. Gut. 1996;38:364–9.
42. Travis S, Menzies IS. Intestinal permeability: functional assessment and significance. Clin Sci. 1992;82:471–88.
43. Menzies IS, Pounder R, Heyer S et al. Abnormal intestinal permeability to sugars in villus atrophy. Lancet. 1979;2:1107–9.
44. Cobden I, Rothwell J, Axon ATR. Intestinal permeability and screening tests for coeliac disease. Gut. 1980;21:512–18.
45. Juby LD, Rothwell J, Axon ATR. Lactulose/mannitol test. An ideal screening test for coeliac disease. Gastroenterology. 1989;96:79–85.
46. Fotherby KJ, Wraight KJ, Neale G. ^{51}CrEDTA/^{14}C mannitol intestinal permeability test. Clinical use in screening for coeliac disease. Scand J Gastroenterol. 1988;23:171–7.
47. Juby LD, Rothwell J, Axon ATR. Cellobiose/mannitol sugar test: a sensitive tubeless test for coeliac disease. Results on 1010 unselected patients. Gut. 1989;30:476–80.
48. Bjarnason I, Peters TJ, Veall N. A persistent defect of intestinal permeability in coeliac disease as demonstrated by a ^{51}Cr-labelled EDTA absorption test. Lancet. 1983;1:323–5.
49. Bjarnason I, Marsh MN, Price A, Levi AJ, Peters TJ. Intestinal permeability in patients with coeliac disease and dermatitis herpetiformis. Gut. 1986;26:1214–19.
50. Hamilton I, Cobden I, Axon ATR. Intestinal permeability in coeliac disease: the response to gluten withdrawal and single dose gluten challenge. Gut. 1982;23:202–10.

51. Ukabam SO, Cooper BT. Small intestinal permeability as an indicator of jejunal mucosal recovery in patients with coeliac sprue on a gluten free diet. J Clin Gastroenterol. 1985;7:232–6.
52. Stenhammer L, Stromberg S. Intestinal permeability to lactulose/L-rhamnose in children with coeliac disease and other gastrointestinal disorders. J Pediatr Gastroenterol Nutr. 1988;7:304–6.
53. Stenhammer L, Falth-Magnusson K, Jansson G, Magnusson KE, Sundqvist T. Intestinal permeability to inert sugars and different-sized polyethyleneglycols in children with celiac disease. J Pediatr Gastroenterol Nutr. 1989;9:281–9.
54. Hetzel DAS, Labrody TJ, Bellon M. The [51]CrEDTA absorption test in coeliac patients treated with a gluten free diet. Int Res Communic J Med Sci. 1986;14:1183–5.
55. Cummins AG, Penttila IA, Labrooy JT, Robb TA, Davidson GP. Recovery of the small intestine in coeliac disease on a gluten-free diet: changes in intestinal permeability, small bowel morphology and T-cell activity. J Gastroenterol Hepatol. 1991;6:53–7.
56. Bjarnason I, O'Morain C, Levi AJ, Peters TJ. The absorption of ^{51}Cr EDTA in inflammatory bowel disease. Gastroenterology. 1983;85:318–22.
57. Ukabam SO, Clamp JR, Cooper BT. Abnormal intestinal permeability to sugars in patients with Crohn's disease of the terminal ileum and colon. Digestion. 1982;27:70–4.
58. O'Morain C, Abelon AC, Chervli LR, Fleischner GM, Das KM. [51]CrEDTA: a useful test in the assessement of inflammatory bowel disease. J Lab Clin Med. 1986;108:430–5.
59. Jenkins RT, Jones DB, Goodacre RL et al. Reversibility of increased intestinal permeability to [51]CrEDTA in patients with gastrointestinal inflammatory bowel disease. J Rheumatol. 1987;82:1159–1164.
60. Pironi L, Miglioli M, Ruggeri E et al. Relationship between intestinal permeability to (^{51}Cr) EDTA and inflammatory activity in asymptomatic patients with Crohn's disease. Dig Dis Sci. 1990;35:582–8.
61. Turck D, Ythier H, Maquet E et al. Increased intestinal permeability to [51]CrEDTA in children with Crohn's disease and coeliac disease. J Pediatr Gastroenterol Nutr. 1987;6:535–7.
62. Howden CW, Robertson C, Duncan A, Morris AJ, Russell RI. Comparison of different measurements of intestinal permeability in inflammatory bowel disease. Am J Gastroenterol. 1991;86:1445–9.
63. Sanderson IR, Boulton P, Menzies IS, Walker-Smith JA. Improvement of abnormal lactulose/rhamnose permeability in active Crohn's disease of the small bowel by an elemental diet. Gut. 1987;28:1073–6.
64. Teahon K, Smethurst P, Levi AJ, Bjarnason I. The effect of elemental diet on intestinal permeability and inflammation in Crohn's disease. Gastroenterology. 1991;101:84–9.
65. Teahon K, Smethurst P, Macpherson AJ, Levi AJ, Menzies IS, Bjarnason I. Intestinal permeability in Crohn's disease and its relation to disease activity and relapse following treatment with elemental diet. Eur J Gastroenterol Hepatol. 1993;5:79–84.
66. Wyatt J, Vogelsang H, Hubl W, Waldhoer T, Lochs H. Intestinal permeability and the predictor of relapse in Crohn's disease. Lancet. 1993;341:1437–9.
67. Noone C, Menzies IS, Banatvala JE, Scopes JW. Intestinal permeability and lactulose hydrolysis in human rotaviral gastroenteritis assessed simultaneously by non-invasive differential sugar permeation. Eur J Clin Invest. 1986;16:217–25.
68. Forget P, Sodoyez-Goffaux F, Zapitelli A. Permeability of the small intestine to [51]CrEDTA in children with acute gastroenteritis or eczema. J Pediatr Gastroenterol Nutr. 1985;4:393–6.
69. Ford RPK, Menzies IS, Phillips AD, Walker-Smith JA, Turner MW. Intestinal sugar permeability: relationship to diarrhoeal disease and small bowel morphology. J Pediatr Gastroenterol Nutr. 1985;4:568–74.
70. Behrens R, Northrop C, Lunn P, Neale G, Hanlon P. Factors affecting the integrity of intestinal mucosa in Gambian children. Proc Nutr Soc. 1986;45:67A.
71. Ukabam SO, Homeda MA, Cooper BJ. Small intestinal permeability in Sudanese subjects: evidence of tropical enteropathy. Trans R Soc Trop Med Hyg. 1986;40:204–7.
72. Behrens RH, Lunn PG, Northrop CA, Hanlon PW, Neale G. Factors affecting the integrity of the intestinal mucosa of Gambian children. Am J Clin Nutr. 1987;45:1433–41.
73. Svartz N. Sulphasalazine. II. Some notes on the discovery and development of salazopyrin. Am J Gastroenterol. 1988;83:497–503.
74. Wood NC, Hamilton I, Axon ATR et al. Abnormal intestinal permeability. An aetiological factor in chronic psychiatric disorders? Br J Psychiatry. 1987;150:853–6.

75. Hollander D, Vadheim C, Brettholz E *et al.* Increased intestinal permeability in patients with Crohn's disease and their relatives. Ann Intern Med. 1986;105:883–5.
76. Teahon K, Smethurst P, Levi AJ, Menzies IS, Bjarnason I. Intestinal permeability in patients with Crohn's disease and their first degree relatives. Gut. 1992;33:320–3.
77. Ruttenberg D, Young GO, Wright JP, Isaacs S. PEG 400 excretion in patients with Crohn's disease, their first degree relatives, and healthy volunteers. Dig Dis Sci. 1992;37:705–8.
78. Munkholm P, Langholz E, Hollander D *et al.* Intestinal permeability in patients with Crohn's disease and ulcerative colitis and their first degree relatives. Gut. 1994;35:68–72.
79. Ainsworth M, Eriksen J, Rasmussen JW, Schaffalitzkydemuckadel OB. Intestinal permeability of ^{51}Cr-labelled ethylenediaminetetraacetic acid in patients with Crohn's disease and their first degree relatives. Scand J Gastroenterol. 1989;24:993–8.
80. Katz KD, Hollander D, Vadheim CM *et al.* Intestinal permeability in patients with Crohn's disease and their healthy relatives. Gastroenterology. 1989;97:927–31.
81. May GR, Sutherland LR, Meddings JB. Is small intestinal permeability really increased in relatives of patients with Crohn's disease? Gastroenterology. 1993;104:1627–32.
82. Hollander D. Permeability in Crohn's disease – altered barrier function in healthy relatives? Gastroenterology. 1993;104:1848–51.
83. Yacyshyn BR, Meddings JB. CD45RO expression on circulating CD19+B cells in Crohn's disease correlates with intestinal permeability. Gastroenterology. 1995;108:132–7.
84. Bjarnason I, Hayllar J, Macpherson AJ, Russell AS. Side effects of nonsteroidal anti-inflammatory drugs on the small and large intestine. Gastroenterology. 1993;104:1832–47.
85. Mahmud T, Somasundaram S, Sigthorsson G, Jacob M, Wrigglesworth J, Bjarnason I. Pathogenesis of NSAID enteropathy: differential effects of R and S flurbiprofen in the rat. (Submitted).
86. Mahmud T, Rafi SS, Scott DL, Wrigglesworth JM, Bjarnason I. Nonsteroidal antiinflammatory drugs and uncoupling of mitochondrial oxidative phosphorylation. Arthritis Rheum. 1996;39:1998–2003.
87. Somasundaram S, Rafi S, Hayllar J *et al.* Mitochondrial damage: a possible mechanism of the 'topical' phase of NSAID-induced injury to the rat intestine. Gut. 1997(In press).
88. Somasundaram S, Rafi S, Jacob M *et al.* Intestinal tolerability of nitroxybutyl-flurbiprofen in rats. Gut. 1997(In press).
89. Somasundaram S, Hayllar J, Rafi S, Wrigglesworth J, Macpherson A, Bjarnason I. The biochemical basis of NSAID-induced damage to the gastrointestinal tract: a review and a hypothesis. Scand J Gastroenterol. 1995;30:289–99.
90. Bjarnason I, Williams P, So A *et al.* Intestinal permeability and inflammation in rheumatoid arthritis; effects of non-steroidal anti-inflammatory drugs. Lancet. 1984;2:1171–4.
91. Bjarnason I, Williams P, Smethurst P, Peters TJ, Levi AJ. The effect of NSAIDs and prostaglandins on the permeability of the human small intestine. Gut. 1986;27:1292–7.
92. Bjarnason I, Smethurst P, Fenn GC, Lee CF, Menzies IS, Levi AJ. Misoprostol reduces indomethacin induced changes in human small intestinal permeability. Dig Dis Sci. 1989;34:407–11.
93. Bjarnason I, Smethurst P, Clarke P, Menzies IS, Levi AJ, Peters TJ. Effect of prostaglandins on indomethacin induced increased intestinal permeability in man. Scand J Gastroenterol. 1989;29(Suppl. 164):97–103.
94. Bjarnason I, Smethurst P, Macpherson A *et al.* Glucose and citrate reduce the permeability changes caused by indomethacin in humans. Gastroenterology. 1992;102:1546–50.
95. Auer IO, Habscheid W, Hiller S, Gerhards W, Eilles C. Nicht-steroidale antiphlogistika erhohen die darmpermeabilitat. Dtsch Med Wochenschr. 1987;112:1032–7.
96. Jenkins RT, Rooney PJ, Jones DB, Bienenstock J, Goodacre RL. Increased intestinal permeability in patients with rheumatoid arthritis. A side effect of nonsteroidal antiinflammatory drug therapy. Br J Rheumatol. 1987;26:103–7.
97. Aabakken L, Osnes M. ^{51}Cr-ethylenediaminetetraacetic acid absorption test. Effects of naproxen, a non-steroidal, antiinflammatory drug. Scand J Gastroenterol. 1990;25:917–24.
98. Bjarnason I, Fehilly B, Smethurst P, Menzies IS, Levi AJ. The importance of local versus systemic effects of non-steroidal anti-inflammatory drugs to increase intestinal permeability in man. Gut. 1991;32:275–7.

99. Bjarnason I, Smethurst P, Menzies IS, Peters TJ. The effect of polyacrylic acid polymers (carbopol) on small intestinal function and permeability changes caused by indomethacin. Scand J Gastroenterol. 1991;26:685–8.
100. Davies GR, Rampton DS. The pro-drug sulindac may reduce the risk of intestinal damage associated with the use of conventional non-steroidal anti-inflammatory drugs. Aliment Pharmacol Ther. 1991;5:593–8.
101. Aabakken L, Larsen S, Osnes K. Sucralfate for prevention of naproxen-induced mucosal lesions. Scand J Rheumatol. 1989;18:361–8.
102. Aabakken L, Larsen S, Osnes M. Cimetidine tablets or suspension in the prevention of gastrointestinal mucosal lesions caused by nonsteroidal anti-inflammatory drugs. Scand J Rheumatol. 1989;18:647–55.
103. Bjarnason I, Zanelli G, Smith T et al. Nonsteroidal antiinflammatory drug induced intestinal inflammation in humans. Gastroenterology. 1987;93:480–9.
104. Segal AW, Isenberg DA, Hajirousow V, Tolfree S, Clark J, Snaith ML. Preliminary evidence for gut involvement in the pathogenesis of rheumatoid arthritis? Br J Rheumatol. 1986;25:162–6.
105. Rooney PJ, Jenkins RT, Smith KM, Coates G. 111-Indium-labelled polymorphonuclear scans in rheumatoid arthritis – an important clinical cause of positive results. Br J Rheumatol. 1986;15:167–70.
106. Morris AJ, Wasson LA, Mackenzie JF. Small bowel enteroscopy in undiagnosed gastrointestinal blood loss. Gut. 1992;33:887–9.
107. Bjarnason I, Zanelli G, Smethurst P et al. Clinico-pathological features of nonsteroidal antiinflammatory drug induced small intestinal strictures. Gastroenterology. 1988;94:1070–4.
108. Siber GR, Mayer RJ, Levin MJ. Increased gastrointestinal absorption of large molecules in patients after 5-fluorourasil therapy for metastatic colon carcinoma. Cancer Res. 1980;40:3430–6.
109. Selby P, McElwain TJ, Crofts M, Lopes N, Mundy J. 51CrEDTA test for intestinal permeability. Lancet. 1984;2:39.
110. Pearson ADJ, Craft AW, Pledger JV, Eastham EJ, Laker MF, Pearson CS. Small bowel function in acute lymphoblastic leukemia. Arch Dis Child. 1984;59:460–5.
111. Pledger JV, Pearson ADJ, Craft AW, Laker MF, Eastham EJ. Intestinal permeability during chemotherapy for childhood tumors. Eur J Pediatr. 1988;147:123–7.
112. Selby PJ, Lopes N, Mundy J, Crofts M, Millar JL, McElwain TJ. Cyclophosphamide priming reduces intestinal damage in man following high dose melphalan chemotherapy. Br J Cancer. 1987;55:531–3.
113. Mansi J, Ellis E, Viner C et al. Gut protection by cyclophosphamide 'priming' in patients receiving high-dose melphalan – effect of drug scheduling. Cancer Chemother Pharmacol. 1992;30:149–51.
114. Bjarnason I, Ward K, Peters TJ. The leaky gut of alcoholism: possible route of entry for toxic compounds. Lancet. 1984;1:179–82.
115. Smethurst P, Menzies IS, Levi AJ, Bjarnason I. Is alcohol directly toxic to the small bowel mucosa? Clin Sci. 1988;75:50–1P.
116. Robinson GM, Orrego H, Israel Y, Deveny P, Kapur BM. Low-molecular weight polyethylene glycol as a probe of gastrointestinal permeability after alcohol ingestion. Dig Dis Sci. 1981;26:23–32.
117. Nissom JA. Reduction of intestinal absorption by synthetic chemicals. Nature. 1960;185:222–4.
118. Utter O. Om Sakaros-toleransch och avsandringen. I. Hos barn. Finska Laksakksk Handl. 1927;69:613–19.
119. Wheeler PG, Menzies IS, Creamer B. Effect of hyperosmolar stimuli and coeliac disease on the permeability of the human gastrointestinal tract. Clin Sci Mol Med. 1978;54:495–501.
120. Laker MF, Menzies IS. Increase in human intestinal permeability following ingestion of hypertonic solutions. J Physiol (Lond). 1977;273:881–94.
121. Smethurst P, Menzies IS, Levi AJ, Bjarnason I. Intestinal permeability: osmolarity revisited. Gut. 1988;29:A1479–80.
122. Launiala K. The effect of unabsorbed sucrose- or mannitol-induced accelerated transit on absorption in the human small intestine. Scand J Gastroenterol. 1969;4:25–32.
123. Laws JW, Neale G. Radiological diagnosis of disaccharidase deficiency. Lancet. 1966;2:139–43.

124. Kiil F. Molecular mechanisms of osmosis. Am J Physiol. 1989;256:R801–8.
125. Ussing HH, Andersen B. The relation between solvent drag and active transport of ions. Zool Chim. 1955:434–40.
126. Ferraris RP, Yasharpour S, Kent Lloyd KC, Mirzayan R, Diamond JM. Luminal glucose concentrations in the gut under normal conditions. Am J Physiol. 1990;259:G822–37.
127. Fine KD, Santa Ana CA, Porter JL, Fordtran JS. Effect of D-glucose on intestinal permeability and its passive absorption in human small intestine *in vivo*. Gastroenterology. 1993;105:1117–26.
128. Fordtran JS, Rector FC, Ewton MF, Soter N, Kinney J. Permeability characteristics of the human small intestine. J Clin Invest. 1965;12:1935–44.
129. Fordtran JS, Rector FC, Locklear TW, Ewton MF. Water and solute movement in the small intestine of patients with sprue. J Clin Invest. 1967;46:287–98.
130. Fordtran JS. Speculation of the pathogenesis of diarrhoea. Fed Proc. 1967;26:1405–14.
131. Krejs G, Fordtran JS. Physiology and pathophysiology of ion and water movement in the human intestine. In: Sleisenger MH, Fordtran JS, Ingelfinger FJ, (editors). Gastrointestinal disease, 2nd edn. Philadelphia, PA: WB Saunders; 1978:297–313.
132. Caparo V. Permeability and related phenomena: basic concepts. In: Csaky TZ, (editors). Pharmacology of intestinal permeation. I. Berlin: Springer-Verlag; 1984:61–9.
133. Pappenheimer JR, Reiss KZ. Contribution of solvent drag through intercellular junctions to absorption of nutrients by the small intestine of the rat. J Membr Biol. 1987;100:123–36.
134. Pappenheimer JR. Paracellular intestinal absorption of glucose, creatinine, and mannitol in normal animals: relation to body size. Am J Physiol. 1990;259:G290–9.
135. Davin JC, Forget P, Mahieu PR. Increased intestinal permeability to (^{51}Cr)EDTA is correlated with IgA immune complex-plasma levels in children with IgA-associated nephropathies. Acta Pediatr Scand. 1988;77:118–24.
136. Ramage JK, Stanisz A, Scicchitano R, Hunt RH, Perdue MH. Effects of immunologic reactions on rat intestinal epithelium. Correlation of increased intestinal permeability to chromium 51 labelled ethylenediaminetetraacetic acid and ovalbumin during acute inflammation and anaphylaxis. Gastroenterology. 1988;94:1368–75.
137. Ferry DM, Butt TJ, Broom MF, Hunter J, Chadwick VS. Bacterial chemotactic oligopeptides and the intestinal mucosal barrier. Gastroenterology. 1989;97:61–7.
138. Vellenga L, Wensing T, Egberts HJA, van Dijk JE, Mouwen JMVM, Breukink HJ. Intestinal permeability to polyethylene glycol 4000 and porcine albumin in piglets infected with transmissible gastroenteritis virus. Vet Res Comm. 1989;13:467–74.
139. Westrom B, Svendsen J, Tageson C. Intestinal permeability to polyethyleneglycol 600 in relation to macromolecular 'closure' in the neonatal pig. Gut. 1984;25:520–5.
140. Blomquist L, Oman H, Henrriksson K, Johansson SGO. Increased absorption of polysucrose, a marker of intestinal paracellular permeability, in Crohn's disease. Eur J Gastroenterol. 1993;5:913–17.
141. Oman H, Akerblom E, Richter W, Johansson SGO. Chemical and physiological properties of polysucrose, a new marker of intestinal permeability to macromolecules. Int Arch Allergy Immunol. 1992;98:220–6.
142. Oman H, Blomquist L, Henriksson AEK, Johansson SGO. Comparison of polysucrose 1500, ^{51}Cr-labelled ethylenediaminetetraacetic acid, and ^{14}C-mannitol as markers of intestinal permeability in man. Scand J Gastroenterol. 1995;30:1172–7.
143. Parrili G, Cumo R, Nardone G, Maio G, Izzo CM, Budillon G. Investigation of intestinal function during acute viral hepatitis using combined sugar load. Gut. 1987;28:1439–44.
144. Baradona E, Lindenbaum J. Metabolic effect of alcohol on the small intestine. In: Lieber CS, (editors). Metabolic aspects of alcoholism. Baltimore, MD: University Park Press; 1977:81–116.
145. Mezey E, Jow E, Slavin RE, Tobon F. Pancreatic function and intestinal absorption in chronic alcoholism. Gastroenterology. 1970;59:657–64.
146. Wilson FA, Hoyumpa AM. Ethanol and intestinal transport. Gastroenterology. 1979;76:388–403.
147. Lindenbaum J, Lieber CS. Effect of chronic ethanol administration on intestinal absorption in man in the absence of nutritional deficiency. Ann NY Acad Sci. 1975;252:228–34.
148. Roggin CM, Iber FL, Kater RHM, Tobon F. Malabsorption in chronic alcoholics. Johns Hopkins Med J. 1969;125:321–30.

149. Aabakken L. ^{51}Cr ethylenediaminetetraacetic acid absorption test. Methodological aspects. Scand J Gastroenterol. 1989;24:351–8.
150. Budillon G, Parrilli G, Pacella M, Cuomo R, Menzies IS. Investigation of intestine and liver function in cirrhosis using combined sugar oral loads. J Hepatol. 1985;1:513–24.
151. Romiti A, Merli M, Martorano M et al. Malabsorption and nutritional abnormalities in patients with liver cirrhosis. Ital J Gastroenterol. 1990;22:118–23.
152. Bac DJ, Swart R, van der Berg JWO, Wilson JHP. Small bowel wall function in patients with advanced liver cirrhosis and portal hypertension: studies on permeability and luminal bacterial overgrowth. Eur J Gastroenterol Hepatol. 1993;5:383–7.
153. Harris CE, Griffiths RD, Freestone N, Billington D, Atherton ST, Macmillan RR. Intestinal permeability in the critically ill. Intensive Care Med. 1992;18:38–41.
154. Ohri SK, Somasundaram S, Koak Y et al. The effect of intestinal hypoperfusion during cardiopulmonary bypass surgery on saccharide permeation and intestinal permeability in man. Gastroenterology. 1993;106:318–23.
155. Riddington DW, Venkatesh B, Boivin CM et al. Intestinal permeability, gastric intramucosal pH, and systemic endotoxemia in patients undergoing cardiopulmonary bypass. J Am Med Assoc. 1996;275:1007–12.
156. Roumen RM, van der Vliet JA, Wevers RA, Goris RJ. Intestinal permeability is increased after major vascular surgery. J Vasc Surg. 1993;17:734–7.
157. Wicks C, Somasundaram S, Bjarnason I et al. Comparison of enteral feeding and total parenteral nutrition after liver transplantation. Lancet. 1993;344:837–40.
158. Pape HC, Dwenger A, Regel G et al. Increased gut permeability after multiple trauma. Br J Surg. 1994;81:850–2.
159. Ziegler TR, Smith RJ, O'Dwyer ST, Demling RH, Wilmore DW. Increased intestinal permeability associated with infection in burn patients. Arch Surg. 1988;123:1313–19.
160. LeVoyer T, Cioffi WG, Pratt L et al. Alterations in intestinal permeability after thermal injury. Arch Surg. 1992;127:26–9.
161. O'Dwyer SJ, Michie HR, Ziegler TR, Revhaug A, Smith RJ, Wilmore DW. A single dose of endotoxin increases intestinal permeability in healthy humans. Arch Surg. 1988;123:1459–64.
162. Magnusson M, Magnusson KE, Sundqvist T, Denneberg T. Urinary excretion of differently sized polyethylene glycols after intravenous administration in uremic and control rats: effects of low- and high-protein diets. Nephron. 1990;56:312–16.
163. Magnusson M, Magnusson KE, Sundqvist T, Denneberg T. Increased intestinal permeability to differently sized polyethylene glycols in uremic rats: effects of low- and high-protein diets. Nephron. 1990;56:306–11.

4
Bacterial translocation

R. D. BERG

INTRODUCTION

Indigenous and non-indigenous bacteria colonizing the gastrointestinal (GI) tract of humans and animals can pass through the intestinal mucosal barrier to appear in extraintestinal sites such as the lymph, mesenteric lymph node (MLN) complex, liver, spleen, kidneys, peritoneal cavity, and blood stream. Viable GI bacteria were cultured from the livers, spleens, and kidneys of various animals and humans as early as 1900[1]. Later it was discovered that the portal blood and livers of presumably healthy dogs also contain viable GI bacteria[2-5]. Even though these and other reports suggested that indigenous GI bacteria could pass from the intestines to extraintestinal sites, no systematic investigations were undertaken of this phenomenon.

Persorption, transmural migration, and translocation are terms that have been used to describe the passage of particles, viruses, and bacteria across the intestinal mucosal barrier (Table 1). Translocation seems the most appropriate of these terms, since it simply describes the relocation of microorganisms from the GI tract to extraintestinal sites without implying anything concerning the actual mechanisms, whereas transmural migration suggests active movement initiated by the microorganism, and persorption is easily confused with the term absorption[6].

Utilizing a variety of animal models we have identified three major mechanisms that promote bacterial translocation from the GI tract: (a) intestinal bacterial overgrowth, (b) increased intestinal permeability or damage to the intestinal mucosa, and (c) compromised host immune defences[7-14] (Table 2). In some animal models of translocation only one mechanism is operating to promote bacterial translocation; in other models several mechanisms are operating to synergistically promote translocation.

BACTERIAL TRANSLOCATION PROMOTED BY INTESTINAL BACTERIAL OVERGROWTH

Various bacterial species readily translocate from the GI tract when their populations attain abnormally high levels, i.e. exhibit intestinal overgrowth. Intestinal

47

Table 1 Terms used to describe the passage of particles or microorganisms from the GI tract across the intestinal barrier

Term	Description	Reference
Persorption	Large solid particles to blood (micrometer range)	Volkheimer et al. Digestion. 1968;1:78–80.
Phage translocation	*Bacillus megaterium* phage to blood	Keller and Engley Proc Soc Exp Biol Med. 1958;18:577–80.
Phage translocation	*Escherichia coli* phage T_1 to lymph	Hildebrand and Wolochow Proc Soc Exp Biol Med. 1962;109:193–5.
Transmural migration	*Escherichia coli* to peritoneum	Frank *et al.* Ann Surg. 1948;128:561–608. Schweinburg, *et al.* Proc Soc Exp Biol Med. 1949;71:150–3.
Bacterial translocation	*Serratia marcescens* to MLN	Wolochow *et al.* J Infect Dis. 1966;116:523–8.
Bacterial translocation	*Streptococcus faecalis* to liver	Fuller and Jayne-Williams Res Vet Sci. 1970;11:368–74.
Bacterial translocation	Indigenous GI bacteria to MLN	Berg and Garlington Infect Immun. 1979;23:403–11.

Table 2 Animal models demonstrating the three major mechanisms promoting translocations

Intestinal bacterial overgrowth
Mice given oral antibiotics
Monoassociated gnotobiotic (ex-germ-free) mice
Starvation
Protein malnutrition
Parenteral alimentation
Enteral alimentation
Bowel obstruction
Bile duct ligation
Streptozotocin-induced diabetes
Endotoxaemia

Physical damage to intestinal mucosa
Oral ricinoleic acid (castor oil)
Endotoxaemia
Injection of zymosan
Thermal injury
Haemorrhagic shock

Impaired host immune defences
Mice injected with immunosuppressive agents
Thymectomy
Athymic (*nu/nu*) mice
CD4/CD8 T cell depletion
Beige/nude (*bg/bg*; *nu/nu*) mice
Lymphoma
Leukaemia
Streptozotocin-induced diabetes
Endotoxaemia
Thermal injury
Haemorrhagic shock

bacterial overgrowth often occurs in humans and animals receiving oral anti-biotics that disrupt the ecological balance in the intestines and allow certain indigenous bacteria resistance to these antibiotics to increase in GI population levels. This ecological disruption by oral antibiotics can also cause the host to lose 'colonization resistance' and thereby enable more pathogenic exogenous bacteria resistant to these antibiotics to colonize the GI tract.

Caecal populations of indigenous Enterobacteriaceae increase dramatically when mice are given oral antibiotics, such as penicillin, metronidazole or clin-damycin[15]. For example, in mice given oral penicillin for only 4 days, the caecal populations of indigenous obligate anaerobes decrease 1000-fold, allowing the caecal populations of Enterobacteriaceae to increase 10 000-fold. This abnormal increase in Enterobacteriaceae caecal populations promotes the translocation of Enterobacteriaceae from the GI tract to the MLN. Even though the oral anti-biotics are discontinued after only 4 days, normal intestinal microecology is not reestablished until approximately 30 days later, and Enterobacteriaceae continue to translocate from the GI tract during this time.

Patients receiving oral antibiotics are also at increased risk to bacterial translocation due to intestinal bacterial overgrowth. The results in animal models suggest that patients may be at risk to bacterial translocation for a con-siderable period even after antibiotic therapy has been discontinued. Clinical sit-uations other than oral antibiotic therapy, such as the administration of a liquid elemental diet or parenteral alimentation, also often lead to intestinal bacterial overgrowth and promote the translocation of bacteria from the GI tract[16].

In subsequent studies we demonstrated a direct cause-and-effect relationship between the caecal populations of certain Enterobacteriaceae and the transloca-tion of Enterobacteriaceae from the GI tract. For example, *E. coli* C25 transloca-tion in gnotobiotic (ex-germ-free) mice monoassociated with *E. coli* C25 was compared with *E. coli* C25 translocation in gnotobiotic mice colonized with *E. coli* C25 plus the entire indigenous GI microflora[17] (Table 3). The strepto-mycin-resistant *E. coli* C25 can be cultured separately from the streptomycin-sensitive *E. coli* strains indigenous to mice. In gnotobiotes monoassociated with *E. coli* C25, the *E. coli* C25 populations remained at 10^9/g caecum during the entire test period, and *E. coli* C25 translocated to 100% of the MLN tested. In gnotobiotes inoculated with *E. coli* C25 and then 1 week later given the whole indigenous GI microflora, *E. coli* C25 caecal populations decreased 100-fold by

Table 3 Antagonism of *E. coli* C25 by indigenous anaerobes

Day	Gnotobiotes (E. coli C25)		Gnotobiotes (E. coli C25 + GI flora)		
	E. coli C25: caecum	E. coli C25: MLN	Anaerobes: caecum	E. coli C25: caecum	E. coli C25: MLN
1	3.2×10^9	5/5	6.3×10^{11}	5.0×10^9	6/7
2	2.5×10^9	5/5	2.5×10^{10}	4.0×10^7	7/7
3	3.2×10^9	5/5	3.2×10^9	6.3×10^6	4/7
4	4.0×10^9	5/5	5.0×10^9	2.5×10^7	0/7
7	6.3×10^9	5/5	3.2×10^9	3.2×10^6	0/7
14	3.2×10^9	5/5	2.0×10^9	2.0×10^6	0/7

day 2 and 1000-fold by day 3. *E. coli* C25 translocation to the MLN ceased by day 4. Thus, when *E. coli* is the only microorganism present in the GI tract it maintains abnormally high population levels of 10^9/g caecum (i.e. intestinal overgrowth) and readily translocates to the MLN. *E. coli* translocation ceases, however, when *E. coli* caecal populations are antagonized by indigenous strict anaerobes to $< 10^8$ *E. coli*/g caecum. To ensure that these results were not due to some abnormality of the germ-free state, the experiments were repeated with identical results in antibiotic-decontaminated mice monoassociated with *E. coli*[18].

The relationship between caecal population levels of Enterobacteriaceae and the translocation of Enterobacteriaceae from the GI tract is even more dramatically demonstrated in gnotobiotic mice triassociated with indigenous *E. coli*, *Klebsiella pneumoniae*, and *Proteus mirabilis*[19]. The gnotobiotes were sacrificed at 1, 3, 5, 8 and 12 weeks after triassociation, and the caecum and MLN cultured for each bacterial species. The percentages of each bacterial species in the caecum and MLN were calculated in relation to the total numbers of bacteria cultured from the caecum and MLN. In each case the percentage of a bacterial species in the caecum was the same as the percentage of that bacterial species in the MLN. The means from all test days are presented in Fig. 1. *E. coli* comprised 25% of the bacteria isolated from the caecum and 32% of the bacteria cultured from the MLN; statistically similar percentages. Similarly, 66% of the caecal bacteria were *K. pneumoniae* and 54% of the MLN cultures were *K. pneumoniae*. *P. mirabilis* comprised 10% of the caecal cultures and 14% of the MLN cultures. These results demonstrate that for each bacterial species the number translocating to the MLN is directly related to its caecal populations.

In the intestinal bacterial overgrowth model, and other animal models in which the intestinal epithelium is not physically damaged, the route of translocation of indigenous bacteria from the GI tract is through the intestinal epithelial

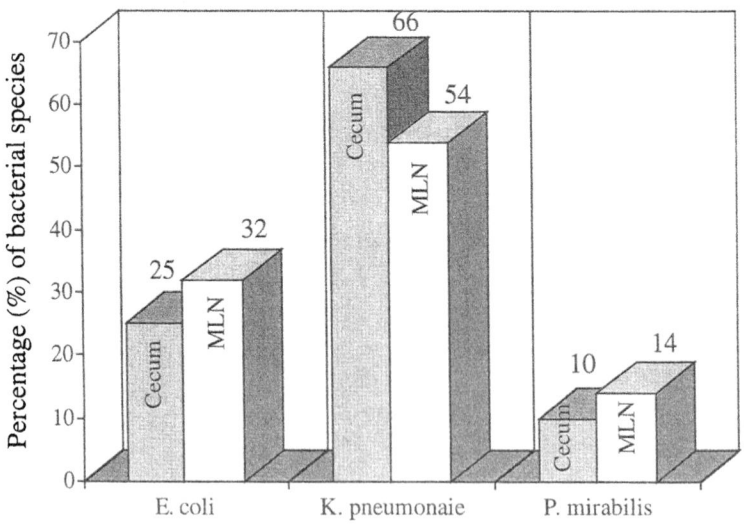

Figure 1 Proportion of bacterial species in caecum and MLN of triassociated gnotobiotic mice

cells (i.e. an intracellular route) rather than between the enterocytes via the tight junctions (i.e. an extracellular route). Even overtly pathogenic microorganisms, such as *Salmonella typhimurium*[20] and *Candida albicans*[21], are seen by microscopy to translocate the intestinal mucosa intracellularly through the intestinal epithelial cells. Once in the lamina propria, translocating bacteria in the intestinal overgrowth model travel by a lymphatic route to the MLN. If the epithelial cell tight junctions or intestinal epithelium are physically damaged – as often occurs after thermal injury, endotoxic shock, or haemorrhagic shock – indigenous bacteria are then able to pass directly through the denuded or ulcerated areas to the lamina propria[13,14]. In these shock models exhibiting physical damage to the mucosal barrier, translocating indigenous bacteria can travel by a vasculature route directly to the liver, in addition to the usual lymphatic route to the MLN.

BACTERIAL TRANSLOCATION PROMOTED BY INCREASED INTESTINAL PERMEABILITY OR PHYSICAL DAMAGE TO THE INTESTINAL MUCOSA

The intact intestinal mucosa provides a physical barrier preventing bacteria colonizing the GI tract from translocating to extraintestinal sites. Translocation of indigenous GI bacteria readily occurs when the intestinal barrier is compromised by chemical agents. For example, ricinoleic acid (12-hydroxy-9-octadecenoic acid), the pharmacologically active constituent of castor oil, when given once intragastrically to mice, severely damages the intestinal mucosa and readily promotes the translocation of indigenous GI bacteria to the MLN[22]. Massive exfoliation of columnar epithelial cells in the proximal small intestine occurs within 2 h after ricinoleic acid administration, and 30% of the MLN cultures are positive for translocating facultatively anaerobic bacteria, such as *P. mirabilis* and *Staphylococcus epidermidis* (Table 4). The incidence of translocation of both facultatively anaerobic and obligately anaerobic bacteria reaches a peak at 4 days following the ricinoleic acid administration. The intestinal mucosa heals and bacterial translocation to the MLN ceases by 7 days after ricinoleic acid administration. This is one of the very few animal models in which indigenous

Table 4 Translocation of indigenous facultatively anaerobic and obligately anaerobic bacteria from the GI tract to the MLN following intragastric inoculation with ricinoleic acid

Time following rincinoleic acid administration (intragastric 1×)	Facultatively anaerobic MLN (percentage positive)	Obligate anaerobes MLN (percentage positive)
0 h	0	0
2 h	30*	15
6 h	37*	30*
2 days	40*	50*
4 days	7*	95*
7 days	0	0

* Denotes significantly different ($p < 0.05$) from 0 h. Ricinoleic acid (50 mg) given intragastrically one time, at time 0.

obligately anaerobic bacteria are seen to translocate at significant levels from the GI tract.

The ischaemia/reperfusion that occurs following haemorrhagic shock, endo-toxic shock, or the shock following thermal injury also physically damages the intestinal epithelium and allows the translocation of indigenous bacteria from the GI tract[23-30]. Examination by microscopy of intestinal tissues from shocked animals reveals ileal and caecal subepithelial oedema and disruption of epithelial cell tight junctions. The injury to the intestinal mucosa during ischaemia/reper-fusion is due, at least partially, to xanthine oxidase-generated, oxygen-free radi-cals. Both intestinal mucosal damage and bacterial translocation in shocked animals are reduced by treatment with: (a) allopurinol, a xanthine oxidase inhibitor; (b) dimethylsulphoxide, a hydroxyl scavenger; (c) deferoxamine, an iron chelator; or (d) feeding animals a tungsten-supplemented, molybdenum-free diet for 2 weeks prior to shock, to deplete intestinal xanthine oxidase.

Failure of the gut barrier in conjunction with liver dysfunction is hypothe-sized to promote or potentiate multiple organ failure, a newly recognized syn-drome leading to death in a variety of patients[31]. Although endotoxin is released in large amounts during the usual lysis of indigenous Gram-negative bacteria in the GI tract, only very small amounts of endotoxin are actually absorbed from the GI tract, and this absorbed endotoxin is readily detoxified by the liver. Shock increases intestinal mucosal permeability and allows the translocation of both endotoxin and bacteria. Patients suffering from severe trauma with associated haemorrhagic shock, endotoxic shock, or thermal injury commonly exhibit intestinal mucosal injury, and are at significant risk to translocation of both bacteria and endotoxin.

BACTERIAL TRANSLOCATION PROMOTED BY COMPROMISED HOST IMMUNE DEFENCES

Resident macrophages are positioned strategically in the MLN to defend against bacterial translocation from the GI tract via the lymphatic route. Consequently, non-specific immunostimulation of macrophages by the injection of formalin-killed *Propionibacterium acnes* (formerly classified as *Corynebacterium parvum*) reduces bacterial translocation to the MLN[32]. For example, *P. acnes* vaccination decreases both the incidence of MLN positive for translocating *E. coli* (75% to 41%) and the numbers of translocating *E. coli* per gram of MLN (1860/g MLN to 304/g MLN) (Table 5). *P. acnes* vaccination has no effect on *E. coli* caecal population levels. In further studies plastic-adherent, *P. acnes*-stimulated spleen or MLN cells (predominantly macrophages) reduced *E. coli* translocation when adoptively transferred to non-vaccinated recipients[33]. Adoptively transferred, non-adherent control cells (predominantly lymphocytes) did not decrease *E. coli* translocation. Macrophages therefore appear to be important effector cells in the host defence against bacterial translocation.

It also has been suggested, however, that macrophages and polymorphonu-clear leucocytes can engulf bacteria at mucosal surfaces and transport them to extraintestinal sites, such as abscesses or even lymph nodes[34]. In this case macrophages would promote bacterial translocation rather than inhibit transloca-

Table 5 Non-specific stimulation of macrophages reduces *E. coli* translocation to the MLN

E. coli C25 monoassociated mice	Spleen weight (g)	CFU/g caecum	Percentage positive MLN (positive/total)	CFU/g MLN
Controls non-vaccinated	0.10	1.65×10^9	75	1860
P. acnes vaccinated*	0.57	2.24×10^9	41 ($p = 0.002$)	304 ($p = 0.009$)

* Mice antibiotic-decontaminated with penicillin plus streptomycin for 4 days and then injected intraperitoneally with 1.4 mg formalin-killed *P. acnes* 1 week (one time) prior to colonization with *E. coli* C25.

tion. More investigation is therefore required to delineate the roles of macrophages and polymorphonuclear leucocytes in the pathogenesis of bacterial translocation under various clinical conditions.

Thymectomy of mice readily promotes the translocation of indigenous GI tract bacteria to 28% of MLN, spleen, liver, and kidneys compared with 3% positive organs in sham-thymectomized control mice[35] (Table 6). Genetically athymic (*nu/nu*) mice also exhibit 'spontaneous' translocation of indigenous GI bacteria, such as *E. coli* and *Lactobacillus acidophilus*, to 50% of their MLN, spleen, liver, and kidneys[36]. Only 5% of these organs in euthymic (*nu/+*) mice contain viable indigenous bacteria. Grafting thymuses to these athymic (*nu/nu*) mice reduces bacterial translocation to that found in control *nu/+* mice. Thus, T cell-mediated immunity appears to be an important component in the host defence against bacterial translocation from the GI tract.

The importance of T cells in the host defence against translocation was subsequently proved by deleting specific T cells to promote bacterial translocation and then adoptively transferring specific T cells back to T cell-depleted mice to inhibit bacterial translocation. Mice were depleted of CD4 and/or CD8 T cells by two intraperitoneal injections of either anti-CD4 or anti-CD8 monoclonal antibodies[37]. This protocol completely depletes CD4 and CD8 T cells in the intestinal epithelium, lamina propria, MLN, and spleen, as demonstrated by flow cytometry. Either CD4 T cell or CD8 T cell depletion readily promotes the translocation of *E. coli* to the MLN. Adoptive transfer of either CD4 T cells, CD8 T cells, or both, from donor mice to T cell-depleted recipients inhibits *E. coli* translocation to the MLN[38].

Table 6 Bacterial translocation in animal models lacking T-cell-mediated immunity*

Organ	nu/nu homozygous nude	nu/+ heterozygous	nu/nu thymus-grafted	+/+ thymectomized	+/+ sham-thymectomized
MLN	40	20	18	46	5
Spleen	56	0	6	29	0
Liver	40	0	0	24	5
Kidneys	60	0	6	12	0
All organs	50	5	8	28	3

* Percentage positive organ cultures (indigenous GI bacteria).

These results provided convincing evidence that T cell-mediated immunity is important in the host defence against bacterial translocation. Since T cells cannot kill bacteria directly, it seems logical that macrophages and/or polymorphonuclear leucocytes are the host effector cells. Bacterial translocation probably occurs in both athymic nude mice and in euthymic mice specifically depleted of T cells because the effector macrophages are not receiving T cell help. Since the development of secretory immunity is also T cell dependent, the lack of secretory IgA in the intestinal secretions of athymic mice and T cell-depleted mice may also be important in allowing bacterial translocation from the GI tract. Unfortunately, the role of specific secretory IgA in the defence against the bacterial translocation has not been examined to date. Secretory IgA reduces the penetration into the lamina propria of non-indigenous overt pathogens, such as *Vibrio cholerae*[39] and *Salmonella enteritidis*[40]. Consequently, it is likely that specific secretory IgA would inhibit the close association of indigenous GI bacteria with the intestinal epithelial cells that must occur just prior to the penetration of the intestinal mucosa by translocating bacteria.

Serum immunoglobulins act as opsonins to increase the effectiveness of phagocytosis and subsequent killing of bacteria by macrophages. Surprisingly, the intravenous injection of anti-*E. coli* IgG into mice does not decrease the numbers of *E. coli* translocating from the GI tract to the MLN, but does reduce the spread of translocating *E. coli* from the MLN to the spleen, liver, kidney, and blood[41]. Thus, serum antibodies appear to be more effective in reducing the spread of translocating bacteria that have already penetrated the intestinal barrier than inhibiting the initial passage of bacteria across the intestinal mucosa.

Probably all components of the host immune system, such as mucosal immunity (secretory IgA), cell-mediated immunity (macrophages and T cells), and humoral immunity (serum immunoglobulins) are involved in the immune defence against bacterial translocation. The injection of mice with immunosuppressive agents, such as cyclophosphamide or prednisolone, readily promotes the translocation of indigenous bacteria to organs such as the MLN, spleen, liver, and kidneys[42]. Bacterial translocation has also been demonstrated in a variety of animal models that exhibit deficiencies in host immune defences, such as animal models of diabetes[10], leukaemia[43], endotoxaemia[24], thermal injury[44,45], and haemorrhagic shock[23]. Patients with compromised immune defences are undoubtedly at risk to bacterial translocation from their GI tracts, and are especially vulnerable to the spread of translocating bacteria from the MLN to other extraintestinal sites. More research is required to delineate the relative roles of the major immune compartments, and to identify the exact immune mechanisms responsible for killing translocating microorganisms.

BACTERIAL TRANSLOCATION INDUCED BY A COMBINATION OF PROMOTING MECHANISMS

More than one mechanism is operating to promote bacterial translocation from the GI tract in complex animal models such as endotoxic shock, haemorrhagic shock, thermal injury, and streptozotocin-induced diabetes[11-14]. To determine whether these mechanisms might operate synergistically to promote bacterial

Table 7 Combination of intestinal bacterial overgrowth plus immunosuppression synergistically promotes bacterial translocation from the GI tract

Antibiotic	Immunosuppressive agent	MLN (percentage positive)	Peritoneal cavity (percentage positive)
Penicillin*		100	0
	Prednisolone†	46	0
Pencillin	Prednisolone	95	75

* Penicillin (1500 U/ml) given *ad libitum* in drinking water for 7 days.
† Prednisolone (100 mg/kg body weight) injected intraperitoneally four times over 7 days.

translocation, mice were given a combination of an oral antibiotic (penicillin) to induce intestinal bacterial overgrowth of Enterobacteriaceae together with an immunosuppressive agent (prednisolone) to compromise host immune defences[46]. Mice given penicillin alone exhibit translocating indigenous bacteria in 100% of the MLN cultures, but the translocating bacteria do not spread systemically to the peritoneal cavity (Table 7). Mice injected with prednisolone alone also exhibit bacterial translocation to the MLN, but to a lesser degree than do mice given only penicillin. The combination of a penicillin plus prednisolone, however, not only promotes bacterial translocation to the MLN, but the translocating bacteria spread systemically to 75% of the peritoneal cavities. In other studies, mice given the combination of clindamycin plus prednisolone died within 14 days due to septicaemia caused by indigenous GI bacteria (primarily *E. coli*, *K. pneumoniae*, *P. mirabilis* and *E. aerogenes*) translocating from their GI tracts. The combination of an oral antibiotic plus an immunosuppressive agent therefore synergistically promotes bacterial translocation from the GI tract, specifically allowing the systemic spread of translocating bacteria from the MLN to other extraintestinal sites.

The synergistic promotion of bacterial translocation by multiple mechanisms has also been demonstrated in other animal models. For example, protein malnutrition results in histological atrophy of the mucosa of the small bowel and caecum, but surprisingly does not induce bacterial translocation[47]. The combination of protein malnutrition plus injection of endotoxin, however, produces intestinal ulcerations with concomitant bacterial translocation[48]. Similarly, a 30% total body surface area burn plus endotoxin injection synergistically promotes intestinal mucosal damage and bacterial translocation[47]. Studies are in progress to delineate the relationships among increased intestinal permeability, intestinal mucosal injury, bacterial translocation, and lethal sepsis in these complex animal models.

CONCLUSIONS

The various species of indigenous bacteria do not all translocate from the GI tract to the MLN or other extraintestinal sites at the same efficiency. The bacteria that translocate at the greatest efficiency from the GI tract to the MLN of monoassociated ex-germ-free mice are the Gram-negative, facultatively anaerobic Enterobacteriaceae, such as *K. pneumoniae*, *E. coli*, and *P. mirabilis*[49]

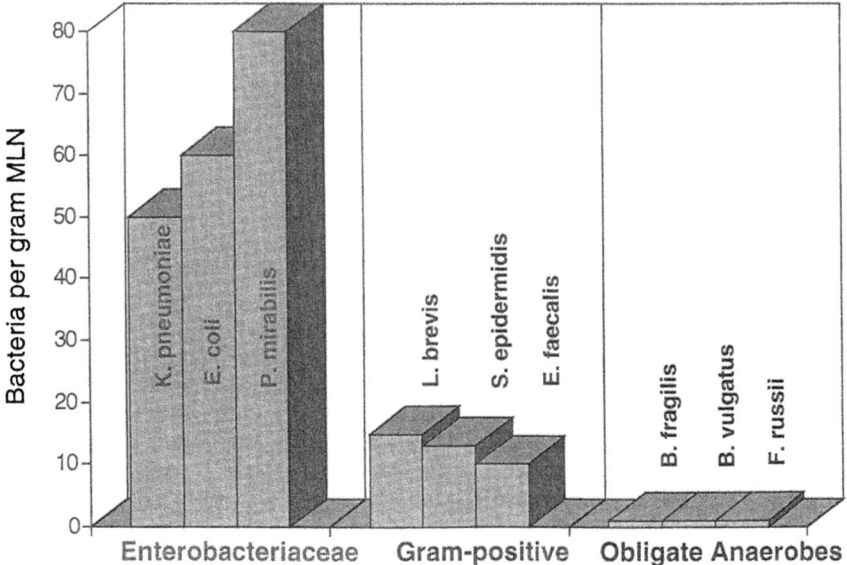

Figure 2 Translocation efficiencies of various species of indigenous bacteria in monoassociated gnotobiotic mice

(Fig. 2). Gram-positive, oxygen-tolerant bacteria, such as *Lactobacillus brevis*, *Staphylococcus epidermidis*, and *Enterococcus faecalis*, translocate at an intermediate level. Interestingly, obligately anaerobic bacteria, such as *Bacteroides fragilis*, *Bacteroides vulgatus*, and *Fusobacterium russii*, are the least effective at translocating from the GI tract, even though they colonize the GI tract at the highest level of any indigenous bacteria (10^{10-11}/g caecum). There appears to be a relationship between the efficiency of translocation of certain obligate indigenous anaerobes and their sensitivity to killing by oxygen. Interestingly, *Enterobacteriaceae* are the bacterial types that translocate most efficiently from the GI tract in the intestinal overgrowth model and in other animal models of translocation, and the Enterobacteriaceae are the most important cause of septicaemia in debilitated patients.

The pathogenesis of bacterial translocation from the GI tract occurs in several discrete stages (Fig. 3). In the healthy adult animal, various indigenous bacteria are translocating continuously from the GI tract in very low numbers. They are usually killed en route or *in situ* in the MLN by the host immune defences, and indigenous bacteria are not normally cultured from the MLN or other extra-intestinal sites from healthy animals. Intestinal overgrowth by certain indigenous bacteria, however, increases their rate of translocation to the MLN. In this first stage of translocation pathogenesis the translocating bacteria are usually confined to the MLN, and do not spread systemically to other organs and sites. Thus, the host shows no clinical signs of infection. The consequences can be more severe, however, if the host is colonized by more virulent non-indigenous

56

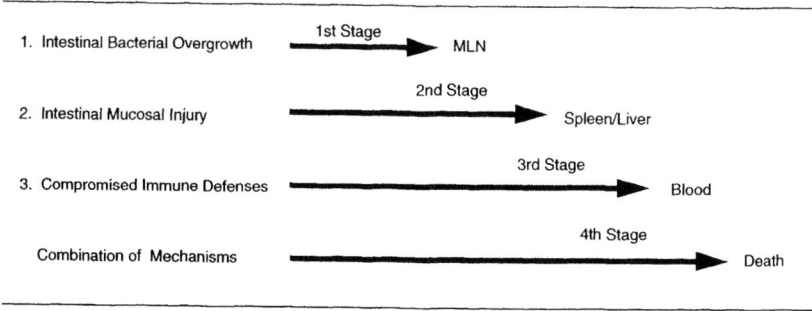

Figure 3   Stages in the pathogenesis of bacterial translocation from the GI tract

bacteria. In the second stage of translocation, often promoted by intestinal mucosal injury, bacteria can translocate by both the lymphatic and vascular routes to the MLN, liver, and spleen. The third stage of translocation pathogenesis occurs when the translocating bacteria spread systemically to the peritoneal cavity and/or blood stream. The host may still recover from this infection, depending upon the virulence properties of the translocating bacteria and the degree of host injury or immunodeficiency. The promotion of bacterial translocation by a combination of two or three major mechanisms brings about the fourth and final stage of translocation pathogenesis. Whether or not the host recovers from this infection, or succumbs to lethal sepsis, depends again upon the level of intestinal bacterial overgrowth, the degree of host immune deficiency, the extent of intestinal mucosal injury, and the pathogenic properties of the translocating microorganisms.

Although bacterial translocation has been studied primarily in animal models, there are several studies demonstrating bacterial translocation in humans. Surveillance cultures of faecal samples from patients with leukaemia or other immunosuppressive disorders demonstrate an association between the bacterial biotype/serotype present at the highest population level in the patient's faeces and the bacterial biotype/serotype most likely to cause subsequent septicaemia in that patient[50]. Rush et al.[51] cultured indigenous GI bacteria directly from the blood of patients with haemorrhagic shock when their systolic blood pressure decreased to < 80 mmHg. Translocating bacteria have also been cultured from the MLN of patients with bowel obstruction[52,53], colorectal cancer[53,54], Crohn's disease[55], ulcerative colitis[56], and inflammatory bowel disease[53].

Selective antibiotic decontamination of debilitated patients to eliminate certain bacteria that are particularly efficient at translocating from the GI tract, such as the Enterobacteriaceae, may eventually prove of benefit. The pathogenesis of bacterial translocation from the GI tract, and the development of opportunistic GI infections, will not be fully understood, however, until more information becomes available concerning the complex ecological interrelationships between the host and its indigenous GI microflora.

References

1. Ford WW. The bacteriology of healthy organs. Trans Assoc Am Phys. 1900;15:389–415.
2. Wolbach SB, Saiki T. A new anaerobic spore-bearing bacterium commonly present in the livers of healthy dogs, and believed to be responsible for many changes attributed to aseptic autolysis of liver tissue. J Med Res. 1909;21:267–78.
3. Ellis JC, Dragstedt LR. Liver autolysis *in vivo*. Arch Surg. 1930;20:8–16.
4. Chau AYS, Goldbloom VC, Gurd FN. *Clostridia* infection as a cause of death after ligation of the hepatic artery. Arch Surg. 1951;63:390–402.
5. Schatten WF. The role of intestinal bacteria in liver necrosis following experimental excision of the hepatic arterial supply. Surgery. 1954;36:256–69.
6. Berg RD, Garlington AW. Translocation of certain indigenous bacteria from the gastrointestinal tract to the mesenteric lymph nodes and other organs in a gnotobiotic mouse model. Infect Immun. 1979;23:403–11.
7. Berg RD. Mechanisms confining indigenous bacteria to the gastrointestinal tract. Am J Clin Nutr. 1980;33:2472–84.
8. Berg RD. Factors influencing the translocation of bacteria from the gastrointestinal tract. In: Sasaki S, Ogawa, A, Hashimoto, K, editors. Recent advances in germfree research. Tokyo: Tokai University Press; 1981:411–18.
9. Berg RD. Translocation of the indigenous bacteria from the intestinal tract. In: Hentges D, editor. The intestinal microflora in health and disease. New York: Academic Press; 1983:333–52.
10. Berg RD. Bacterial translocation from the intestines. Exp Anim. 1985;34:1–16.
11. Berg RD. Bacterial translocation from the gastrointestinal tract. J Med. 1992;23:217–44.
12. Berg RD. Translocation and the indigenous gut flora. In: Fuller R, editor. Probiotics: the scientific basis. London: Chapman & Hall;1992:55–85.
13. Berg RD. Translocation of enteric bacteria in health and disease. In: Cottier H, Kraft R, editors. Gut-derived infectious–toxic shock (GITS). A major variant of septic shock. Current Studies in Hematology and Blood Transfusion. Basel: Karger; 1992;59:44–65.
14. Berg RD. Bacterial translocation from the gastrointestinal tract. Trends Microbiol. 1995;3:149–54.
15. Berg RD. Promotion of the translocation of enteric bacteria from the gastrointestinal tracts of mice by oral treatment with penicillin, clindamycin, or metronidazole. Infect Immun. 1981;33:854–61.
16. Spaeth G, Berg RD, Specian RD, Deitch EA. Food without fiber promotes bacterial translocation from the gut. Surgery. 1990;108:240–7.
17. Berg RD, Owens WE. Inhibition of translocation of viable *Escherichia coli* from the gastrointestinal tract to the mesenteric lymph nodes and other organs in a gnotobiotic mouse model. Infect Immun. 1979;25:820–7.
18. Berg RD. Inhibition of *Escherichia coli* translocation from the gastrointestinal tract by the normal cecal flora in gnotobiotic or antibiotic-decontaminated mice. Infect Immun. 1980;29:1073–81.
19. Steffen EK, Berg RD. Relationship between cecal population levels of indigenous bacteria and translocation to the mesenteric lymph nodes. Infect Immun. 1983;39:1252–9.
20. Takeuchi A. Electron microscope studies of experimental *Salmonella* infection. Am J Pathol. 1967;50:109–36.
21. Alexander JW, Boyce ST, Babcock GF *et al.* The process of microbial translocation. Arch Surg. 1990;212:496–512.
22. Morehouse J, Specian R, Stewart J, Berg RD. Promotion of the translocation of indigenous bacteria of mice from the GI tract by oral ricinoleic acid. Gastroenterology. 1986;91:673–82.
23. Baker JW, Deitch EA, Berg R, Ma L. Hemorrhagic shock impairs the mucosal barrier resulting in bacterial translocation from the gut and sepsis. Surg Forum. 1987;37:73–4.
24. Deitch EA, Berg R, Specian R. Endotoxin promotes the translocation of bacteria from the gut. Arch Surg. 1987;122:185–90.
25. Baker JW, Deitch EA, Ma L, Berg R. Hemorrhagic shock promotes the systemic translocation of bacteria from the gut. J Trauma. 1988;28:896–906.
26. Deitch EA, Bridges W, Baker *et al.* Hemorrhagic shock-induced bacterial translocation is reduced by xanthine oxidase inhibition or inactivation. Surgery. 198;104:191–8.

27. Deitch EA, Ma W-J, Ma L, Berg R, Specian R. Endotoxin-induced bacterial translocation: a study of mechanisms. Surgery. 1989;106:292–300.
28. Deitch EA, Taylor M, Grisham M, Ma L, Bridges W, Berg R. Endotoxin induces bacterial translocation and increases xanthine oxidase activity. J Trauma. 1989;29:1679–83.
29. Deitch EA, Bridges W, Ma L, Berg R, Specian R, Granger DN. Hemorrhagic shock-induced bacterial translocation: the role of neutrophils and hydroxyl radicals. J Trauma. 1990;30:942–52.
30. Deitch EA, Specian RD, Berg RD. Endotoxin-induced bacterial translocation and mucosal permeability: role of xanthine oxidase, complement activation and macrophage products. Crit Care Med. 1991;19:785–91.
31. Carrico CJ, Meakins JL, Marshall JC, Fry D, Maier RV. Multiple organ failure syndrome. Arch Surg. 1986;121:196–208.
32. Fuller KG and Berg RD. Inhibition of bacterial translocation from the gastrointestinal tract by nonspecific immunostimulation. In: Wostmann BS, Pleasants JR, Pollard M, Teah BA and Wagner M, editors. Germfree research: microflora control and its application to the biomedical sciences. New York: Alan R. Liss; 1985:195–8.
33. Gautreaux MD, Deitch EA, Berg RD. Immunological mechanisms preventing bacterial translocation from the gastrointestinal tract. Microecol Ther. 1990;20:31–4.
34. Wells CL, Maddus MA, Simmons RL. Role of the macrophage in the translocation of intestinal bacteria. Arch Surg. 1987;122:48–53.
35. Owens WE, Berg RD. Bacterial translocation from the gastrointestinal tracts of thymectomized mice. Curr Microbiol. 1982;7:169–74.
36. Owens WE, Berg RD. Bacterial translocation from the gastrointestinal tract of athymic (nu/nu) mice. Infect Immun. 1980;27:461–7.
37. Gautreaux M, Deitch E, Berg RD. T-cells in the host defense against bacterial translocation from the gastrointestinal tract. Infect Immun. 1994;62:2874–84.
38. Gautreaux M, Gelder F, Jennings S, Deitch E, Berg RD. Adoptive transfer of T-cells to T-cell depleted mice inhibits bacterial translocation from the gastrointestinal tract. Infect Immun. 1995;63:3827–34.
39. Apter FM, Lencer WI, Finkelstein RA, Mekalanos JJ, Neutra MR. Monoclonal immunoglobulin A antibodies directed against cholera toxin prevent the toxin- induced chloride secretory response and block toxin binding to intestinal epithelial cells *in vitro*. Infect Immun. 1993;61:5271–8.
40. Michetti P, Mahan MJ, Slauch JM, Mekalanos JJ, Neutra MR. Monoclonal secretory immunoglobulin A protects mice against oral challenge with the invasive pathogen *Salmonella typhimurium*. Infect Immun. 1992;60:1786–92.
41. Gautreaux MD, Deitch EA, Berg RD. Immunological mechanisms preventing bacterial translocation from the gastrointestinal tract. Microecol Ther. 1990;20:31–4.
42. Berg RD. Bacterial translocation from the gastrointestinal tracts of mice receiving immunosuppressive chemotherapeutic agents. Curr Microbiol. 1983;8:285–92.
43. Penn RL, Maca RD, Berg RD. Leukemia promotes the translocation of indigenous bacteria from the gastrointestinal tract to the mesenteric lymph nodes and other organs. Microecol Ther. 1986;15:85–91.
44. Maejima K, Deitch EA, Berg RD. Promotion by burn stress of the translocation of bacteria from the gastrointestinal tracts of mice. Arch Surg. 1984;119:166–72.
45. Maejima K, Deitch EA, Berg RD. Bacterial translocation from the gastrointestinal tract of rats receiving thermal injury. Infect Immun. 1984;43:6–10.
46. Berg RD, Wommack E, Deitch EA. Immunosuppression and intestinal bacterial overgrowth synergistically promote bacterial translocation. Arch Surg. 1988;123:1359–64.
47. Deitch EA, Berg R. Bacterial translocation from the gut: a mechanism of infection. J Burn Care Rehab. 1987;8:475–82.
48. Ma L, Specian RD, Berg RD, Deitch EA. Effects of protein malnutrition and endotoxin on the intestinal mucosal barrier to the translocation of indigenous flora in mice. J Parent Ent Nutr. 1989;13:572–8.
49. Steffen EK, Berg RD, Deitch EA. Comparison of the translocation rates of various indigenous bacteria from the gastrointestinal tract to the mesenteric lymph nodes. J Infect Dis. 1988;157:1032–7.
50. Tancrede CH, Andremont AO. Bacterial translocation and gram-negative bacteremia in patients with hematological malignancies. J Infect Dis. 1985;152:99–103.

51. Rush BF, Sori AJ, Murphy TF, Smith S, Flanagan JJ, Machiedo GW. Endotoxemia and bacteremia during hemorrhagic shock: the link between trauma and sepsis? Ann Surg. 1988;207:549–54.
52. Deitch EA. Simple intestinal obstruction causes bacterial translocation in man. Arch Surg. 1989;123:699–701.
53. Sedman PC, Macfie J, Sagar P, Mitchell CJ, May J, Mancey-Jones B, Johnstone D. The prevalence of gut translocation in humans. Gastroenterology. 1994;107:643–9.
54. Vincent P, Colombel JF, Lescut D *et al*. Bacterial translocation in patients with colorectal cancer. J Infect Dis. 1988;158:1395–6.
55. Ambrose MS, Johnson M, Burdon DW, Keighley MRB. Incidence of pathogenic bacteria from mesenteric lymph nodes and ileal serosa during Crohn's disease surgery. Br J Surg. 1984;71:623–5.
56. Peitzman AB, Udekwu AO, Ochoa J. Bacterial translocation in trauma patients. J Trauma. 1991;31:1083–7.

5
Intestinal permeability in inflammatory bowel disease

K. R. GARDINER

INTRODUCTION

The gastrointestinal tract has important endocrine, metabolic, immunological and barrier functions as well its better-known role in nutrient absorption. As a barrier the intestinal mucosa separates potentially harmful microorganisms, carcinogens and food antigens in the intestinal lumen from the body's internal environment[1]. The intestinal mucosal barrier is a multi-tiered defence and comprises both non-immunological and immunological components[2]. The intestinal commensal flora inhibits the growth of pathogens, and secretions such as mucus and secretory immunoglobulin A inhibit adhesion and invasion of the mucosa by bacteria (Fig. 1). The epithelial layer consists of the lipid cell membrane of intestinal cells and the paracellular junctional areas[1]. The immune cells within the epithelial and subepithelial layers, and in the intestinal lymph nodes, identify and remove antigens that penetrate through the physical epithelial barrier[3]. The hepatic and splenic reticuloendothelial cells act as a reserve system to filter antigens that manage to penetrate the barrier[3].

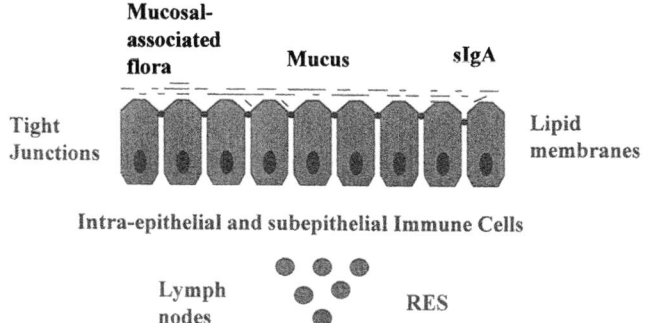

Figure 1   The gut mucosal barrier. sIgA = secretory immunoglobulin A; RES = reticuloendothelial system

FUNCTION OF THE GUT MUCOSAL BARRIER

The maintenance of normal epithelial cell structure prevents transepithelial migration of particles from the gut lumen, and the preservation of tight junctions between cells prevents movements through the paracellular channels[4]. However, the tight junction is an active and dynamic space between cells which opens and closes, and allows relatively large amounts of fluids, nutrients and medium-sized compounds to enter through it into the lamina propria of the intestine. The tight junction appears to open after the ingestion of food, and to serve as a portal for absorption of nutrients through the paracellular route, bypassing the transcellular route.

Even under normal circumstances there is evidence that luminal macromolecules are absorbed to a small extent by the small intestine. Horseradish peroxidase (MW 40 000) and intact bovine serum albumin (MW 68 000) are transported by enterocytes into the portal vein and intestinal lymphatics[5]. Trace amounts of endotoxin have been detected in portal and systemic venous blood samples in healthy humans, but it appears that any endotoxin that escapes from the intestinal lumen is rapidly cleared by the reticuloendothelial system[6]. There is also evidence that intact bacteria can be transported by specialized intestinal epithelial cells (M cells) to macrophages within Peyer's patches of healthy rodents[7]. Intact colonic mucosa is believed to provide an effective barrier to the absorption of potentially toxic, immunogenic or proinflammatory products of luminal commensal bacteria[8].

DYSFUNCTION OF THE GUT MUCOSAL BARRIER

Dysfunction of the mucosal barrier results from an imbalance between aggressive and defensive factors on the intestinal mucosa[9]. Colonization with enteric pathogens, ingestion of non-steroidal anti-inflammatory analgesics and the use of broad-spectrum antibiotics predispose the mucosa to ulceration[10]. Maintenance of mucosal blood flow, supply of oxidative fuels and a normal intestinal bacterial flora protect against barrier dysfunction[11].

Failure of the intestinal mucosal barrier results in penetration of the intestinal wall by microbial and dietary antigens. Dysfunction of the mucosal barrier may be identified by the demonstration of extraintestinal migration of gut bacteria or endotoxin (translocation) or by increased passive penetration of the intestinal barrier by non-charged macromolecules (permeability)[4,11]. Demonstration of increased faecal clearance of α_1-antitrypsin and albumin are also indicative of increased intestinal permeability[12].

Bacterial translocation occurs transcellularly[13], and may be assessed by quantitative and qualitative culture of mesenteric lymph nodes, liver, spleen and blood, by detection of [14]C- or FITC-tagged bacteria or indirectly by measuring urinary nitrate excretion[11,14]. Uptake of endotoxin can be assessed using the chromogenic *Limulus* assay, or by measurement of plasma radioactivity after administration of [3]H-, [125]I- or ^{14}C-labelled endotoxin[11].

Intestinal permeability is usually assessed by measuring the urinary excretion of orally administered non-metabolized macromolecules such as sugars (lactulose, mannitol, rhamnose, cellobiose), inert polymers (polyethylene glycol, FITC-dextran) or radiolabelled compounds (^{51}CrEDTA, ^{99m}TcDTPA)[15]. Alternatively the probes may be administered into a segment of small intestine by intubation[12]. These probes, which are much smaller ($r = 0.63$ nm) than typical antigens ($r > 1$ nm), penetrate the intestinal mucosa through tight junctions or mucosal ulcers. There is an inverse relationship between intestinal permeability and the size of hydrophilic molecules, with permeation decreasing as molecular size increases[16].

Although there is some evidence that increases in mucosal permeability to hydrophilic probes occur in parallel with increases in extent of macromolecular translocation, these phenomena occur by different pathways and are probably unrelated[11].

GUT MUCOSAL BARRIER DYSFUNCTION IN EXPERIMENTAL INFLAMMATORY BOWEL DISEASE (IBD)

Translocation of enteric bacteria to extraintestinal sites has been reported in a hapten-induced model of colitis and found to correlate positively with the severity of the colonic inflammation[17]. Systemic endotoxaemia has also been observed in experimental models of colitis in the mouse (dextran sulphate sodium)[18], rat (hapten-, acetic acid- and ethanol-induced models)[19,20], rabbit (carrageenan- and formalin/lipopolysaccharide-induced)[21,22] and dog (spontaneous haemorrhagic enterocolitis)[23]. Systemic endotoxaemia has been found to correlate positively with severity of the colitis (acetic acid rat model, trinitrobenzenesulphonic acid (TNBS) rat model, carrageenan rabbit model) and of the systemic response (TNBS rat model). In addition, there is evidence of a specific systemic antibody response to endotoxin in the TNBS rat model of colitis[24]. Colonic permeability to hydrophilic probes is also increased in rat (TNBS, acetic acid), guinea-pig (carrageenan) and rabbit (immune complex) models of colitis[20,25–27]. A significant positive correlation was found between severity of colonic inflammation and colonic permeability[20]. Yamada et al.[28] have shown rapid and significant increases in colonic mucosal permeability (blood-lumen clearance of ^{51}Cr-EDTA) within 2 h of intracolonic instillation of acetic acid, ethanol or TNBS/E. Increased intestinal permeability to ^{51}Cr-EDTA has also been found after induction of experimental enteritis with ethanol, cetrimide or methotrexate[29].

Induction of intestinal inflammation is therefore seen to result in systemic endotoxaemia, bacterial translocation and increased permeability suggesting that gut barrier dysfunction is a feature of intestinal inflammation irrespective of animal species or inducing agent.

GUT MUCOSAL BARRIER FUNCTION IN CLINICAL IBD

There is both direct and indirect evidence that gut mucosal barrier dysfunction is a feature of IBD.

Direct evidence

Bacterial translocation

Three main mechanisms are thought to promote bacterial translocation: disruption of the ecology of the indigenous gut flora resulting in intestinal bacterial overgrowth, physical damage of the intestinal mucosa and impaired host defence[30]. At least two of these factors are features of IBD, with an obvious physical disruption of the epithelial barrier by inflammation and ulceration and a disturbed bacterial flora[31]. It is therefore not surprising that bacterial translocation has been observed in patients with active IBD. In patients undergoing surgery for IBD, enteric bacteria were cultured from the ileal serosa in 27% of patients, mesenteric lymph nodes in 33%, portal blood in 24% and liver biopsies in 11%[32–34]. Eade and Brooke[34] reported that the incidence of positive blood culture correlated with the severity of the disease.

Endotoxaemia

There is limited information on portal endotoxaemia in patients with IBD, with only 13 reports of portal sampling in patients with ulcerative colitis (UC), of which five were positive; and no reports regarding Crohn's disease (CD)[6,35,36]. Systemic endotoxaemia has been repeatedly documented in both CD and UC, and has been shown to correlate positively with clinical and biochemical activity in IBD[37–42], as well as radiological extent[38,42]. Reduction in systemic endotoxaemia is associated with resolution of disease relapse[37,39,41]; with restoration to normal of plasma protein and serum iron concentrations[39,43]; and with reduction in indices of disease activity[39].

Intestinal permeability

Increased intestinal permeability to hydrophilic probes has been reported in patients with CD[44–49]. Variable results have been reported for smaller probes such as PEG 400 and 600, with results being more consistent for larger molecules such as ^{51}Cr-EDTA and lactulose[50]. Most studies have assumed that excretion of these permeability markers reflects small intestinal absorption as no increase in permeability to orally administered sugars or PEG 400 was demonstrated in patients with UC[51,52]. However, studies in which the probe ^{51}Cr-EDTA is administered rectally have revealed that there is also a significant increase in colonic permeability in active UC or CD[53,54]. Significant absorption of orally administered ^{51}Cr-EDTA and of ^{99m}Tc-DTPA has also been demonstrated in patients with colonic inflammation[46,47].

The degree of intestinal permeability correlates positively with both disease extent[47] and activity[46,47,55] in patients with IBD. Serial measurements of intestinal permeability in IBD have shown that a return of permeability to normal is associated with clinical remission and a reduction in intestinal inflammation[56].

Intestinal protein loss

Beeken et al.[57] have shown a correlation between gastrointestinal protein loss and length of affected bowel in CD. Logan et al.[58] have shown that as patients with small bowel CD respond to treatment their gastrointestinal protein loss reduces.

Indirect evidence

Indirect evidence for mucosal barrier dysfunction in patients with IBD is provided by reports of increased concentrations of antibodies to dietary and bacterial antigens, of circulating immune complexes and the improvement in disease activity in CD that follows bowel rest.

Antibody response to enteric bacteria and bacterial products

Systemic concentrations of antibodies to enteric bacteria are increased in patients with IBD[59–62] and correlate with disease severity[60]. There are also reports of an increased antibody response to components of the bacterial cell wall (endotoxin core, lipid A and peptidoglycans) in patients with CD[42,49,63–66] and to a lesser extent UC[66]. There was a positive correlation between the plasma concentration of endotoxin core-antibody and systemic endotoxaemia in patients with active CD[42]. An association between lipid A antibody concentration and disease activity has been described in CD[65] and between IgA antibody to peptidoglycans and extraintestinal inflammation in UC[66].

Antibacterial antibody studies have shown that there is increased plasma cell exposure to intestinal bacteria or their products in IBD patients, which suggests that bacteria are translocating across the intestinal wall. The occurrence of antibodies against multiple different species and different serotypes suggests that no one bacterial species or strain is implicated.

Antibody response to dietary antigens

Raised systemic concentrations of antibody to a variety of dietary antigens (casein, gluten, maize, bovine serum albumin, β-lactoglobulin A and B, gliadin, yeast cell wall mannan, *Saccharomyces cerevisiae*) have been reported in UC and CD[67–71], though reports in the literature are not consistent[71–73]. Brignola *et al.*[74] found that there were more positive reactions (RAST) against specific IgE to 10 selected foodstuffs in patients with UC and CD than in healthy controls.

There was also evidence that circulating antibody concentrations against bovine serum albumin correlated with disease activity[68,69]. In addition, high titres of circulating antibodies to whole milk were associated with multiple relapses of UC during a trial period[75]. The increased antibody production to dietary antigens found in patients with IBD suggests that there is increased penetration of the intestinal mucosa by dietary antigens.

Circulating immune complexes

Significantly elevated concentrations of circulating immune complexes have been reported in IBD[76–82], but not consistently[83,84]. There is evidence that the titre of immune complexes correlates with disease activity[77,85], with extraintestinal manifestations[76], and is higher in patients with colonic rather than small intestinal CD [76]. These immune complexes were heterogeneous[79], suggesting that they represented a secondary phenomenon, possibly a response to increased intestinal permeability[76,81,86].

Bowel rest

Further indirect evidence that dysfunction of the intestinal mucosal barrier occurs in patients with IBD, and contributes to disease activity, is provided by reports of reduced disease activity or remission induced by bowel rest. In patients with CD, most studies have found that bowel rest achieved by faecal stream diversion[87,88], administration of an elemental diet[56,58,89–92] or by administration of total parenteral nutrition (TPN)[93,94] is beneficial (reduced disease activity, reduction in intestinal protein loss, reduction in intestinal permeability, suppression of circulating immune complexes)[56,58,91,92]. However, Lochs et al.[95], in a randomized controlled trial in patients with CD, found that the combination of TPN and total bowel rest resulted in a similar improvement to that found with TPN alone. Administration of elemental diet or of TPN appears to be more beneficial in patients with small bowel CD than in large bowel disease[56,94]. Reintroduction of small bowel effluent into the defunctioned colon of patients ($n = 22$) with CD treated by split ileostomy resulted in a detectable clinical response in seven patients and relapse in one[96]. Rutgeerts et al.[97] showed that patients with CD who had undergone ileocolonic resection and a diverting ileostomy developed relapse of disease only after restoration of intestinal continuity.

However, in patients with severe UC, bowel rest either by TPN[98,99] or by faecal diversion[87] had no significant beneficial effects[100].

It is not clear why bowel rest is effective in CD (possibilities include a reduction in dietary antigen load, modification of faecal flora and improved nutritional status) but not in UC[100].

CLINICAL SIGNIFICANCE OF GUT BARRIER DYSFUNCTION IN IBD

Therefore there is both direct and indirect evidence that intestinal mucosal barrier dysfunction occurs in patients with IBD, that the severity of this dysfunction correlates with disease extent and activity, and that resolution of disease relapse is associated with a reduction in intestinal permeability, gastrointestinal protein loss and systemic endotoxaemia. The next logical question is whether the gut barrier dysfunction found in patients with IBD is of clinical significance (either as a primary event or an aggravating factor) or is an epiphenomenon. The evidence for each of these possibilities will be discussed in turn.

Barrier dysfunction as a primary event

It has been proposed that an increase in intestinal permeability as a result of a genetic predisposition[45] or due to a transient insult (intestinal infection, use of non-steroidal anti-inflammatory analgesics or antibiotics) results in activation of gut-associated lymphoid tissue by luminal antigens, inducing a state of hyperactivity and persistent inflammation. In favour of such a hypothesis are the following:

1. Evidence of microscopic and cytochemical abnormalities in macroscopically normal intestinal mucosa in CD[101]. In particular abnormal epithelial tight junctions have been described, with increased separation between cells and abnormalities in the structural strands of the tight junction[102,103].
2. Both *in-vitro* and clinical evidence of increased permeability in apparently unaffected jejunal mucosa in patients with CD[104,105].
3. The finding that patients with clinically inactive CD who have increased intestinal permeability are more likely to suffer a clinical relapse during the succeeding 6–12 months[56,106].
4. An increased prevalence (5–10%) of IBD has been observed among first-degree relatives of affected patients[107]. It has been reported that a subgroup of first-degree relatives of patients with CD have increased intestinal permeability[45,108]. It was therefore suggested that an inherited defect in the intestinal mucosal barrier predisposed an individual to the subsequent development of IBD. However not all studies of relatives have found abnormal intestinal permeability[48,109–112].
5. Intestinal infections, antibiotics and non-steroidal anti-inflammatory drugs are all recognized factors leading to relapse of IBD[113–117]. It is interesting, therefore, that intestinal permeability is increased both in association with intestinal infections[118–120] and with the use of non-steroidal anti-inflammatory analgesics[121].

Against a primary dysfunction is the fact that intestinal permeability often returns to normal with resolution of the disease process[47,91,122]. The abnormalities in structure (microscopic and cytochemical) in macroscopically normal intestine and in function (elevated hydrophilic probe excretion) in patients during remission and in first-degree relatives may reflect subclinical disease activity or structural and/or functional mucosal changes as a consequence of previous inflammation[47,106], rather than a pre-existing abnormality[3].

Barrier dysfunction as an aggravating factor

The hypothesis here is that an increase in intestinal mucosal permeability as a result of intestinal inflammation allows penetration of the intestinal wall by dietary or bacterial antigens, which contribute to the local intestinal inflammation or the systemic features of IBD or both[8,123].

There is no direct evidence that translocating luminal antigens contribute to *intestinal inflammation* seen in IBD. However, there is some indirect evidence:

1. Intestinal macrophages in patients with UC have an augmented expression of CD14 receptors, suggesting an increased exposure to translocating lipopolysaccharide and providing a mechanism for aggravating intestinal inflammation[124].
2. Systemic administration of endotoxin results in increased intestinal permeability in human volunteers and increased permeability and bacterial translocation in experimental animals[125,126].
3. Systemic or intestinal intramural injection of bacterial cell wall polymers in experimental animals results in a chronic granulomatous intestinal inflammation[127,128] in association with increased mucosal permeability[128].

4. In an experimental model of colitis induced in rabbits by intrarectal administration of formalin and lipopolysaccharide, only mild transient changes occurred in the absence of lipopolysaccharide, and a second challenge with lipopolysaccharide prolonged the colits[22].

5. The IL-2 knockout mouse and the HLA B27 transgenic rat models of colitis show attenuation or elimination of colitis when the experimental animals are raised in a germ-free environment, implicating commensal bacteria in the aetiology of the colitis[129,130].

6. Disease activity is reduced in patients with CD following administration of antibiotics[131,132] or an elemental diet, bowel rest, or whole-gut irrigation[39]. However, it is not possible to assert that these luminal antigens are exerting a toxic effect on the intestinal mucosa as a result of penetration of the intestinal barrier.

In addition, it has been suggested that translocation of enteric bacteria and their products would explain *systemic* immune activation, disturbances in hepatic function, the pathogenesis of abscesses and fistulas, extraintestinal manifestations, and the high incidence of sepsis following elective surgery in IBD patients[32-34,37,38]. There is evidence that both systemic endotoxaemia and intestinal permeability correlate positively with acute-phase protein response in IBD. In addition, Lange et al.[18] have shown that when dextran-sulphate sodium colitis is induced in lps gene-defective mice there was a less severe systemic inflammatory response, less bacteraemia and lower mortality than in mice with a normal sensitivity to lipopolysaccharide. This would support a role for translocating endotoxin in the development of systemic infection, septic shock and death in this model of colitis.

Barrier dysfunction as an epiphenomenon

An alternative hypothesis is that the finding of extraintestinal bacteria and bacterial products in patients with IBD may simply reflect a generalized increase in intestinal permeability as a result of intestinal inflammation, and not be clinically significant. Indeed, there is enhanced uptake of macromolecules in experimental models of colitis irrespective of the inducing agent[8,20,25,27], as well as in infective intestinal disorders[118-120,133]. Serum agglutinins to numerous enteric bacteria are demonstrable in healthy volunteers and in patients with coeliac disease[62,68], as well as in patients with IBD.

CONCLUSIONS

There is strong direct and indirect evidence to show that deranged intestinal mucosal barrier function is a feature of active IBD. There is good support for a pathogenic role of barrier dysfunction in IBD:

1. Episodes of intestinal infection and the use of NSAIDs are associated with increased intestinal permeability and relapses of disease.
2. Bowel rest/faecal diversion can lead to disease remission.
3. Impaired barrier function is predictive of relapse.

There is insufficient evidence to support a primary role for intestinal mucosal barrier dysfunction in the pathogenesis of IBD.

These conclusions carry implications for both monitoring and treatment of patients with IBD. Persistently increased intestinal permeability is predictive of relapse in patients with CD[106]. Reduction in intestinal permeability could be used as a marker of efficacy of therapy[12]. When it comes to treatment, these findings would suggest that, in addition to traditional treatment to reduce host response (salicylates, corticosteroids, azathioprine), patients with IBD may also benefit from treatment to reduce the intestinal antigen load (whole-gut irrigation, elemental diet, reflorastration, adsorbents) and to enhance intestinal healing (selective gut nutrients, growth factors, mucosal protection agents)[39,134-137].

References

1. Hollander D. The intestinal permeability barrier. A hypothesis as to its regulation and involvement in Crohn's disease. Scand J Gastroenterol. 1992;27:721–6.
2. Langkamp-Henken B, Glezer JA, Kudsk KA. Immunologic structure and function of the gastrointestinal tract. Nutr Clin Pract. 1992;7:100–8.
3. Hollander D. Permeability in Crohn's disease: altered barrier failure functions in healthy relatives? Gastroenterology. 1993;104:1848–51.
4. van Leeuwen PAM, Boermeester MA, Houdijk APJ et al. Clinical significance of translocation. Gut. 1994;35:S28–34.
5. Warshaw AL, Walker WA, Cornell R, Isselbacher KJ. Small intestinal permeability to macromolecules. Lab Invest. 1971;25:675–84.
6. Engström L, Törngren S, Rohdin-Alm C. Peroperative endotoxin concentrations in portal and peripheral venous blood in patients undergoing right hemicolectomy for carcinoma. Eur J Surg. 1992;158:301–5.
7. Owen RL, Pierce NF, Apple RT, Cray WC Jr. M cell transport of *Vibrio cholerae* from the intestinal lumen into Peyer's patches: a mechanism for antigen sampling and for microbial transepithelial migration. J Infect Dis. 1986;153:1108–18.
8. Hobson CH, Butt TJ, Ferry DM, Hunter J, Chadwick VS, Broom MF. Enterohepatic circulation of bacterial chemotactic peptide in rats with experimental colitis. Gastroenterology. 1988;94:1006–13.
9. Sartor RB. Role of intestinal microflora in initiation and perpetuation of inflammatory bowel disease. Can J Gastroenterol. 1990;4:271–7.
10. Berg RD. Promotion of the translocation of enteric bacteria from the gastrointestinal tract of mice by oral treatment with penicillin, clindamycin or metronidazole. Infect Immun. 1981;33:854–61.
11. Gardiner KR, Kirk SJ, Rowlands BJ. Novel substrates to maintain gut integrity. Nutr Res Rev. 1995;8:43–66.
12. Franchimont D, Louis E, Simon S, Belaiche J. Intestinal permeability in Crohn's disease. Acta Gastroenterol Belg. 1996;59:15–19.
13. Wells CL, Jechorek RP, Olmsted SB, Erlandsen SL. Effect of LPS on epithelial integrity and bacterial uptake in the polarised human enterocyte-like cell line Caco-2. Circ Shock. 1993;40:276–88.
14. Oudenhoven IMJ, Klaasen HLBM, Lapré JA, Weerkamp AH, van der Meer R. Nitric oxide-derived urinary nitrate as a marker of intestinal bacterial translocation in rats. Gastroenterology. 1994;107:47–53.
15. Editorial. Intestional permeability. Lancet 1985;1:256–8.
16. Jenkins RT, Bell RA. Molecular radii of probes used in studies of intestinal permeability. Gut. 1987;28:110–11.
17. Gardiner KR, Erwin PJ, Anderson NH, Barr JG, Halliday MI, Rowlands BJ. Colonic bacteria and bacterial translocation in experimental colitis. Br J Surg. 1993;80:512–16.
18. Lange S, Delbro DS, Jennische E, Mattsby-Baltzer I. The role of the lps gene in experimental ulcerative colitis in mice. APMIS. 1996;104:823–33.

19. Gardiner KR, Anderson NH, McCaigue MD, Erwin PJ, Halliday MI, Rowlands BJ. Adsorbents as anti-endotoxin agents in experimental colitis. Gut. 1993;34:51–5.
20. Gardiner KR, Anderson NH, Rowlands BJ, Barbul A. Colitis and colonic mucosal barrier dysfunction. Gut. 1995;37:530–5.
21. Aoki K. A study of endotoxemia in ulcerative colitis and Crohn's disease. II. Experimental study. Acta Med Okayama. 1978;32:207–16.
22. Hotta T, Yoshida N, Yoshikawa T, Sugino S, Kondo M. Lipopolysaccharide-induced colitis in rabbits. Res Exp Med. 1986;186:61–9.
23. Wessels BC, Gaffin SL. Anti-endotoxin immunotherapy for canine parvovirus endotoxaemia. J Small Animal Pract. 1986;27:609–15.
24. Neilly PJD, Gardiner KR, Kirk SJ et al. Endotoxaemia and cytokine production in experimental inflammatory bowel disease. Br J Surg. 1995;82:1479–82.
25. Seidman EG, Hanson DG, Walker WA. Increased permeability to polyethylene glycol 4000 in rabbits with experimental colitis. Gastroenterology. 1986;90:120–6.
26. Delahunty T, Recher L, Hollander D. Intestinal permeability changes in rodents: a possible mechanism for degraded carrageenan-induced colitis. Fd Chem Toxicol. 1987;25:113–18.
27. Gaginella TS, Chadwick VS, Debongie J-C, Lewis JC, Phillips SF. Perfusion of rabbit colon with ricinoleic acid: dose-related mucosal injury, fluid secretion, and increased permeability. Gastroenterology. 1977;73:95–101.
28. Yamada T, Marshall S, Specian RD, Grisham MB. A comparative analysis of two models of colitis in rats. Gastroenterology. 1992;102:1524–34.
29. Bjarnason I, Smethurst P, Levi AJ, Peters TJ. Intestinal permeability to ^{51}Cr-EDTA in rats with experimentally induced enteropathy. Gut. 1985;26:579–85.
30. Deitch EA. The immunocompromised host. Surg Clin Am. 1988;68:181–90.
31. Ambrose NS, Young D, Burdon DW, Keighley MRB. Changes in intestinal flora in Crohn's disease. Br J Surg. 1982;69:681.
32. Ambrose NS, Johnson M, Burdon DW, Keighley MRB. Endogenous intraperitoneal contamination without enterotomy in surgery for Crohn's disease. Br J Surg. 1983;70:301.
33. Ambrose NS, Johnson M, Burdon DW, Keighlty MRB. Incidence of pathogenic bacteria from mesenteric lymph nodes and ileal serosa during Crohn's disease surgery. Br J Surg. 1984;71:623–5.
34. Eade MN, Brooke BN. Portal bacteraemia in cases of ulcerative colitis submitted to colectomy. Lancet. 1969;1:1008–9.
35. Jacob AI, Goldberg PK, Bloom N, Degenshein GA, Kozinn PJ. Endotoxin and bacteria in portal blood. Gastroenterology. 1977;72:1268–70.
36. Palmer KR, Duerden BI, Holdsworth CD. Bacteriological and endotoxin studies in cases of ulcerative colitis submitted to surgery. Gut. 1980;21:851–4.
37. Aoki K. A study of endotoxemia in ulcerative colitis and Crohn's disease. I. Clinical study. Acta Med Okayama. 1978;32:147–58.
38. Colin R, Grancher T, Lemeland J-F et al. Recherche d'une endotoxinemie dans les enterocolites inflammatoires cryptogenetiques. Gastroenterol Clin Biol. 1979;3:15–19.
39. Wellmann W, Fink PC, Schmidt FW. Whole-gut irrigation as anti-endotoxinaemic therapy in inflammatory bowel disease. Hepatogastroenterology. 1984;31:91–3.
40. Wellmann W, Fink PC, Benner F. Endotoxinamie bei entzundlichen Darmerkrankungen. Verh Ges Inn Med. 1984;90:827–9.
41. Fink PC, Suin de Boutemard C, Haeckel R, Wellmann W. Endotoxaemia in patients with Crohn's disease: a longitudinal study of elastase α1-proteinase inhibitor and Limulus–Amoebocyte–lysate reactivity. J Clin Chem Clin Biochem. 1988;26:117–22.
42. Gardiner KR, Halliday MI, Barclay GR, et al. The significance of systemic endotoxaemia in inflammatory bowel disease. Gut. 1995;36:897–901.
43. Kirkin BV, Fomin SA, Ivanov AF et al. Efficiency of hemosorption in treatment of patients with ulcerative colitis. Biomater Artif Cells Artif Org. 1987;15:271–9.
44. Bjarnason I, O'Morain C, Levi AJ, Peters TJ. Absorption of [51]chromium-labelled ethylenediaminetetraacetate in inflammatory bowel disease. Gastroenterology. 1983;85:318–22.
45. Hollander D, Vadheim CM, Brettholz E, Petersen GM, Delahunty T, Rotter JI. Increased intestinal permeability in patients with Crohn's disease and their relatives. A possible etiologic factor. Ann Intern Med. 1986;105:883–5.

46. Casellas F, Aguadé S, Soriano B, Accarino A, Molero J, Guarner L. Intestinal permeability to ^{99m}Tc DTPA in inflammatory bowel disease. Am J Gastroenterol. 1986;81:767–70.
47. Jenkins RT, Jones DB, Goodacre RL *et al.* Reversibility of increased intestinal permeability to ^{51}Cr-EDTA in patients with gastrointestinal inflammatory diseases. Am J Gastroenterol. 1987;82:1159–64.
48. Katz KD, Hollander D, Vadheim CM *et al.* Intestinal permeability in patients with Crohn's disease and their healthy relatives. Gastroenterology. 1989;97:927–31.
49. Oriishi T, Sata M, Toyonaga A, Sasaki E, Tanikawa K. Evaluation of intestinal permeability in patients with inflammatory bowel disease using lactulose and measuring antibodies to lipid A. Gut. 1995;36:891–6.
50. Daum F. Is intestinal permeability really a genetic marker for Crohn's disease? J Pediatri Gastroenterol Nutr. 1993;16:340–1.
51. Cobden I, Rothwell J, Axon ATR. Intestinal permeability and screening tests for coeliac disease. Gut. 1980;21:512–18.
52. Jenkins RT, Goodacre RL, Rooney PJ, Bienenstock J, Sivakumaran T, Walker WHC. Studies of intestinal permeability in inflammatory bowel diseases using polyethylene glycol 400. Clin Biochem. 1986;19:298–302.
53. Rask-Madsen J, Schwartz M. Absorption of 51 CrEDTA in ulcerative colitis following rectal instillation. Scand J Gastroenterol. 1970;5:361–8.
54. O'Morain CA, Chervu LR, Milstein DM, Das KM. Chromium 51 ethylenediaminetetraacetate test: a useful test in the assessment of inflammatory bowel disease. J Lab Clin Med. 1986;108:430–5.
55. Murphy MS, Eastham EJ, Nelson R, Pearson AD, Laker MF. Intestinal permeability in Crohn's disease. Arch Dis Child. 1989;64:321–5.
56. Teahon K, Smethurst P, Levi AJ, Bjarnason I. The effect of elemental diet on intestinal inflammation and permeability in Crohn's disease. Gastroenterology. 1991;101:84–9.
57. Beeken WL, Baseh MJ, Sylvester DL. Intestinal protein loss in Crohn's disease. Gastroenterology. 1971;62:207.
58. Logan RFA, Gillon J, Ferrington C, Ferguson A. Reduction of gastrointestinal protein loss by elemental diet in Crohn's disease of the small bowel. Gut. 1981;22:383–7.
59. Thayer WR, Brown M, Sangree MH, Katz J, Hersh T. *Escherichia coli* 0:14 and colon hemagglutinating antibodies in inflammatory bowel disease. Gastroenterology. 1969;57:311–18.
60. Brown WR, Lee EM. Radioimmunologic measurements of bacterial antibodies. II. Human serum antibodies reactive with *Bacteroides fragilis* and *Enterococcus* in gastrointestinal and immunologic disorders. Gastroenterology. 1974;66:1143–53.
61. Tabaqchali S, O'Donoghue DP, Bettelheim KA. *Escherichia coli* antibodies in patients with inflammatory bowel disease. Gut. 1978;19:108–13.
62. Matthews N, Mayberry JF, Rhodes J *et al.* Agglutinins to bacteria in Crohn's disease. Gut. 1980;21:376–80.
63. Schüßler P, Kruis W, Marget W. Lipod-A-Antikörpertiter bei Morbus Crohn. Klin Wochenschr. 1976;54:1055–6.
64. Ramadori G, Hopf U, Galanos C, Eckhardt R, Meyer zum Büschenfelde KH. Demonstration of circulating antibodies against lipid A in patients with chronic diseases of liver and gut. Hepatogastroenterology. 1980;27:305.
65. Kruis W, Schüßler P, Weinzierl M. Circulating lipid A antibodies and their relationship to different clinical conditions of patients with Crohn's disease. Hepatogastroenterology. 1987;34:123–6.
66. Sartor RB, Cleland DR, Catalano CJ, Schwab JH. Serum antibody to bacterial cell wall peptidoglycan in inflammatory bowel disease patients. Gastroenterology. 1985;88:1571A.
67. Taylor KB, Truelove SC. Circulating antibodies to milk proteins in ulcerative colitis. Br Med J. 1961;2:924–9.
68. Falchuk KR, Isselbacher KJ. Circulating antibodies to bovine albumin in ulcerative colitis and Crohn's disease. Gastroenterology. 1976;70:5–8.
69. Lerner A, Rossi TM, Park B, Albini B, Lebenthal E. Serum antibodies to cow's milk proteins in pediatric inflammatory bowel disease. Crohn's disease versus ulcerative colitis. Acta Paediatr Scand. 1989;78:384–9.

70. McKenzie H, Main J, Pennington CR, Parratt D. Antibody to selected strains of *Saccharomyces cerevisiae* (baker's and brewer's yeast) and *Candida albicans* in Crohn's disease. Gut. 1990;31:536–8.
71. Lindberg E, Magnusson KE, Tysk C, Jarnerot G. Antibody (IgG, IgA, and IgM) to baker's yeast (*Saccharomyces cerevisiae*), yeast mannan, gliadin, ovalbumin and betalactoglobulin in monozygotic twins with inflammatory bowel disease. Gut. 1992;33:909–13.
72. Taylor KB, Truelove SC, Wright R. Serological reactions to gluten and cow's milk proteins in gastrointestinal disease. Gastroenterology. 1964;46:99–108.
73. Jewell DP, Truelove SC. Circulating antibodies to cow's milk proteins in ulcerative colitis. Gut. 1972;13:796–801.
74. Brignola C, Miniero R, Campieri M *et al*. Dietary allergy evaluated by PRIST and RAST in inflammatory bowel disease. Hepatogastroenterology. 1986;33:128–30.
75. Wright R, Truelove SC. Circulating antibodies to dietary proteins in ulcerative colitis. Br Med J. 1965;2:142–4.
76. Hodgson HJF, Potter BJ, Jewell DP. Immune complexes in ulcerative colitis and Crohn's disease. Clin Exp Immunol. 1977;29:187–96.
77. Fiasse R, Lurhuma AZ, Cambiaso CL, Masson PL, Dive C. Circulating immune complexes and disease activity in Crohn's disease. Gut. 1978;19:611–17.
78. Nielsen H, Hyltoft-Peterson P, Svehag SE. Circulating immune complexes in ulcerative colitis. II. Correlation with serum protein concentrations and complement conversion products. Clin Exp Immunol. 1978;31:81.
79. Pallone F, Montano S, Rocci R, Iavicoli M, Di Mario U. New evidence of circulating immune complexes in Crohn's disease using two sensitive methods. J Clin Lab Immunol. 1981;5:23–5.
80. Hobbiss J, Cooper KM, Moore M, Gowland E, Schofield PF. Limitations of immune complex measurements in colorectal disease. Br J Surg. 1983;70:473–7.
81. Danis TA, Harries AD, Heatley RV. Antigen–antibody complexes in inflammatory bowel disease. Scand J Gastroenterol. 1984;19:603–6.
82. Bartoloni C, Guidi L, Pili R *et al*. Assay, isolation and characterization of circulating immune complexes from serum of gastrointestinal cancer, stage III and IV melanoma and chronic inflammatory bowel disease patients. Oncology. 1993;50:27–34.
83. Soltis RD, Hasz D, Morris MJ, Wilson ID. Evidence against the presence of circulating immune complexes in chronic inflammatory bowel disease. Gastroenterology. 1979;76:1380–5.
84. Knoflach P, Vladutiu AO, Swierczynska Z, Weiser MM, Albini B. Lack of circulating immune complexes in inflammatory bowel disease. Int Arch Allergy Appl Immunol. 1986;80:9–16.
85. Jewell DP, MacLennan KP, Truelove SC. Circulating immune complexes in ulcerative colitis and Crohn's disease. Gut. 1972;13:139.
86. Hodgson HJF. Immunological aspects of inflammatory bowel diseases of the human gut. Agents Actions. 1992; Special Conference Edition: C27–C31.
87. Truelove SC, Ellis H, Webster CU. Place of a double-barrelled ileostomy in ulcerative colitis and Crohn's disease of the colon: a preliminary report. Br Med J. 1965;1:150–3.
88. Burman JH, Thompson H, Cooke WT, Williams JA. The effects of diversion of intestinal contents on the progress of Crohn's disease of the large bowel. Gut. 1971;12:11–15.
89. Voitk AJ, Echave V, Feller JH, Brown RA, Gurd FN. Experience with elemental diet in the treatment of inflammatory bowel disease. Is this primary therapy? Arch Surg. 1973;107:329–33.
90. O'Morain C, Segal AM, Levi AJ. Elemental diet in treatment of acute Crohn's disease. Br Med J. 1980;281:1173–5.
91. Sanderson IR, Boulton P, Menzies I, Walker-Smith JA. Improvement of abnormal lactulose/rhamnose permeability in active Crohn's disease of the small bowel by an elemental diet. Gut. 1987;28:1073–6.
92. O'Keefe SJ, Ogden J, Rund J, Potter P. Steroids and bowel rest versus elemental diet in the treatment of patients with Crohn's disease: the effects of protein metabolism and immune function. J Parent Ent Nutr. 1989;13:455–60.
93. Vogel CM, Corwin TR, Baue AE. Intravenous hyperalimentation in the treatment of inflammatory diseases of the bowel. Arch Surg. 1974;108:460–7.
94. Greenberg GR, Fleming CR, Jeejeebhoy KN, Rosenberg IH, Sales D. Tremaine WJ. Controlled trial of bowel rest and nutritional support in the management of Crohn's disease. Gut. 1988;29:1309–15.

95. Lochs H, Meryn S, Marosi L, Ferenci P, Hörtnagl H. Has total bowel rest a beneficial effect in the treatment of Crohn's disease. Clin Nutr. 1983;2:61–4.
96. Harper PH, Lee ECG, Kettlewell MGW, Bennett MK, Jewell DP. Role of the faecal stream in the maintenance of Crohn's colitis. Gut. 1985;26:279–84.
97. Rutgeerts P, Goboes K, Peeters M et al. Effect of faecal stream diversion on recurrence of Crohn's disease in the neoterminal ileum. Lancet 1991;2:771–4.
98. McIntyre PB, Powell-Tuck J, Wood SR et al. Controlled trial of bowel rest in the treatment of severe acute colitis. Gut. 1986;27:481–4.
99. Dickinson RJ, Ashton MG, Axon ATR, Smith RC, Yeung CK, Hill GL. Controlled trial of intravenous hyperalimentation and total bowel rest as an adjunct to the routine therapy of ulcerative colitis. Gastroenterology. 1980;79:1199–204.
100. Rhodes J, Rose J. Does food affect acute inflammatory bowel disease? The role of parenteral nutrition, elemental and exclusion diets. Gut. 1986;27:471–4.
101. Thyberg J, Graf W, Klingenström P. Intestinal fine structure in Crohn's disease. Virchows Arch [Pathol Anat]. 1981;391:141–52.
102. Dvorak AM, Dickersin GR. Crohn's disease: transmission electron microscopic studies. I. Barrier function. Possible changes related to alterations of cell coat, mucus coat, epithelial cells and paneth cells. Human Pathol. 1980;11:561–71.
103. Marin ML Greenstein AJ, Geller RE, Gordon RE, Aufses AH. A freeze fracture study of Crohn's disease of the terminal ileum: changes in epithelial tight junction organization. Am J Gastroenterol. 1983;78:537–47.
104. Dawson DJ, Lobley RW, Burrows PC, Notman JA, Mahon M, Holmes R. Changes in jejunal permeability and passive permeation of sugars in intestinal biopsies in coeliac disease and Crohn's disease. Clin Sci. 1988;74:427–31.
105. Teahon K, Somasundaram S, Smith T, Menzies I, Bjarnason I. Assessing the site of increased intestinal permeability in coeliac disease and inflammatory bowel disease. Gut. 1996;38:864–9.
106. Wyatt J, Vogelsang H, Hubl W, Waldoer T, Lochs H. Intestinal permeability and the prediction of relapse in Crohn's disease. Lancet. 1993;341:1437–9.
107. Tytgat GNJ, Mulder CJJ. The aetiology of Crohn's disease. Int J Colorectal Dis. 1986;1:188–92.
108. May GR, Sutherland LR, Meddings JB. Is small intestinal permeability really increased in relatives of patients with Crohn's disease? Gastroenterology. 1993;104:1627–32.
109. Ruttenberg D, Young GO, Wright JP, Isaacs S. PEG-400 excretion in patients with Crohn's disease, their first-degree relatives, and healthy volunteers. Dig Dis Sci. 1992;37:705–8.
110. Ainsworth M, Eriksen J, Waever-Rasmussen I, Schaffalitzky DE, Mucadel OB. Intestinal permeability of ^{51}Cr-labelled ethylenediaminetetraacetic acid in patients with Crohn's disease and their healthy relatives. Scand J Gastroenterol. 1989;24:993–8.
111. Munkholm P, Langholz E, Hollander D et al. Intestinal permeability in patients with Crohn's disease and ulcerative colitis and their first degree relatives. Gut. 1994;35:68–72.
112. Lindberg E, Söderholm JD, Olaison G, Tysk C, Järnerot G. Intestinal permeability to polyethylene glycols in monozygotic twins with Crohn's disease. Scand J Gastroenterol. 1995;39:780–3.
113. Mee AS, Jewell DP. Factors inducing relapse in inflammatory bowel disease. Br Med J. 1978;2:801–2.
114. Rampton DS, Sladen GE. Relapse of ulcerative proctocolitis during treatment with nonsteroidal anti-inflammatory drugs. Postgrad Med J. 1981;57:297–9.
115. Rampton DS, McNeil NI, Sarner M. Analgesic ingestion and other factors preceding relapse in ulcerative colitis. Gut. 1983;24:187–9.
116. Isgar B, Harman M, Whorwell PJ. Factors preceding relapse of ulcerative colitis. Digestion. 1983;26:236–8.
117. Schumacher G, Kollberg B, Sandstedt B et al. A prospective study of first attacks of inflammatory bowel disease and non-relapsing colitis. Scand J Gastroenterol. 1993;28:1077–85.
118. Forget P, Sodoyez-Goffaux F, Zappitelli A. Permeability of the small intestine to [51Cr]EDTA in children with acute gastroenteritis or eczema. J Pediatr Gastroenterol Nutr. 1985;4:393–6.
119. Ford RPK, Menzies IS, Phillips AD, Walker-Smith JA, Turner MW. Intestinal sugar permeability: relationship to diarrhoeal disease and small bowel morphology. J Pediatr Gastroenterol Nutr. 1985;4:568–74.

120. Noone C, Menzies IS, Banatvala JE, Scopes JW. Intestinal permeability and lactose hydrolysis in human rotaviral gastroenteritis assessed simultaneously by non-invasive differential permeation. Eur J Clin Invest. 1986;16:217–25.
121. Jenkins AP, Trew DR, Crump BJ et al. Do non-steroidal anti-inflammatory drugs increase colonic permeability? Gut. 1991;32:66–9.
122. Adenis AQ, Colombel J-F, Lecouffe P, Wallaert B, Hecquet B, Marchandise X, Cortot A. Increased pulmonary and intestinal permeability in Crohn's disease. Gut. 1992;33:678–82.
123. Baldassano RN, Schreiber S, Johnston RB et al. Crohn's disease monocytes are primed for accentuated release of toxic oxygen metabolites. Gastroenterology. 1993;105:60–6.
124. Grimm MC, Pavli P, Van der Pol E, Doe WF. Evidence for a CD14+ population of monocytes in inflammatory bowel disease mucosa – implications for pathogenesis. Clin Exp Immunol. 1995;100:291–7.
125. O'Dwyer ST, Michie HR, Ziegler TR, Revhaug A, Smith RJ, Wilmore DW. A single dose of endotoxin increases intestinal permeability in healthy humans. Arch Surg. 1988;123:1459–64.
126. Fink MP. Gastrointestinal mucosal injury in experimental injury in experimental models of shock, trauma and sepsis. Crit Care Med. 1991;19:627–41.
127. Sartor RB, Cromartie WJ, Powell DW, Schwab JH. Granulomatous enterocolitis induced in rats by purified bacterial cell wall fragments. Gastroenterology. 1985;89:587–95.
128. Yamada T, Sartor RB, Marshall S, Specian RD, Grisham MB. Mucosal injury and inflammation in a model of chronic granulomatous colitis in rats. Gastroenterology. 1993;104:759–71.
129. Sadlack B, Merz H, Schorle H, Schimpl A, Feller AC, Horak I. Ulcerative colitis-like disease in mice with a disrupted interleukin-2 gene. Cell. 1993;75:253.
130. Taurog JD, Richardson JA, Croft JT et al. The germfree state prevents development of gut and joint inflammatory disease in HLA-B27 transgenic mice. J Exp Med. 1994;180:2359–64.
131. Saverymuttu S, Hodgson HJF, Chadwick VS. Controlled trial comparing prednisolone with an elemental diet plus non-absorbable antibiotics in active Crohn's disease. Gut. 1985;26:994–8.
132. Sutherland L, Singleton J, Sessions J et al. Double-blind, placebo controlled trial of metronidazole in Crohn's disease. Gut. 1991;32:1071–5.
133. Magliulo E, Scevola D, Fumarola D, Vaccaro R, Bertotto A, Burberi S. Clinical experience in detecting endotoxemia with the Limulus test in typhoid fever and other Salmonella infections. Infection. 1976;4:21–4.
134. McCann ML. Reflorastation therapy for inflammatory bowel disease (IBD), both Crohn's disease (CD) and ulcerative colitis (UC). J Allergy Clin Immunol. 1993;91:230.
135. Bass P, Luck MS. Effect of epidermal growth factor on experimental colitis in the rat. J Pharmacol Exp Ther. 1993;264:984–90.
136. Procaccino F, Reinshagen M, Hoffmann P et al. Protective effect of epidermal growth factor in an experimental model of colitis in rats. Gastroenterology. 1994;107:12–17.
137. Dugan MER, McBurney MI. Luminal glutamine perfusion alters endotoxin-related changes in ileal permeability of the piglet. J Parent Ent Nutr. 1995;19:83–7.

6
Intestinal absorption of small particles

J. SEIFERT

The first description of the absorption of particles from the gut which was 150 years ago by E. F. G. Herbst[1], caused a sensation, because this observation was in contradiction to physiological doctrine. This publication was not, of course, agreed with by most well-known scientists, and it would be probably forgotten, if a number of confirmatory publications had not appeared, during subsequent years[2]. One of the best known scientists studying the absorption of particles is G. Volkheimer; he has written a lot about the subject[3–6], but his interpretation of the observation that starch particles can be found in blood after enteral application was that the absorption of particles was a physiological accident rather than a physiological rule. So the question must be asked: 'Is the absorption of intact particles from the gastrointestinal tract really only an accident, or are there rules of which we are presently unaware'?

If the absorption of particles from the gut obeys certain rules, and is not a physiological accident, then absorption can be regulated and possibly used therapeutically.

To discover whether the absorption of particles does obey rules, two factors must be taken into consideration. On one hand the wall of the gut and its barriers must be investigated; on the other hand the physical, chemical, and biological properties of the particles must be known. Dr Bjarnasson and Dr Gardiner have considered intestinal permeability under physiological and physiopathological conditions in detail. I will therefore restrict myself to some basic investigations which demonstrate that the absorption of particles follows certain rules.

Every study of absorption must be performed with regard to the fact that absorbed particles or substances are transported after absorption along two different routes. On the one hand they can be transported via the portal venous blood, and on the other hand there is also transport via the lymphatics.

Particles and macromolecules are mainly absorbed via the lymphatic vessels. This was described by Owen and colleagues[7,8]; therefore the thoracic duct was cannulated in our investigations, since it is known that this vessel is the reservoir for the lymph of the gastrointestinal tract.

Initially we should discover whether or not there is a relationship between the absorption of particles and the age of the organism. Morris and Morris[9], and other authors[10] have reported that young animals can absorb macromolecules better than older animals.

Therefore three groups of rats, with different but defined ages, were investigated. One group was 6–8 weeks old with a mean body weight of 150 g; the second group was 5 months old with a mean body weight of 280 g; in the last group were animals older than 9 months with a mean body weight of 450 g.

The thoracic duct was cannulated in all animals according to the method of Bollmann et al.[11], and the lymph was collected at 1 h intervals over a period of 6 h. After the intragastric application of 3.7×10^9 FITC labelled 1 μm polystyrol particles via a tube, the collected lymph was investigated with optical fluorescence methods to find the absorbed particles. As shown in Fig. 1, observation of particles in the lymph is an irregular and rare event.

If the absorption of particles is correlated with the age of the animals it becomes obvious (as shown in Fig. 2) that only a few particles can be found in the lymph of young animals. Most particles were absorbed in the group of middle-aged animals. In old animals the absorption of particles again decreases. This finding was unexpected with reference to the literature. It corresponds, however, fairly well with the efficiency of the gastrointestinal tract with regard to the digestive and absorptive functions of other nutrients in correlation with the age of the organism.

In the same animal model a further consideration was tested; namely the correlation between the number of particles absorbed and the dose of particles originally applied. For this purpose one group of rats were treated with a low dose of 3.7×10^5 particles. A second group received 3.7×10^7 and a third group was treated intragastrically with 3×10^9 particles.

Figure 3 shows that there obviously exists a dose-dependent absorption of particles. The more particles which are enterally offered, the more particles could be found in the collected lymph. Nevertheless further increases in the enterally applied doses of particles did not significantly increase the absorbed

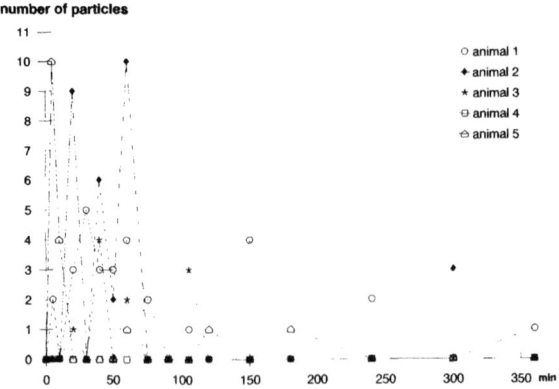

Figure 1 Number of particles in the lymph of the thoracic duct after the intraduodenal administration of 3.7×10^9 FITC-labelled polystyrol particles (1 μm)

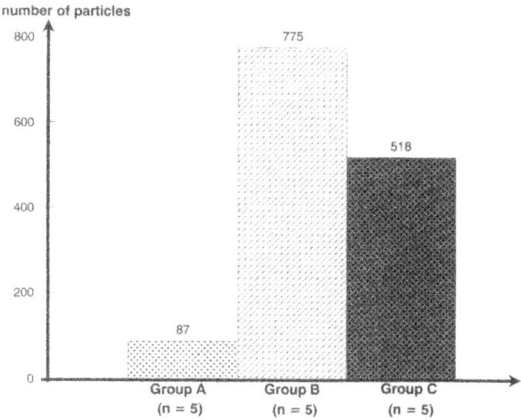

Figure 2   Number of particles absorbed within 6 h in relation to age of animals. Group A, young rats; group B, middle-aged rats; group C, old rats

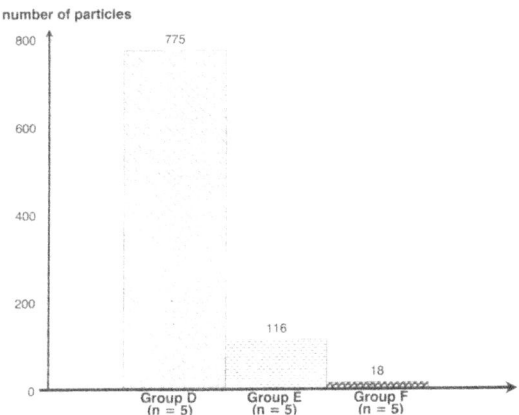

Figure 3   Number of absorbed particles in relation to the dose. In group D 3.7×10^9 particles, in group E 3.7×10^7 particles, and in group; F 3.7×10^5 particles were administered intraduodenally

particles. These observations demonstrate that the absorption of particles obeys certain rules, and is by no means a simple physiological accident.

The main entrance for the absorption of particles from the gut seems to be the M cells of the Peyer's patches. Peyer's patches are accumulations of lymph follicles in the gut, mainly in the jejunum and ileum. Their surface makes direct contact with the lumen of the gut. Using a magnification of 20 000, polystyrol particles can be observed on the surface of the M cell (Fig. 4). Using an even higher magnification it could be shown (Fig. 5) that the microfolds cover one particle and at the same time the M cell is sinking from the normal level of the lumen to deeper regions. It is known that M cells are mobile cells. Investigating the underlying region of the dome of the lymph follicle one finds particles fixed

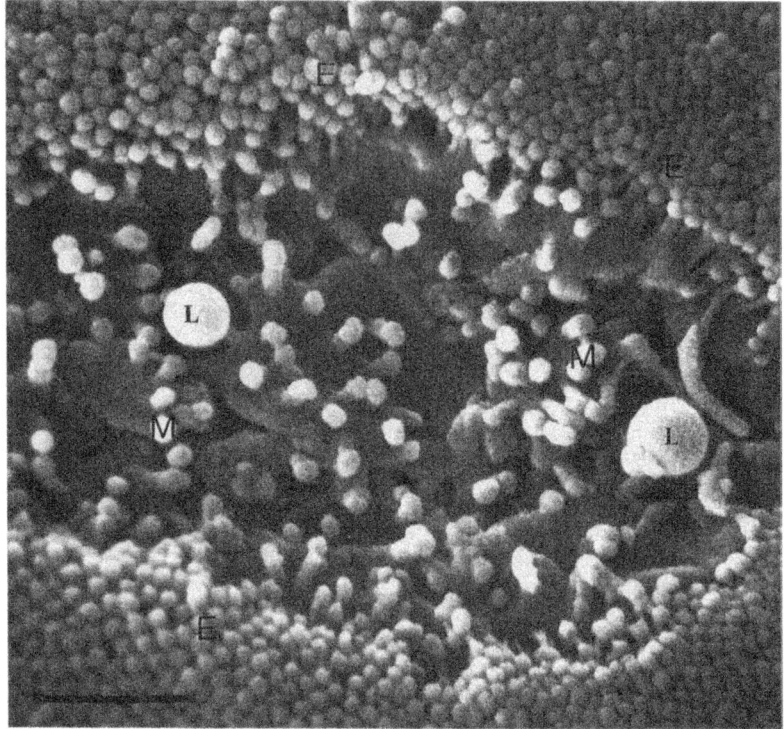

Figure 4 M cell of a Peyer's plaque with two latex beads (L) on the surface. The M cell is surrounded by enteroabsorptive cells (E). The microfolds are a characteristic feature of the M cells (M). (Scale bar = 1 μm)

or possibly incorporated on macrophages (Fig. 6). Using intravital microscopy combined with videotechnique it could be shown that two different absorption mechanisms are important. One mechanism is a very fast absorption which is finished within 8 s; the second mechanism is longer lasting; it is finished after 34 s. For both mechanisms a binding to the M cell is necessary. The observation that the absorption of particles is not a continuous but a cyclic event, with long-lasting and very short absorption mechanisms, correlates very well with the number of particles in the lymph, which was shown in Fig. 1.

Very similar results with regard to the absorption mechanism, but also with regard to the kinetics of the absorption, were detected after the enteral application of microorganisms. Also, after the enteral application of *Pseudomonas aeruginosa*, microorganisms could be found on the surface of the M cells (Fig. 7). Investigations of the portal venous blood revealed an initial increase of the microorganism within 15 min (Fig. 8). This figure also shows that therapeutic substances can influence the absorption of microorganisms, which are in this case handled like particles. The lower curve indicates that cyclosporin A is able to almost completely prevent the absorption of *Ps. aeruginosa*. Changes in the

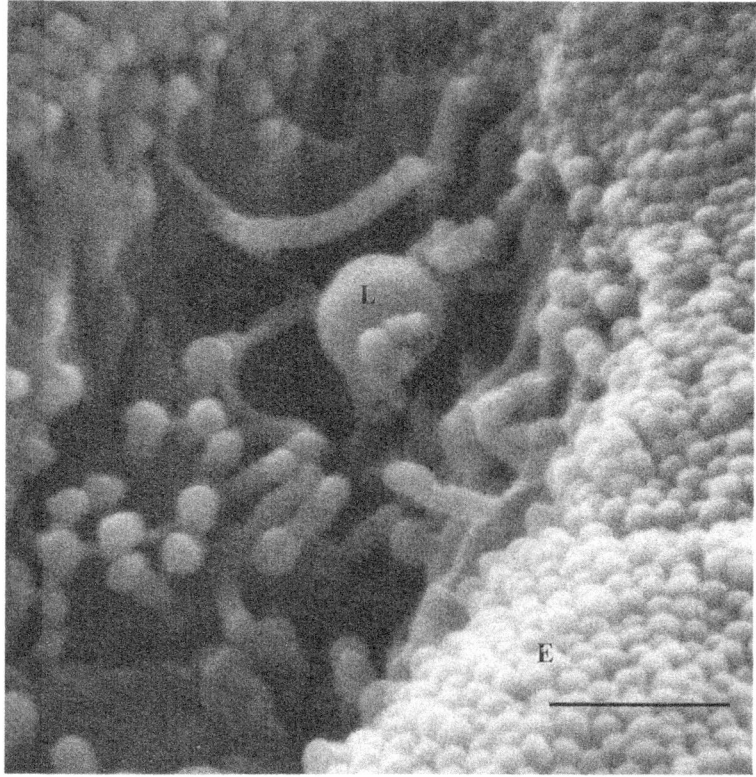

Figure 5   M cell of a Peyer's plaque (scale bar = 0.5 μm). Microfolds seem to fix the particles (L) and to settle down from the normal level of the lumen. E = enteroabsorptive cell

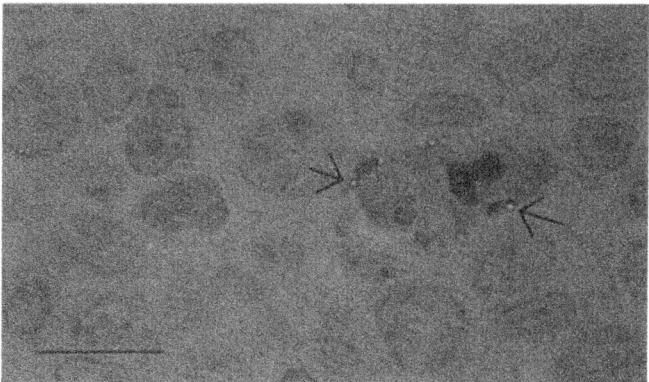

Figure 6   Particles associated with macrophages 10 min after application. Light micrograph from a lymphoid follicle of a Peyer's patch. (Scale bar = 10 μm)

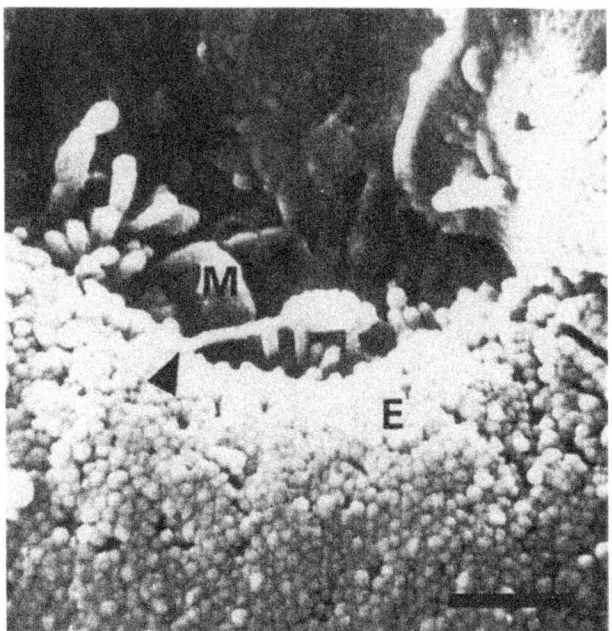

Figure 7 M cell with microfolds (M) surrounded by an enteroabsorptive cell (E). The arrow marks a *Ps. aeruginosa* with its characteristic polar tail

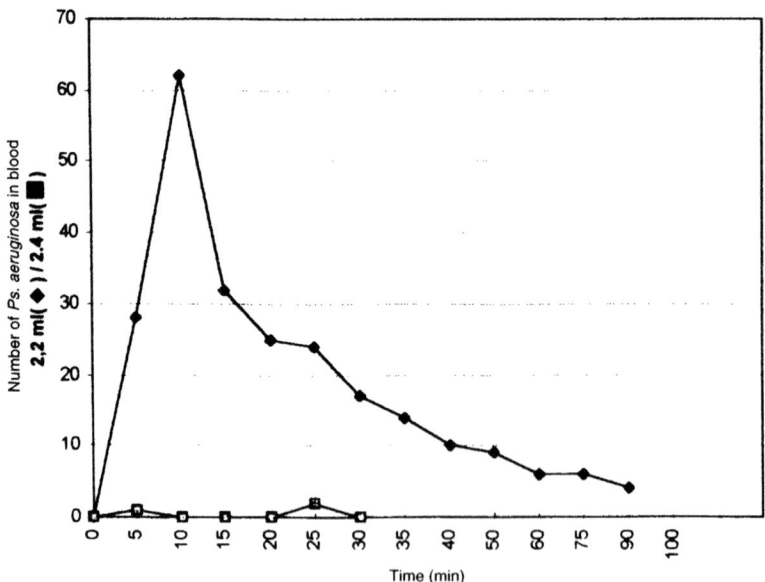

Figure 8 Number of microorganisms (*Ps. aeruginosa*) in portal venous blood after oral application of 3.5×10^9 *Ps. aeruginosa* (♦) in rats. Pretreatment with cyclosporin A reduced the number significantly (□)

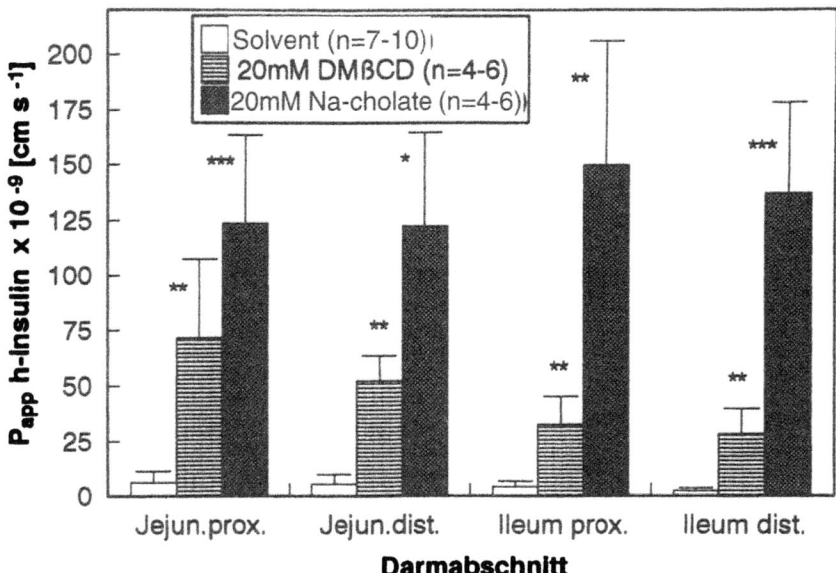

Figure 9 An improvement of the absorption of particles could be induced by dimethyl-β-cyclodextrin and sodium-cholate. Insulin served as an indicator; it was encapsuled in microemulsion particles. $^* p < 0.05;\ ^{**} p < 0.01;\ ^{***} p < 0.001$

shape of M cells induced by cyclosporin A are probably responsible for this decrease in absorption. Scanning electron microscopic pictures verify a reduction of microfolds and a clumping of the cells.

Apart from the impairment of absorption there are also substances which can improve the uptake of particles. Of many substances investigated the results of two are shown in Fig. 9. In this experiment the everted gut sac method[12] was utilized for absorption studies. Insulin was incorporated in the particles of a microemulsion. This was used as an indicator for the uptake of particles. As shown, a marked improvement of the absorption of particles can be obtained by using dimethyl-β-cyclodextrin, and an even more marked improvement with sodium-cholate.

Neither the influence of therapeutic medicaments on the absorption of particles nor the influence of substances which are produced in the body is clarified. There is, however, great interest in improving the absorption of particles, because microparticles can be used as a vehicle for the transport of medicaments.

The absorption of particles is negligible for the energy supply of the living organism. However, it seems to play a major role in immunological mechanisms such as the recognition of foreign antigens and the induction of an immune response. Although the amount of absorbed particles is low under normal conditions, it is a fact that particle absorption follows physical, biological and biochemical rules, and is certainly not a physiological accident.

References

1. Herbst EFG. Das Lymphgefäβsystem und seine Verrichtungen. Göttingen: Vandenhoek u Ruprecht Verlag; 1844.
2. Hirsch R. Über das Vorkommen von Stärkekörnern in Blut und Urin. Z Exp Pathol Ther. 1906;3:390–2.
3. Volkheimer G, Schulz FH. The phenomenon of persorption. Digestion. 1968;1:213–18.
4. Volkheimer G, Schulz, FH, Aurich I, Strauch S, Benthin K, Wendland H. Persorption of particles. Digestion. 1968;1:78–80.
5. Volkheimer G, Schulz FH. Lindenau A, Beitz U. Persorption of metallic iron particles. Gut. 1969;10:32–3.
6. Volkheimer G. Passage of particles through the wall of the gastrointestinal tract. Environ Health Perspect. 1974;9:215–25.
7. Owen RL, Nemanic P. Antigen processing structures of the mammalian intestinal tract: an SEM study of lymphoepithelial organs. Scan Elect Microsc. 1978;11:367–78.
8. Owen RL, Jones AL. Epithelial cell specialization within human Peyer's patches: an ultrastructural study of intestinal lymphoid follicles. Gastroenterology. 1974;66:189–203.
9. Morris B, Morris R. Fractionation studies on the absorption of labelled immunoglobulin-G by the gut of young rats. J Physiol. 1977;265:429–42.
10. Hemmings WA, Williams EW. Quantitative and visualization studies of the transport of rat and bovine IgG and ferritin across the segments of small intestine of the suckling rat. Proc R Soc Lond B. 1977;197:425–40.
11. Bollmann JL, Cain JC, Grindley JH. Technique for the collection of lymph from the thoracic duct of the rat. J Lab Clin Med. 1948;33:1349–52.
12. Schilling RJ, Mitra AK. Intestinal transport of insulin. Int J Pharmacol. 1990;62:53–64.

Section III
Bile acid, amino acid and drug metabolism – it's not only the liver, it may be the gut

7
Bile acids and intestinal bacteria: peaceful coexistence versus deadly warfare

A. F. HOFMANN and L. R. HAGEY

INTRODUCTION

The interaction of intestinal bacteria with primary bile acids generates modified bile acids that are in part absorbed. As a result the liver is continuously exposed to a flux of modified bile acids originating from the intestine. Generally these modified bile acids are well tolerated or, if toxic, are detoxified by hepatic enzymes. The result is a 'peaceful coexistence' between the germ-free liver and the germ-laden intestine. Under conditions in which the flux of modified bile acids is altered qualitatively or quantitatively, or in which the liver has increased sensitivity or decreased detoxification ability, liver damage may result. When this occurs, and is sufficiently severe to kill the host, peaceful coexistence changes to 'deadly warfare'. In this chapter we will describe the interactions between bile acids and bacteria, and give examples of both peaceful coexistence and deadly warfare. From an evolutionary point of view, interaction between bile acids and bacteria has received relatively little attention. Because experimental data are quite limited in some areas, parts of this chapter will necessarily be of a speculative nature. More detailed reviews of several of the topics considered here are available[1-5].

This chapter will also advance two additional hypotheses. The first is that bile acids influence the symbiotic relationship between intestinal bacteria and their vertebrate host. In the proximal small intestine of most mammals, bile acids are present in high, micellar concentrations and bacterial action on bile acids or nutrients is minimal. Bile acids may in fact inhibit the growth of bacteria by their bacteriostatic action and/or inhibit bacterial adhesion by their detergent properties. In the large intestine, in contrast, the opposite condition is present. The bacterial flora is increased in concentration by several orders of magnitude, and the bile acid concentration is decreased greatly, well below that required for micelle formation. Because not only bile acids but also water is absorbed in the distal small intestine, the concentration of bile acids entering the large intestine is still quite high. The rapid decrease in the concentration of bile acids is a direct result of bacterial action. Bacterial enzymes render bile acids less soluble (by deconjugation and dehydroxylation); this effect is enhanced by the lower pH of the caecum. Some of the bacterially modified bile acids adsorb to bacteria; others are absorbed by the colonic epithelium and join the circulating bile acids. Others may precipitate from solution. These multiple events cause an overall decrease in monomeric bile acid concentration by at least one order of magnitude. The result precludes micelle formation and allows bacteria to flourish.

The second hypothesis is that bacterial modification of bile acids has played a key role in bile acid evolution. Bacteria remove the hydroxy group at C-7 from chenodeoxycholic acid, resulting in the formation of lithocholic acid, a toxic bile acid. A number of biological adaptations have occurred that either prevent the formation of lithocholic acid or result in its rapid elimination. Among these adaptations are the formation of trihydroxy bile acids by hydroxylation of chenodeoxycholic acid or a precursor in its biosynthetic pathway. Thus, the evolution of trihydroxy bile acids may be considered a response to bacterial 7-dehydroxylation of chenodeoxycholic acid.

GUT DESIGN

The essential function of the gut is to absorb nutrients, vitamins, minerals, and water, as well as to serve as an excretory conduit for materials excreted in bile. To mediate these functions the gut begins with a stomach that serves as an acidifying reservoir (to mediate both pre-digestion and sterilization of the ingested foodstuffs). The stomach empties into the intestine, a digestive absorptive tube whose end discharges food residues, bacteria, and secreted molecules to the outside. At the proximal end of the small intestine, gastric content is neutralized by pancreatic bicarbonate, and admixed with bile and pancreatic enzymes. Pancreatic and surface enzymes mediate the absorption of carbohydrates and proteins; efficient lipid absorption requires hydrolysis of ester bonds by lipases and esterases followed by solubilization of the products by bile acid micelles.

In some species, digestion of dietary nutrients is mediated not only by the hydrolytic action of gastric, pancreatic, and enterocyte brush-border enzymes, but also by bacterial enzymes. Digestion catalysed by endogenous secretions may be termed 'endolytic', and that catalysed by bacterial enzymes may be termed 'xenolytic'. The fraction of calories provided by endolytic digestion varies widely but, in general, endolytic digestion is likely to predominate in carnivores, whereas xenolytic digestion is likely to predominate in herbivores.

Xenolytic digestion may occur either in the foregut or hindgut. In ruminants (foregut fermenters), an anaerobic pre-stomach converts cellulose and plant lipids to short-chain fatty acids (SCFA) and saturated long-chain fatty acids (LCFA). The SCFA are absorbed from the rumen, and the saturated LCFA are subsequently solubilized by bile acid micelles and absorbed from the small intestine. The rumen ends in a true acidic stomach which sterilizes rumen contents before they are emptied into the small intestine. In hindgut fermenters, fermentation of cellulose and other non-absorbable carbohydrates occurs in the anaerobic caecum. Again, SCFA are formed and absorbed. For some animals, such as horses, hindgut fermentation is the major source of dietary calories and is therefore essential for life[6,7]. Bile acids are not present in rumen contents, and are present at only minuscule concentrations in the anaerobic caecum. Accordingly, the solubilizing action of bile acids is important for endolytic digestion of lipids, and not for xenolytic digestion, whose major substrates are carbohydrates and proteins.

CHEMISTRY OF PRIMARY CHOLANOIDS

In vertebrates, cholesterol is degraded to bile alcohols or bile acids, which in their conjugated form are water-soluble and surface-active. The term 'bile salt' was used by Haslewood[8] for such compounds in their conjugated form, but it seems preferable to use the term 'cholanoid', which applies to all bile alcohols or bile acids irrespective of their conjugation[9]. The term 'primary' indicates that the molecule was synthesized from cholesterol by the action of tissue enzymes. Primary cholanoids are the substrates for bacterial enzymes.

Cholanoids may be subdivided into three great classes according to the terminal polar group of the side-chain – the C_{27} bile alcohols, the C_{27} bile acids, and the C_{24} bile acids. We have suggested that it is useful to define three 'default' cholanoids; that is, the cholanoids corresponding to these three side-chain structures, and possessing in addition, a 3α-hydroxy and a 7α-hydroxy group[10]. The rationale for this suggestion is that all cholanoids must have a hydroxyl group at C-3 (from cholesterol) and most cholanoids have an additional hydroxyl group at C-7, as hydroxylation at C-7 (either of cholesterol or a later intermediate) is an early step in the biosynthesis pathway of bile acids. Since the preponderance of natural cholanoids have an A/B ring juncture in *cis* conformation, the hydrogen at C-5 is in the β configuration. With these three default cholanoids as building blocks it is possible to describe the structure of most primary bile alcohols and bile acids by additional hydroxylations on the steroid nucleus and/or side-chain of the default structures. [There are a small number of exceptions. These consist of bile acids with 3β- or 7β-hydroxy groups, or bile acids in which the A/B ring juncture is *trans* (5α- or allo-bile acids)].

The C_{27} bile alcohols occur in ancient fish (jawless and cartilaginous) as well as in herbivorous bony fish[8,10–12]. They also occur in amphibia and in five ancient mammals (elephant, manatee, rhinoceros, hyrax, and horse). One additional hydroxylation (besides C-3, C-7, and C-27) may occur on the nucleus; sites identified to date are C-12, C-6, C-16, and C-2. Additional hydroxylation also occurs on the side-chain (at C-26, C-25, C-24, and C-23). Generally not more than two or three additional hydroxylations occur; consequently, most C_{27} bile alcohols are pentols or hexols. All C_{27} bile alcohols isolated from the bile of healthy vertebrates have been conjugated, and conjugation has been solely with sulphate. The sulphate is present esterified to the terminal hydroxy group of the side-chain (C-27)[12].

The C_{27} bile acids occur in amphibians (frogs), reptiles (crocodilians, turtles, and lizards) as well as in ancient birds[8,10–13]. Additional hydroxylation on the steroid nucleus has been reported to occur at C-12 or at C-16, but more sites of nuclear hydroxylation are likely to be found. Side-chain hydroxylation occurs at C-22, C-24, C-25, and C-26. Most C_{27} bile acids have only a single hydroxy group on the side-chain, but bile acids with two hydroxy groups on the side-chain have been reported. To date, all C_{27} bile acids isolated from bile have been conjugated, and conjugation has been exclusively with taurine. Such conjugates are termed N-acyl (or aminoacyl) amidates. The term 'amidates' is frequently used as a convenient name to distinguish taurine and glycine conjugates from bile acids conjugated with other molecules such as sulphate or glucuronate[9].

The C_{24} bile acids occur in bony (ray-finned) fish, in lizards and snakes, in birds, and in mammals. One additional nuclear hydroxy group is normally present. Common sites of hydroxylation are C-12 (α), C-6 (α or β), or C-16 (α). Less common sites of hydroxylation are C-1 (α or β), C-15, and C-5 (β). Side-chain hydroxylation occurs at C-23 (α carbon) or at C-22 (β carbon). Usually the sum of nuclear and side-chain hydroxy groups does not exceed three[10,11]. In humans there are two primary bile acids: cholic acid ($3\alpha,7\alpha,12\alpha$- trihydroxy) and chenodeoxycholic acid ($3\alpha,7\alpha$-dihydroxy; CDCA)

Bile acids – both C_{27} and C_{24} – are conjugated with taurine or taurine derivatives (such as N-methyltaurine or cysteinolic acid). C_{24} bile acids are also conjugated with glycine in mammals and some species of pigeons. Conjugation of bile acids is not always complete. Small proportions of cholic acid occur in unconjugated form in many species, and in several Australian marsupials most of the bile acids are present in unconjugated form[14].

MODIFICATION OF PRIMARY CHOLANOIDS BY BACTERIAL ENZYMES

Deconjugation

Hydrolysis of bile alcohol sulphates has received little study to date. Sulphatase is not present in pancreatic secretions, and it is unlikely that endolytic cleavage of bile alcohol sulphates occurs. Microorganisms capable of hydrolysing bile alcohol sulphates have been reported[15].

Amidates of C_{27} bile acids are cleaved by mixed bacterial cultures[16], but as yet a single bacterial species capable of hydrolysing such cholestanoic acid conjugates has not been identified. Analyses of faecal bile acids from the alligator[17] indicate that some deconjugation (and 7-dehydroxylation) occurs in these reptiles. However, the extent of deconjugation of C_{27} bile acids has received little study.

Much more is known about the deconjugation (deamidation) of C_{24} amidates. A great variety of bacterial species capable of hydrolysing the common natural bile acid conjugates have been identified[18]. It is unlikely that gastric, pancreatic, and glycocalyx enzymes can deconjugate bile acid amidates because faecal bile acids of germ-free animals remain entirely in conjugated form. In addition, C_{24} bile acid amidates do not undergo deconjugation when incubated with pancreatic juice or mucosal homogenates[19]. Therefore, because deconjugation is mediated solely by bacterial enzymes, the site at which it occurs is determined by the colonization pattern of the intestine.

Dehydroxylation at C-7

The key biotransformation of cholanoids by bacterial enzymes is 7-dehydroxylation, since this step generates new bile acids with new physicochemical and physiological properties. Hylemon and his colleagues have elucidated the multiple biochemical steps involved in 7-dehydroxylation of cholic acid to form deoxycholic acid ($3\alpha,12\alpha$-dihydroxy, DCA) and CDCA to form lithocholic acid (3α-hydroxy)[20]. It is likely that the pathway described by these workers applies to all C_{24} and all C_{27} bile acids that undergo 7-dehydroxylation. The first step is formation of a coenzyme A thio-ester[21]. Such cannot occur with a bile alcohol, and does not readily occur with a glycine or taurine amidate, because of their lower pK_a values. Accordingly, the prevailing opinion is that 7-dehydroxylation requires prior deconjugation. The strongest lines of evidence in support of this belief are: (a) the resistance of N-methyl bile acids to 7-dehydroxylation[22,23]; and (b) the resistance to 7-dehydroxylation of a series of bile acid sulphonates in which the terminal carboxyl group was replaced by a sulphonic acid group[24].

Subsequent steps in 7-dehydroxylation involve the formation of an intermediate, from which the C-7 hydroxy group is eliminated[20].

Side-chain topology is also important in 7-dehydroxylation as nor (C_{23}) and dinor (C_{22}) bile acids do not undergo this reaction. (P. Hylemon and A. F. Hofmann; unpublished observations). It is also thought that bile acids with a hydroxyl group at C-23 (α-hydroxy bile acids) do not undergo 7-dehydroxylation because the 7-deoxy derivatives of these bile acids have never been identified in bile. It is likely that α-hydroxy bile acids do not readily form a CoA derivative because such acids are relatively strong acids with a pK_a of 4.2[25]. Pellicciari, Roda, and their colleagues have synthesized a large number of bile acids with modified side-chains that are resistant to 7-dehydroxylation[26,27].

There has been little systematic examination of the rate at which 7-dehydroxylation proceeds for the spectrum of C_{27} and C_{24} bile acids occurring in vertebrates. Among the C_{24} bile acids, cholic acid, CDCA, and hyocholic acid ($3\alpha,6\alpha,7\alpha$-trihydroxy) are readily 7-dehydroxylated. In the hamster[28] and human[29], β-muricholic ($3\alpha,6\beta,7\beta$-trihydroxy) does not undergo 7-dehydroxylation. Whether β-hyocholic ($3\alpha,6\alpha,7\beta$-trihydroxy; also termed ω-muricholic) and α-muricholic ($3\alpha,6\beta,7\alpha$-trihydroxy) undergo 7-dehydroxylation has not been studied. Figure 1 shows a chromatogram of faecal bile acids of the Chinese Monal pheasant *Lophophorus ihllysii*. In this sample, 7-dehydroxylation did not occur with three uncommon trihydroxy bile acids ($1\beta,3\alpha,7\alpha$-trihydroxy, $3\alpha,5\beta,7\alpha$-trihydroxy, and $3\alpha,4\beta,7\alpha$-trihydroxy). These data suggest that such bile acids are resistant to bacterial 7-dehydroxylation, in contrast to cholic acid and hyocholic acid, which are also formed in this species.

Intestinal site of deconjugation and 7-dehydroxylation

No information is available as to the site and extent of deconjugation of bile alcohol sulphates. It would be reasonable to propose that for animals such as the elephant, in which caecal fermentation of dietary cellulose is an essential digestive process, deconjugation of bile alcohol sulphates would begin in the small intestine and be completed in the large intestine. For herbivorous fish, which

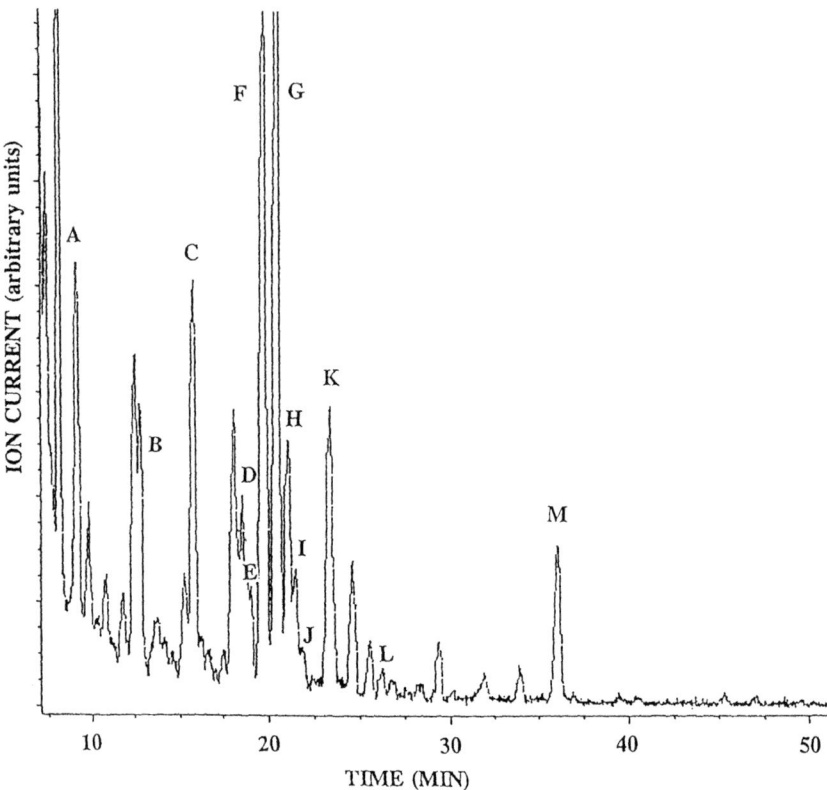

Figure 1 Gas chromatography/mass spectrum of faecal bile acids and sterols of the Chinese Monal pheasant (*Lophophorus ihllysii*). Bile acids were deconjugated by alkaline hydrolysis, esterified with methanol, and converted to trimethylsilyl derivatives. The identities of the peaks percentage composition (normalized to 100%) were as follows: **A**, 1-hexacosanol, 8.5%; **B**, 5β-cholestan-3β-ol, 4.8%; **C**, cholesterol, 11.4%; **D**, cholic acid, 2.6%; **E**, allolithocholic acid, 1.6%; **F**, lithocholic acid, 20.1%; **G**, chenodeoxycholic acid, 26.1%; **H**, hyocholic acid, 6.5%; **I**, 5β-hydroxychenodeoxycholic acid, 2.5%; **J**, murideoxycholic acid, 0.8%; **K**, a mixture of 1β-hydroxychenodeoxycholic acid, 5.3%, and β-sitosterol, 3.6%; **L**, 4β-hydroxychenodeoxycholic acid, 0.6% and **M**, 3α-hydroxy-7-oxo-5β-cholan-24-oic acid, 4.8%. The absence of 7-deoxy products in bile acids with a third hydroxy group at C-5β (**I**), C-1β (**L**), or C-4β (**L**) indicates that these bile acids, in contrast to cholic acid and hyocholic acid, have not undergone 7-dehydroxylation by enteric flora

may have a relatively short intestine, deconjugation of bile alcohol sulphates might not occur at all.

To assess the site and extent of deconjugation of bile acids one can sample intestinal content directly. Unfortunately, such an approach gives only a minimal estimate of deconjugation, because unconjugated bile acids are rapidly absorbed from the small intestine after they are formed. One can determine the turnover of the steroid and amino acid moieties of a conjugated bile acid by labelling each moiety and determining the specific activity decay curve[30]. This gives a value for the extent to which the steroid moiety is deconjugated, returned to the liver, and reconjugated. If assumptions are made about the number of times that the pool circulates per day, and if it is assumed, in addition, that all bile acids lost from the enterohepatic circulation are deconjugated, one can estimate the amount of deconjugation occurring per day using compartmental analysis[31].

For C_{27} bile acids the presence of 7-deoxy bile acids in the faeces of the alligator[17] indicates that 7-dehydroxylation (after deconjugation) is extensive. However, there is virtually no information available on the extent of 7-dehydroxylation of C_{27} bile acids in amphibians, reptiles, and ancient birds.

For C_{24} bile acids, deconjugation has been shown to occur to a considerable extent in the small intestine in the rat[32], the rabbit[33], and to a moderate extent in humans[34–36].

Since faecal bile acids are predominantly in unconjugated form in humans, rat, and hamster, it is likely that bile acid deconjugation proceeds to completion during large intestinal transit in all species in which the large intestine is heavily colonized by bacteria. The only instances in which deconjugation does not occur is the germ-free animal[37] and in the panda (both the red and the giant panda) species, in whom the dietary intake is rich in fibre and the intestine has a very short transit time.

Dehydroxylation of bile acids at C-7, in contrast to deconjugation, is mediated solely by a relatively small number of anaerobic bacterial species[2]. Dehydroxylation can therefore occur only in the anaerobic caecum or during disease conditions such as the stagnant loop syndrome in which anaerobic pockets develop in the small intestine because of extreme stasis. It is a reasonable speculation that 7-dehydroxylation occurs in all animals with an anaerobic caecum.

METABOLISM AND SIGNIFICANCE OF BACTERIAL MODIFICATION OF CHOLANOIDS

Physicochemical properties of unconjugated cholanoids

Little is known about the physicochemical properties of unsulphated bile alcohols. Goto et al.[38] examined the solubility of 5α-cyprinol, the bile alcohol of the Asiatic carp. The molecule had a limited aqueous solubility (≈ 300 μmol/L), and did not form micelles at this concentration. If other bile alcohols have similar solubility properties, deconjugation would result in loss of function, since the liberated bile alcohol is insufficiently amphipathic to self-associate and form micelles. Deconjugation would also result in loss from the enterohepatic circulation, since bile alcohols are poorly absorbed from the intestine.

The physicochemical properties of unconjugated C_{27} bile acids have not been examined, but it seems reasonable to predict that these molecules should behave in a manner similar to that of their corresponding C_{24} homologues. All unconjugated bile acids with an unsubstituted side chain have a pK_a of ≈ 5.0[39]. For C_{24} unconjugated bile acids the aqueous solubility of the protonated form of most dihydroxy bile acids is quite low (10–30 μmol/L). The solubility of trihydroxy bile acids is several-fold greater[39]. The solubility of unconjugated bile acids, as that of any weak acid, rises logarithmically with increasing pH[40].

Absorption of unconjugated bile acids from the intestine

Unconjugated bile acids, whether C_{27} or C_{24}, will be absorbed passively from the small and large intestine[5]. Whether carrier-mediated absorption of unconjugated bile acids also occurs is not known.

No experimental data dealing with the absorption of C_{27} bile acids are available, but the principles applying to the absorption of C_{24} bile acids are also likely to apply to the absorption of C_{27} bile acids. For C_{24} bile acids the absorption rate is the product of the permeability, the monomeric concentration, and the surface area. The amount absorbed will be the product of the rate of absorption and time of exposure. Mathematically,

$$Q_{abs} = P \cdot C \cdot A \cdot T$$

where Q_{abs} is the amount of bile acid absorbed, P is permeability (amount absorbed in relation to concentration) (cm/s); C is the monomeric concentration (μmol/L) of the protonated species; A is surface area (cm^2); and T is exposure time (in seconds).

In the small intestine the monomeric concentration will be influenced by the pH of the microclimate, as acidic pH increases protonation. The presence of micelles will diminish the monomeric concentration of bile acids if bile acid molecules adsorb to micelles. As noted above, precipitation from solution and adsorption to bacteria are also likely to occur. The major determinant of P is the number of hydroxy groups, since P for most small molecules is correlated inversely with the polar surface area[41]. Monohydroxy and dihydroxy bile acids are absorbed rapidly. Cholic acid is absorbed considerably more slowly, and it is unclear whether cholic acid absorption is entirely passive or in part carrier-mediated (cf. ref. 42).

The intraluminal pH decreases from about 7.5 in the distal ileum to about 5.5 in the caecum, probably because of short-chain fatty acid production by anaerobic bacteria. As a result of this decreased pH, the solubility of unconjugated bile acids will decrease about 100-fold. The unconjugated bile acids may precipitate from solution, adsorb to bacteria, or be passively absorbed. The principles that were summarized above for the absorption of unconjugated bile acids from the small intestine also apply to the absorption of unconjugated bile acids from the large intestine. There are, however, some differences between the large and small intestine in addition to the much lower monomeric concentration that should influence the rate of bile acid absorption: (a) the surface area of the large intestine is probably smaller than that part of the small intestine available to unconjugated bile acids and (b) the transit time of the large intestine is several times greater than that of the small intestine. Simulations of bile acid metabolism in humans suggest that absorption of unconjugated bile acids from the large intestine is considerably less than that from the small intestine if expressed as mmol/day[43,44].

Bile acids are not appreciably biotransformed during enterocyte passage. Passage of hydrophobic bile acids (monohydroxy and dihydroxy bile acids) across the basolateral membrane is likely to be passive. Cholic acid transport may be passive and/or carrier-mediated.

Unconjugated bile acids are transported to the liver in portal blood. Lymphatic absorption is negligible. Hepatic uptake involves both passive and active mechanisms[45].

Metabolism of unconjugated bile acids in the liver

Unconjugated bile acids are 'repaired' during transit through the hepatocyte.

Nuclear repair involves epimerization of 3β-hydroxy bile acids to 3α-hydroxy bile acids via a 3-oxo intermediate. The 3-oxo bile acids are reduced to 3α-hydroxy bile acids, but the reduction is not always complete; 7-oxo bile acids are reduced stereospecifically to 7-hydroxy bile acids. The reduction may be incomplete or complete, and whether 7α-hydroxy or 7β-hydroxy bile acids are formed is species-dependent[3].

The 7-deoxy bile acids that are absorbed from the intestine may undergo no, partial, or complete rehydroxylation at C-7. Because many species of vertebrates have biliary bile acids containing appreciable proportions of deoxycholic acid, it is obvious that 7-rehydroxylation is frequently absent or partial. In some species hydroxylation occurs at a site other than C-7 (see below).

Side-chain repair involves reamidation, that is reconjugation with taurine or glycine. In humans, lithocholic acid is not only reamidated but, in addition, undergoes sulphation at C-3 to form a sulpholithocholyl amidate[46].

If the side-chain of a bile acid is shortened by a single methylene group the resulting 'nor' compound does not undergo amidation, but instead is conjugated with glucuronate[47]. Glucuronidation, a microsomal process, occurs instead of amidation because such C_{23} bile acids are poor substrates for the enzymes involved in bile acid amidation. For C_{24} bile acids the absence in biliary bile acids of appreciable proportions of glucuronides suggests that the amidation process for unconjugated bile acids entering the hepatocyte is highly efficient, and occurs before the unconjugated bile acids partition into the microsomal compartment. Accordingly, hydroxylation (either at C-7 or elsewhere), which also occurs in the microsomal compartment, must occur after reamidation. Because a carrier mechanism is required for an amidated bile acid to enter and exit the microsomal compartment, microsomal transporters for bile acids are likely to be present.

An overall scheme of bile acid metabolism in vertebrates is shown in Fig. 2.

BIOLOGICAL SIGNIFICANCE OF BACTERIAL MODIFICATIONS OF BILE ACIDS

Deconjugation

Bile acid deconjugation in the small intestine is unlikely to have any important physiological effects in most healthy vertebrates for several reasons. First, most nutrient absorption occurs in the proximal small intestine, and deconjugation is more likely to occur in the distal small intestine. Second, unconjugated bile acids are not much more toxic than their corresponding amidates. Third, unconjugated primary bile acids have been fed to many animal species, and at least

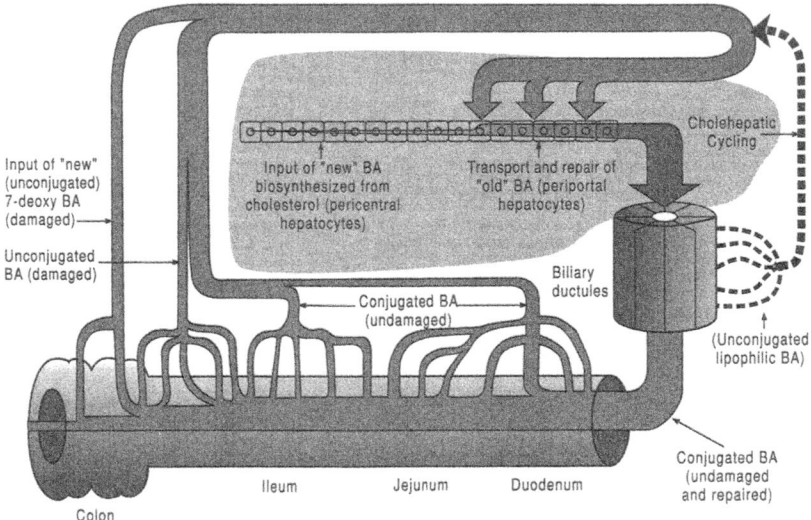

Figure 2 Metabolism and enterohepatic cycling of bile acids in vertebrates possessing a caecum. The liver is denoted by the stippled solid above; the intestine is denoted by the tube below. Dark stippling indicates the flux of bile acids. Bile acids are synthesized from cholesterol in the pericentral hepatocytes. A recycling pool accumulates because of intestinal conservation involving both active and passive mechanisms. Bile acids are deconjugated in the distal small intestine, and some of the unconjugated bile acids (termed 'damaged') are absorbed. In the colon, bile acids undergo 7-dehydroxylation and some of these 7-deoxy bile acids are absorbed. The periportal cells repair the damaged bile acids, and transport them, together with undamaged bile acids that have been returned from the intestine, into the canaliculus. Dihydroxy bile acids, if secreted in unconjugated form, can be absorbed from the biliary ductules and undergo cholehepatic shunting; however, there is no evidence that conjugation is incomplete in any healthy vertebrate

with doses similar to the biosynthesis rate, toxicity is uncommon (but see below). The physiological effect of deconjugation is to decrease the intraluminal concentration of bile acids, because unconjugated bile acids are absorbed rapidly and passively from the small intestine. Another consideration is that intraluminal pH increases in the distal small intestine. As a result, unconjugated bile acids should be present in their ionized and water-soluble form. Their anions can join conjugated bile acid anions in micelle formation and thereafter function as effectively as conjugated bile acid anions in the solubilization of lipolysis products. It can even be argued that deconjugation of bile acids is beneficial for the host, in that it enhances bile acid conservation from the small intestine. Passive intestinal absorption of unconjugated bile acids diminishes the requirement for carrier-mediated absorption of conjugated bile acids.

In the large intestine, deconjugation appears to be much more important from an ecological standpoint, at least in those species with an anaerobic caecum. First, deconjugation decreases bile acid solubility markedly at the pH conditions prevailing in the caecum (pH 5–6)[40]. This effect, together with enhanced passive absorption, should decrease the bacteriostatic action of bile acids, permitting bacterial flora to flourish. Second, deconjugation is a prerequisite for 7-dehydroxylation, which also contributes to a decreased aqueous concentration of bile acids, since 7-deoxy unconjugated bile acids are less soluble than their 7-hydroxy precursors.

Deconjugation–dehydroxylation appears to influence colonic morphology by an unknown mechanism. The germ-free mouse has a very large caecum, whose size diminishes when cholestyramine is administered[48]. It may be that, in the germ-free animal, conjugated bile acids stimulate colonic secretion because of their elevated intraluminal concentration[49], and that such stimulation of secretion causes morphological changes. Factors other than, or in addition to, bile acids may also be involved.

Dehydroxylation

Toxicity of exogenous 7-deoxy bile acids

In health, 7-dehydroxylation of bile acids does not cause hepatotoxicity because the input of toxic bile acids is small enough that it can be completely detoxified. When intestinal bacteria are provided with an increased amount of a precursor of a toxic bile acid, or when there is increased microbial 7-dehydroxylation activity, input of 7-deoxy bile acids from the large intestine increases. When this occurs, the role of the bacteria changes from peaceful coexistence to deadly warfare.

The chronic toxicity of 7-deoxy bile acids has been shown by numerous studies in which these bile acids or their precursors have been added to the diet. Toxicity is dose-related and species-dependent. Toxicity results from direct damage to hepatocytes or cholangiocytes (necrosis and/or apoptosis)[50] or precipitation of the calcium salt of the administered compound (or a metabolite) in the biliary system[51]. Other toxic effects, such as bile duct proliferation, have also been observed[52]. The order of toxicity is as follows: lithocholic acid > deoxycholic acid $\geqslant$ chenodeoxycholic acid.

Lithocholic acid is toxic in the chicken, mouse, rat, rabbit, and rhesus monkey[52–54]. CDCA, which is metabolized to lithocholic acid, is toxic in the rabbit[54,55], rat[56] rhesus monkey[57] and baboon[58]. Ursodeoxycholic acid ($3\alpha,7\beta$-dihydroxy; UDCA), which is also metabolized to lithocholic acid, is toxic in the rabbit[55,59]. If lithocholic acid accumulates during UDCA feeding then it is toxic in the rhesus monkey[57], but not if it does not accumulate[60]. Toxicity of CDCA may be prevented by antibiotic administration[61], or by administration of deconjugation-resistant forms of CDCA or UDCA such as the N-methylglycine or N-methyltaurine amidates[59]. Because of the ability of the human liver to detoxify lithocholic acid it is probably not toxic in humans, but this has not been tested experimentally, for ethical reasons.

Deoxycholic acid is less toxic than lithocholic acid, but toxicity is readily shown in the rat if a sufficiently high dose is given[62,63]. In guinea pigs, administration of cholyltaurine (taurocholate) leads to accumulation of deoxycholic acid and its 3-oxo derivative, and results in death[64]. In rabbits, if cholestanol is added to the diet, it is absorbed and converted in the liver to allocholic acid (the 5α, A/B *trans* isomer of cholic acid). Allocholic acid is then conjugated with glycine in the hepatocyte and secreted into bile. In the intestine allocholylglycine undergoes bacterial deconjugation – dehydroxylation to form allodeoxycholic acid, which is absorbed from the colon, and amidated with glycine in the hepatocyte. In the biliary tract, allodeoxycholylglycine precipitates as its insoluble calcium salt. Such precipitation leads to secondary biliary cirrhosis, and ultimately to the death of the cholestanol-fed rabbit[65]. Administration of antibiotics decreases the formation of allodeoxycholic acid and abolishes the formation of concrements in the biliary tract[66]. In humans, administration of deoxycholic acid at a dose of 15 mg/kg for periods of a few weeks has been reported to cause hepatotoxicity in a few patients[67] but, in general, hepatotoxicity has not been observed when deoxycholic acid, or cholic acid, its precursor, is administered at this dosage.

Other 7-deoxy bile acids appear to be less toxic. Hyodeoxycholic acid ($3\alpha,6\alpha$-dihydroxy) has been administered to rats, hamsters, and prairie dogs without toxicity being reported[68]. Murideoxycholic acid ($3\alpha,6\beta$-dihydroxy) has been reported to form concrements composed of the calcium salt of the anion of its taurine conjugate in cholesterol-fed prairie dogs; this compound is much less soluble at body temperature than hyodeoxycholic acid[69].

CDCA, the primary bile acid, has physicochemical properties that are similar to those of deoxycholic acid. Its toxicity is readily shown in acute infusion studies in rodents[70], but chronic feeding studies in animals that possess a caecum are not straightforward because administered CDCA is converted by bacteria to lithocholic acid. There are two notable exceptions. One is the squirrel monkey, a species that lacks a caecum and therefore does not form lithocholic acid; CDCA is not toxic in this species[71]. The second is the human, that detoxifies lithocholic acid by sulphation. In humans, CDCA is mildly hepatotoxic[72], but UDCA is not[73]. Both are converted to lithocholic acid, and probably administration of either bile acid results in increased input of lithocholic acid into the enterohepatic circulation[74]. It seems reasonable to attribute the hepatotoxicity observed during CDCA administration to gallstone patients to CDCA *per se*, and not to invoke an additional effect of lithocholic acid[75].

Adaptations preventing toxicity of endogenous 7-deoxy bile acids in health

The input of 7-deoxy bile acids from the colon cannot cause significant liver toxicity in the healthy animal, by definition. Yet it is clear that CDCA is converted to lithocholic acid in most species possessing a caecum, and that lithocholic acid is a toxic bile acid. A number of biological adaptations appear to have evolved to prevent lithocholic acid toxicity. These adaptations which either prevent the formation of lithocholic acid or permit its efficient detoxification are summarized in Table 1.

To prevent the formation of lithocholic acid, the hepatocyte can make a trihydroxy bile acid with substituents at C-3, C-7, and at a third carbon atom (denoted X). When such a $3\alpha,7\alpha$,X-trihydroxy bile acid undergoes 7-dehydroxylation, it is converted to a 7-deoxy bile acid having the structure of a 3α,X-dihydroxy bile acid. A variant on this scheme is to insert a hydroxy group at C-23 on the side-chain. Such α-hydroxy bile acids are dehydroxylated slowly or not at all. A second preventive adaptation at the hepatic level is to form a conjugate that is resistant to bacterial deconjugation–dehydroxylation. In some angel fish, bile acids are conjugated with N-methyl taurine[11]. In marine mammals and

Table 1 Biological adaptations preventing lithocholic acid accumulation or hepatotoxicity in animals synthesizing C_{24} bile acids

Organ site	Mechanism	Species example	Comment
I. Prevention of formation			
Liver	Nuclear hydroxylation of CDCA	Many	7-dehydroxylation forms 3,X dihydroxy bile acid rather than lithocholic acid
Liver	C-23 (α) hydroxylation of CDCA	Marine mammals, birds	C-23 OH conjugates deconjugated more slowly than those of corresponding conjugates with unsubstituted side-chain. Unconjugated C-23 OH bile acids resistant to 7-dehydroxylation
Liver	Conjugation with N-methyltaurine	Angel fish	Conjugates resistant to deconjugation and dehydroxylation
Intestine (colon)	Absence of caecum	Squirrel monkey	Little 7-dehydroxylation occurs
Intestine (colon)	Absence of 7-dehydroxylating flora	Giant panda	Rapid transit and diet rich in fibre may contribute
II. Detoxification			
Liver	7-Rehydroxylation of LCA	Hamster, guinea pig, prairie dog	
Liver	Hydroxylation of LCA at site other than C-7	Pig, rat, hamster, guinea pig	
Liver	3-Sulphation of LCA	Human	Sulphation prevents conservation by intestinal transporters

CDCA, chenodeoxycholic acid; LCA, lithocholic acid

wading birds, α-hydroxy CDCA is formed and conjugated with taurine. The taurine conjugate of α-hydroxy CDCA is more resistant to deconjugation than the taurine amidate of CDCA[76].

At an intestinal level a preventive adaptation is to fail to develop a caecum, as occurs in the squirrel monkey. As noted above, in pandas, 7-dehydroxylation does not occur in the caecum. Possible reasons are rapid colonic transit or the absence of organisms that mediate 7-dehydroxylation.

Detoxification adaptations occur in the hepatocyte, and include efficient repair and/or conversion to a conjugate which is rapidly excreted. Efficient rehydroxylation occurs in species such as the guinea pig[64], hamster[77], and prairie dog[78]. In other species, hydroxylation of lithocholic acid at a site other than C-7 occurs[79]. In the human and the brush rabbit, lithocholic acid undergoes sulphation at C-3[46]. Such sulphation results in rapid faecal excretion, as the sulphated amidate is not a substrate for the intestinal bile acid transporters and the molecule is not absorbed passively.

As a result of any or all of these adaptations, the proportion of lithocholic acid in biliary bile acids is less than 5% in all species examined.

Moderate proportions ($< 40\%$) of DCA appear to be well tolerated in many mammalian species. The proportion in biliary bile acids is a function of input of newly formed deoxycholic acid, to what extent it is rehydroxylated, and its turnover rate.

In humans the proportion of deoxycholic acid in biliary bile acids varies greatly, ranging from 0% to 60%[80]. The variation is attributable to variable input of newly formed deoxycholic acid from the colon, because the turnover rate of DCA is identical to that of CDCA[34]. In most animals DCA constitutes $< 40\%$ of biliary bile acids. The only animals identified to date in which deoxycholic acid exceeds 80% of biliary bile acids are the rabbit and the sperm whale[11].

For CDCA the story is unclear, because formation of a trihydroxy bile acid by hydroxylation of a CDCA intermediate (such as 7α-hydroxy-cholest-4-ene-3-one) or CDCA *per se* not only decreases the substrate for lithocholic acid formation, but also decreases the proportion of CDCA *per se* in bile. In addition, some species have only CDCA in their biliary bile acids (vultures, cranes, lemurs)[11].

It can be argued that hydroxylation of bile acids during biosynthesis at sites other than C-12 to form trihydroxy bile acids that do not undergo 7-dehydroxylation is an adaptation preventing the formation of deoxycholic acid. Examples of such bile acids are shown in Fig. 1.

Evidence for toxicity of endogenous deoxycholic acid in patients with cholesterol gallstones

There is a considerable volume of evidence that in some patients with cholesterol gallstones the input of deoxycholic acid from the colon is increased, and that this increased input of deoxycholic acid causes increased biliary cholesterol secretion and induces the formation of gallstones[81]. Berr and his colleagues have identified a subset of patients with cholesterol gallstones who rapidly convert cholic acid to deoxycholic acid, apparently because of increased 7-dehydroxylating activity, and in whom the input of deoxycholic acid from the colon is increased. Administration of ampicillin decreased the input of deoxycholic acid and decreased the cholesterol saturation of bile[82].

MODULATION OF SMALL INTESTINAL FLORA BY BILE ACIDS

Evidence for bile acids modulating small intestinal flora

A remaining question is whether bile acids suppress bacterial growth or bacterial translocation (to lymph nodes) in the small intestine. Several studies have shown that bile duct ligation results in bacterial invasion and translocation to lymph nodes[83–88]. In patients with cirrhosis, in whom bile acid secretion into the intestine is decreased, an increase in the bacterial colonization of the small intestine has been reported to occur[89]. In a canine model, administration of a formula diet increased the extent of bacterial translocation[88], and there is one report that oral bile acid administration decreased bacterial translocation caused by bile duct ligation[87].

If an increased bacterial concentration in the small intestine leads to increased deconjugation, the bile acid concentration will decrease still more because of the passive absorption of unconjugated bile acids. Thus, there is a delicate balance between micellar concentrations of bile acids suppressing bacterial deconjugation (and promoting lipid absorption), and increased deconjugation causing bile acids to decrease below their critical micellization concentration and bacteria to proliferate and invade the intestinal mucosa. How these putative bacteriostatic and anti-invasive effects of bile acids are mediated has not been clarified.

Therapeutic and evolutionary implications

This chapter has assembled the arguments that suggest that the evolution from CDCA to trihydroxy bile acids occurred as a response to the toxicity of lithocholic acid. It is advantageous for the host to have high concentrations of bile acids in the small intestine to enhance lipid absorption and decrease bacterial density. It is also advantageous for the host that derives calories from its large intestine to have a low concentration of bile acids there, so that bacterial fermentation can proceed with vigour, generating calories. In disease conditions such as ileal resection, in which there is a decreased bile acid concentration[90] and possibly an increased bacterial concentration in the small intestine, it may be desirable to administer a deconjugation–dehydroxylation-resistant bile acid such as cholylsarcosine[91]. In principle, restoration of the bile acid concentration to a micellar level should enhance lipid absorption and decrease bacterial invasion. Experiments to test this idea are in the planning stage.

Acknowledgements

The authors' work is supported by the National Institutes of Health (DK 21506), by a grant-in-aid from the Falk Foundation e. V., Freiburg, Germany, and by the Zoological Society of San Diego. This paper is dedicated to the late Erwin H. Mosbach, PhD, with whom A. F. H. collaborated for three decades on the interactions between bacteria and bile acids. Carolina Cerrè PhD reviewed the manuscript and made many helpful criticisms. Phyllis Crosthwaite created Fig. 2.

References

1. Macdonald IA, Bokkenheuser VD, Winter J, McLernon AM, Mosbach EH. Degradation of steroids in the human gut. J Lipid Res. 1983;24:675–700.
2. Hylemon PB. Metabolism of bile acids in intestinal microflora. In: Danielsson H, Sjövall J, editors, Sterols and bile acids. New York: Elsevier; 1985:331–43.
3. Elliott WH: Metabolism of bile acids in liver and extrahepatic tissues. In: Danielsson H, Sjövall J, editors. Sterols and bile acids. Amsterdam; Elsevier; 1985:303–29.
4. Hofmann AF. Enterohepatic circulation of bile acids. In: Schultz SG, editor. Handbook of physiology. Section on the gastrointestinal system. Bethesda: American Physiological Society; 1989:567–96.
5. Hofmann AF. Intestinal absorption of bile acids and biliary constituents: the intestinal component of the enterohepatic circulation and the integrated system. In: Johnson LR, Alpers DH, Christensen J, Jacobson ED, Walsh JH, editors. Physiology of the gastrointestinal tract. New York: Raven Press; 1994:1845–65.
6. Stevens CE. Evolution of vertebrate herbivores. Acta Vet Scand. 1989;86 (Suppl.):9–19.
7. Udèn P. Comparative aspects of fiber fermentation in mammals. Acta Vet Scand. 1989;86 (Suppl.):35–45.
8. Haslewood GAD. The biological importance of bile salts. Amsterdam: North-Holland; 1978.
9. Hofmann AF, Sjövall J, Kurz G et al. A proposed nomenclature for bile acids. J Lipid Res. 1992;33:599–604.
10. Hofmann AF, Schteingart CD, Hagey LR. Species differences in bile acid metabolism. In: Paumgartner G, Beuers U, editors. Bile acids in liver diseases. Boston: Kluwer; 1995:3–30.
11. Hagey LR. Bile acid biodiversity in vertebrates: chemistry and evolutionary implication. PhD thesis, University of California, San Diego; 1992.
12. Hoshita T. Bile alcohols and primitive bile acids. In: Danielsson H, Sjövall J, editors. Sterols and bile acids. Amsterdam: Elsevier; 1985:279–302.
13. Une M, Hoshita T. Natural occurrence and chemical synthesis of bile alcohols, higher bile acids, and short side chain bile acids. Hiroshima J Med Sci. 1994;43:37–67.
14. Lee SP, Lester R, St Pyrek J. Vulpecholic acid ($1\alpha,3\alpha,7\alpha$-trihydroxy-5β-cholan-24-oic acid): a novel bile acid of a marsupial, *Trichosurus vulpecula* (Lesson). J Lipid Res. 1987;28:19–31.
15. Huijghebaert SM, Eyssen HJ. Specificity of bile salt sulfatase activity from *Clostridium* sp. strains S1. Appl Environ Microbiol. 1982;44:1030–4.
16. Batta AK, Salen G, Cheng FW, Shefer S. Cleavage of the taurine conjugate of $3\alpha,7\alpha,12\alpha$-trihydroxy-5β-cholestan-26-oic acid by rat fecal bacteria. J Biol Chem. 1979;254:11907–9.
17. Tint GS, Dayal B, Batta AK et al. The fecal bile acids and sterols of *Alligator mississippiensis*. Gastroenterology. 1981;80:114–19.
18. Shimada K, Brickness KS, Finegold SM. Deconjugation of bile acids by intestinal bacteria: review of literature and additional studies. J Infect Dis. 1969;119:73–81.
19. Huijghebaert SM, Hofmann AF. Pancreatic carboxypeptidase hydrolysis of bile acid-amino acid conjugates: selective resistance of glycine and taurine amidates. Gastroenterology. 1986;90:306–15.
20. Coleman JP, White WB, Egestad B, Sjövall J, Hylemon PB. Biosynthesis of a novel bile acid nucleotide and mechanism of 7α-dehydroxylation by an intestinal *Eubacterium* species. J Biol Chem. 1987;262:4701–7.
21. Mallonee DH, Adams JL, Hylemon PB. The bile acid-inducible baiB gene from *Eubacterium* sp. strain VPI 12708 encodes a bile acid-coenzyme A ligase. J Bacteriol. 1992;174:2065–71.
22. Batta AK, Salen G, Shefer S. Substrate specificity of cholylglycine hydrolase for the hydrolysis of bile acid conjugates. J Biol Chem. 1984;259:15035–9.
23. Schmassmann A, Angellotti MA, Ton-Nu HT et al. Transport, metabolism, and effect of chronic feeding of cholylsarcosine, a conjugated bile acid resistant to deconjugation and dehydroxylation. Gastroenterology. 1990;98:163–74.
24. Kihira K, Okamoto A, Ikawa S et al. Metabolism of sodium $3\alpha,7\alpha$-dihydroxy-5β-cholane-24-sulfonate in hamsters. J Biochem (Japan). 1991;109:879–81.

25. Roda A, Grigolo B, Minutello A, Pellicciari R, Natalini B. Physicochemical and biological properties of natural and synthetic C-22 and C-23 hydroxylated bile acids. J Lipid Res. 1990;31:289–98.
26. Roda A, Grigolo B, Aldini R et al. Bile acids with a cyclopropyl-containing side chain. IV. Physicochemical and biological properties of the four diastereoisomers of $3\alpha,7\alpha$-dihydroxy-22, 23-methylene-5β-cholan-24-oic acid. J Lipid Res. 1987;28:1384–97.
27. Roda A, Cerrè C, Manetta AC, Cainelli G, Umani-Ronchi A, Panunzio M. Synthesis and physicochemical, biological, and pharmacological properties of new bile acids amidated with cyclic amino acids. J Med Chem. 1996;39:2270–6.
28. Miki S, Mosbach EH, Cohen BI et al. Metabolism of β-muricholic acid in the hamster and prairie dog. J Lipid Res. 1993;34:1709–16.
29. Sacquet E, Parquet M, Riottot M, Raizman A, Nordlinger B, Infante R. Metabolism of β-muricholic acid in man. Steroids. 1985;45:411–26.
30. Hepner GW, Hofmann AF, Thomas PJ. Metabolism of steroid and amino acid moieties of conjugated bile acids in man. I. Cholylglycine. J Clin Invest. 1972;51:1889–97.
31. Hoffman NE, Hofmann AF. Metabolism of steroid and amino acid moieties of conjugated bile acids in man. IV. Description and validation of a multicompartmental model. Gastroenterology. 1974;67:887–97.
32. Zhang R, Barnes S, Diasio RB. Differential intestinal deconjugation of taurine and glycine bile acid N-acyl amidates in rats. Am J Physiol. 1992;262:G351–8.
33. Hellström K, Sjövall J. Turnover of deoxycholic acid in the rabbit. J Lipid Res. 1962;3:397–404.
34. Hepner GW, Hofmann AF, Thomas PJ. Metabolism of steroid and amino acid moieties of conjugated bile acids in man. II. Glycine-conjugated dihydroxy bile acids. J Clin Invest. 1972;51:1898–905.
35. Hepner GW, Sturman JA, Hofmann AF, Thomas PJ. Metabolism of steroid and amino acid moieties of conjugated bile acids in man. III. Cholyltaurine (taurocholic acid). J Clin Invest. 1973;52:433–40.
36. Northfield TC, McColl I. Postprandial concentrations of free and conjugated bile acids down the length of the normal human small intestine. Gut. 1973;14:513–18.
37. Madsen D, Beaver M, Chang L, Bruckner-Kardoss E, Wostmann B. Analysis of bile acids in conventional and germfree rats. J Lipid Res. 1976;17:107–11.
38. Goto T, Holzinger F, Hagey LR et al. Physicochemical and physiological properties of 5α-cyprinol sulfate, the biliary surfactant of the carp: why bile acids evolved from bile alcohols. Hepatology. 1997;26:296A.
39. Roda A, Fini A. Effect of nuclear hydroxy substituents on aqueous solubility and acidic strength of bile acids. Hepatology. 1984;4 (Suppl.):72–6S.
40. Hofmann AF, Mysels KJ. Bile acid solubility and precipitation in vitro and in vivo: the role of conjugation, pH, and Ca^{2+} ions. J Lipid Res. 1992:33:617–26.
41. Palm K, Luthman K, Ungell AL, Strandlund G, Artursson P. Correlation of drug absorption with molecular surface properties. J Pharm Sci. 1996;85:32–9.
42. Gurantz D, Hofmann AF. Influence of bile acid structure on bile flow and biliary lipid secretion in the hamster. Am J Physiol. 1984;247:G736–48.
43. Molino G, Hofmann AF, Cravetto C, Belforte G, Bona B. Simulation of the metabolism and enterohepatic circulation of endogenous chenodeoxycholic acid in man using a physiological pharmacokinetic model. Eur J Clin Invest. 1986;16:397–414.
44. Hofmann AF, Cravetto C, Molino G, Belforte G, Bona B. Simulation of the metabolism and enterohepatic circulation of endogenous deoxycholic acid in man using a physiological pharmacokinetic model for bile acid metabolism. Gastroenterology. 1987;93:693–709.
45. Muller M, Jansen PLM. Molecular aspects of hepatobiliary transport. Am J Physiol. 1997;35:G1285–303.
46. Cowen AE, Korman MG, Hofmann AF, Cass OW. Metabolism of lithocholate in healthy man. I. Biotransformation and biliary excretion of intravenously administered lithocholate, lithocholylglycine, and their sulfates. Gastroenterology. 1975;69:59–66.
47. Yeh HZ, Schteingart CD, Hagey LR et al. Effect of side chain length on biotransformations, hepatic transport, and choleretic properties of chenodeoxycholyl homologues in the rodent: Studies with dinor- (C_{22}), nor- (C_{23}), and chenodeoxycholic acid (C_{24}). Hepatology. 1997;26:374–85.

48. Asano T. Modification of cecal size in germfree rats by long-term feeding of anion exchange resin. Am J Physiol. 1969;217:911–18.
49. Mekhjian HS, Phillips SF, Hofmann AF. Colonic secretion of water and electrolytes induced by bile acids: perfusion studies in man. J Clin Invest. 1971;50:1569–77.
50. Spivey JR, Bronk SF, Gores GJ. Glycochenodeoxycholate-induced lethal hepatocellular injury in rat hepatocytes. J Clin Invest. 1993;92:17–24.
51. Hofmann AF. Animal models of calcium cholelithiasis. Hepatology. 1984;4:209–11S.
52. Palmer RH. Toxic effects of lithocholate on the liver and biliary tree. In: Taylor W, editor. The hepatobiliary system. Fundamental and pathological mechanism. New York: Plenum; 1976:227–40.
53. Palmer RH. Bile acids, liver injury, and liver disease. Arch Intern Med. 1972;30:606–17.
54. Fischer CD, Cooper NS, Rothschild MA, Mosbach EH. Effect of dietary chenodeoxycholic acid and lithocholic acid in the rabbit. Am J Dig Dis. 1974;18:877–86.
55. Cohen BI, Hofmann AF, Mosbach EH et al. Differing effects of nor-ursodeoxycholic or ursodeoxycholic acid on hepatic histology and bile acid metabolism in the rabbit. Gastroenterology. 1986;91:189–97.
56. Shefer S, Zaki FG, Salen G. Early morphologic and enzymatic changes in livers of rats treated with chenodeoxycholic and ursodeoxycholic acids. Hepatology. 1983;3:201–8.
57. Dyrszka H, Chen T, Salen G, Mosbach EH. Toxicity of chenodeoxycholic acid in the Rhesus monkey. Gastroenterology. 1975;69:333–7.
58. Morissey KP, McSherry CK, Swarm RL, Nieman WH, Deitrick JE. Toxicity of chenodeoxycholic acid in the nonhuman primate Surgery. 1975;77:851–60.
59. Schmassmann A, Hofmann AF, Angellotti MA et al. Prevention of ursodeoxycholate hepatotoxicity in the rabbit by conjugation with N-methyl amino acids. Hepatology. 1990;11:989–96.
60. Sarva RP, Fromm H, Farivar S et al. Comparison of the effects between ursodeoxycholic and chenodeoxycholic acid on liver function and structure and on bile acid composition in the Rhesus monkey. Gastroenterology. 1980;79:629–36.
61. Salen G, Dyrszka H, Chen T, Saltzman WH, Mosbach EH. Prevention of chenodeoxycholic acid toxicity with lincomycin. Lancet. 1975;1:1082.
62. Delzenne NM, Calderon PB, Taper HS, Roberfroid MB. Comparative hepatotoxicity of cholic acid, deoxycholic acid and lithocholic acid in the rat: in vivo and in vitro studies. Toxicol Lett. 1992;61:291–304.
63. Shefer S, Kren BT, Salen G. et al. Regulation of bile acid synthesis by deoxycholic acid in the rat: different effects on cholesterol 7α-hydroxylase and sterol 27-hydroxylase. Hepatology. 1995;22:1215–21.
64. Crombie DL, Hagey LR, Lillienau J, Miyai K, Hofmann AF. Toxicity of orally administered cholytaurine in the guinea pig: discovery of a rodent that cannot detoxify deoxycholic acid. Gastroenterology. 1992;102:A922.
65. Hofmann AF, Mosbach EH. Identification of allodeoxycholic acid as the major component of gallstones induced in the rabbit by 5α-cholestan-3β-ol. J Biol Chem. 1964;239:2813–21.
66. Hofmann AF, Bokkenheuser V, Hirsch RL, Mosbach EH. Experimental cholelithiasis in the rabbit induced by cholestanol feeding: effect of neomycin treatment on bile composition and gallstone formation. J Lipid Res. 1968;9:244–53.
67. LaRusso NF, Szczepanik PA, Hofmann AF, Coffin SB. Effect of deoxycholic acid ingestion on bile acid metabolism and biliary lipid secretion in normal subjects. Gastroenterology. 1977;72:132–40.
68. McSherry CK, Mosbach EH, Cohen BI, Une M, Stenger RJ, Singhal AK. Hyodeoxycholic acid: a new approach to gallstone prevention. Am J Surg. 1985;149:126–32.
69. Cohen BI, Ayyad N, Mosbach EH et al. Replacement of cholesterol gallstones by murideoxycholyl taurine gallstones in prairie dogs fed murideoxycholic acid. Hepatology. 1991;14:158–68.
70. Miyai K, Price VM, Fisher MM. Bile acid metabolism in mammals. Ultrastructural studies on the intrahepatic cholestasis induced by lithocholic and chenodeoxycholic acids in the rat. Lab Invest. 1971;24:292–302.
71. Suzuki H, Hamada M, Kato F. Metabolism of lithocholic and chenodeoxycholic acids in the squirrel monkey. Gastroenterology. 1985;89:631–6.
72. Schoenfield LJ, Lachin JM, the Steering Committee, the National Cooperative Gallstone Study Group. Chenodiol (chenodeoxycholic acid) for dissolution of gallstones: the National Cooperative Gallstone Study. Ann Intern Med. 1981;95:257–82.

73. Fromm H, Malavolti M. Dissolving gallstones. Adv Intern Med. 1988;33:409–30.
74. Hofmann AF. Pharmacology of ursodeoxycholic acid, an enterohepatic drug. Scand J Gastroenterol. 1994;29:1–15.
75. Fisher RL, Hofmann AF, Converse JL, Rossi SS. Lan SP. The lack of relationship between hepatotoxicity and lithocholic acid sulfation in biliary bile acids during chenodiol therapy in the National Cooperative Gallstone Study. Hepatology. 1991;14:454–63.
76. Merrill JR, Schteingart CD, Hagey LR *et al.* Hepatic biotransformation in rodents and physico-chemical properties of 23(R)-hydroxychenodeoxycholic acid, a natural α-hydroxy bile acid. J Lipid Res. 1995;37:98–112.
77. Emerman S, Javitt NB. Metabolism of taurolithocholic acid in the hamster. J Biol Chem 1967;242:661–4.
78. Cohen BI, Singhal AK, Mongelli J, Rothschild MA, McSherry CK, Mosbach EH. Hydroxylation of secondary bile acids in the perfused prairie dog liver. Lipids. 1983;18:909–12.
79. Einarsson K. On the formation of hyodeoxycholic acid in the rat. J Biol Chem. 1966;241:534–9.
80. Hofmann AF, Grundy SM, Lachin JM *et al.* Pretreatment biliary lipid composition in white patients with radiolucent gallstones in the National Cooperative Gallstone Study. Gastroenterology. 1982;83:738–52.
81. Marcus SN, Heaton KW. Intestinal transit, deoxycholic acid and the cholesterol saturation of bile – three inter-related factors. Gut. 1986;27:550–8.
82. Berr F, Kullak-Ublick GA, Paumgartner G, Münzing W, Hylemon PB. Alteration of intestinal microflora may cause cholesterol gallstones by excessive input of deoxycholic acid in man. Gastroenterology. 1996;111:1116–20.
83. Reynolds JV, Murchan P, Leonard N, Clarke P, Keane FB, Tanner WA. Gut barrier failure in experimental obstructive jaundice. J Surg Res. 1996;62:11–16.
84. Parks RW, Clements WD, Pope C, Halliday MI, Rowlands BJ, Diamond T. Bacterial transloca-tion and gut microflora in obstructive jaundice. J Anat. 1996;189:561–5.
85. Cakmakci M, Tirnaksiz B, Hayran M, Belek S, Gurbuz T, Salek I. Effects of obstructive jaun-dice and external biliary diversion on bacterial translocation in rats. Eur J Surg. 1996;162:567–71.
86. Kalambaheti T, Cooper GN, Jackson GDF. Role of bile in non-specific defence mechanisms of the gut. Gut. 1994;35:1047–52.
87. Ding JW, Andersson R, Soltesz V, Willen R, Bengmark S. The role of bile and bile acids in bac-terial translocation in obstructive jaundice in rats. Eur Surg Res. 1993;25:11–19.
88. Chuang JH, Chen WJ, Lo SK, Chang NK. Adverse metabolic and microbiological effects of tube feeding in experimental canine obstructive jaundice. J Parent Ent Nutr. 1997;21:36–40.
89. Morencos FC, de las Heras Casano G, Martin Ramos L, Lopez Arias MJ, Ledesma F, Pons Romero F. Small bowel bacterial overgrowth in patients with alcoholic cirrhosis. Dig Dis Sci. 1995;40:1252–6.
90. Poley JR, Hofmann AF. Role of fat maldigestion in pathogenesis of steatorrhea in ileal resection. Fat digestion after two sequential meals with or without cholestyramine. Gastroenterology. 1976;70:1125–9.
91. Schmassmann A, Fehr HF, Locher J *et al.* Cholylsarcosine, a new bile acid analogue: metabo-lism and effect on biliary secretion in humans. Gastroenterology. 1993;104:1171–81.

8
Gastric first-pass metabolism of alcohol: interaction with ammonia and associated gastritis

C. S. LIEBER

INTRODUCTION

That alcohol can disappear from the stomach has been known for a long time, and was considered to be part of the absorption of alcohol from the gastrointestinal tract. It was quantitated postprandially by Cortot et al.[1] in seven healthy subjects. They concluded that 'Of the ingested alcohol, $39.4 \pm 4.1\%$ was absorbed through the stomach wall during the first postprandial hour and $73.2 \pm 4.2\%$ during the total postcibal period whereas only $24 \pm 3\%$ was absorbed during the same time in the duodenum.' It was also known that, when alcohol is taken orally, blood levels achieved are generally lower than those obtained after administration of the same dose intravenously[2,3], so-called first-pass metabolism (FPM). Many drugs undergo FPM, which usually reflects hepatic metabolism. The observation that the gastric mucosa contains significant amounts of alcohol dehydrogenase (ADH), however, raised the possibility that the stomach may contribute to the FPM. Evidence obtained in experimental animals and in humans, both *in vivo* and *in vitro*, have now supported this contention. In addition, gastric FPM of ethanol was shown to be of significance for alcohol–drug interactions and for its impact on blood alcohol levels, as well as for various pathological states and physiological conditions of the stomach. It may also interact with *Helicobacter pylori* in the pathogenesis of gastritis.

GASTRIC FIRST-PASS METABOLISM OF ETHANOL AND ITS INTERACTIONS WITH OTHER DRUGS

Gastric ADH and its role in first-pass metabolism

The human gastric mucosa possesses several ADH isoenzymes[4,5], one of which (class IV ADH or sigma-ADH) is not present in the liver (Fig. 1). This enzyme has now been purified[6], its full-length cDNA obtained, the complete amino acid

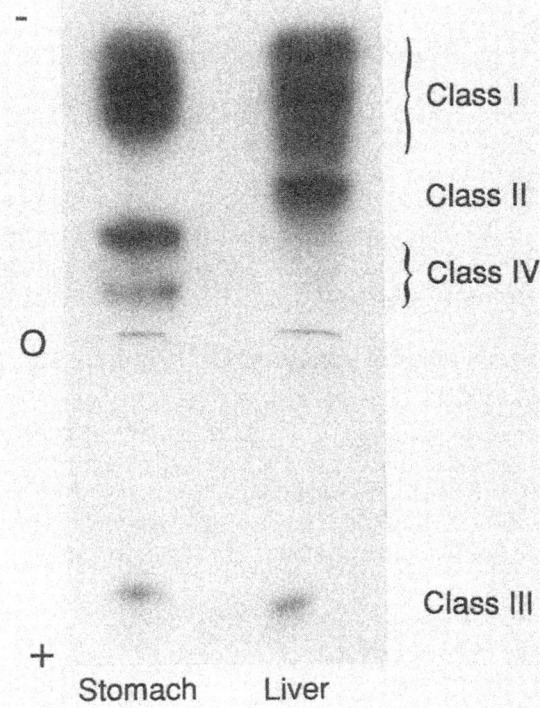

Figure 1 ADH isoenzymes in cytosol from gastric mucosa and liver obtained during surgery. Two bands of activity with slow cathodic mobility on starch gel electrophoresis were present in the gastric mucosa, but not in the liver. They correspond to what has been called μ- or σ-ADH (from ref. 5)

sequence deduced[7,8], and its gene cloned and localized to chromosome 4[9]. Gastric ADH is responsible for a large portion of ethanol metabolism found in cultured rat[10] and human[11] gastric cells. Its *in-vivo* effect is reflected by the FPM of ethanol. The relative contribution of gastric and hepatic ethanol metabolism to FPM is still the subject of debate[12–15]. Specifically, the question was raised whether the difference between blood alcohol levels after oral or intravenous administration[2,3] truly represents FPM or simply reflects slower absorption of alcohol and, if there is FPM, is it mainly of gastric or hepatic origin. To study this, rats were given the same dose of alcohol (1 g/kg) either by intragastric intubation or by intravenous, intraportal, and intraduodenal infusions at a rate that mimicked the loss of alcohol from the stomach. Higher blood alcohol concentration (BAC) levels after intravenous than intragastric alcohol were observed, indicating true FPM. Higher levels after intraportal or intraduodenal infusions (in fact, comparable to those obtained with the intravenous route) demonstrated negligible FPM when the route of delivery bypassed the stomach, yet included the liver. Furthermore, rats that had developed portosystemic shunts after ligation of the portal vein exhibited blood alcohol curves and FPM equivalent to those of sham-operated controls, indicating that FPM is not dependent on first-pass flow through the liver, but reflects gastric metabolism[16]. The absence of significant hepatic FPM was attributed to the saturation of hepatic ADH by recirculating alcohol, resulting in no appreciable increase in metabolism secondary to newly absorbed alcohol. Finally, the *in-vivo* gastric metabolism of alcohol in pylorus-ligated rats was demonstrated by significantly lower BAC values when alcohol was administered intragastrically than when an amount identical to that lost from the ligated stomach was given intraportally. Thus, the lower BAC values with oral, as opposed to intravenous, alcohol are not simply a consequence of slow absorption, but result from FPM occurring predominantly in the stomach, and the role of gastric ethanol metabolism in this FPM has now been firmly established experimentally[16,17].

Effect of chronic alcohol consumption, ethnicity and gender

FPM is partly lost in the alcoholic[18], together with decreased gastric ADH activity. Moreover, FPM disappears after gastrectomy[19]. Sigma-ADH is also absent or markedly decreased in activity in a large percentage of Japanese subjects[20], and their FPM is reduced correspondingly[21], in keeping with a predominant role for sigma-ADH in human FPM. Thus, the FPM represents some kind of 'protective barrier' against the systemic effects of ethanol, including attenuation of liver damage[22,23].

Women have a greater vulnerability than men to the development of organ damage after chronic alcoholic abuse, both in terms of liver disease[24–27] and brain damage[28]. It is noteworthy that, in Caucasians, gastric ADH activity is lower in women than in men[29], with associated higher blood alcohol levels, at least below the age of 50 years[30], an effect much more striking in alcoholic than in non-alcoholic women[29]. These gender differences were obvious at levels of social drinking. Furthermore, in women, the alcohol consumed is distributed in a 12% smaller water space[29] because of a difference in body composition (more fat and less water) Women may also have a higher central nervous system sensitivity to ethanol[31]. In the latter study, first-pass metabolism was not pronounced, but interpretation of these results is difficult in view of the extreme variability in terms of the concentration for half-maximal velocity (K_m) and other parameters of ethanol metabolism. A further complication was the simultaneous oral and intravenous administration. Moreover, the single dose of alcohol used was comparatively large (0.6 g/kg) and it has been shown that the relative importance of the FPM decreases progressively with increase in alcohol dose[2,3,18].

Effect of concentration, interactions with other drugs and diurnal variations

Gastric ADH isozymes require a relatively high ethanol concentration for optimal activity. Therefore, the concentration of alcoholic beverages affects the amount metabolized[32], with lesser FPM and higher blood levels after beer than whiskey[33] for equivalent amounts of ethanol. Fasting also strikingly decreases FPM[18], most probably because of accelerated gastric emptying, resulting in shortened exposure of ethanol to gastric ADH, and its more rapid intestinal absorption. Commonly used drugs, such as aspirin[34], and some H$_2$-blockers[4,35], but not omeprazole[36], decrease gastric ADH activity *in vitro* and/or accelerate gastric emptying[37]; they produce increased blood alcohol levels *in vivo*, particularly at low alcohol doses, equivalent to social drinking. Although questioned at first, such increases in blood levels have now been confirmed[38,39] for the low ethanol dose of 0.15 g/kg. The H$_2$-blocker action on blood alcohol levels has also been shown using higher doses of ethanol[40–43] with an associated increase in intoxication scores[43], but these effects with larger amounts of ethanol are still the subject of controversy, in part because large alcohol doses can overwhelm FPM (see above). Furthermore, some of the negative investigations used dilute concentrations of alcohol[44], at which gastric FPM is minimal[32]. Moreover, not all subjects display significant FPM[45], and published negative reports with H$_2$-blockers do not specify whether FPM was present to begin with. The studies in which there was clear documentation of a pre-existing FPM before the administration of H$_2$-blockers, both cimetidine[46] and ranitidine[40,47] treatments, resulted in significant decreases in FPM and increases in BAC values after postprandial consumption of 0.3 g/kg alcohol dose. The effects on blood alcohol levels of a single dose of H$_2$-receptor antagonists[48–50], or those after a very short treatment period (1$^1/_2$ days)[51], have been studied with high doses of ethanol. These studies reported negative results, as expected under those conditions, especially since all except one[50] were carried out in the fasting state. Two other negative studies, one after 3 days of cimetidine administration in male and female patients with peptic ulcer[38], and another after 6 days of ranitidine (300 and 600 mg/day) in normal men[52], used a combination of fasting and postprandial alcohol administration amounting to 0.67 and 0.5 g/kg, respectively. Again, no assessment of baseline FPM was reported.

It has been suggested that FPM could have diurnal variations[38], but no significant differences in FPM, peak BAC, values or areas under the curve (AUC) were found when alcohol was given in the morning and in the evening to the same subjects 1 h after the same standard meal[46].

Quantification of alcohol FPM

Traditionally, comparison of the AUC obtained after oral and intravenous administration of a drug has been used to estimate FPM. In contrast to most other drugs, however, alcohol follows Michaelis–Menten rather than first-order kinetics[53,54]; thus comparison of AUC is applicable only when BAC values are very low and the rate of alcohol elimination is approximately proportional to concentration. To measure FPM at higher concentrations, and to take into account the known pharmacokinetics of alcohol, the quantities of alcohol reaching the systemic blood by both the oral and intravenous routes can be calculated by integration of the Michaelis–Menten formula over the entire blood alcohol curve[32]. Confirmation that the quantity entering the blood by the intravenous route approximates the dose validates the procedure. FPM is then defined as the difference between the quantity of alcohol that reaches the systemic circulation by the intravenous route and the quantity that enters by the oral route. The integration method is not influenced by rate of infusion[16,55] and, in contrast to AUC, it is applicable to a wide range of alcohol doses. Typically, healthy male social drinkers given a 300 mg/kg dose of 10% wt/vol alcohol (equivalent to a generous drink) after a standard meal exhibit a mean FPM equal to 85 ± 9 mg/kg, or about 28% of the dose[46], but numerous factors can affect this amount (see above).

Functional implications

Use of drugs and social drinking are likely to occur concurrently. Therefore, one should be concerned whether the changes in blood alcohol levels produced by some of these drugs may result in unexpected impairment in performing operations that require a high degree of attention, judgement and/or motor coordination, such as automobile driving. Some studies aimed at reaching levels associated with gross intoxication have been carried out, with single doses as large as 1.5 g/kg[56]. With such amounts the contribution of the FPM to the blood levels is minimal (see above) and the lack of effect of cimetidine could have been anticipated. However, in some of the studies using 0.75–0.8 g/kg[41–43], the blood alcohol levels after treatment with H_2-receptor antagonists exceeded the legal limits established for driving in many countries, including some states in the USA[57], and a significant rise in intoxication scores associated with the cimetidine-induced increase in BAC was documented[43]. The legal limits of intoxication have been progressively decreasing, as the evidence for clinically significant impairment has been obtained at low blood alcohol levels: altered performance of complex psychomotor tasks has been reported at BAC as low as 15 mg/dl, or 3.33 mmol/L[58,59] and impaired judgement has been documented at 25 mg/dl or 5.4 mmol/L[60]. Thus, if we consider the data by DiPadova *et al.*[40], on average, an individual taking some H_2-blockers will reach BAC values above those at which altered judgement was detected, and such impairment to perform complex tasks will persist for a longer time than when the same dose of alcohol (0.3 g/kg) is imbided in the absence of the drug. These findings represent minimal estimates because they do not fully reproduce the most common setting of social drinking, in which alcoholic beverages are imbided repeatedly in small amounts over a prolonged period of time. When the social drinking situation was simulated by giving small drinks (0.15 g/kg) at 30-min intervals, the effect of cimetidine on BAC values was shown to be cumulative[61] (Fig. 2). As a result, BAC values associated with impaired mental function and driving capacity were reached sooner, and maintained for a longer time, than in the absence of the drug.

ALCOHOLIC GASTRITIS

Clinical observations

A large dose of alcohol taken acutely damages the gastric mucosa, with mucosal erythema and superficial ulcerations, as shown in an endoscopic study by Palmer[62]. In a prospective study in humans, Gottfried *et al.*[63] documented that alcohol causes endoscopically visible antral erythema and friability, and microscopic mucosal haemorrhage. Various mechanisms for the pathogenesis of these

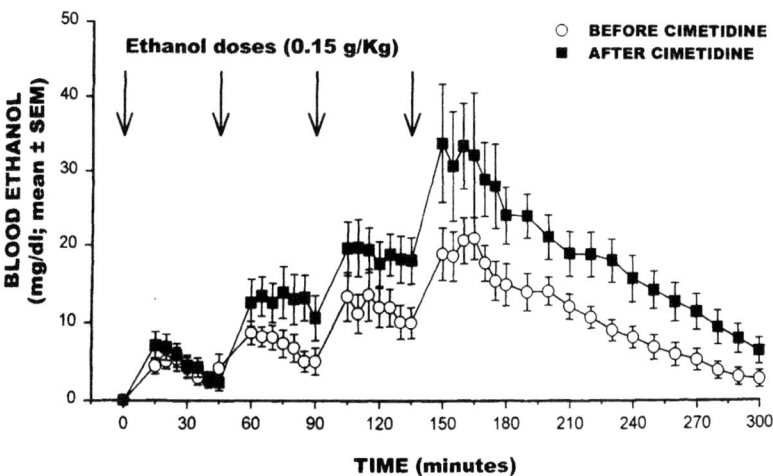

Figure 2 Mean (± SE) blood alcohol levels after repeated oral consumption of small doses of ethanol. Nine volunteers were given four small doses of ethanol (each dose 0.15 g/kg body weight, which is less than one drink) before and after the administration of cimetidine (400 mg twice a day for 7 days). In all nine subjects the blood alcohol levels increased after the administration of cimetidine, and in two subjects the peak level exceeded 50 mg/dl. The effect of cimetidine on repeated drinking was significant ($p < 0.01$ by two-way analysis of variance for repeated measures) (modified from ref. 61)

acute gastric lesions have been proposed, and are discussed elsewhere[64]. The present brief review focuses only on chronic gastritis, defined as inflammation of the mucosa, assessed histologically. It is common in the alcoholic[64] but its pathogenesis is still debated. On the one hand, some ethanol is metabolized in the stomach (see above), and the resulting toxic acetaldehyde could be incriminated in the pathogenesis of chronic gastric pathology, the same way it was shown to play a major role in chronic liver disease[64]. On the other hand, the pathology and symptomatology of chronic gastritis in the alcoholic is similar to those of patients infected with *Helicobacter pylori*. Indeed, compared to non-alcoholic subjects the alcoholic patients were found to have a higher incidence of chronic gastritis of the antrum[65], a lesion now known to be commonly associated with *H. pylori*. Furthermore, *H. pylori* infection is more common in heavy drinkers[66], as shown in a prospective study of 144 patients which revealed a statistically significant relationship between high alcohol consumption and the presence of *H. pylori*, whereas there was no correlation with smoking. This raised the question of the respective role of alcohol and *H. pylori* in the pathogenesis of gastritis in the alcoholic, an issue of practical therapeutic importance. Moreover, in the case of gastroduodenal ulcer, it is now accepted[67] that *H. pylori* is a main aetiological agent, that the production of ammonia (NH₃) from urea plays a pathogenic role, and that anti-*H. pylori* therapy is effective. By contrast, *H. pylori's* contribution to gastritis, especially the alcoholic variety, is still debated or even ignored, and such gastritis is not yet included in the accepted indications for antibiotic therapy.

Aetiology of chronic gastritis in the alcoholic

Role of alcohol

Much controversy has surrounded the question of whether alcohol can cause chronic gastritis in humans. Wolff[68], using a blind biopsy technique, detected no relationship between alcohol intake and histological evidence of atrophic gastritis, confirming earlier observations by Palmer[62]. However, chronic gastritis in the alcoholic, like that associated with *H. pylori*[69], is usually of the 'B' type[70], namely it predominates in the antrum and therefore may have been missed with the early rigid endoscopic instruments. Indeed, later studies documented a connection between alcoholism and chronic gastritis[71-73]. Dinoso *et al.*[74] found that only 50% of alcoholics had normal fundic histology compared to 85.7% of the controls. In the antrum only 15.6% had a normal biopsy, and 65% had antral atrophic gastritis.

Role of H. pylori *and NH₃*

As mentioned above, the prevailing view is that *H. pylori* infection is more common in alcoholics than in non-alcoholics[66], although no unanimity[75] has been reached on this point. In any event, in addition to the direct effect of alcohol, *H. pylori* could also play a role in the pathogenesis of the gastritis. Indeed, *H. pylori* may adversely affect the stomach because of its high urease activity, which converts urea into NH_3, the causticity of which was shown in cultured rat gastric cells[76]. Moreover, in rats, dietary ammonia loading for 2 weeks or longer resulted in a 1.5–2-fold increase in the weight and mucosal thickness of the stomach and proximal duodenum, with evidence of mild gastritis and enterochromaffin-like cell hyperplasia[77]. Thus, the pathogenic role of NH_3 in gastritis, long suspected, is now more firmly documented, despite some opposite views originally expressed. Fitzgerald and Murphy[78] suggested that the ammonia may even have a protective function by neutralizing gastric acidity. This concept was based on the observation that administration of urea, in amounts sufficient to raise temporarily the blood urea level by 12 mg per cent, was followed by a decrease of gastric acidity. However, Burke and Page[79] were unable to confirm these findings. Indeed, the acid-neutralizing capacity of NH_3 is significant only in the presence of uraemia and its associated very high gastric ammonia levels (Fig. 3) which can neutralize the acid (Fig. 4)[80,81]. In patients undergoing haemodialysis the sudden reappearance of the acid upon correction of the uraemia may have precipitated gastrointestinal ulcerations and bleedings[82]. With the advent of H_2-blockers and their routine administration in such patients, this complication is now under control.

The issue of the pathogenic role of NH_3 in the gastritis was addressed directly in non-alcoholic *H. pylori*-positive patients with chronic renal failure[81], in whom it was expected that a high urea level and, accordingly, elevated NH_3 concentration, might amplify the changes. Gastric urea and ammonia were measured, and the severity of gastritis was evaluated histologically by counting mononuclear and polymorphonuclear cells. High gastric ammonia and low urea in *H. pylori*-positive patients, and the converse in *H. pylori*-negative subjects, were observed. There was a significant correlation ($p < 0.025$) between gastric ammonia and

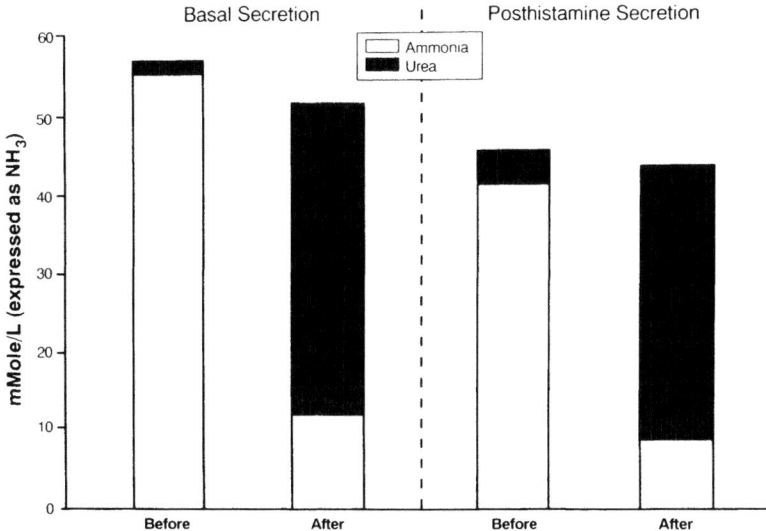

Figure 3 Mean gastric ammonia and urea in six uraemic patients. Concentrations in basal and post-histamine secretions are shown before and after 1 week of treatment with oxytetracycline (20 mg/kg per day p.o.) which produced about an 80% reduction of gastric ammonia ($p < 0.05$), replaced by an equivalent amount of unsplit urea, illustrating the suppression of gastric urease activity (data from ref. 80)

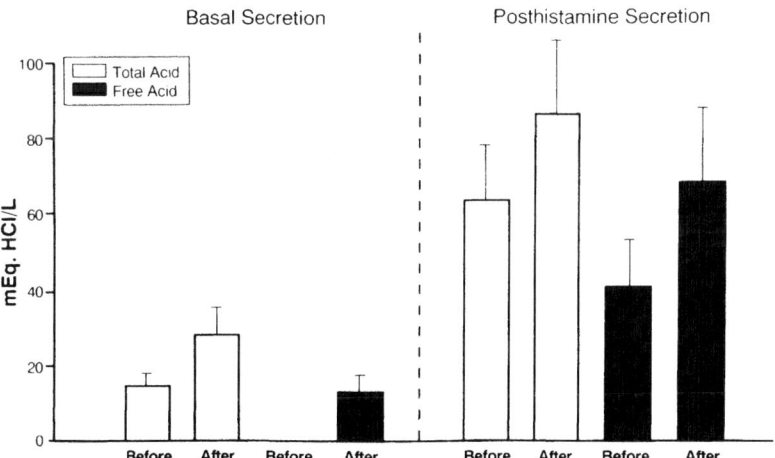

Figure 4 Gastric total and free acid in the six uraemic subjects of Fig. 3. The suppression of ammonia was associated with a restoration of free acid, as well as an increase of total acid in basal secretion and corresponding changes of the post-histamine response (data from ref. 80)

interstitial polymorphonuclear leucocyte infiltration, suggesting a causal link[81]. Indeed, myeloperoxidase from neutrophils produces hypochlorous acid[83] which, in the presence of ammonia, yields monochloramine, found to be very toxic in cultured rat gastric cells[76]. Furthermore, suppression of *H. pylori* was associated with a decrease in NH_3 and an increase of urea, with a corresponding improvement in morphology[81]. The significant correlation between the severity of gastric inflammation and the gastric juice NH_3 concentration suggested that NH_3 plays a pathogenic role in the gastric injury, thereby also incriminating *H. pylori*, since NH_3 is a reliable marker of gastric bacterial infection. As early as 1957, measurement of gastric juice NH_3 (derived from urea) was considered a likely reflection of bacterial infection when it was found, for the first time, that an antibiotic (namely oxytetracycline) strikingly decreases gastric urease activity and NH_3 production in non-uraemic subjects (Fig. 5) as well as in uraemic subjects[84], an observation confirmed shortly thereafter in a larger group of both non-uraemic and uraemic patients (Fig. 3)[80,85] or in cirrhotics (Fig. 6)[86]. The validity of gastric juice NH_3 measurement as a marker of *H. pylori* infection was reaffirmed more recently[87]. Since spirochaete-like organisms had been described on the human gastric mucosa[88,89], it was postulated at that time[84] that the most likely explanation for the suppression of gastric NH_3 (and its replacement by unsplit urea) after oxytetracycline was the eradication of urease-producing microorganisms known to exist in the stomach. Indeed, urease activity had been found in the stomach in 1924 by Luck and Seth[90], but they believed it to be intrinsic to the mucosal cells. Accordingly, the alternative hypothesis was raised that the tetracycline may not have been acting as an antibiotic, but rather in some direct chemical way on a 'constitutive' urease present in the gastric cell. To address this objection, four additional antibiotics were used. Two of them (ampicillin and neomycin) were found to also decrease the urease activity[80,91], although they differed structurally from oxytetracycline. It was thus apparent that their effect reflected an antibacterial mechanism, indirectly confirming the bacterial nature of the gastric urease. Nevertheless, Aoyagi *et al.*[92] and others rejected such a view, despite the additional key observation that urease was detected when bacteria were present, but not in germ-free animals[93].

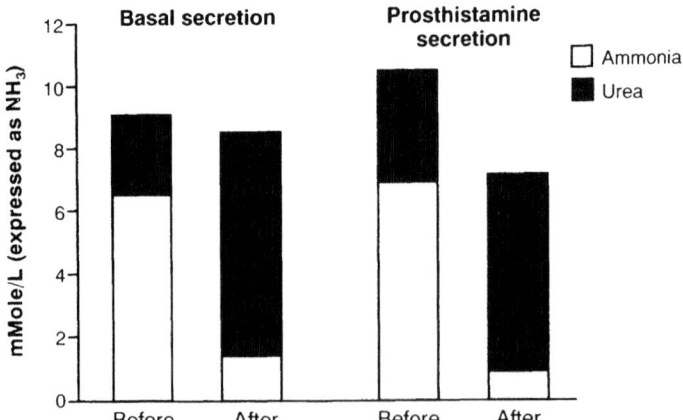

Figure 5 Mean gastric ammonia and urea in six non-uraemic subjects. Concentrations in basal and post-histamine secretions are shown before and after 1 week of treatment with oxytetracycline (20 mg/kg per day p.o.) which resulted in a significant decrease in gastric ammonia and corresponding increase in urea (data from ref. 84)

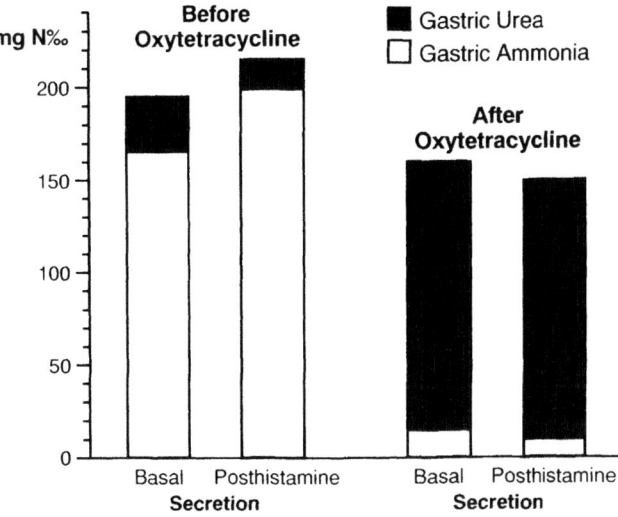

Figure 6 Effect of oxytetracycline on gastric ammonia and urea in a patient with liver cirrhosis. After 5 days of antibiotic treatment (20 mg/kg per day), there was a striking decrease of gastric ammonia (from ref. 86)

The possible link between gastric infection and gastritis was brought up again by the association between 'active' gastritis and Gram-negative bacteria[94], episodes of 'epidemic gastritis' with hypochlorhydria[95,96], the description of 'unidentified curved bacilli' associated with chronic gastritis[97] and their culture, and differentiation from corresponding animal bacterial species[98]. The predominant organism involved was identified as '*Campylobacter*' (now reclassified as *Helicobacter pylori*) and its contribution to gastritis[99] and to the urease activity[100] was recognized. More recently, a larger and prospective study[101] confirmed the role of *H. pylori* in chronic gastritis.

Symptomatology of chronic gastritis

The link between histological gastritis and symptoms has remained a rather elusive problem. Indeed, an age-related rise in *H. pylori* gastritis occurs without an apparent increase in symptoms, and even asymptomatic subjects may have signs of gastritis in their biopsy specimens[102]. However, some reported a significant correlation between the infiltration of antral mucosa with polymorphonuclear leucocytes and symptoms in patients with non-ulcer dyspepsia[103]. Furthermore, it was noted 40 years ago that, in patients with uraemia, gastric ammonia suppression with antibiotics (Fig. 3) results in restoration of gastric acid secretion (Fig. 4). However, the question of the amelioration of gastritis-associated symptoms has been more elusive. Some investigators observed a significant reduction in complaints[104–106], whereas others found no symptomatic difference between placebo and agents with antibacterial activity against *H. pylori*[107–109]. These disparate results may have been due to more effective clearance of *H. pylori* in some studies than in others, or the contribution of aggravating factors, such as smoking and anxiety, as well as inadequate follow-up.

Respective role of alcohol, NH_3, and their interactions in the pathogenesis of gastritis

To resolve the question of the relative role of alcohol and NH_3 (hence *H. pylori*) in the pathogenesis of the gastritis, a study was conducted in 18 alcoholics with dyspepsia[110]. *H. pylori* was found in 14 individuals and was associated with chronic antral gastritis, whereas gastric biopsy specimens were normal in the four *H. pylori*-negative alcoholics. Assessments were repeated 3–4 weeks after controlled abstinence during hospitalization. There was no change in histological findings, indicating that alcohol itself was not the major causative agent (Fig. 7). Next, in 10 *H. pylori*-positive alcoholics, *H. pylori* was suppressed with antibiotics, which resulted in almost complete normalization of histological findings. Four control *H. pylori*-positive subjects who received only antacids showed no improvement (Fig. 8). Dyspeptic symptoms were quantified by a 'total dyspepsia score' based on severity of epigastric pain, nausea, vomiting, heartburn, halitosis, burping, postprandial bloating, and flatulence. They significantly improved after antibiotic treatment and elimination of *H. pylori*, whereas there was no change with antacid treatment alone (Fig. 9). Because the clearance of *H. pylori* correlated with resolution of the dyspeptic symptoms and histological improvement, it was concluded that *H. pylori* played a predominant role in the pathogenesis and symptomatology of the chronic gastritis in these alcoholics[110].

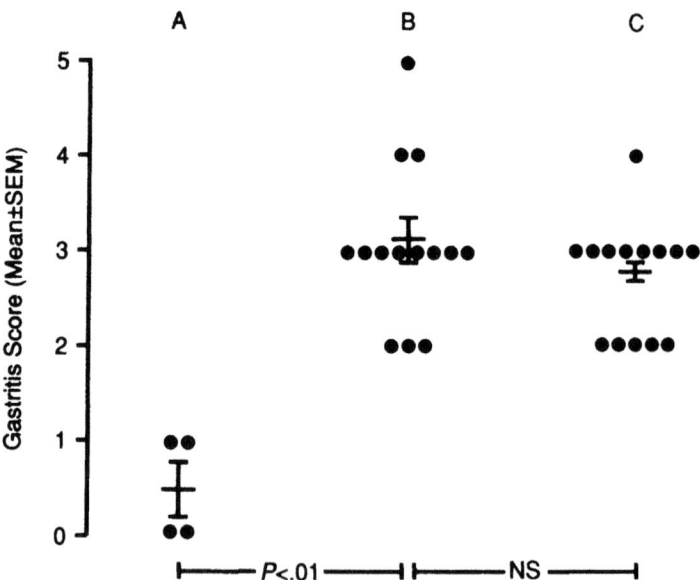

Figure 7 Histological gastritis scores in *H. pylori*-negative and *H. pylori*-positive alcoholics, and effect of abstinence. **A** indicates *H. pylori*-negative; **B**, *H. pylori*-positive, before abstinence; and **C**, *H. pylori*-positive, after abstinence. The 3–4 weeks of abstinence did not result in a significant change. NS indicates not significant (from ref. 110)

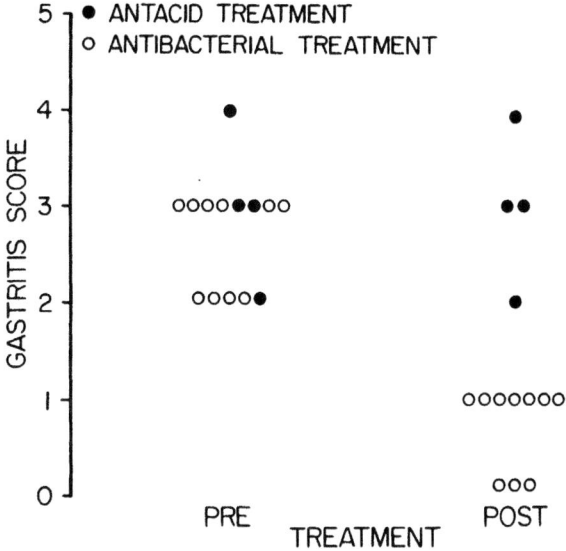

Figure 8 Effect of antibiotic treatment on gastritis scores in *H. pylori*-positive alcoholics. Closed circles indicate antacid treatment; open circles, antibacterial treatment consisting of bismuth subsalicylate, amoxycillin, and metronidazole. $p < 0.01$ for scores before and after antibacterial treatment (from ref. 110)

As already mentioned, the severity of *H. pylori*-induced gastric injury was also found to correlate with gastric juice ammonia[81], but the mechanism of the interaction between alcohol and NH_3 in the pathogenesis and severity of alcoholic gastritis has not as yet been elucidated. Since both ethanol and *H. pylori*-generate NH_3 activate cysteine proteases[111], they could potentiate each other's gastric toxicity. Conceivably, this observation could lead to some interesting novel therapeutic approaches (through corresponding enzyme inhibitors) and might explain, at least in part, why *H. pylori* infection is more common in alcoholics than in non-alcoholics[66]. It is also possible that the alcohol (or acetaldehyde)-induced mucosal injury, in turn, may favour implantation of *H. pylori* or its persistence in the stomach. Furthermore, *H. pylori* contains alcohol dehydrogenase activity[112]. Thus, the presence of the substrate alcohol can be expected to promote production of the toxic metabolite acetaldehyde. However, in human antral gastric mucosa, *H. pylori* infection is associated with a significant decrease in mucosal alcohol dehydrogenase activity[113,114], at least in the antrum[115]. It was also suggested that ADH of bacterial origin (such as *H. pylori*) does not contribute significantly to gastric ethanol metabolism[116]. At present the net effect of *H. pylori* infection on gastric ethanol metabolism and acetaldehyde production has not yet been fully clarified.

Role of *H. pylori* in hepatic encephalopathy

Encephalopathy in patients with cirrhosis was known to be associated with elevated arterial blood ammonia[86,117] and, in such subjects, reduction of gastric

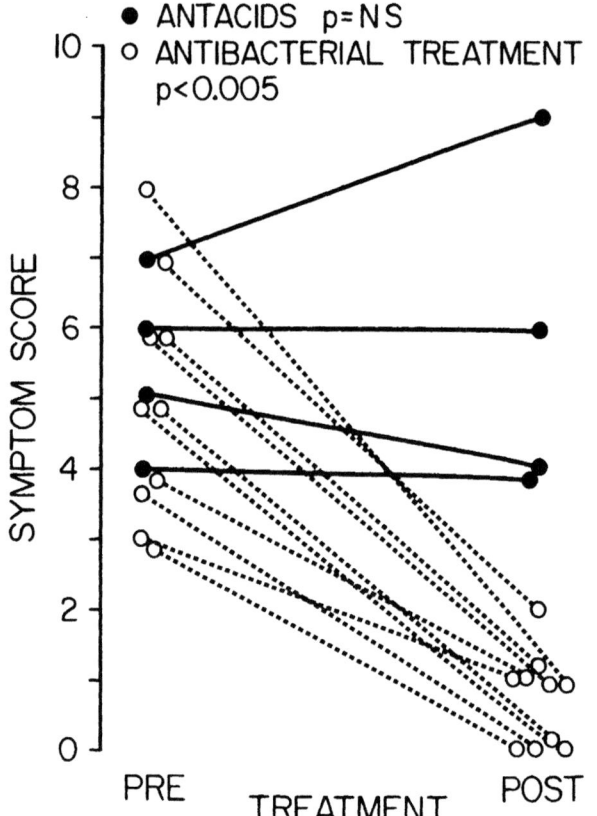

Figure 9 Effect of treatment on symptom scores in *H. pylori*-positive alcoholics. Closed circles indicate antacid treatment; open circles, antibacterial treatment. $p < 0.005$ for scores before and after antibacterial treatment; not significant for scores before and after antacid treatment. Whereas antibacterial treatment significantly improved the symptomatology, there was no such effect after antacid therapy alone (from ref. 110)

ammonia with oxytetracycline was achieved (Fig. 6) with associated improvement in symptomatology[86]. It was pointed out at that time that such therapy with elimination of gastric ammonia production may be of special practical importance in patients with liver disease who also have azotaemia and hence exhibit strikingly elevated gastric ammonia[80]. The exacerbation, by the NH_3 derived from urea, of the encephalopathy in patients with underlying liver disease, especially when renal insufficiency develops, and their successful antibacterial treatment was attributed to the fact that 'these antibiotics prevent urea splitting by interfering with urease activity of bacterial origin'[118]. Since, in patients with uraemia, gastrointestinal ammonia formation might reach very high levels, uraemia, even of a moderate degree, appears as a potential danger for patients with liver disease. This entity was named the 'renal–hepatic syndrome' and prevention of this complication with antibiotics was suggested, based on case reports of the successful therapeutic use of oxytetracycline in cirrhotics with encephalopathy[117], associated with a striking inhibition of ammonia production from gastric urea (Fig. 6). Subsequently, a greater urease activity in the stomach of patients with cirrhosis (compared to normals) was also demonstrated[119]. Furthermore, it was shown that patients with acute, moderate or severe alcoholic hepatitis have a high *H. pylori* infection rate (as determined by serology), and that those infected are at higher risk for portosystemic encephalopathy[120]. Gastric ammonia production from *H. pylori* was quantitated, its contribution to systemic ammonia documented experimentally[121], and amelioration of the encephalopathy in patients with liver disease through *H. pylori* eradication was verified recently[122]. Thus, anti-*H. pylori* therapy should now be considered routinely in the treatment of patients with hepatic encephalopathy, in addition to other therapeutic modalities, such as corticosteroids. The latter are now recommended for the treatment of patients with alcoholic hepatitis and encephalopathy[123], but their mode of action is not yet elucidated; in addition to dampening the inflammatory response, corticosteroids may act by reducing circulating NH_3 levels, as documented in an experimental model of chronic hepatic encephalopathy in Eck fistula dogs[124].

Therapeutic and diagnostic implications

In aggregate, the weight of the studies reviewed here should now be sufficient to consider antibiotics for the treatment of alcoholic gastritis, the same way that they are now accepted therapy for the ulcer pathology caused by *H. pylori*[67]. Indeed, 40 years have now elapsed since the first elimination of gastric urease-producing bacteria by the use of antibiotics in humans[84], and a casual link between *H. pylori* and gastritis has been shown by the landmark experiments of Marshall *et al.*[98–100,125], Morris and Nicholson[126], as well as the prospective studies of antibacterial treatment for chronic antral gastritis by Rauws *et al.*[127] and others. It now appears warranted to complete the trials needed to finally establish gastritis as an indication for antibiotic treatment. As a corollary, wider diagnostic efforts are warranted. Thus far, diagnosis of *H. pylori* infection has been based on histological detection of the organism or of its urease activity (e.g. Clo test) in biopsies of gastric mucosa[128], immunological detection of circulating antibodies to *H. pylori*[129], as well as measurement of exhaled products of urea hydrolysis[130,131]. Assessment of urease activity by the measurement of NH_3 (relative to urea) present in the gastric juice provides a technically simpler, yet as accurate, diagnostic tool, as recently reported[87].

SUMMARY AND CONCLUSIONS

1. The stomach contributes to the metabolism of ethanol and provides a protective barrier against its penetration into the body.
2. This effect is attenuated by drugs.
3. Patients should be warned of the corresponding increase in blood alcohol levels.
4. Oxidation of ethanol generates acetaldehyde, a toxic metabolite causing tissue injury.

5. Alcohol abuse also favours colonization by *H. pylori*.
6. *H. pylori* produces ammonia that contributes to chronic gastritis.
7. Antibiotics eliminate gastric ammonia, and should be considered for the treatment of chronic gastritis, including that of the alcoholic.
8. In patients with hepatic encephalopathy, *H. pylori* eradication may also be beneficial.

Acknowledgements

Original personal studies reviewed here were supported by the Department of Veterans Affairs and the US Public Health Service. Skilful typing of the manuscript by Ms Diana Moises is gratefully acknowledged.

References

1. Cortot A, Jobin G, Fucrot F, Aymes C, Giraudeaux V, Modigliani R. Gastric emptying and gastrointestinal absorption of alcohol ingested with a meal. Dig Dis Sci. 1986;31:343–8.
2. Julkunen RJK, DiPadova C, Lieber CS. First pass metabolism of ethanol a gastrointestinal barrier against the systemic toxicity of ethanol. Life Sci. 1985;37:567–73.
3. Julkunen RJK, Tannenbaum L, Baraona E, Lieber CS. First pass metabolism of ethanol: an important determinant of blood levels after alcohol consumption. Alcohol. 1985;2:437–41.
4. Hernández-Muñoz R, Caballeria J, Baraona E, Uppal R, Greenstein R, Lieber CS. Human gastric alcohol dehydrogenase: its inhibition by H_2-receptor antagonists, and its effect on the bioavailability of ethanol. Alcoholism: Clin Exp Res. 1990;14:946–50.
5. Baraona E, Gentry RT, Lieber CS. Bioavailability of alcohol: role of gastric metabolism and its interaction with other drugs. Dig Dis. 1994;12:351–67.
6. Stone CL, Thomason HR, Bosron WF, Li T-K. Purification and partial amino acid sequence of a high activity human stomach alcohol dehydrogenase. Alcoholism: Clin Exp Res. 1993;17:911–18.
7. Yokoyama H, Baraona E, Lieber CS. Molecular cloning of human class IV alcohol dehydrogenase. Biochem Biophys Res Commun. 1994;203:219–24.
8. Farrés J, Moreno A, Crosas B et al. Alcohol dehydrogenase of class IV (δADH) from human stomach; cDNA sequence and structure/function relationships. Eur J Biochem. 1994;224:549–57.
9. Yokoyama H, Baraona E, Lieber CS. Molecular cloning and chromosomal localization of ADH7 gene encoding human class IV ADH. Genomics. 1996;31:243–5.
10. Mirmiran-Yazdy SA, Haber PS, Korsten MA et al. Metabolism of ethanol in rat gastric cells and its inhibition by cimetidine. Gastroenterology. 1995;108:737–42.
11. Haber PS, Gentry T, Mak KM, Mirmiran-Yazdy AA, Greenstein RJ, Lieber CS. Metabolism of alcohol by human gastric cells: relation to first pass metabolism. Gastroenterology. 1996;111:863–70.
12. Levitt MD, Levitt DG. The critical role of the rate of ethanol absorption in the interpretation of studies purporting to demonstrate gastric metabolism of ethanol. J Pharmacol Exp Ther. 1994;269:297–304.
13. Lieber CS, Gentry RT, Baraona E. First pass metabolism of ethanol. In: Saunders JB, Whitfield JB, editors. The biology of alcohol problems. UK Elsevier; 1996:315–26.
14. Sato N, Kitamura T. First-pass metabolism of ethanol: an overview. Gastroenterology 1996;111:1143–4.
15. Smith T, DeMaster EG, Furne JK, Springfield J, Levitt MD. First-pass gastric mucosal metabolism of ethanol is negligible in the rat. J Clin Invest. 1992;89:1801–6.
16. Lim Jr RT, Gentry RT, Ito D, Yokoyama H, Baraona E, Lieber CS. First pass metabolism of ethanol in rats is predominantly gastric. Alcoholism: Clin Exp Res. 1993;17:1337–44.
17. Caballeria J, Baraona E, Lieber CS. The contribution of the stomach to ethanol oxidation in the rat. Life Sci. 1987;41:1021–7.
18. DiPadova C, Worner TM, Julkunen RJK, Lieber CS. Effects of fasting and chronic alcohol consumption on the first pass metabolism of ethanol. Gastroenterology. 1987;92:1169–73.

19. Caballeria J, Frezza M, Hernandez-Munoz R et al. The gastric origin of first pass metabolism of ethanol in humans: effect of gastrectomy. Gastroenterology. 1989;97:1205–9.
20. Baraona E, Yokoyama A, Ishii H et al. Lack of alcohol dehydrogenase isoenzyme activities in the stomach of Japanese subjects. Life Sci. 1991;49:1929–34.
21. Dohmen K, Baraona E, Ishibadsshi H et al. Ethnic differences in gastric sigma alcohol dehydrogenase activity and ethanol first pass metabolism. Alcoholism: Clin Exp Res. 1996;20:1569–76.
22. Battiston L, Moretti M, Tulissi P et al. Hepatic glutathione determination after ethanol administration in rat: evidence of the first-pass metabolism of ethanol. Life Sci. 1994;56:241–8.
23. Imuro Y, Bradford BU, Forman DT, Thurman RG. Glycine prevents alcohol-induced liver injury by decreasing alcohol in the rat stomach. Gastroenterology. 1996;110:1536–42.
24. Morgan MY, Sherlock S. Sex-related differences among 100 patients with alcoholic liver disease. Br Med J. 1977;1:939–41.
25. Pequignot G, Tuyns AJ, Berta JL. Ascitic cirrhosis in relation to alcohol consumption. Int J Epidemiol (Lond). 1978;7:113–20.
26. Parrish KM, Dufour MC, Stinson FS, Harford TC. Average daily alcohol consumption during adult life among decedents with and without cirrhosis: the 1986 National Mortality Followback Survey. J Studies Alcohol. 1993;54:450–6.
27. Becker U, Deis A, Sorenson TIA, et al. Prediction of risk of liver disease by alcohol intake, sex, and age: a prospective population study. Hepatology. 1996;23:1025–9.
28. Mann K, Batra A, Günthner A, Schroth G. Do women develop alcoholic brain damage more readily than men? Alcoholism: Clin Exp Res. 1992;16:1052–6.
29. Frezza, M, Di Padova C, Pozzato G, Terpin M, Baraona E, Lieber CS. High blood alcohol levels in women. The role of decreased gastric alcohol dehydrogenase activity and first-pass metabolism. N Engl J Med. 1990;322:95–9.
30. Seitz HK, Egerer G, Simanowski UA et al. Human gastric alcohol dehydrogenase activity: effect of age, gender and alcoholism. Gut. 1993;34:1433–7.
31. Ammon E, Schäfer C, Hofmann U, Klotz U. Disposition and first-pass metabolism of ethanol in humans: is it gastric or hepatic and does it depend on gender? Clin Pharmacol Ther. 1996;59:503–13.
32. Roine RP, Gentry RT, Lim Jr RT, Baraona E, Lieber CS. Effect of concentration of ingested ethanol on blood alcohol levels. Alcoholism: Clin Exp Res. 1991;15:734–8.
33. Roine RP, Gentry RT, Lim Jr RT, Heikkonen E, Salaspuro M, Lieber CS. Comparison of blood alcohol concentrations after beer and whiskey. Alcoholism: Clin Exp Res. 1993;17:709–11.
34. Roine RP, Gentry RT, Hernández-Muñoz R, Baraona E, Lieber CS. Aspirin increases blood alcohol concentrations in human after ingestion of ethanol. J Am Med Assoc. 1990;264:2406–8.
35. Caballeria J, Baraona E, Rodamilans M, Lieber CS. Effects of cimetidine on gastric alcohol dehydrogenase activity and blood ethanol levels. Gastroenterology. 1989;96:388–92.
36. Roine RP, Hernández-Muñoz R, Baraona E, Greenstein R, Lieber CS. Effect of omeprazole on gastric 'first pass metabolism' of ethanol. Dig Dis Sci. 1992;37:891–6.
37. Amir I, Anwar N, Baraona E, Lieber CS. Ranitidine increases the bioavailability of imbibed alcohol by accelerating gastric emptying. Life Sci. 1996;58:511–18.
38. Palmer RH, Frank WO, Nambi P, Wetherington JD, Fox MJ. Effects of various concomitant medications on gastric alcohol dehydrogenase and first-pass metabolism of ethanol. Am J Gastroenterol. 1991;86:1749–55.
39. Fraser AG, Hudson M, Sawyer AM, Rosalki SM, Pounder RE. Short report: the effect of ranitidine on post-prandial absorption of a low dose of alcohol. Aliment Pharmacol Ther. 1992;6:267–71.
40. DiPadova C, Roine RP, Frezza M, Gentry RT, Baraona E, Lieber CS. Effects of ranidine on blood alcohol levels after ethanol ingestion: comparison with other H_2-receptor antagonists. J Am Med Assoc. 1992;267:83–6.
41. Seitz HK, Veith S, Czygan P, Bösche J, Simon B, Gugler R, Kommerell B. In vivo interactions between H_2-receptor antagonists and ethanol metabolism in man and in rats. Hepatology. 1984;4:1231–4.
42. Guram M, Howden CW, Holt S. Further evidence for an interaction between alcohol and certain H_2-receptor antagonists. Alcoholism: Clin Exp Res. 1991;15:1084–5.

43. Feely J, Wood AJ. Effect of cimetidine on the elimination and actions of ethanol. J Am Med Assoc. 1982;247:2219–21.

44. Raufman JP, Notar-Francesco V, Raffaniello RD, Strauss EW. Histamine-2 receptor antagonists do not alter serum ethanol levels in fed, non-alcoholic men. Ann Intern Med. 1993;118:488–94.

45. Sharma R, Gentry RT, Lim Jr RT, Lieber CS. First pass metabolism of alcohol: absence of diurnal variation and its inhibition by cimetidine after an evening meal. Dig Dis Sci. 1995;40:2091–7.

46. Sharma R, Gentry RT, Lim RT, Lieber CS. First pass metabolism of alcohol: absence of diurnal variation and its inhibition by cimetidine after an evening meal. Am J Gastroenterol. 1992;87:1276.

47. Fiatarone Jr, Bennett MK, Kelly P, James OFW. Ranitidine but not gastritis or female sex reduces the first pass metabolism of ethanol. Gut. 1991;31:A594.

48. Borgmann von H, Papke J, Dökert B, Barthels K, Krause D. Einfluβ von Cimetidin auf die Ethanolkinetik. Z Klin Med. 1989;44:781–4.

49. Papke J, Borgmann von H, Dökert B, Barteles H, Krause D. Cimetidin und Ethanol. Z Gesamte Inn Med. 1989;44:731–3.

50. Dauncey H, Chesher GB, Palmer RH. Cimetidine and ranitidine: lack of effect on the pharmacokinetics of an acute ethanol dose. J Clin Gastroenterol. 1993;17:189–94.

51. Norpoth T, Kneip M, Oehmichen M, Staak M, Iffland R, Käferstein. Alkolkinetik undpsychophysische Leistungfähigkeit unter der Applikation von H$_2$Rezeptoren-Blockern. Beiträge zur gerichd Medizin. 1986;44:1–4.

52. Kleine M, Ertl D. Comparative trial in volunteers to investigate possible ethanol-ranitidine (R) interaction. Ann Pharmacother. 1993;27:841–5.

53. Wilkinson PK. Pharmacokinetics of ethanol: a review. Alcoholism: Clin Exp Res. 1980;4:6–21.

54. Wagner JG, Wilkinson PK, Ganes DA. Parameters V_m and K_m for elimination of alcohol in young male subjects. Alcohol Alcoholism. 1989;24:555–64.

55. Gentry RT, Sharma R, Lim RT, Baraona E, Dipadova C, Lieber CS. A new method to quantify first metabolism of alcohol: application to the effects of H$_2$-blockers on alcohol bioavailability. Gastroenterology. 1992;102:811 (abstract).

56. Johnson KI, Fenzl E, Hein B. Einfluβ von Cimetidin auf den Abbau und die Wirkung des Alkohols. Arzneim Forsch. 1984;34:734–6.

57. Holt S. Alcohol and H$_2$-receptor antagonists: over the counter, under the table? Am J Gastroenterol. 1990;85:516–17.

58. Klein KE, Breuker K, Brüner H, Wegmann HM. Blutalkohol und Fluguntüchtigkeit. Versuch einer Erarbeitung von Richtwerten für die allgemeine Luftfahrt. Int Z ngew Physiol. 1967;24:254–7.

59. Moskowitz H, Burns MM, Williams AF. Skill performance at low blood alcohol levels. J Stud Alcohol. 1985;46:482–5.

60. Modell JG, Mountz JM. Drinking and flying – the problem of alcohol use in pilots. N Engl J Med. 1990;323:455–61.

61. Gupta AM, Baraona E, Lieber CS. Significant increase of blood alcohol by cimetidine after repetitive drinking of small alcohol doses. Alcoholism: Clin Exp Res. 1995;19:1083–7.

62. Palmer ED. Gastritis: a reevaluation. Medicine. 1954;33:199–290.

63. Gottfried EB, Korsten MA, Lieber CS. Alcohol-induced gastric and duodenal lesions in man. Am J Gastroenterol. 1978;70:587–92.

64. Lieber CS. Medical and nutritional complications of alcoholism: mechanisms and management. New York: Plenum Press; 1992:579.

65. Parl FF, Lev R, Thomas E, Pitchumoni CS. Histologic and morphometric study of chronic gastritis in alcohol patients. Hum Pathol. 1979;10:45–56.

66. Pateron D, Fabre M, Ink O et al. C. Influence de l'alcool et de la cirrhose sur la présence de Helicobacter pylori dans la muqueuse gastrique. Gastroenterol Clin Biol. 1990;14:555–68.

67. NIH Consensus Conference. Helicobacter pylori in peptic ulcer disease. NIH Consensus Development Panel on Helicobacter pylori in peptic ulcer disease. J Am Med Assoc. 1994;272:65–9.

68. Wolff G. Does alcohol cause chronic gastritis? Scand J Gastroenterol. 1970;4:289–91.

69. Hazell SL, Hennessy WB, Borody TJ et al. Campylobacter pyloridis gastritis II: distribution of bacteria and associated inflammation in the gastroduodenal environment. Am J Gastroenterol. 1987;82:297–301.

70. Strickland RG, Mackay IR. A reappraisal of the nature and significance of chronic atrophic gastritis. Dig Dis. 1973;18:426–37.
71. Joske RA, Fineki ES, Wood LJ. Gastric biopsy: A study of 1000 consecutive biopsies. Q J Med. 1955;48:269–94.
72. Roberts DM. Chronic gastritis, alcohol and non-ulcer dyspepsia. Gut. 1972;13:768–74.
73. Pitchumoni GS, Glass GBJ. Alcohol injury to the gastrointestinal mucosa. In: Glass GBJ, editor. Progress in gastroenterology. New York: Grune & Stratton; 1977:717–58.
74. Dinoso VP, Chey WY, Braverman SP. Gastric secretion and gastric mucosal morphology in chronic alcoholics. Arch Intern Med. 1972;130:715–20.
75. Laine L. *Helicobacter pylori*, gastric ulcer, and agents noxious to the gastric mucosa. Gastroenterol Clin N Am. 1993;22:117–25.
76. Dekigai H, Murakami M, Kita T. Mechanism of *Helicobacter pylori*-associated gastric mucosal injury. Dig Dis Sci. 1995;40:1332–9.
77. Lichtenberger LM, Dial EJ, Romero JJ, Lechago J, Jarboe LA, Wolfe MM. Role of luminal ammonia in the development of gastropathy and hypergastrinemia in the rat. Gastroenterology. 1995;108:320–9.
78. Fitzgerald O, Murphy P. Studies on the physiological chemistry and clinical significance of urease and urea with special reference to the stomach. Irish J Med Sci. 1950;6:97–159.
79. Burke JO, Page SG. The effects of orally administered urea on healthy subjects and their gastric secretory response to histamine. Gastroenterology. 1954;26:503–5.
80. Lieber CS, Lefèvre A. Ammonia as a source of gastric hypoacidity in patients with uremia. J Clin Invest. 1959;38:1271–7.
81. Triebling AT, Korsten MA, Dlugosz JW, Paronetto F, Lieber CS. Severity of *Helicobacter*-induced gastric injury correlates with gastric juice ammonia. Dig Dis Sci. 1991;36:1089–96.
82. Verbanck M, Toussaint C, Lieber CS, Lefèvre A. Gastroduodenal bleeding complicating acute anuria during treatment by artificial kidney. Acta Gastroenterol Belg. 1957;20:798–809.
83. Murakami M, Asagoe K, Dekigai H, Kusaka S, Saita H, Kita T. Products of neutrophil metabolism increase ammonia-induced gastric mucosal damage. Dig Dis Sci. 1995;40:268–73.
84. Lieber CS, Lefèvre A. Effect of oxytetracycline on acidity, ammonia and urea in gastric juice in normal and uremic subjects. CR Soc Biol (Paris). 1957;151:1038–42.
85. Lieber CS, Lefèvre A. Effects of antibiotics on gastric juice in normal and uremic subjects: ammonia as source of hypoacidity in uremic patients. In: Proc World Congress Gastroenterology. Baltimore, MD: Williams & Wilkins; 1959;1:117–18.
86. Lieber CS, Lefèvre A. Ammonia and intermediary metabolism in hepatic coma: value of the determination of blood ammonia in the diagnosis and management of cirrhosis. Acta Clin Belg. 1958;13:328–57.
87. Mokuolu AO, Sigal SH, Lieber CS. Gastric juice urease activity as a diagnostic test for *Helicobacter pylori* infection. Am J Gastroenterol. 1997;92:644–8.
88. Doenges JL. Spirochetes in the gastric glands of *Macacus rhesus* and of man without related disease. Arch Pathol Lab Med. 1939;27:469–77.
89. Freedburg AS, Barron LE. The presence of spirochetes in human gastric mucosa. Am J Dig Dis. 1940;7:443–5.
90. Luck JM, Seth TN. Gastric urease. Biochem J. 1924;18:1227–31.
91. Meyers S, Lieber CS. Reduction of gastric ammonia by ampicillin in normal and azotemic subjects. Gastroenterology. 1976;70:244–7.
92. Aoyagi T, Engstrom GW, Evans WB, Summerskill WHJ. Gastrointestinal urease in man. Gut. 1966;7:631–5.
93. Delluva AM, Markley K, Davies RE. The absence of gastric urease in germ-free animals. Biochim Biophys Acta. 1968;151:646–50.
94. Steer HW, Colin-Jones DG. Mucosal changes in gastric ulceration and their response to carbenoxolone sodium. Gut. 1975;16:590–7.
95. Ramsey EJ, Carey KV, Peterson WL et al. Epidemic gastritis with hypochlorhydria. Gastroenterology. 1979;76:1449–57.
96. Graham DY, Alpert LC, Smith JL, Yoshimura HH. Iatrogenic *Campylobacter pylori* infection is a cause of epidemic achlorhydria. Am J Gastroenterol. 1988;83:974–80.
97. Warren JR. Unidentified curved bacilli on gastric epithelium in active chronic gastritis. Lancet. 1983;1:1273.
98. Marshall BJ. Unidentified curved bacilli on gastric epithelium in active chronic gastritis. Lancet. 1983;1:1273–5.

99. Marshall BJ, Armstrong JA, McGechie DB, Glancy RJ. Attempts to fulfil Koch's postulates for pyloric *Campylobacter*. Med J Aust. 1985;142:436–9.

100. Marshall BJ, Langton SR. Urea hydrolysis in patients with *Campylobacter pyloridis* infection. Lancet. 1986;1:965–6.

101. Kudo M, Asaka M, Kato M *et al*. Role of *Helicobacter pylori* in chronic gastritis: a prospective study. J Clin Gastroenterol. 1995;2:S174–8.

102. Kreuning J, Bosman FT, Kuiper G, Wal AM, Lindeman J. Gastric and duodenal mucosa in healthy individuals. J Clin Pathol. 1978;31:69–77.

103. Toukan AU, Kamal MF, Amr SS, Arnaout MS, Abu-Romiyeh AS. Gastroduodenal inflammation in patients with non-ulcer dyspepsia. Dig Dis Sci. 1985;30:313–20.

104. Lambert JR, Borromeo M, Kormam MG, Hansky J. Role of *Campylobacter pyloridis* in non-ulcer dyspepsia: a randomized controlled trial. Gastroenterology. 1987;92:1488 (abstract).

105. Borody T, Daskalopoulos G, Brandl S, Carrick J, Hazell S. Dyspeptic symptoms improve following eradication of gastric *Campylobacter pyloridis*. Gastroenterology. 1987;92:1324 (abstract).

106. Rokkas T, Pursey C, Uzoechina E *et al*. Non-ulcer dyspepsia and short term De-Nol therapy: a placebo controlled trial with particular reference to the role of *Campylobacter pylori*. Gut. 1988;29:1386–91.

107. McNulty CA, Gearty JC, Crump B *et al*. *Campylobacter pyloridis* and associated gastritis: investigator-blind, placebo controlled trial of bismuth salicylate and erythromycin ethylsuccinate. Br Med J. 1986;293:645–9.

108. Glupczynski Y, Burette A, Labbe M, Deprez C, DeReuck M, Deltenre M. *Campylobacter pyloridis*-associated gastritis: a double blind placebo controlled trial with amoxicillin. Am J Gastroenterol. 1988;83:365–71.

109. Loffeld RJFL, Potters HVHP, Stobberingh E, Flending JA, Van Spreeuwel JP, Arends JW. *Campylobacter pyloridis* associated gastritis in patients with non-ulcer dyspepsia: a double blind placebo controlled trial with colloidal bismuth subcitrate. Gut. 1989;30:1206–12.

110. Uppal R, Lateef SK, Korsten MA, Paronetto F, Lieber CS. Chronic alcoholic gastritis: roles of alcohol and *Helicobacter pylori*. Arch Intern Med. 1991;151:760–4.

111. Nagy L, Kussststche S, Hauschka PV, Szabo S. Role of cysteine proteases and protease inhibitors in gastric mucosal damage induced by ethanol or ammonia in the rat. J Clin Invest 1996;98:1047–54.

112. Salmela KS, Salaspuro M, Gentry RT, Methuen T, Hook-Nikanne J, Kosunen, Roine RP. *Helicobacter* infection and gastric ethanol metabolism. Alcoholism: Clin Exp Res. 1994;18:1294–9.

113. Roine RP, Salmela KS, Salaspuro M. Alcohol metabolism in *Helicobacter pylori*-infected stomach. Ann Med. 1995;27:583–8.

114. Brown ASJM, Fiatarone JR, Wood P *et al*. The effect of gastritis on human gastric alcohol dehydrogenase activity and ethanol metabolism. Aliment Pharmacol Ther. 1995;9:57–61.

115. Thuluvath P, Wojno KJ, Yardley JH, Mezey E. Effects of *Helicobacter pylori* infection and gastritis on gastric alcohol dehydrogenase activity. Alcoholism: Clin Exp Res. 1994;18:795–8.

116. Yin S-H, Liao C-S, Wu C-W *et al*. Human stomach alcohol and aldehyde dehydrogenases: comparison of expression pattern and activities in alimentary tract. Gastroenterology. 1997;112:766–76.

117. Lefevre A, Lustman F, Lieber CS. Total plasma ammonia and pNH3 in patients with hepatic precoma and coma. Rev Franc Etud Clin Biol. 1963;8:455–64.

118. Lieber CS, Davidson CS. Complications resulting from renal failure in patients with liver disease. Arch Intern Med. 1960;106:749–52.

119. Rappaport WJ, Kern F, Jr. Gastric urease activity in normal subjects and in subjects with cirrhosis. J Lab Clin Med. 1963;61:550–9.

120. Gubbins GP, Mortiz TE, Marsano LS, Talwalkar R, McClain CJ, Mendenhall CL. *Helicobacter pylori* is a risk factor for hepatic encephalopathy in acute alcoholic hepatitis: the ammonia hypothesis revisited. Am J Gastroenterol. 1993;88:1906–10.

121. Ito S, Kohli Y, Kato T, Abe Y, Ueda T. Significance of ammonia produced by *Helicobacter pylori*. Eur J Gastroenterol Hepatol. 1994;6:167–74.

122. Dasani BM, Sigal SH, Lieber CS. The role of *Helicobacter pylori* in the pathogenesis and treatment of chronic hepatic encephalopathy. Hepatology. 1995;22:161 (abstract).

123. Ramond MJ, Poynard T, Rueff B *et al.* A randomized trial of prednisolone in patients with severe alcoholic hepatitis. N Engl J Med. 1992;326:507–12.

124. Lieber CS, Lefévre A, Lustman Fr. Effect of prednisolone on the increased ammonia blood level in Eck fistula dogs. Revue Bel Pathol. 1958;26:414–25.

125. Marshall BJ, McGechie DB, Rogers PA, Glancy RJ. Pyloric *Campylobacter* infection and gastroduodenal disease. Med J Aust. 1985;142:439–44.

126. Morris A, Nicholson G. Ingestion of *Campylobacter pyloridis* causes gastritis and raised fasting pH. Am J Gastroenterol. 1987;82:192–9.

127. Rauws EAJ, Langenberg W, Houthoff HJ, Zanen HC, Tytgat GNJ. *Campylobacter pyloridis*-associated chronic active antral gastritis: a prospective study of its prevalence and the effects of antibacterial and antiulcer treatment. Gastroenterology. 1988;94:33–40.

128. Cutler AF, Havstad S, Ma CK, Blaser MJ, Perez-Perez GI, Schubert TT. Accuracy of invasive and noninvasive tests to diagnose *Helicobacter pylori* infection. Gastroenterology. 1995;109:136–41.

129. Marchildon PA, Ciota LM, Zamaniyan FZ, Peacock JS, Graham DY. Evaluation of three commercial enzyme immunoassays compared with the ^{13}C urea breath test for detection of *Helicobacter pylori* infection. J Clin Microbiol. 1996;34:1147–52.

130. Slomianski A, Schubert T, Cutler AF. [^{13}C] Urea breath test to confirm eradication of *Helicobacter pylori*. Am J Gastroenterol. 1995;90:224–6.

131. Klein PD, Malaty HM, Martin RF, Graham KS, Genta RM, Graham DY. Noninvasive detection of *Helicobacter pylori* infection in clinical practice: the ^{13}C urea breath test. Am J Gastroenterol. 1996;91:690–94.

9
Ethanol oxidation and acetaldehyde production by colonic microbes

M. SALASPURO, K. JOKELAINEN and T. NOSOVA

INTRODUCTION

After its oral intake alcohol is absorbed to the portal blood from the stomach and upper part of the small intestine. Thereafter it is rapidly transported by blood circulation to other organs including the large bowel. Ethanol is evenly distributed to the water phase of all organs, and accordingly, after the distribution phase, ethanol levels in the terminal ileum[1] and colon[2] are equal to those of the blood and liver. There is more and more evidence that alcohol is not merely an innocent bystander in the large bowel. Ethanol can be metabolized to acetaldehyde by many intracolonic microbes and also by colonic mucosal cells. However, as compared to the liver, the intracolonic oxidation of accetadehyde is limited. This results in strikingly high intracolonic levels of reactive, toxic and carcinogenic acetaldehyde. Therefore intracolonic acetaldehyde derived from microbial oxidation of ethanol is a possible candidate in the pathogenesis of alcohol-related gastrointestinal symptoms and diseases such as diarrhoea, colon polyps and cancer, and alcoholic liver injury[3,4].

COLONIC FLORA

The most richly colonized site of the digestive tract is the large intestine. More than 400 different bacterial species and 10^{14} individual bacteria inhabit a single human colon at a given time[5]. Accordingly, the number of intestinal bacteria is ten-fold as compared to the number of cells in the human host[6]. The metabolic capability of the colonic microflora has been estimated to be at least as great as that of the liver[7], or even to exceed that of the whole human body[8]. The volume of the large intestine is about 540 ml, and it receives approximately 1.5 kg of material from the small bowel each day. Most of this is water, which is rapidly absorbed. The adult large gut contains around 220 g of contents[9], with an average daily faecal output[10] of 120 g. Bacteria are the major component of faeces, comprising approximately 55% of solids[11].

ALCOHOLIC FERMENTATION BY INTESTINAL MICROBES

A number of bacteria and yeasts possess alcohol dehydrogenase (ADH) activity[12]. Under anaerobic conditions these microbes are capable of producing energy through fermentation[13]. In alcoholic fermentation the end-product is ethanol, which is derived from acetaldehyde in a reductive reaction mediated by bacterial alcohol dehydrogenase[14]. The reaction runs as follows:

Alcoholic fermentation

$$\text{Glucose} \xrightarrow{\text{ADH}} \text{Acetaldehyde} \leftrightarrow \text{Ethanol}$$

Due to the alcoholic fermentation, small amounts of ethanol have earlier been found in the contents of the alimentary tract and portal blood of normal rats[15]. An enhanced production of endogenous ethanol as a result of bacterial overgrowth has been demonstrated in jejunal blind-loop contents of rats[16]. In humans significant endogenous ethanol levels have been found in jejunal aspirates of patients with tropical sprue[17], and in venous blood of patients after jejunoileal bypass for morbid obesity[18]. Thirty-nine cases of intragastrointestinal alcohol fermentation syndrome, manifesting as alcohol intoxication after a high carbohydrate diet in patients with gastrointestinal abnormalities and associated overgrowth of *Candida albicans*, have been described in Japan[19]. Endogenous blood alcohol levels up to 90 mg% could be demonstrated in these patients.

ACETALDEHYDE PRODUCTION IN THE LARGE INTESTINE BY COLONIC BACTERIA

As shown above, the last reaction catalysed by microbial alcohol dehydrogenase in alcoholic fermentation can also run in the opposite direction, with acetaldehyde as an end-product. An example of this type of reversed reaction is acetaldehyde production *in vitro* by human mouth washings and bronchopulmonary washings[20].

The reversed microbial ADH reaction also produces striking amounts of acetaldehyde when human colonic contents are incubated *in vitro* at 37°C with increasing ethanol concentrations[21]. It should be emphasized that this reaction is already active at comparatively low (10–100 mg%) ethanol concentrations known to exist in the colon during normal drinking[21,22]. Moreover, intracolonic acetaldehyde formation takes place at a pH value normally found in the colon, and is rapidly reduced with lowering of the pH[21]. It remains to be established whether lactulose or high-fibre diet, which can decrease faecal pH, might also be able to decrease colonic acetaldehyde production from ethanol *in vivo*.

After an acute dose of ethanol to rats, acetaldehyde levels higher than in the liver or in the blood have been demonstrated in colonic mucosa[23]. Since, in that study, mucosal acetaldehyde levels were significantly lower in germ-free than in normal animals, mucosal acetaldehyde was suggested to be generated at least in part through bacterial ethanol oxidation[23]. Our recent *in vivo* studies in pigs demonstrate that intracolonic acetaldehyde levels increase in parallel with increasing blood and intracolonic ethanol concentrations[22].

ALCOHOL AND ALDEHYDE DEHYDROGENASES OF THE BACTERIA REPRESENTING HUMAN COLONIC FLORA

There are marked differences in the alcohol dehydrogenase activity and acetaldehyde-producing capacity among the aerobic bacteria representing the normal human colonic flora[24]. The mean cytosolic alcohol dehydrogenase activity of some bacteria can be up to 30 times higher than that of the rat liver when determined at similar conditions (Fig. 1)[24]. The highly significant positive correlation between bacterial alcohol dehydrogenase activity and their acetaldehyde-producing capacity from ethanol strongly suggests the catalytic role of microbial alcohol dehydrogenase in the production of acetaldehyde from ethanol[24].

Alcohol dehydrogenases of the so-far-tested bacteria representing human colonic flora show a variety of K_m values for ethanol ranging from 0.06 to 29.9 mmol/L[25]. These values are comparable with the ethanol concentrations found in the large intestine during moderate drinking. Under these circumstances bacterial alcohol dehydrogenases are able to metabolize ethanol to acetaldehyde with a velocity close to maximal and, accordingly, to produce marked amounts of acetaldehyde[25]. On the other hand the rather high K_m values for ethanol of some bacterial alcohol dehydrogenases[25] explain the close association between increasing intracolonic acetaldehyde and ethanol levels found in our earlier *in-vivo* study[22].

Acetaldehyde administered intracolonically to pigs is rapidly eliminated, and this is associated with an increase in intracolonic acetate and ethanol levels (Fig. 2)[22]. Obviously intracolonic acetaldehyde is effectively metabolized partly by colonic mucosal cells and partly by intracolonic microbes. Indeed, many aerobic bacteria representing the normal flora of the human large intestine possess significant cytosolic $NADP^+$- and NAD^+-dependent aldehyde dehydrogenase activity[26]. Furthermore, these bacteria metabolize acetaldehyde to acetate effectively *in vitro*[26]. Individual variation in the capability of colonic flora to produce or to remove acetaldehyde may thus be one factor regulating intracolonic

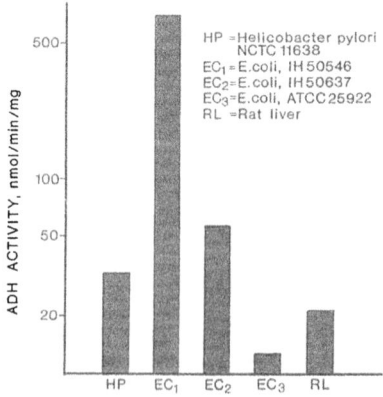

Figure 1 Alcohol dehydrogenase (ADH) activity of some bacteria representing the human gut flora as compared to ADH activity of rat liver. Adapted from Jokelainen *et al.*[24]

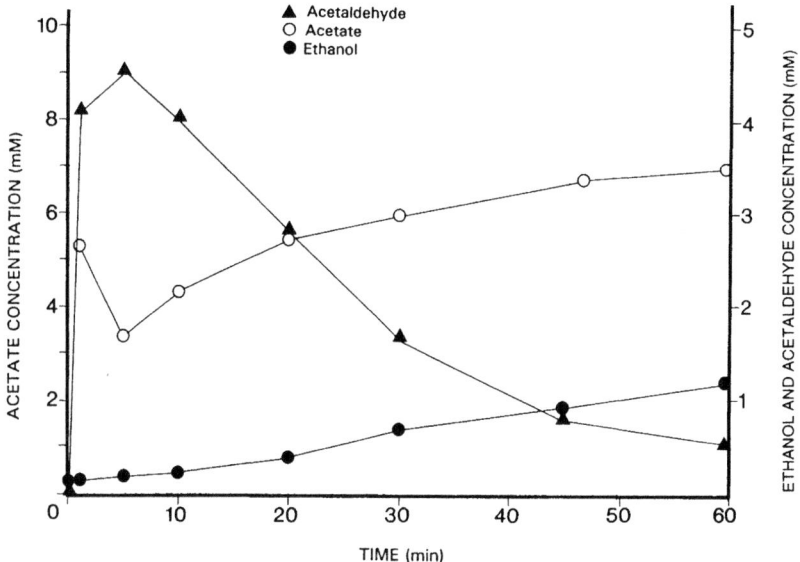

Figure 2 Metabolism of acetaldehyde in the large intestine: 500 ml of 5 mmol/L acetaldehyde solution was introduced intracolonically to piglets within 10 min. Adapted from Jokelainen et al.[22]

acetaldehyde levels during ethanol oxidation. In addition, acetaldehyde is easily absorbed from the colon to the portal blood[27] and, accordingly, may also be metabolized further in the liver.

BACTERIOCOLONIC PATHWAY FOR ETHANOL OXIDATION

Our results suggest the existence of a bacteriocolonic pathway for ethanol oxidation:

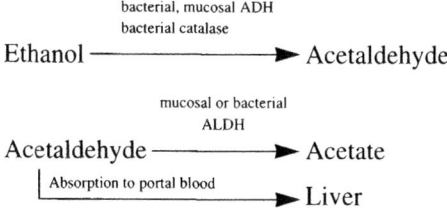

Via this pathway, intracolonic ethanol is at first oxidized to acetaldehyde in a reaction catalysed by bacterial or colonic mucosal alcohol dehydrogenase. Moreover, our most recent results obtained in incubations of human colonic contents *in vitro* indicate that a significant proportion of microbial acetaldehyde production from ethanol is mediated by microbial catalase[28]. In a subsequent reaction acetaldehyde is oxidized by colonic mucosal or bacterial aldehyde dehydrogenase to acetate. Furthermore, acetaldehyde may be metabolized by

127

some other so-far-undertermined microbial pathways existing even in other microbes to a variety of substrates. Acetate is further metabolized by either colonic mucosal cells or by bacteria, or it may be excreted via the faecal route. An additional possibility is that part of intracolonically produced acetaldehyde and/or acetate is absorbed to the portal blood and is metabolized further in the liver[27].

The rate-limiting steps of the bacteriocolonic pathway for ethanol oxidation remain to be established in future studies. However, according to our most recent results the reduction of rat colonic flora and faecal alcohol dehydrogenase activity with ciprofloxacin decreases ethanol elimination rate by 9%[29]. More importantly, ciprofloxacin treatment totally abolishes the alcohol-induced enhancement in ethanol elimination rate[30]. Ciprofloxacin, however, did not inhibit hepatic alcohol dehydrogenase activity or the microsomal ethanol-oxidizing system in the liver. These findings suggest that the role of the bacterio-colonic pathway in total ethanol elimination is quantitatively important, and may explain most of the extrahepatic metabolism of ethanol which has been known, for decades, to exist[31-33]. Moreover, the bacteriocolonic pathway appears to be the major inducible pathway for ethanol elimination during chronic alcohol consumption.

It should be noted that the anaerobic conditions prevailing in the colon may not in general favour the oxidation of ethanol and acetaldehyde by bacterial enzymes. It is well known that in faecal flora anaerobic organisms outnumber facultative organisms by a factor of 1000. However, due to the diffusion of oxygen from the colonic mucosa, the mucosa-associated flora contains as many, or even more, aerobes than anaerobes[34]. Therefore, the higher oxygen tension of the mucosal surface and its flora may favour the oxidation of ethanol to acetaldehyde and acetaldehyde to acetate also *in vivo*.

As compared to the metabolism of ethanol in the liver, the bacterio-colonic pathway for ethanol oxidation differs in some important respects. Mitochondrial and cytosolic aldehyde dehydrogenase activities of rat colonic mucosa are approximately six times lower than corresponding activities in the liver[35]. Aldehyde dehydrogenase activity of the colonic mucosa may thus be sufficient for the removal of acetaldehyde produced by colonic mucosal alcohol dehydrogenase during ethanol oxidation, but it may be insufficient for the removal of acetaldehyde produced by intracolonic bacteria. This favours the accumulation of acetaldehyde in the colon during ethanol oxidation. Indeed, we have recently been able to demonstrate variable and sometimes strikingly high intracolonic acetaldehyde levels, up to 2.7 mmol/L, after a moderate dose (1.5 g/kg body weight) of ethanol to rats. The great variability in intracolonic acetaldehyde levels during ethanol oxidation most probably can be explained by individual variations in alcohol- and acetaldehyde-metaboliz-ing enzymes of the intestinal microbes. Since intracolonic ethanol is partly oxidized in the colon by bacterial enzymes, all ethanol calories may not become available for the human body. Part of the ethanol-derived calories may be excreted via the faecal route; therefore the bacteriocolonic pathway offers a new explanation for the well-known disappearance of a proportion of ethanol calories[36].

CONCLUSIONS AND CLINICAL ASSOCIATIONS

The main characteristics and possible clinical associations of the bacteriocolonic pathway for ethanol oxidation are presented in Table 1. As reviewed above, the bacteriocolonic pathway results in strikingly high intracolonic acetaldehyde levels. High intracolonic acetaldehyde levels in the large intestine could act as a local irritant. Diarrhoea and flatulence are the most frequent gastrointestinal symptoms in chronic alcoholics[37], but their pathogenesis has so far, by and large, been unknown. Ethanol has been demonstrated to decrease both the frequency and amplitude of basal motility waves in the rectosigmoid in humans[38], and in alcoholics with diarrhoea there is a rapid oral–caecal transit time[39]. Histological and ultrastructural specimens of rectal mucosa of heavy drinkers reveal marked pathological changes[40]. On light microscopy there is a decrease in the number of goblet cells both in the surface epithelium and in the crypts. In addition, the lamina propria may be heavily infiltrated with mononuclear cells. Electron microscopy reveals swollen and distorted mitochondria and dilated vesicular endoplasmic reticulum. These abnormalities disappear after 2 weeks' abstinence[40].

The pathogenesis of endotoxaemia induced by alcohol and/or liver injury is unknown[41]. One possibility is that chronic alcoholism increases the intestinal permeability of the gut[42]. In this process elevated intracolonic acetaldehyde

Table 1 The main characteristics and possible clinical associations of the bacteriocolonic pathway for ethanol oxidation

Characteristics of the pathway	Clinical associations
Variability in the K_m values and other characteristics of microbial alcohol and aldehyde dehydrogenases	Variability in the levels of endogenous acetaldehyde in the large bowel. Positive correlation between intracolonic ethanol and acetaldehyde levels. Diarrhoea associating with positive faecal culture for *Hafnia alvei*
High intracolonic acetaldehyde level	Diarrhoea and flatulence of chronic alcoholics. Changes in gut motility and rapid oral–caecal transit time in alcoholics. Histological and ultrastructural changes in the rectal mucosa of heavy drinkers. Leakage of endotoxins to portal circulation. Increased susceptibility of heavy drinkers to colon polyps and cancer. May be an important determinant of blood acetaldehyde level. Extrahepatic acetaldehyde via portal blood may contribute to the hepatotoxicity of alcohol
Induction of the bacteriocolonic pathway for ethanol oxidation	Explains the enhanced rate of ethanol elimination associating with chronic alcohol consumption. During chronic alcohol consumption: (a) the shifting of a larger part of ethanol oxidation from the liver to the large bowel may protect the liver; or (b) the formation and absorption of some hepatotoxic factor, i.e. acetaldehyde and/or endotoxin from the colon, may contribute to the pathogenesis of alcohol-related liver injury

levels could be an important pathogenetic factor. Alternatively, heavy drinking may also alter the composition of the intestinal[43] or faecal flora.

The induction of the bacteriocolonic pathway for the ethanol oxidation during chronic alcohol administration may explain the enhanced rate of ethanol elimination observed even in the presence of relatively severe alcoholic liver injury[44,45].

The variability in the characteristics of different microbial alcohol dehydrogenases may also have some clinical implications. For instance the very low K_m of the ADH of *Hafnia alvei* for ethanol (0.06 mmol/L)[25] allows it to metabolize intracolonic endogenous ethanol (0.4–0.6 mmol/L) to acetaldehyde. Accordingly, the increased colonic endogenous acetaldehyde levels might explain, at least in part, the pathogenesis of *H. alvei*-associated diarrhoea[46]. Furthermore, the large variation in the levels of endogenous acetaldehyde[22] may reflect individual variability in the kinetics of microbial alcohol and aldehyde dehydrogenases.

Acetaldehyde is a highly reactive compound, that has been linked to several organ-toxic effects of ethanol[47]. Acetaldehyde binds covalently with macromolecules and proteins, thus forming acetaldehyde adducts[48,49]. Acetaldehyde binding with tissue proteins may initiate several biochemical and immunological reactions, which have been related especially to the pathogenesis of alcoholic liver injury[50,51]. Furthermore, acetaldehyde may enhance lipid peroxidation by several mechanisms[47]. Accordingly, acetaldehyde of extrahepatic origin, i.e. acetaldehyde formed by bacterial alcohol dehydrogenase in the colon from ethanol, may contribute to the pathogenesis of alcoholic liver injury. This is supported by our recent findings indicating that a low dose of acetaldehyde delivered to rats, in drinking water, may produce microvesicular fatty infiltration of the liver even in the absence of ethanol[27].

Chronic ethanol consumption enhances 1,2-dimethylhydrazine- and acetoxymethylmethylnitrosamine-induced rectal carcinogenesis[23,52] and selectively stimulates rectal cell proliferation in rats[53]. Furthermore, chronic ethanol feeding enhances rectal hyperregeneration, which is age-dependent[54,55]. According to the International Agency for Research on Cancer there is sufficient evidence for the carcinogenicity of acetaldehyde to experimental animals[56]. Most recent epidemiological studies suggest an association between alcohol consumption and the risk of colorectal polyps and cancer also in humans[56–60]. Since ethanol itself is not a carcinogen, acetaldehyde produced by colonic microbes could at least in part explain the above-mentioned findings.

It can be concluded that there is increasing evidence that the large bowel is an important organ for ethanol metabolism and acetaldehyde production. Under normal conditions up to 10% of ethanol may be metabolized by this extrahepatic pathway. More importantly, the bacteriocolonic pathway for ethanol oxidation appears to be the major inducible pathway for ethanol elimination during chronic alcohol consumption. The existence of this acetaldehyde-producing pathway in the large bowel may explain, at least in part, the increased gastrointestinal morbidity such as diarrhoea and increased risk of colon polyps and cancer, among heavy drinkers. Furthermore, intracolonically produced acetaldehyde may be an important determinant of blood acetaldehyde level and a potential hepatotoxin. Many alcohol-related diseases may thus be of bacterial origin.

Acknowledgements

This work has been financially supported by grants from Yrjö Jahnsson Foundation, the Finnish Foundation for Gastroenterological Research, the Finnish–Norwegian Foundation for Medicine, Mary and George C. Ehrnrooth Foundation, Research-Foundation of Orion Corp., the Finnish Medical Foundation, HUCH-Foundation and the Finnish Foundation for Alcohol Studies. The skilful technical assistance of Ms Tuula Moisio is greatly acknowledged. The authors also thank Dr Hannele Jousimies-Somer, and Dr Anja Siitonen, National Public Health Institute, for providing the bacterial strains.

References

1. Halstedt CH, Robles EA, Mezey E. Distribution of ethanol in the human gastrointestinal tract. Am J Clin Nutr. 1973;26:831–4.
2. Levitt MD, Doizaki W, Levine AS. Hypothesis: metabolic activity of the colonic bacteria influences organ injury from ethanol. Hepatology. 1982;2:598–600.
3. Salaspuro M. Bacteriocolonic pathway for ethanol oxidation: characteristics and implications. Ann Med. 1996;28:195–200.
4. Salaspuro M. Microbial metabolism of ethanol and acetaldehyde and clinical consequences. Addiction Biol. 1997;2:35–46.
5. Luckey TD. Bicentennial overview of intestinal microecology. Am J Clin Nutr. 1977;30:1753–61.
6. Savage DC. Microbial ecology of the gastrointestinal tract. Ann Rev Microbiol. 1977;31:107–33.
7. Bingham SA. Meat, strach, and nonstarch polysaccharides and large bowel cancer. Am J Clin Nutr. 1988;48:762–7.
8. Cummings JH. Fermentation in the human large intestine: evidence and implications for health. Lancet. 1983;1:1206–9.
9. Banwell JG, Branch WJ, Cummings JH. The microbial mass in the human large intestine. Gastroenterology. 1981;80:1104.
10. Macfarlane GT, Macfarlane S. Human colonic microbiota: ecology, physiology and metabolic potential of intestinal bacteria. Scand J Gastroenterol. 1997;32(Suppl. 222):3–9.
11. Stephen AM, Cummings JH. The microbial contribution to human faecal mass. J Med Microbiol. 1980;13:45–56.
12. Reid MF, Fewson CA. Molecular characterization of microbial alcohol dehydrogenase. Crit Rev Microbiol. 1994;20:13–56.
13. Zeikus JG. Chemical and fuel production by anaerobic bacteria. Annu Rev Microbiol. 1980;34:423–64.
14. Neale AD, Scopes RK, Kelly JM, Wettenhall REH. The two alcohol dehydrogenases of *Zymomonas mobilis*. Purification by differential dye ligand chromatography, molecular characterisation and physiological roles. Eur J Biochem. 1986;154:119–24.
15. Krebs HA, Perkins JR. The physiological role of liver alcohol dehydrogenase. Biochem J. 1970;118:635–44.
16. Baraona E, Julkunen R, Tannenbaum L, Lieber CS. Role of intestinal bacterial overgrowth in ethanol production and metabolism in rats. Gastroenterology. 1986;90:103–10.
17. Klipstein FA, Holdeman LV, Corcino JJ, Moore WEC. Enterotoxigenic intestinal bacteria in tropical sprue. Ann Intern Med. 1973;79:632–41.
18. Mezey E, Imbembo AL, Potter JJ, Rent KC, Lombardo L, Holt PR. Endogenous ethanol production and hepatic disease following jejunoileal bypass for morbid obesity. Am J Clin Nutr. 1975;28:1277–83.
19. Kaji H, Asanuma Y, Yahara O et al. Intragastrointestinal alcohol fermentation syndrome: report of two cases and review of the literature. J Forensic Sci Soc. 1984;24:461–71.
20. Miyakawa H, Baraona E, Chang JC, Lesser MD, Lieber CS. Oxidation of ethanol to acetaldehyde by bronchopulmonary washings: role of bacteria. Alcohol Clin Exp Res. 1986;10:517–20.
21. Jokelainen K, Roine RP, Väänänen H, Färkkilä M, Salaspuro M. *In vitro* acetaldehyde formation by human colonic bacteria. Gut. 1994;35:1271–4.

22. Jokelainen K, Matysiak-Budnik T, Mäkisalo H, Höckerstedt K, Salaspuro M. High intracolonic acetaldehyde values produced by a bacteriocolonic pathway for ethanol oxidation in piglets. Gut. 1996;39:100–4.

23. Seitz HK, Simanowski UA, Garzon FT et al. Possible role of acetaldehyde in ethanol-related rectal cocarcinogenesis in the rat. Gastroenterology. 1990;98:406–13.

24. Jokelainen K, Siitonen A, Jousimies-Somer H, Nosova T, Heine R, Salaspuro M. In vitro alcohol dehydrogenase-mediated acetaldehyde production by aerobic bacteria representing the normal colonic flora in man. Alcohol Clin Exp Res. 1996;20:967–72.

25. Nosova T, Jousimies-Somer H, Kaihovaara P, Jokelainen K, Heine R, Salaspuro M. Characteristics of alcohol dehydrogenases of certain aerobic bacteria representing human colonic flora. Alcohol Clin Exp Res. 1997;21:489–94.

26. Nosova T, Jokelainen K, Kaihovaara P et al. Aldehyde dehydrogenase activity and acetate production by aerobic bacteria representing the normal flora of human large intestine. Alcohol Alcoholism. 1996;31:555–64.

27. Matysiak-Budnik T, Jokelainen K, Kärkkäinen P, Mäkisalo H, Ohisalo J, Salaspuro M. Hepatotoxicity and absorption of extrahepatic acetaldehyde in rats. J Pathol. 1996;178:469–74.

28. Tillonen J, Kaihovaara P, Salaspuro M. Role of catalase in in vitro acetaldehyde formation by colonic bacteria. Alcohol Alcoholism 1997;32:407.

29. Jokelainen K, Nosova T, Koivisto T, et al. Inhibition of bacteriocolonic pathway for ethanol oxidation by ciprofloxacin in rats. Life Sci. 1997;61:1755–62.

30. Nosova T, Jokelainen K, Väkeväinen S, Salaspuro M. Bacteriocolonic pathway for ethanol oxidation is induced by chronic alcohol administration. J Hepatol. 1997;26(Suppl. 1):58.

31. Larsen JA. Extrahepatic metabolism of ethanol in man. Nature. 1959;184:1236.

32. Larsen JA, Tygstrup N, Winkler K. The significance of the extrahepatic elimination of ethanol in determination of hepatic blood flow by means of ethanol. Scand J Clin Lab Invest. 1961;13:116–21.

33. Huang M-T, Huang C-C, Chen M-Y. In vivo uptake of ethanol and release of acetate in rat liver and GI. Life Sci. 1993;53:165–70.

34. Hill MJ. The normal gut bacterial flora. In: Hill MJ, editor. Role of gut bacteria in human toxicology and pharmacology. Basingstoke: Burgess Science Press; 1995:3.

35. Koivisto T, Salaspuro M. Aldehyde dehydrogenases of the rat colon: comparison with other tissues of the alimentary tract and the liver. Alcohol Clin Exp Res. 1996;20:551–5.

36. Lieber CS. Do alcohol calories count? Am J Clin Nutr. 1991;54:976–82.

37. Fields JZ, Turk A, Durkin M, Ravi NV, Keshavarzian A. Increased gastrointestinal symptoms in chronic alcoholics. Am J Gastroenterol. 1994;89:382–6.

38. Berenson MM, Avner DL. Alcohol inhibition of rectosigmoid motility in humans. Digestion. 1981;22:210–15.

39. Keshavarzian A, Iber FL, Dangleis MD, Cornish R. Intestinal transit and lactose intolerance in chronic alcoholics. Am J Clin Nutr. 1986;44:70–6.

40. Brozinsky S, Fani K, Grosberg SJ, Wapnick S. Alcohol ingestion-induced changes in the human rectal mucosa: light and electron microscopic studies. Dis Col Rectum. 1978;21:329–35.

41. Schenker S, Bay MK. Alcohol and endotoxin: another path to alcoholic liver injury? Alcohol Clin Exp Res. 1995;19:1364–6.

42. Bjarnason I, Ward K, Peters TJ. The leaky gut of alcoholism: possible route of entry for toxic compounds. Lancet. 1984;1:179–82.

43. Bode JC, Bode C, Heidelbach R, Durr HK, Martini GA. Jejunal microflora in patients with chronic alcohol abuse. Hepatogastroenterology. 1984;31:30–4.

44. Ginestal-da-Cruz A, Correia JP, Menezes L. Ethanol metabolism in liver cirrhosis and chronic alcoholism. Acta Hepatogastroenterol. 1975;22:369–74.

45. Ugarte G, Iturriaga H, Pereda T. Possible relationship between the rate of ethanol metabolism and the severity of hepatic damage in chronic alcoholics. Am J Dig Dis. 1977;22:406–10.

46. Ridell J, Siitonen A, Paulin L, Mattila L, Korkeala H, Albert MJ. Hafnia alvei in stool specimens from patients with diarrhea and healthy controls. J Clin Microbiol. 1994;32:2335–7.

47. Lauterburg BH, Bilzer M. Mechanisms of acetaldehyde hepatotoxicity. J Hepatol. 1988;7:384–90.

48. Lin RC, Smith SR, Lumeng L. Detection of protein–acetaldehyde adduct in the liver of rats fed alcohol chronically. J Clin Invest. 1988;81:615–19.

49. Holstege A, Bedosa P, Poynard T, *et al.* Acetaldehyde-modified epitopes in liver biopsy specimens of alcoholic and nonalcoholic patients: localization and association with progression to liver fibrosis. Hepatology. 1994;19:367–74.
50. Worrall S, deJersey J, Nicholls R, Wilce P. Acetaldehyde/protein interactions: are they involved in the pathogenesis of alcoholic liver disease? Dig Dis. 1993;11:265–77.
51. Niemelä O. Acetaldehyde adducts of proteins: diagnostic and pathogenetic implications in diseases caused by excessive alcohol consumption. Scand J Clin Chem. 1993;213:45–54.
52. Seitz HK, Czykan P, Wahldherr R *et al.* Enhancement of 1,2-dimethylhydrazine-induced rectal carcinogenesis following chronic ethanol consumption in the rat. Gastroenterology. 1984;86:886–91.
53. Simanowski UA, Seitz HK, Baier B, Kommerell B, Schmidt-Gayak H, Wright NA. Chronic ethanol consumption selectively stimulates rectal cell proliferation in the rat. Gut. 1986;27:278–82.
54. Simanowski UA, Suter P, Russell RM *et al.* Enhancement of ethanol induced rectal mucosal hyper regeneration with age in F344 rats. Gut. 1994;35:1102–6.
55. Simanowski UA, Stickel F, Maier H, Gärtner U, Seitz HK. Effect of alcohol on gastrointestinal cell regeneration as a possible mechanism in alcohol-associated carcinogenesis. Alcohol. 1995;12:111–15.
56. International Agency For Research on Cancer. Working Group on the Evaluation of the Carcinogenic Risk of Chemicals to Humans. Acetaldehyde. 1985; IARC Monographs 36:101–32.
57. Kearney J, Giovannucci E, Rimm EB *et al.* R, Diet, alcohol, and smoking and the occurrence of hyperplastic polyps of the colon and rectum. Cancer Causes Control. 1995;6:45–56.
58. Martinez ME, McPherson RS, Annegers JF, Levin B. Cigarrete smoking and alcohol consumption as risk factors for colorectal adenomatous polyps. J Natl Cancer Inst. 1995;87: 274–9.
59. Giovannucci E, Rimm EB, Ascherio A, Stampfer MJ, Colditz GA, Willett WC. Alcohol, low-methionine–low-folate diets, and risk of colon cancer in men. J Natl Cancer Inst. 1995;87:265–73.
60. Longnecker MP. Alcohol consumption and risk of cancer in humans: an overview. Alcohol. 1995;12:87–96.

10
Adaptation of liver cell function to enteral resorption: role of liver cell hydration

D. HÄUSSINGER, F. SCHLIESS, A.-K. KURZ,
U. WARSKULAT, S. HEINRICH, M. WETTSTEIN and
S. VOM DAHL

INTRODUCTION

The liver is the first organ which comes into contact with enterally absorbed nutrients. Here, nutrient delivery from the intestine is sensed, and this information is not only distributed to other organs, but is also used to trigger an adaptation of liver function in order to augment the effective hepatic processing of nutrients. Adaptation of liver cell function to enterally resorbed nutrients involves neural and endocrine mechanisms, as well as direct substrate effects on liver parenchymal and non-parenchymal cells. Although gastrointestinal distension exerts some influence on hepatic blood flow, the well-preserved metabolic response of transplanted livers to a nutrient load argues against a major role of neural mechanisms, and points to a superiority of endocrine and substrate-induced regulation.

Much effort has been devoted to the understanding of hormone action, substrate transport and the allosteric regulation of hepatic enzymes. Recent data suggest that alterations of liver cell hydration under the influence of hormones and substrates present another important and novel mechanism by which liver cell function can adapt to intestinal resorption. It appears that hepatocyte swelling and shrinkage trigger opposing functional patterns of hepatic metabolism and gene expression. Liver cell hydration changes are the result of an altered activity of ion and substrate transport systems in the plasma membrane of the hepatocyte, which give rise to osmotic water shifts into or out of the cell. Such water shifts lead to an activation of intracellular signal transduction pathways, which mediate the adaptation of metabolic liver cell function and gene expression. In addition, some components of intracellular signal transduction can respond directly to an increased substrate concentration. For example, an increased amino acid load to the liver induces cell swelling, which in turn activates mitogen-activated protein kinases and other as-yet-unknown signalling systems. The functional consequence is an inhibition of proteolysis and glycogenolysis, a stimulation of protein and glycogen synthesis, as well as an increase in bile acid secretion. Simultaneously, in the longer term, the expression of several genes, which are involved in amino acid metabolism, is altered. Thus, amino acid-induced liver cell swelling is a simple and elegant means to adapt metabolic liver function to an increased substrate load. This chapter summarizes some aspects on this topic, and for a detailed analysis the reader is referred to recent reviews[1-4].

PHYSIOLOGICAL MODULATORS OF LIVER CELL HYDRATION

Liver cell hydration is dynamic, and can change within minutes under the influence of substrates, hormones, oxidative stress and aniso-osmotic environments. Aniso-osmotic exposure may primarily be seen as an experimental tool to study the functional consequences of liver cell hydration changes, but one should keep in mind that, during intestinal absorption of water, portal venous blood may become slightly hypotonic[5]. Further, clinically relevant aniso-osmotic states (220–400 mOsmol/L) due to hypo- and hypernatraemia have been documented[6,7]. Physiological modulators of cell hydration can induce hydration changes of up to 20%, and changes of extracellular osmolarity by up to 100 mOsmol/L are required to mimic such effects (Table 1).

Cumulative substrate uptake

Na^+-dependent amino acid transporters in the plasma membrane can cause intra/extracellular amino acid concentration gradients of up to 20-fold. Na^+ entering the hepatocyte together with the amino acid is extruded in exchange for K^+ by the electrogenic Na^+/K^+-ATPase (Fig. 1). The cellular accumulation of amino acids and K^+ leads to hepatocyte swelling, which in turn triggers volume regulatory K^+ efflux[8-10]. This regulatory volume decrease, however, only prevents cell swelling from becoming excessive, and the hepatocytes remain in a swollen state as long the amino acid load continues[10]. Cessation of amino acid delivery is followed by rapid cell shrinkage, and a regulatory volume increase finally brings back cell volume to the starting level[10]. Importantly, amino acid-induced cell swelling and volume-regulatory responses occur upon exposure to amino acids in the physiological concentration range, and physiological fluctuations of the portal amino acid concentration are accompanied by parallel alterations of liver cell volume. The degree of amino acid-induced cell swelling seems largely related to the steady-state intra/extracellular amino acid concentration gradient. This gradient, and accordingly the degree of cell swelling, is modified by hormones and the nutritional state in a complex way through effects on the expression of plasma membrane transport systems, the electrochemical Na^+ gradient as a driving force for Na^+ coupled transport, and alterations of intracellular amino acid metabolism. For example, insulin and starvation, which are known to stimulate amino acid transport via system A, enhance glycine-induced hepatocyte swelling[11,12]. Conjugated bile acids also induce cell swelling[13], but the osmotic effects of bile acids accumulating inside the cell may

Table 1 Effectors on cell volume in perfused rat liver (percentage change of intracellular water)

Insulin (35 nmol/L)	+12 ± 1 (15)
*Insulin (35 nmol/L)	+5 ± 1 (4)
Insulin (35 nmol/L) + bumetanide (5 μmol/L)	+6 ± 1 (3)
Insulin (35 nmol/L) + glucagon (100 nmol/L)	+3 ± 3 (4)
Phenylephrine (5 μmol/L)	+8 ± 1 (4)
Bradykinin (100 nmol/L	+8 ± 1 (4)
Glucagon (100 nmol/L)	−14 ± 3 (6)
Dibutyryl-cAMP (50 μmol/L)	−9 ± 1 (4)
Adenosine (50 μmol/L)	−6 ± 3 (3)
Vasopressin (15 nmol/L)	−2 ± 2 (4)
ATP (20 μmol/L)	−6 ± 2 (6)
Serotonin (5 μmol/L)	−5 ± 1 (4)
Vasopressin (15 nmol/L) + glucagon (100 nmol/L)	−23 ± 3 (4)
Vasopressin (35 nmol/L) + cAMP (50 μmol/L)	−16 ± 1 (6)
Adenosine (50 μmol/L) + phenylephrine (5 μmol/L)	−1 ± 3 (3)
Insulin (35 nmol/L) + cAMP (50 μmol/L)	−4 ± 2 (3)
Glutamine (1 mmol/L)	+6 ± 1 (3)
Glutamine (3 mmol/L)	+10 ± 2 (3)
Glycine (2 mmol/L)	+5 ± 0 (3)
*Glycine (2 mmol/L)	+11 ± 0 (3)
Glycine (2 mmol/L) + glutamine (2 mmol/L)	+12 ± 1 (3)
Alanine (2 mmol/L)	+6 ± 0 (7)
*Alanine (2 mmol/L)	+14 ± 2 (6)
Taurochloate (100 μmol/L)	+11 ± 1 (7)
Benzylamine (0.5 mmol/L)	−14 ± 1 (4)
t-Butylhydroperoxide (0.2 mmol/L)	−10 ± 2 (4)
Ethanol (100 mmol/L)	+9 ± 1 (4)
Ethanol in presence of 4-methylpyrazole (0.1 mmol/L)	−6 ± 1 (4)
Acetaldehyde (5 mmol/L)	+9 ± 1 (4)
Hypo-osmotic (265 mOsmol/L)	+10 ± 1 (4)
Hypo-osmotic (225 mOsmol/L)	+16 ± 1 (4)
Hyperosmotic (345 mOsmol/L)	−5 ± 1 (4)
Hyperosmotic (385 mOsmol/L)	−15 ± 2 (4)

The intracellular water space ('liver cell volume') was determined in the perfused rat liver using a [^{3}H]inulin/[^{14}C]urea washout technique as described in ref. 19. Under normo-osmotic conditions (305 mOsmol/L) the intracellular water space was 559 ± 7 μl/g (n = 88); the data are given as percentage change of intracellular water space, as occurs after a 30-min exposure to hormones and amino acids; i.e. after completion of volume-regulatory ion fluxes. Negative values indicate cell shrinkage, positive values cell swelling. Data are from livers from fed rats, except those marked with an asterisk; these denote 24 h starvation. Data are from refs 12, 13, 17, 19, 26, 27, 32 and 34.

be insufficient to account for this. Here, a bile acid-induced increase in membrane Na[+] permeability[14] could come into play.

Ethanol

Ethanol induces cell swelling in isolated hepatocytes[15,16] and perfused rat liver at concentrations of as small as 5 mmol/L[16]. This effect is not due to ethanol itself, because during inhibition of alcohol dehydrogenases by 4-methylpyrazol

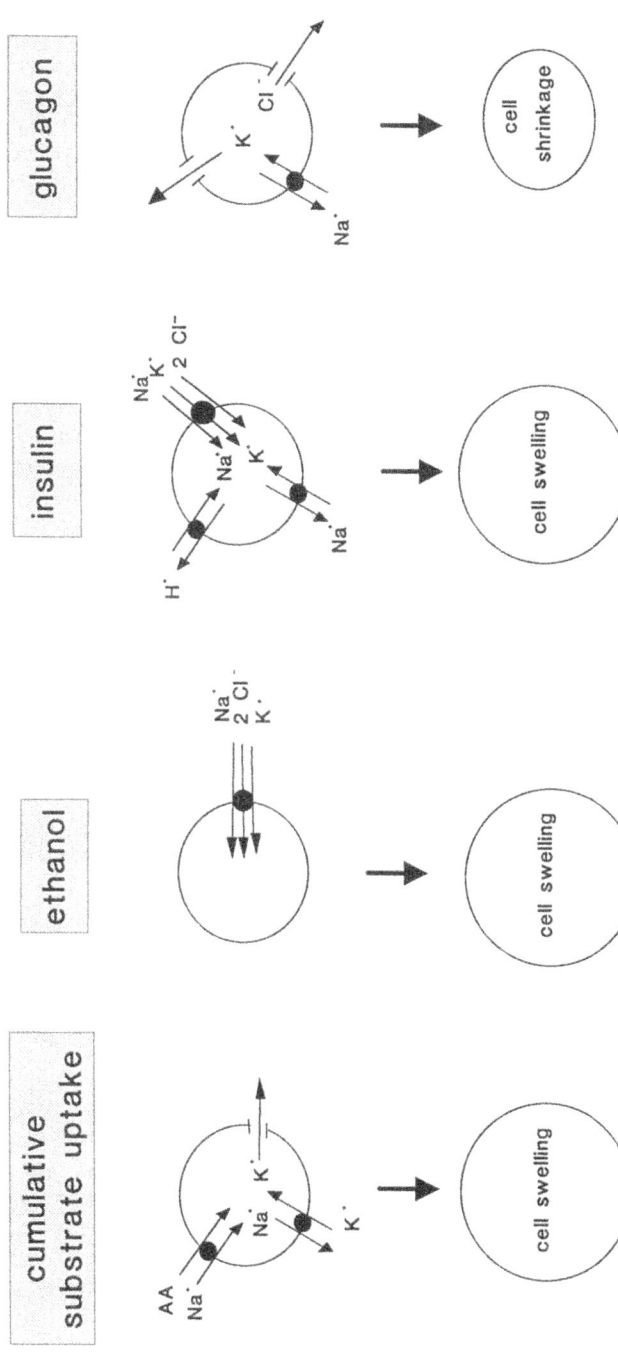

Figure 1 Modulation of hepatocellular hydration by amino acids, ethanol, insulin and glucagon. Amino acids cause cell swelling due to cumulative, Na^+-dependent uptake into the cell. Ethanol activates bumetanide-sensitive Na-K-2Cl transport (or another cation-Cl cotransporter). This transporter is also activated by insulin, which in addition stimulates Na^+/H^+ antiport and Cl^-/HCO_3^- antiport. Cell shrinkage is induced by glucagon due to an opening of K^+ and Cl^- channels

137

addition of ethanol no longer causes cell swelling. It is likely that the swelling potency of ethanol is related to acetaldehyde formation, because acetaldehyde infusion also produces cell swelling. Ethanol/acetaldehyde-induced hepatocyte swelling is completely abolished in the presence of bumetanide, indicating an activation of Na-K-2Cl cotransport, or of another loop diuretic-sensitive cation-chloride cotransporter[16]. It appears that ethanol activates the same bumetanide-sensitive transporter as does insulin (Fig. 1), because the swelling potency of ethanol disappears completely when hepatocytes were pre-exposed to insulin[16].

Insulin and glucagon

Whereas aniso-osmotic exposure and cumulative amino acid transport into hepatocytes lead primarily to cell swelling with secondary activation of volume-regulatory ion transporters, hormones are potent modulators of hepatocyte volume by primarily affecting the activity of volume-regulatory ion transport systems[3,4,17-20] (Fig. 1). Insulin stimulates amiloride-sensitive Na^+/H^+ exchange[21], loop-diuretic-sensitive Na-K-2Cl-cotransport[17,18] and the Na^+/K^+ ATPase[21,22]; i.e. transport systems which are also turned on for regulatory volume increase in hepatocytes and many other cell types (for reviews see refs 1 and 4). The concerted activation of these transporters leads to cellular accumulation of potassium, sodium and chloride, and consequently to cell swelling. Insulin-induced cell swelling and cellular K^+ accumulation is abolished in the presence of bumetanide plus amiloride. Glucagon activates Na^+/K^+-ATPase[4,23], but simultaneously depletes cellular $K^{+17,18}$, probably reflecting the simultaneous opening of K^+ and anion channels[18]. As a result of the cellular depletion of Na^+, K^+, and probably Cl^-, hepatocytes shrink (Fig. 1). The physiological relevance is underlined by the finding that half-maximal effects of insulin and glucagon on liver cell hydration are found at hormone concentrations normally present in portal venous blood in vivo, i.e. at 10^{-9} and 10^{-10}mol/L, respectively[19]. Also other hormones modify hepatocellular hydration[19]. In addition, glucagon and Ca^{2+}-mobilizing hormones were identified as modulators of mitochondrial matrix volume (for review see ref. 24), but may affect the cytosolic and mitochondrial water spaces in opposite directions.

Oxidative stress and urea

Oxidative stress exerted by hydroperoxides induces hepatocellular shrinkage due to an opening of Ba^{2+}-sensitive K^+ channels[25,26]. Cell shrinkage and K^+ channel opening also occur when hydrogen peroxide is generated intracellularly during the oxidation of monoamines. Under these conditions K^+ efflux and cell shrinkage are markedly augmented when H_2O_2 disposal is impaired following inhibition of catalase by aminotriazole, but is abolished by inhibitors of monoamine oxidase, such as pargyline[26]. Thus, the balance between intracellular metabolic H_2O_2 generation and its removal by detoxication systems such as catalase and glutathione peroxidase may be one determinant of hepatocellular K^+ balance and accordingly cell volume[26]. K^+ channel opening under the influence of urea at concentrations found in uraemia also induces cell shrinkage[27].

LIVER CELL HYDRATION AND LIVER CELL FUNCTION

The hepatocellular hydration state is now recognized as an important determinant of cell function. Hormones and nutrients in part exert their effects on metabolism and gene expression in liver by a modification of cell volume. Indeed, long-known adaptations of liver function in response to a protein meal, such as stimulation of protein and glycogen synthesis, inhibition of proteolysis and glycogenolysis or induction of urea cycle enzymes, can also be induced by swelling hepatocytes in hypo-osmotic media. The intracellular signal transduction pathways which are activated in response to cell volume changes, and which mediate the multiple effects of hydration changes on metabolism and gene expression in liver, are complex and only partially characterized[28,30]. Inhibition of these osmosignalling events abolishes the osmosensitivity of some metabolic pathways[29,31]. Control of liver cell function by the hydration state creates an elegant control mechanism which helps to adapt cellular metabolism to alterations of the environment (substrate, tonicity, hormones) and to intestinal nutrient resorption.

Such a regulatory mechanism also implies that the role of Na$^+$ -dependent amino acid transport systems in the plasma membrane is not limited to amino acid translocation. Instead, these transporters also act as transmembrane signalling systems by altering cellular hydration in response to substrate supply (Fig. 2).

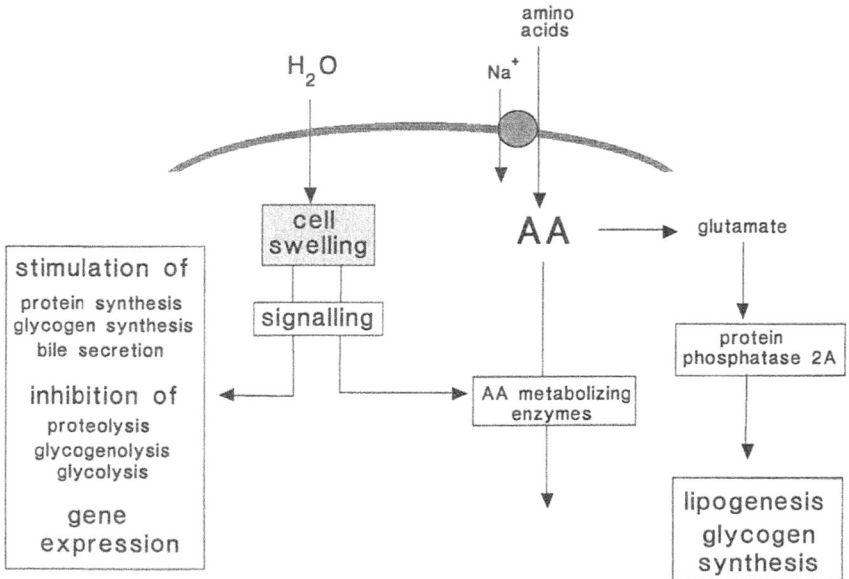

Figure 2 Concentrative amino acid transport and cell function. Na$^+$-dependent amino acid transport systems not only translocate amino acids across the plasma membrane, but simultaneously trigger, via an osmotic water shift into the cell, multiple adaptations of metabolic liver function to the increased nutrient load. In addition to an activation of osmosignalling pathways, glutamate derived from amino acids can directly interfere with protein phosphatases and modulate the basic functional pattern triggered by cell swelling

Likewise, transmembrane ion movements under the influence of hormones are an integral part of hormonal signal transduction mechanisms with alterations of cellular hydration acting as another 'second messenger' of hormone action[1,3,4,18].

The metabolic changes elicited by hepatocyte swelling are listed in Table 2, and in the following sections a few examples are discussed in detail.

Table 2   Effect of hypo-osmotic cell swelling on liver function

---

Increased by hypo-osmotic cell swelling
Protein synthesis
Amino acid uptake
Glutamine breakdown
Glycine oxidation
Urea synthesis from amino acids
Ketoisocaproate oxidation
Glycogen synthesis
Lactate uptake
Pentose phosphate shunt
Acetyl-CoA carboxylase activity
Lipogenesis
Oxygen uptake
MAP-kinase activity
Glutathione (GSH) efflux
Taurocholate excretion into bile
Actin polymerization
Microtubule stability
Exocytosis
pH in vesicular compartments
Transient membrane hyperpolarization

Decreased by cell swelling
Proteolysis
Glutamine synthesis
Urea synthesis from NH_4^+
Glycogenolysis
Glycogenolysis
Glucose-6-phosphatase activity
Carnitine palmitoyl transferase I activity
GSSG in bile
Cytosolic pH, viral replication

Increase of mRNA levels for
c-jun*, ornithine decarboxylase[†], argininosuccinate lyase*[,†]
argininosuccinate synthase*[,†], β-actin[†], tubulin[†], glutaminase*
glutaminase synthase[†]

Decrease of mRNA levels for
Phosphoenolpyruvate carboxykinase*[,†], tyrosine aminotransferase*[,†]
taurine transport (TAUT)*[,†]

Opposite functional patterns are triggered by hyperosmotic cell shrinkage. In general, liver cell swelling acts as an anabolic signal, whereas cell shrinkage is catabolic.
* Effect described in hepatoma cells.
[†] Effect described in rat liver or isolated rat hepatocytes.

LIVER CELL HYDRATION AND PROTEOLYSIS

The long-known antiproteolytic effect of glutamine and glycine in liver is quantitatively mimicked by swelling the cells in hypo-osmotic media to the same extent as in these amino acids (Fig. 3). This indicates that such metabolic effects may be related to the swelling potency of these nutrients.

Indeed, cell hydration is one major mechanism for the control of proteolysis in liver[12,32,33]: cell swelling inhibits, whereas conversely, cell shrinkage stimulates, protein breakdown under conditions in which the proteolytic pathway is not already fully activated. There is a close relationship between the proteolytic activity and the extent of hepatocellular hydration (Fig. 4), regardless of whether the latter is modified by insulin, glucagon, insulin-like growth factor, glutamine, glycine, alanine, ethanol, bile acids, the K^+ channel blocker Ba^{2+} or anisotonic exposure[12,32]. Irrespective of the underlying cause, a 1% increase of hepatocellular hydration gives roughly a 2% inhibition of proteolysis[12,32]. Current evidence suggests that hydration changes are the common mechanism underlying proteolysis control by these effectors in liver: the known antiproteolytic effect of insulin and several (but not all) amino acids is transmitted in large part by

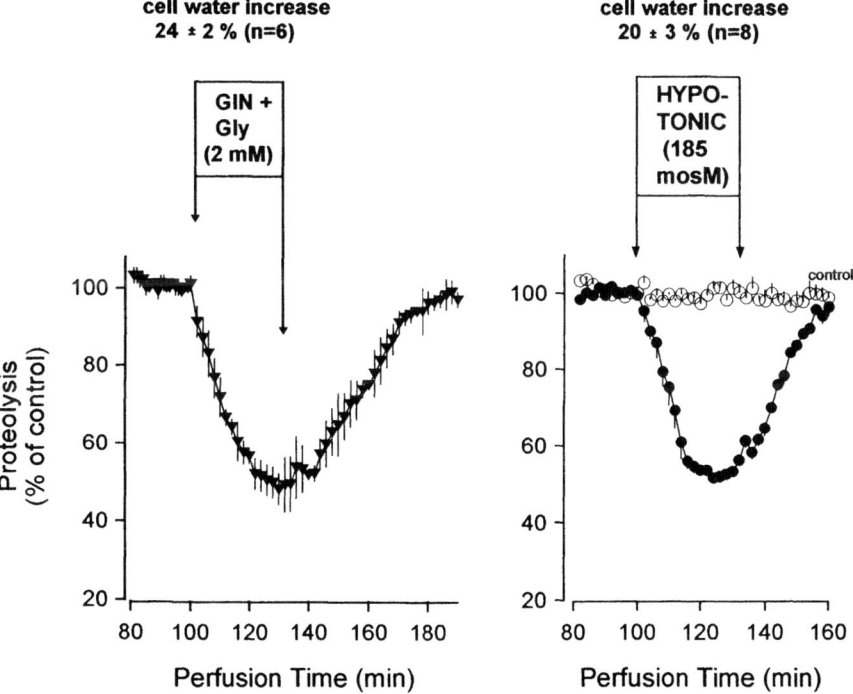

Figure 3 Inhibition of proteolysis in perfused rat liver by glutamine/glycine and hypo-osmotic exposure. The antiproteolytic effect of the amino acids is quantitatively mimicked by swelling the hepatocytes in hypo-osmotic media to the same extent as the amino acids do

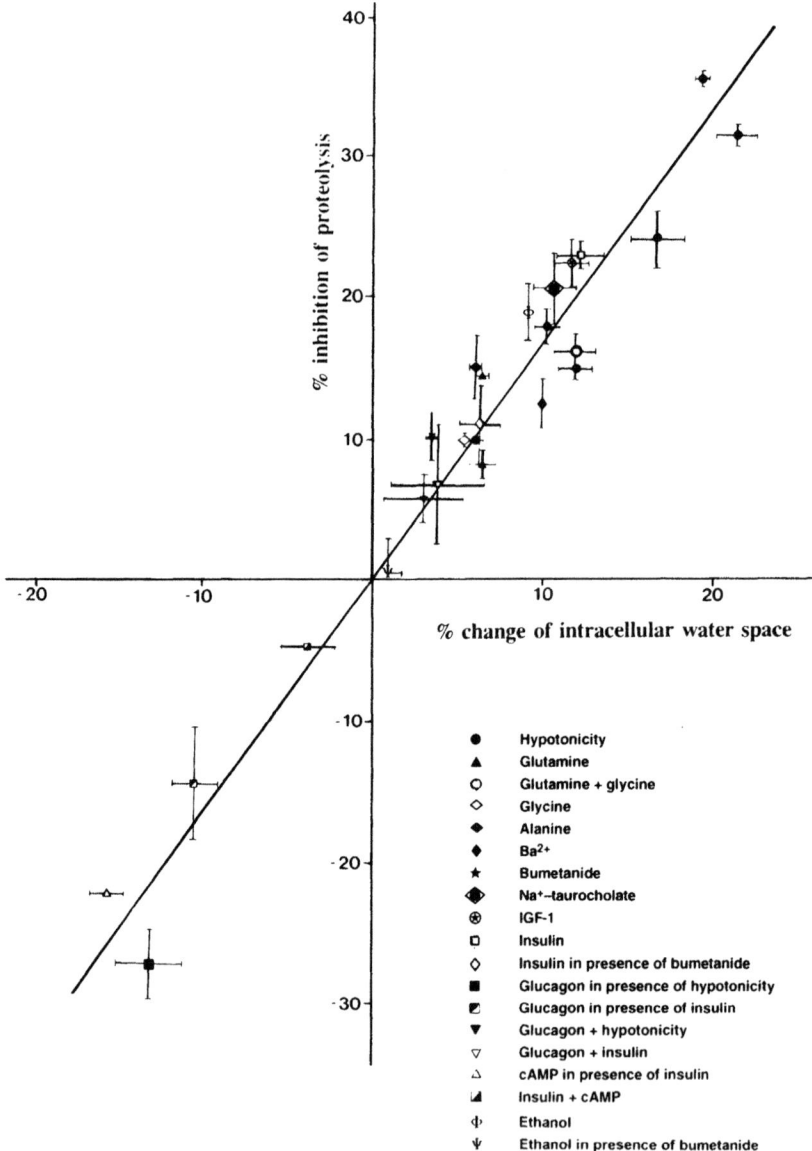

Figure 4 Relationship between cell volume and proteolysis in liver. Cell volume in perfused liver was determined as intracellular water space and proteolysis was assessed as [³H]leucine release in effluent perfusate from perfused livers from rats, which were prelabelled *in vivo* by intraperitoneal injection of [³H]leucine 16 h prior to the perfusion experiment. Cell shrinkage stimulates proteolysis, whereas cell swelling inhibits it. It should be noted that proteolysis is already maximally activated in the absence of hormones and amino acids, and cannot be further stimulated by hyperosmotic or glucagon-induced cell shrinkage. The proteolysis-stimulating effect of these cell-shrinking manoeuvres, however, becomes apparent when proteolysis is preinhibited by either amino acids or insulin. Cell volume changes were induced by insulin, cAMP, glucagon, amino acids, Ba²⁺, taurocholate or aniso-osmotic exposure. Adapted from refs 12 and 32.

agonist-induced cell swelling, whereas stimulation of proteolysis by glucagon is mediated by cell shrinkage[11,12,18,32,34]. Indeed, the antiproteolytic action of insulin disappears, when insulin-induced cell swelling is prevented in the presence of inhibitors of the Na^+/H^+ antiporter and the Na^+-K^+-$2Cl^-$ cotransporter, or is reversed by hyperosmotic shrinkage[11,32]. Likewise, the antiproteolytic effect of ethanol disappears when ethanol-induced cell swelling is inhibited by bumetanide or by 4-methylpyrazole[16]. The nutritional state influences hepatic proteolysis by modifying the swelling potencies of hormones and amino acids[12,33]. For example, in the fed state the anti-proteolytic effect of glycine is only about one-third compared to that found after 24 h starvation due to a 3-fold higher swelling potency of glycine during starvation. The latter is explained by an up-regulation of the glycine-transporting amino acid transport system A in starvation[35]. Similarly, both the swelling potency and the antiproteolytic effect of insulin are diminished in parallel during starvation by 60–70%, probably due to hepatic insulin resistance under these conditions[12].

The mechanisms explaining how cellular hydration exerts control on proteolysis have not been fully established; however, intact microtubular structures are required. Disruption of microtubules by colchicine abolishes the antiproteolytic action of hypo-osmotic, amino acid- or insulin-induced cell swelling in perfused liver[36–38], but not proteolysis control by amino acids, which act via mechanisms other than cell swelling[38]. A requirement for intact microtubules may also explain why hypo-osmotic cell swelling was found to be without effect on proteolysis in freshly isolated rat hepatocytes[38,39]. However, sensitivity of proteolysis to cell volume reappears when cytoskeletal structures are reconstituted in culture[38]. Current evidence suggests that protein phosphorylation may play a role in mediating the volume sensitivity of proteolysis. This regulation could reside at the levels of ribosomal protein S6 phosphorylation[40], acidification of prelysosomal, endocytotic/autophagic vesicular compartments[37,41] and possibly, but not yet proven, at the level of phosphorylation of microtubule-associated proteins.

Liver cell hydration also affects rates of protein synthesis, but in an opposite direction to proteolysis. Hyperosmotic cell shrinkage inhibits, whereas hypo-osmotic cell swelling stimulates, protein synthesis[39,42], and protein synthesis is also stimulated in response to glutamine-induced cell swelling. However, hormone effects on liver protein synthesis cannot consistently be explained on the basis of cell volume changes; here other mechanisms come into play, such as volume-independent hormone signalling towards gene expression.

Liver cell volume also affects amino acid and ammonia metabolism (for reviews see refs 1 and 3). For example glutamine deamidation and glycine oxidation are stimulated in response to hypo-osmotic stress in perfused rat liver[10,43,44], as is glutamine uptake across the plasma membrane[10,45]. Swelling-induced activation of glutaminase and glycine oxidation are most likely due to simultaneous mitochondrial swelling[24], indicating that alterations of amino acid metabolism following aniso-osmotic cell volume changes can at least in part be explained by parallel alterations of mitochondrial matrix volume. The mechanism underlying the activation of glutaminase and glycine cleavage enzyme complex by mitochondrial swelling is not fully understood; however, alterations in mitochondrial membrane fluidity and the attachment of these enzymes to the mitochondrial membrane may play a role.

HEPATOCYTE HYDRATION AND BILE FORMATION

In rat liver, conjugated bile acids are taken up across the sinusoidal plasma membrane by a Na^+-dependent transporter, whereas canalicular excretion is thought to be predominantly accomplished by an ATP-dependent transport system (for reviews see refs 46 and 47) and to represent the rate-controlling step for overall transcellular bile acid transport. In perfused rat liver the rate of transcellular taurocholate transport from the sinusoidal space into the biliary lumen is critically dependent upon the hydration state of the hepatocyte[13,29,48,49]. Cell shrinkage inhibits, whereas cell swelling stimulates, taurocholate excretion into bile, regardless of whether cell volume is modified by anisotonic exposure, amino acids[13] or ethanol. The swelling-induced stimulation of taurocholate excretion into bile is due to an increase of transport capacity[13,29]. An increase of hepatocellular hydration by about 10% leads within minutes to a doubling of the V_{max} of taurocholate excretion into bile. This increase of V_{max} is not explained by changes of cellular ATP content or membrane potential, but is abolished in the presence of colchicine[48,49], indicating the requirement of intact microtubules for the interaction between cellular hydration and taurocholate excretion into bile. From this and the substantial evidence for a transient stimulation of exocytosis as an early response to hypo-osmotic cell swelling[13,48–52], it was postulated that alterations of hepatocellular hydration induce rapid changes of the taurocholate secretion capacity due to a microtubule-dependent insertion/retrieval of canalicular bile acid transporter molecules into/from the canalicular membrane. These transporters may be stored in an intracellular vesicular compartment underneath the canalicular membrane, and could correspond to the known bile acid-containing vesicles, which were seen in the past to reflect 'vesicular transcellular bile acid transport'. Evidence for such an osmodependent insertion/retrieval process of transport ATPases into/out of the canalicular membrane was recently obtained in our laboratory by means of the immunohistochemical localization of MRP2 (cMRP, cMOAT), a canalicular transporter for organic anions[53].

The swelling-induced stimulation of taurocholate excretion is abolished in the presence of tyrosine kinase inhibitors, after pretreatment with cholera or pertussis toxin or in the presence of PD 090859, an inhibitor of mitogen-activated protein (MAP)-kinase kinase (MEK)[28,29,54]. All these inhibitors also interrupt a signal transduction sequence, which mediates a swelling-induced activation of MAP-kinases in rat hepatocytes[28,29,54]. This suggests a causal relationship between swelling-induced MAP-kinase activation and the stimulation of bile acid transport. Interestingly MAP-kinases are also activated by tauroursodeoxycholate, which may explain the stimulation of canalicular bile acid excretion by this compound[54]. However, the upstream signalling events responsible for tauroursodeoxycholate- and swelling-induced MAP-kinase activation are different[54].

Because taurocholate itself increases cellular hydration, a homeostatic feedforward system ensues: an increased bile acid load to the liver induces cell swelling, which in turn augments biliary excretion by triggering the insertion of bile acid transporter molecules into the canalicular membrane. This and the hepatocyte swelling in response to nutrients could help to speed up enterohepatic circulation of bile acids during intestinal absorption.

HEPATOCELLULAR HYDRATION AND GENE EXPRESSION

Cell hydration can also affect hepatic metabolism by modifying gene expression. This involves not only genes coding for osmolyte transporters in Kupffer and sinusoidal endothelial cells, but also the expression of genes which are not necessarily linked to osmoregulation, in parenchymal cells (for review see refs 3 and 4). Examples are argininosuccinate lyase and argininosuccinate synthase (Table 2), whose mRNA levels increase in response to hypo-osmotic exposure and decrease in response to hyperosmotic cell shrinkage[55,56]. This resembles the known induction of urea cycle enzymes in response to protein feeding *in vivo*, and although in this latter situation enzyme induction due to hormonal changes may play an important role, these findings suggest that amino acid-induced hepatocyte swelling may contribute to this adaptation.

Also the mRNA levels of phosphoenolpyruvate carboxykinase (PEPCK) are strongly controlled by hepatocellular hydration; the mRNA levels increase during cell shrinkage and decrease during cell swelling[55,57]. Up-regulation of both PEPCK, a gluconeogenic key enzyme, and of proteolysis in response to hepatocyte shrinkage may be seen as an example for a coordinate adaptation of functionally linked processes by the hydration state. Complementation by an inhibition of glycogen synthesis[58,59] and stimulation of glycogenolysis brings about a glucose-homeostatic response. Osmoregulation of PEPCK mRNA does not involve protein kinase C or changes in cAMP levels[55,57]; it also occurs independently of MAP-kinase activation, but is sensitive to the protein kinase inhibitors H7 and H89[55]. There is some evidence that induction of PEPCK during cell shrinkage is mediated via an activation of Jun-kinases, which also lead to an induction of c-jun mRNA during cell shrinkage, and to a lesser extent during cell swelling[30,60].

CELL VOLUME SENSING AND SIGNALLING

In view of the multiple effects of cell hydration on cell function, the question arises as to how cell volume changes are sensed, and how the signal is transduced to the level of cell function. Little is known about the structures that sense the changes in liver cell hydration, and the issue remains speculative. One hypothesis postulates that the extent of macromolecular crowding, i.e. the cytosolic protein concentration, will determine the tendency of intracellular macromolecules to associate with the plasma membrane and effect their enzymatic activity[61,62]. Other potential candidates for cell volume sensing include the actin cytoskeleton, whose polymerization state increases within 1 min following cell swelling[62], or distinct integral membrane proteins which may act as osmosensors. In line with this, histidine kinases have recently been identified in yeast, which are putative integral membrane proteins and may act as osmosensors[63]. The signal is transduced by autophosphorylation and subsequent phosphate transfer to an aspartate residue in the receiver domain of a cognate response regulator molecule that regulates a MAP-kinase-like protein kinase cascade[64]. As yet, a counterpart in liver has not been identified.

145

The intracellular signalling events which couple changes in liver cell hydration to cell function are known only in part. Different signalling systems are probably activated in parallel following osmotic water flow into or out of the cell. Besides changes in protein phosphorylation, the cytoskeleton and intracellular ions may be involved in linking cell function to cell hydration.

Hypo-osmotic signalling events

In hepatocytes and H4IIE hepatoma cells, hypo-osmotic cell swelling leads within 1 min to an activation of MAP-kinases Erk-1 and Erk-2[28,29]. Erk activation is also observed in response to glutamine-induced cell swelling (unpublished result). MAP-kinases are serine/threonine kinases, which are activated by dual phosphorylation at threonine and tyrosine residues (for review see refs 65 and 66). A signal transduction sequence, which is initiated by the osmotic water shift across the plasma membrane and ultimately leads to changes in cell function, has been identified in rat hepatoma and liver cells[28,29,54]. Here, hypo-osmotic cell swelling results within 1 min in a pertussis toxin-, cholera toxin-, MEK-inhibitor-sensitive and genistein-sensitive, but protein kinase C- and Ca^{2+} independent phosphorylation of the MAP-kinases Erk-1 and Erk-2. This suggests that liver cell swelling leads to a G-protein-mediated activation of a yet-unidentified tyrosine kinase, which acts to activate a pathway towards MEK (MAP-kinase kinase) and MAP-kinases (Fig. 5). The functional significance of this volume-signalling pathway in liver is suggested by the findings that both hypo-osmotic MAP kinase activation and the swelling-induced alkalinization of vesicular compartments[28,31] and stimulation of bile acid excretion[29,4] can be inhibited at upstream events, i.e. at the G-protein or tyrosine kinase or MEK level by suitable inhibitors such as cholera and pertussis toxin, erbstatin, genistein or PD 098059, respectively. The finding that some metabolic responses to hypo-osmotic liver swelling are completely abolished by G-protein, tyrosine kinase and MEK inhibitors indicates that simple dilution of intracellular substrates following the osmotic water shifts cannot explain the cell volume-dependence of metabolism, and suggests that cell volume signalling may start at the plasma membrane. The intracellular signalling cascade which is initiated in response to liver cell swelling (Fig. 5A) resembles that triggered by growth factor receptor activation. This similarity may explain why cell swelling acts like an anabolic signal in liver with respect to protein and carbohydrate metabolism (Table 2). In rat hepatoma cells the swelling-induced MAP kinase activation is accompanied, after an initial transient increase, by a marked and persistent decrease of mRNA levels for MAP-kinase phosphatase-1 (MPK-1). MKP-1 is a dual-specificity protein phosphatase which inactivates MAP-kinases[66] and may contribute to the transient nature of the Erk signal.

MAP-kinases have multiple protein substrates[65,66], such as the microtubule-associated proteins MAP-2 and Tau, other protein kinases, such as S6-kinase and transcription factors such as c-Jun. In fact, the swelling-induced activation of MAP-kinases is followed by an increased phosphorylation of c-Jun, which may explain – due to autoregulation of the c-jun gene – the increase in c-jun mRNA levels 30 min after the onset of cell swelling[28,60]. However, inhibitors of swelling-induced MAP-kinase activation do not abolish the swelling-induced

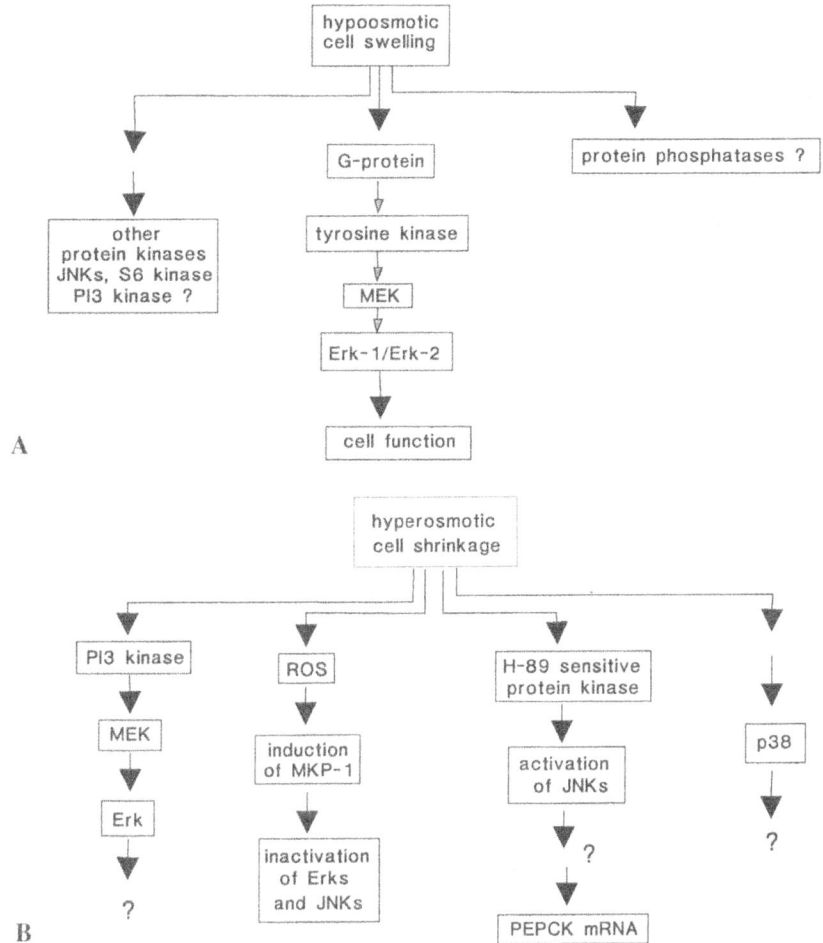

Figure 5 Cell volume signalling in the hepatocyte. The schemes are hypothetical, and it should be kept in mind that the signalling sequences depicted here are far from complete. **A**: Hypo-osmotic signalling; **B**: hyperosmotic signalling. Abbreviations: ROS, reactive oxygen species; Erk, extracellular signal-regulated kinase; JNKs, Jun-kinases; MKP-1, MAP-kinase phosphatase-1

reduction of PEPCK mRNA levels[55]. Accordingly, further, an as-yet-unidentified osmosignalling pathway must be postulated. Microtubules play an important role in transducing some metabolic alterations in response to changes of cellular hydration. For example, disruption of microtubules by colchicine, colcemid or nocodazol abolishes the swelling-induced alkalinization of endocytotic vesicles[37,41], the inhibition of proteolysis[36-38], exocytosis[49] and the stimulation of biliary excretion[48,49,52,67] in liver. It remains to be established to what extent changes in the phosphorylation of microtubule-associated proteins is involved in the microtubule- and MAP-kinase-dependent cell volume signalling.

On the other hand, other pathways which are activated in response to cell swelling, such as stimulation of glycine oxidation or of the pentose phosphate shunt, are not affected following microtubule disruption. Intact microtubules are not required for the swelling-induced activation of MAP-kinases (Schliess F, Häussinger D, unpublished result). This suggests that microtubular structures are required during cell volume signalling at a step downstream of MAP-kinases.

Hyperosmotic signalling

Hyperosmotic cell shrinkage leads within 20 min to an activation of Jun-kinases[30], being followed by a strong induction of c-jun mRNA (Fig. 5B). This could at least in part explain the up-regulation of PEPCK mRNA levels in response to cell shrinkage via modulation of AP-1 transcription factor activity. In line with this speculation is the observation that both hyperosmotic Jun-kinase activation and PEPCK induction are sensitive to inhibition by H89. Hyperosmotic exposure also leads to a weak and delayed wortmannin-sensitive activation of Erks, and an induction of MAP-kinase phosphatase-1 (MKP-1), which acts to terminate the Erk and Jun-kinase signals[30]. MKP-1 induction in response to cell shrinkage can be blocked by antioxidants, indicating that oxidative stress is involved in hyperosmotic signalling[30]. However, little is known about the precise role played by these protein kinase and phosphatase activity changes for specific changes in cell function.

PERSPECTIVE

Current evidence suggests that changes of liver cell hydration in response to nutrients and hormones are an independent and potent signal which helps to adapt metabolic liver function and gene expression to changes in intestinal absorption. It appears that nutrient-induced cell swelling activates signal trans-duction mechanisms which produce an anabolic response, whereas nutrient deprivation-induced cell shrinkage triggers a catabolic state. Apparently, cell hydration changes trigger basic patterns of cell function which can be modified in detail by direct effects of specific nutrients on intracellular signalling path-ways. One example is the finding that hypo-osmotic cell swelling lowers PEPCK mRNA levels, whereas glutamine-induced cell swelling leads to an up-regulation of PEPCKm mRNA levels. Both responses appear meaningful, because an up-regulation of gluconeogenesis should be favoured in response to a portal amino acid load, even when cell swelling switches off hepatic proteolysis. Here apparently substrate-specific regulatory mechanisms come into play which override the signals which are set by hydration changes. Indeed, a glutamate-activated protein phosphatase from the 2A class has recently been identified[68], which also mediates the glutamine-induced increase of lipogenesis.

The complex interplay between cell hydration and the function of liver parenchymal and non-parenchymal cells also has considerable impact on our understanding of liver function in health and disease. These interactions involve not only problems of cholestasis, hepatic protein turnover and viral replication[69], but also mechanisms of liver damage due to the important role of cell hydration for the function of non-parenchymal cells[70-73]. Here, in addition to cell hydration, the availability of osmolytes, such as betaine and taurine, and the expression of the respective osmolyte transporters were shown to have important consequences for the production of mediators of inflammation by these cells and their phagocytotic activity. It is hoped that this review will stimulate further research in this exciting area.

Acknowledgements

Our own work reported herein was supported by Deutsche Forschungsgemeinschaft, the Gottfried-Wilhelm-Leibniz-Prize, the Schilling-Stiftung and the Fonds der Chemischen Industrie.

References

1. Lang F, Häussinger D, editors. Interaction of cell volume and cell function. Heidelberg: Springer Verlag; 1993.
2. Häussinger D. Regulation and functional significance of liver cell volume. Prog Liv Dis. 1996;14:29–53.
3. Häussinger D. The role of cellular hydration for the regulation of cell function. Biochem J. 1996;313:697–710.
4. Graf J, Häussinger D. Ion transport in hepatocytes: mechanisms and correlations to cell volume, hormone actions and metabolism. J Hepatol. 1996;24:53–77.
5. Haberich FJ, Aziz O, Nowacki PE. Flüssigkeitsspeicherung in der Leber nach enteraler Wasserresorption. Pflügers Arch. 1966;285:73–89.
6. Lee JH, Arcinue E, Ross BD. Organic osmolytes in the brain of an infant with hypernatremia. N Engl J Med. 1994;331:439–42.
7. Häussinger D, Laubenberger J, vom Dahl S. et al. Proton magnetic resonance spectroscopic studies on human brain myo-inositol in hypoosmolarity and hepatic encephalopathy. Gastroenterology. 1994;107:1475–80.
8. Bakker-Grunwald T. Potassium permeability and volume control in isolated rat hepatocytes. Biochim Biophys Acta. 1983;731:239–42.
9. Kristensen LO, Folke M. Volume-regulatory K^+ efflux during concentrative uptake of alanine in isolated rat hepatocytes. Biochem J. 1984;221:265–8.
10. Häussinger D, Lang F, Bauers K, Gerok W. Interactions between glutamine metabolism and cell volume regulation in perfused rat liver. Eur J Biochem. 1990;188:689–95.
11. Hallbrucker C, vom Dahl S, Lang F, Gerok W, Häussinger D. Inhibition of hepatic proteolysis by insulin: role of hormone-induced alterations of cellular K^+ balance. Eur J Biochem. 1991;199:467–74.
12. vom Dahl S, Häussinger D. Nutritional state and the swelling-induced inhibition of proteolysis in the perfused rat liver. J Nutr. 1996;126:395–402.
13. Häussinger D, Hallbrucker C, Saha N, Lang F, Gerok W. Cell volume is a major determinant of bile acid excretion. Biochem J. 1992;288:681–9.
14. Wehner F. Taurocholate depolarizes rat hepatocytes in primary culture by increasing cell membrane Na^+ conductance. Pflügers Arch. 1993;424:145–51.
15. Wondergem R, Davis J. Ethanol increases hepatocyte water volume. Alcoholism Clin Exp Res. 1994;18:1230–6.
16. vom Dahl S, Häussinger D, Bumetanide-sensitive cell swelling mediates the inhibitory effect of ethanol on hepatic proteolysis. (Submitted).
17. Hallbrucker C, vom Dahl S, Lang F, Gerok W, Häussinger D. Modification of liver cell volume by insulin and glucagon. Pflügers Arch. 1991;418:519–21.
18. Häussinger D, Lang F. Cell volume and hormone action. Trends Pharmacol Sci. 1992;13:371–3.
19. vom Dahl S, Hallbrucker C, Lang F, Gerok W, Häussinger D. Regulation of liver cell volume by hormones. Biochem J. 1991;280:105–9.

20. Al-Habori M, Peak M, Thomas TH, Agius L. The role of cell swelling in the stimulation of glycogen synthesis by insulin. Biochem J. 1992;282:789–96.
21. Jakubowski J, Jakob A. Vasopressin, insulin and peroxides of vanadate influence Na$^+$ transport mediated by Na$^+$/K$^+$ ATPase or Na$^+$/H$^+$ exchanger of rat liver plasma membrane vesicles. Eur J Biochem. 1990;193:541–9.
22. Fehlmann M, Freychat P. Insulin and glucagon stimulation of Na$^+$/K$^+$ ATPase transport activity in isolated rat hepatocytes. J Biol Chem. 1981;256:7449–53.
23. Moule SK, McGivan JD. Regulation of the plasma membrane potential in hepatocytes – mechanisms and physiological significance. Biochim Biophys Acta. 1990;1031:383–97.
24. Halestrap AP. The regulation of the matrix volume of mammalian mitochondria *in vivo* and *in vitro* and its role in the control of mitochondrial metabolism. Biochim Biophys Acta. 1989;973:355–82.
25. Hallbrucker C, Ritter M, Lang F, Gerok W, Häussinger D. Hydroperoxide metabolism in rat liver: K$^+$ channel activation, cell volume changes and eicosanoid formation. Eur J Biochem. 1992;211:449–58.
26. Saha N, Schreiber R, vom Dahl S, Lang F, Gerok W, Häussinger D. Endogenous hydroperoxide formation, cell volume and cellular K$^+$ balance in perfused rat liver. Biochem J. 1993;296:701–7.
27. Hallbrucker C, vom Dahl S, Ritter M, Lang F, Häussinger D. Effects of urea on K$^+$ fluxes and cell volume in perfused rat liver. Pflügers Arch. 1994;428:552–60.
28. Schliess F, Schreiber R, Häussinger D. Activation of of extracellular signal related kinases Erk-1 and Erk-2 by cell swelling in H4IIE hepatoma cells. Biochem J. 1995;309:13–17.
29. Noé B, Schliess F, Wettstein M, Heinrich S, Häussinger D. Regulation of taurocholate excretion by a hypoosmolarity-activated signal transduction pathway in rat liver. Gastroenterology. 1996;110:858–65.
30. Schliess F, Heinrich S, Häussinger D. Hyperosmotic induction of the mitogen-activated protein kinase phosphatase MKP-1 in H4IIE rat hepatoma cells. Biochem J. (Submitted).
31. Schreiber R, Häussinger D. Characterization of the swelling-induced alkalinization of endocytotic vesicles in fluorescein isothiocyanate-dextran-loaded rat hepatocytes. Biochem J. 1995;309:19–24.
32. Häussinger D, Hallbrucker C, vom Dahl S, Decker S, Schweizer U, Lang F, Gerok W. Cell volume is a major determinant of proteolysis control in liver. FEBS Lett. 1991;283:70–2.
33. Hallbrucker C, vom Dahl S, Lang F, Häussinger D. Control of hepatic proteolysis by amino acids: the role of cell volume. Eur J Biochem. 1991;197:717–24.
34. vom Dahl S, Hallbrucker C, Lang F, Gerok W, Häussinger D. Regulation of liver cell volume and proteolysis by glucagon and insulin. Biochem J. 1991;278:771–7.
35. Hayes MR, McGivan JD. Differential effects of starvation on alanine and glutamine transport in isolated rat hepatocytes. Biochem J. 1982;204:365–8.
36. Häussinger D, Stoll B, vom Dahl S et al. Effect of hepatocyte swelling on microtubule stability and tubulin mRNA levels. Biochem Cell Biol. 1994;72:12–19.
37. Busch GL, Schreiber R, Dartsch PC et al. Involvement of microtubules in the link between cell volume and pH of acidic cellular compartments in rat and human hepatocytes. Proc Natl Acad Sci USA. 1994;91:9165–9.
38. vom Dahl S, Stoll B, Gerok W, Häussinger D. Inhibition of proteolysis by cell swelling in the liver requires intact microtubular structures. Biochem J. 1995;308:529–36.
39. Meijer AJ, Gustafson LA, Luiker JJFP et al. Cell swelling and the sensitivity of autophagic proteolysis to inhibition by amino acids in isolated rat hepatocytes. Eur J Biochem. 1993;215:449–54.
40. Luiken JFP, Blommaart EFC, Boon L, van Woerkom GM, Meijer AJ. Cell swelling and the control of autophagic proteolysis in hepatocytes: involvement of phosphorylation of ribosomal protein S6? Biochem Soc Trans. 1994;22:458–61.
41. Schreiber R, Stoll B, Lang F, Häussinger D. Effects of aniso-osmolarity and hydroperoxides on intracellular pH in isolated rat hepatocytes as assessed by (2′,7′)-bis(carboxyethyl)-5(6)-carboxyfluorescein and fluorescein isothiocyanate-dextran fluorescence. Biochem J. 1994;303:113–20.
42. Stoll B, Gerok W, Lang F, Häussinger D. Liver cell volume and protein synthesis. Biochem J. 1992;287:217–22.
43. Häussinger D, Stoll B, Morimoto Y, Lang F, Gerok W. Anisoosmotic liver perfusion: redox shifts and modulation of α-ketoisocaproate and glycine metabolism. Biol Chem Hoppe-Seyler. 1992;373:723–34.

44. Brosnan JT, Jois M, Hall B. Hormonal regulation of glycine metabolism. In: Lubeck G, Rosenthal GA, editors. Amino acids: biochemistry, biology and medicine. ESCOM Science Publ BV; 1990:869–902.
45. Bode B, Kilberg MS. Amino acid dependent increase of hepatic system N activity is linked to cell swelling. J Biol Chem. 1991;266:7376–81.
46. Boyer JL, Graf J, Meier PJ. Hepatic transport systems regulating pH_i, cell volume and bile excretion. Annu Rev Physiol. 1992;54:415–38.
47. Nathanson MH, Boyer JL. Mechanisms and regulation of bile secretion. Hepatology. 1991;14:551–566.
48. Häussinger D, Saha N, Hallbrucker C, Lang F, Gerok W. Involvement of microtubules in the swelling-induced stimulation of transcellular taurocholate transport in perfused rat liver. Biochem J. 1993;291:355–60.
49. Bruck R, Haddad P, Graf J, Boyer JL. Regulatory volume decrease stimulates bile flow, bile acid excretion and exocytosis in isolated perfused rat liver. Am J Physiol. 1992;262:G806–12.
50. Pfaller W, Willinger C, Stoll B, Hallbrucker C, Lang F, Häussinger D. Structural reaction pattern of hepatocytes following exposure to hypotonicity. J Cell Physiol. 1993;154:248–53.
51. Gratzl R, Gajdzik L, Lassacher R, Graf J. Observations on exocytosis and endocytosis in hepatocytes subjected to osmotic stress. In: Wehner F, Petzinger E, editors. Cell biology and molecular basis of liver transport. Dortmund: Projekt Verlag; 1995:44–51.
52. Keppler D, Kartenbeck J. The canalicular conjugate export pump encoded by the cmrp/cmoat gene. Prog Liv Dis. 1996;14:55–67.
53. Kubitz R, D'Urso D, Keppler D, Häussinger D. Osmodependent dynamic localization of the mrp2 gene-encoded conjugate export pump in the rat hepatocyte canalicular membrane. Gastroenterology. 1997; in press.
54. Schliess F, Kurz AK, vom Dahl S, Häussinger D. Activation of mitogen-activated protein kinases mediates the stimulation of bile acid secretion by tauroursodeyoxycholate in rat liver. Gastroenterology. 1997;113:1306–14.
55. Warskulat U, Newsome WP, Noé B, Stoll B, Häussinger D. Anisoosmotic regulation of hepatic gene expression. Biol Chem Hoppe Seyler. 1996;377:57–65.
56. Quillard M, Husson A, Lavoinne A. Glutamine increases argininosuccinate synthetase mRNA levels in rat hepatocytes. The involvement of cell swelling. Eur J Biochem. 1996;236:56–9.
57. Newsome WP, Warskulat U, Noe B et al. Modulation of phosphoenolpyruvate carboxykinase mRNA levels by the hepatocellular hydration state. Biochem J. 1994;304:555–60.
58. Baquet A, Maisin L, Hue L. Swelling of hepatocytes activates acetyl-CoA carboxylase in parallel to glycogen synthase. Biochem J. 1991;278:887–90.
59. Meijer AJ, Baquet A, Gustafson L, van Woerkom GM, Hue L. Mechanism of activation of liver glycogen synthase by swelling. J Biol Chem. 1992;267:5823–8.
60. Finkenzeller G, Newsome WP, Lang F, Häussinger D. Increase of c-jun mRNA upon hypoosmotic cell swelling of rat hepatoma cells. FEBS Lett. 1994;340:163–6.
61. Minton AP, Colclasure GC, Parker JC. Model for the role of macromolecular crowding in regulation of cellular volume. Proc Natl Acad Sci USA. 1992;89:10504–6.
62. Parker JC. In defense of cell volume? Am J Physiol. 1993;265:C1191–200.
63. Theodoropoulos PA, Stournaras C, Stoll B et al. Hepatocyte swelling leads to rapid actin polymerization and increases actin mRNA levels. FEBS Lett. 1992;311:241–5.
64. Maeda T, Wurgler-Murphy SM, Saito H. A two-component system that regulates an osmosensing MAP kinase cascade in yeast. Nature. 1994;369:242–5.
65. Nishida E, Gotoh Y. The MAP kinase cascade is essential for diverse signal transduction pathways. Trends Biochem Sci. 1993;18:128–31.
66. Waskiewicz AJ, Cooper JA. Mitogen and stress response pathways: MAP kinase cacades and phosphatase regulation in mammals and yeast. Curr Opin Cell Biol. 1995;7:798–805.
67. Boyer JL, Soroka CJ. Vesicle targeting to the apical domain regulates bile excretory function in isolated rat hepatocytes. Gastroenterology. 1995;109:1600–11.
68. Baquet A, Gaussin V, Bollen M, Stalmans W, Hue L. Mechanism of activation of liver acetyl-CoA carboxylase by cell swelling. Eur J Biochem. 1993;217:1083–9.
69. Offensperger WB, Offensperger S, Stoll B, Gerok W, Häussinger D. Effects of anisoosmotic exposure on duck hepatitis B virus replication. Hepatology. 1994;20:1–7.
70. Zhang F, Wettstein M, Warskulat U et al. Hyperosmolarity stimulates prostaglandin synthesis and cyclooxygenase-2 expression in activated rat Kupffer cells. Biochem J. 1995;312:135–43.

71. Warskulat U, Zhang F, Häussinger D. Modulation of phagocytosis by anisoosmolarity and betaine in rat liver macrophages (Kupffer cells) and RAW 264.7 mouse macrophages. FEBS Lett. 1996;391:287–92.
72. Zhang F, Warskulat U, Häussinger D. Modulation of tumor necrosis factor-α release by anisoosmolarity and betaine in rat liver macrophages. FEBS Lett. 1996;391:293–6.
73. Zhang F, Warskulat U, Wettstein M, Häussinger D. Identification of betaine as an osmolyte in rat liver macrophages. Gastroenterology. 1996;110:858–65.

11
Amino acid metabolism in the gut

M. PLAUTH and A.-E. ROSKE

INTRODUCTION

Transport of solutes and water has long been regarded as the major function of intestinal epithelial cells. In recent decades, however, it has been found that the intestinal epithelium is actively involved in the metabolism of xenobiotics[1] or compounds such as heme or bilirubin[2] or the synthesis of lipoproteins[3]. This review will focus on the role of the small intestine in intermediary amino metabolism, particularly that of glutamine.

As early as 1939 ammonia release during osmotic work was thought to originate within the gut wall[4]. Subsequently, transamination by intestinal mucosa of glutamate, aspartate and later also of branched-chain keto acids and aromatic amino acids has been demonstrated[5-11].

GLUTAMINE METABOLISM IN RAT INTESTINE

Uptake of glutamine and release of alanine was observed by Finch and Hird[12] in their studies using intestinal segments; later, Neptune[13] found a rise in CO_2 release from glutamine consumed by intestinal rings, and he suggested that glutamine may be utilized as metabolic fuel.

In a series of pioneering experiments Windmueller and Spaeth[14-18] investigated glutamine metabolism in preparations of isolated perfused intestine or segmental *in-situ* perfusions. From their data it became clear that the intestinal mucosa extracted glutamine from arterial blood at a rate of 25–30%. Within mucosal cells glutamine then was metabolized into CO_2, ammonia, alanine and citrulline as major metabolic products (Fig. 1). Obviously, only about 20–40% of glutamine carbon was oxidized to yield energy and CO_2, whereas the remainder was released in the form of alanine or citrulline. These workers also demonstrated that the K_m value of intestinal glutaminase, the key enzyme for the degradation of glutamine, was 2.2 mmol/L. This value is much closer to arterial glutamine concentrations than the K_m value of 22 mmol/L for hepatic mitochondrial glutaminase[19]. It was also shown that glutamine was utilized predominantly

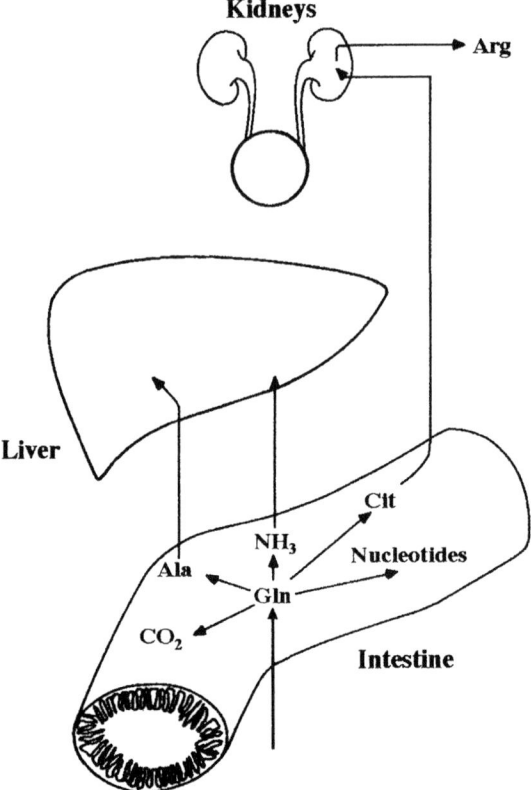

Figure 1 Intestinal metabolism of glutamine into CO_2, alanine (Ala), ammonia (NH_3), citrulline (Cit), and arginine (Arg). Glutamine also serves as the most important nitrogen donor for the biosynthesis of nucleotides or amino sugars

by intestinal mucosal cells, whereas cells of the submucosa or muscularis layer consumed only little glutamine[19]. In cultures of freshly isolated rat enterocytes it was demonstrated that specific functions of intestinal epithelial cells were dependent on glutamine[20].

In the rat, intestinal mucosal cells are the major source of circulating citrulline which, in the kidney, can be converted into arginine[18]. Subsequent observations confirmed the important role of the small intestine for whole-body arginine metabolism and protein synthesis. In rats, inhibition of intestinal citrulline synthesis caused severe growth retardation[21] and arginine became an essential amino acid after extensive resection of small intestine[22].

Glutamine metabolism by intestinal mucosal cells is not dependent on the route of glutamine supply, i.e. from arterial blood or from the intestinal lumen, and the pattern of metabolic products does not vary according to route of administration[15,23].

METABOLISM OF OTHER AMINO ACIDS

From studies in experimental animals there is evidence that not only glutamine, glutamate or aspartate, but also asparagine, glycine (to serine), leucine (to ammonia) and alanine (to ammonia and glutamate) are not only absorbed in intact form but also subject to metabolism by the intestinal mucosa[16,24]. Conversely, transamination of luminally administered keto acids has also been described[25,26].

INTESTINAL GLUTAMINE METABOLISM IN HUMANS

Due to the difficult access to the portal or the mesenteric vein only limited data are available on intestinal glutamine metabolism in humans. For a long time arterial–portal-venous concentration differences obtained during elective surgery in a limited number of patients were the only evidence to confirm a significant net uptake by the intestinal tract also in humans[27–29]. Only recently have these data been extended and reaffirmed[30–32], demonstrating also a release of alanine, ammonia and citrulline[32].

The important role of the small intestine in whole-body glutamine synthesis can be deduced from the following observations. After subtotal resection the whole-body rate of appearance of [^{15}N]glutamine, a measure of substrate turnover, was significantly reduced, whereas that of leucine remained unaltered[33]. After duodenal infusion the extraction of [2-^{15}N]glutamine by the intestinal tract was 54%, indicating an avid 'first-pass' metabolism already during absorption; the extraction of [^{15}N]glutamate (88%) was even higher[34]. In critically ill patients, glutamine release from skeletal muscle was significantly reduced only in those who underwent extensive small bowel resection[35]. This was interpreted as a reduction in the demand of glutamine due to loss of intestinal tissue; in that view the release of glutamine from skeletal muscle would have been governed by intestinal demand.

INTESTINAL GLUTAMINE METABOLISM IN PATHOPHYSIOLOGICAL CONDITIONS

In dogs, after trauma an increase in gut glutamine consumption and a reduction in alanine release has been observed initially[36]. This finding was not fully confirmed in as much as selective catheterization demonstrated a reduction in intestinal, but an increase in splenic, glutamine consumption in operated pigs[37]. This discrepancy may be due to the fact that, in the original study, arterial–venous differences of portal drained viscera, i.e. intestine and spleen and pancreas, rather than selective intestinal arterial–venous differences, were measured.

In sepsis, intestinal glutamine uptake seems to be reduced in experimental animals and in humans[38,39].

In experimental animals, a number of investigations have been performed to study the effect of acidosis on intestinal glutamine metabolism, and results are heterogeneous. In chronically catheterized dogs acidosis was accompanied by an increase in intestinal glutamine uptake and ammonia release[40], that was not reduced after correction of the acidosis. However, in acidotic animals hepatic glutamine balance shifted from uptake to release, and arterial glutamine levels were increased, although muscle release did not change[40]. In perfusions of iso-lated rat intestine, acidosis *per se* did not alter glutamine metabolism[23]; it is therefore likely that during acidosis changes in intestinal glutamine metabolism resulted predominantly from increased substrate availability.

In acidotic animals the increased intestinal glutamine consumption is associ-ated with a change in the pattern of major metabolic products. Ammonia release is increased at the expense of alanine release. This ammonia partitioning is asso-ciated with a decrease in urinary excretion of urea, but an increase in that of ammonia[41]. This phenomenon has been interpreted as an example of metabolic cooperation between intestine and liver, in which the intestine provides the liver with increased amounts of ammonia, thereby favouring hepatic glutamine pro-duction over ureagenesis (Fig. 2). As a result, glutamine would be available in

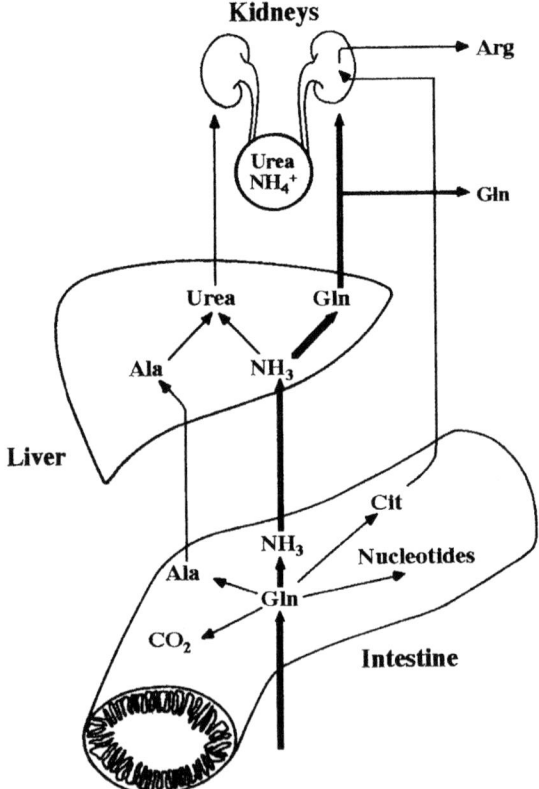

Figure 2   Role of intestinal glutamine metabolism during metabolic acidosis favouring hepatic glu-tamine production from ammonia for renal acid excretion via protonated ammonia. Ala: alanine, Arg: arginine, Cit: citrulline, Glc: glucose, Gln: glutamine

amounts sufficient for renal acid excretion via ammonia[42]. Obviously, portal ammonia concentration seems to be a relevant signal for this change in hepatic glutamine flux[43,44].

For whole-body glutamine metabolism the small intestine and liver, but also skeletal muscle, kidneys and mononuclear cells, are the most relevant tissues. Skeletal muscle provides the largest pool of free glutamine in the body. Skeletal muscle and, according to the prevailing metabolic condition, liver are the major endogenous sources of glutamine. Intestine, mononuclear cells and kidneys are net consumers of glutamine. The central position of intestine and liver in whole-body nitrogen metabolism is illustrated in Fig. 3. Channelling nitrogen flux into ureagenesis leads to irreversible nitrogen loss, whereas hepatic synthesis of glutamine provides the options for either nitrogen retention or nitrogen excretion in the form of urinary ammonia.

METABOLIC COOPERATION OF INTESTINE AND LIVER *IN VITRO*

To study metabolic cooperation between intestine and liver, preparations of isolated rat intestine and liver have been used in a combined perfusion model[45]. This has proved a viable and metabolically stable preparation. Regarding glutamine metabolism, the combined perfusion resulted in stable concentrations of ammonia and alanine in the recirculating perfusate, despite the constant release

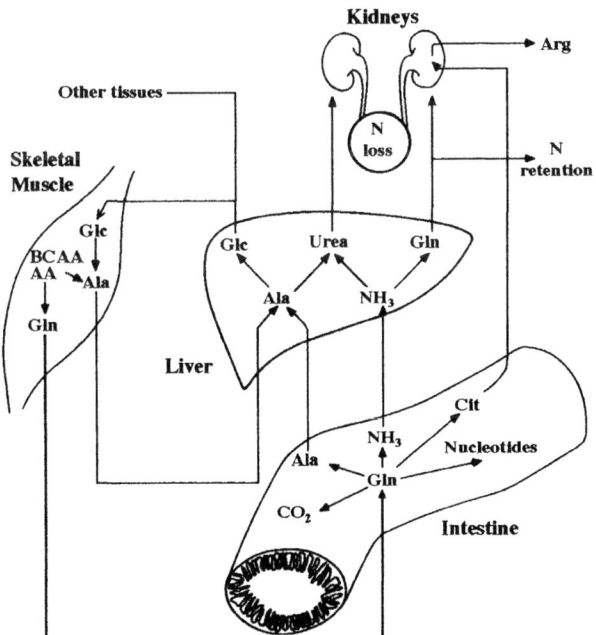

Figure 3 Central position of intestine and liver in interorgan glutamine metabolism. AA: amino acids, Ala: alanine, Arg: arginine, BCAA: branched-chain amino acids, Cit: citrulline, Glc: glucose, Gln: glutamine

of both compounds from intestinal metabolism[45]. As another example of gut–liver interaction in this preparation a switch from hepatic glutamine release to uptake has been shown to occur following luminal perfusion with glucose[46]. In a different preparation with single-pass perfusion and intact nerve supply to liver and intestine, glucose absorption has been shown to increase after portal insulin levels had been raised[47]. These observations illustrate that metabolic cooperation between intestine and liver can also be demonstrated *in vitro*, and that these preparations may serve useful to further clarify the mechanisms involved[48].

POST-FEEDING HYPERAMMONEMIA – A MODEL FOR DISTURBED GUT–LIVER COOPERATION

Hyperammonaemic coma in germ-free animals with a portocaval anastomosis, or after hepatectomy, has puzzled investigators for a long time[49,50]. This situation has been termed 'the germ-free paradox', since according to traditional views hyperammonaemia was due to absorbed ammonia that was generated by the metabolism of colonic bacteria. This 'paradox', however, can easily be explained on the basis of intestinal glutamine metabolism as discussed above[14–17,51]. Indeed, the endogenous ammoniagenesis resulting from small intestinal glutamine utilization was the most obvious cause for hyperammonaemia in these animals.

Based on animal studies it was proposed that 50% of the portal ammonia load was derived from intestinal glutamine metabolism rather than colonic bacterial metabolism[51]. It was also hypothesized that disaccharides or unabsorbable antibiotics might be effective in the treatment of hyperammonaemia by a direct effect on intestinal glutamine metabolism[52]. In perfusion studies of isolated rat small intestine, however, this view could not be confirmed[53]. Moreover, antibiotics were ineffective in preventing hyperammonaemia after blood gavage in dogs, whereas after a blood enema the rise in blood ammonia was prevented by such treatment[54].

Recently, the role of intestinal ammonia generation from arterial and/or luminal glutamine has also been verified in patients with cirrhosis of the liver[55]. In these patients the intestine and the kidneys were the major sources of ammonia in the fasting state. The immediate rise in arterial–mesenteric venous concentration differences after the initiation of duodenal feeding documented that the small intestine was the major source of post-feeding hyperammonaemia in patients with liver cirrhosis and trans-jugular intrahepatic portosystemic shunt.

In healthy humans, the small intestinal mucosa processes compounds such as glutamine for optimal utilization by the liver according to the whole organism's needs. Alanine and ammonia are provided at high concentrations in portal blood, and these substrates can readily be utilized by periportal hepatocytes[56]. On the contrary, dicarboxylic amino acids such as glutamate or aspartate, which can only be taken up by the small population of perivenous hepatocytes[57], are extracted efficiently by the intestine. Thus, one might understand this cooperation in an extended view of splanchnic rather than just hepatic metabolic zona-

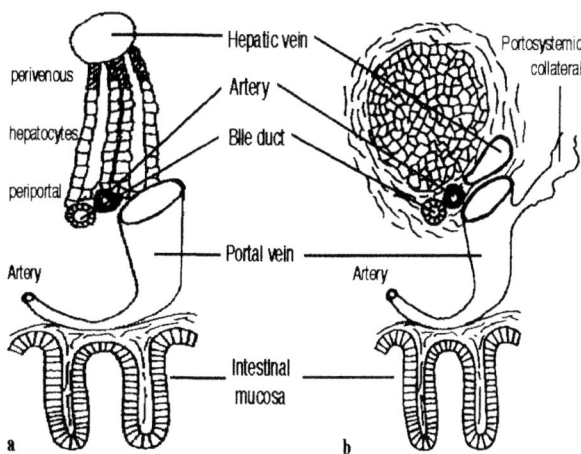

Figure 4   a: Proposed view of the metabolic zonation of splanchnic organs and its role in health, when intestinal metabolism provides periportal hepatocytes with substrates in optimal composition and quantity. This is exemplified by high ammonia and low glutamate or aspartate concentrations in portal blood. **b**: In liver cirrhosis, metabolic zonation of splanchnic organs is disrupted. In the liver, hepatocyte zonation is severely disrupted within pseudolobules. Intra- and extrahepatic porto-systemic collaterals allow products of intestinal metabolism, such as ammonia, to escape into the systemic circulation which were destined exclusively for the liver

tion, or an extended version of functional heterogeneity of splanchnic epithelia (Fig. 4a).

In patients with liver cirrhosis, the beneficial effects of this finely tuned metabolic cooperation between intestine and liver is broken by the occurrence of portosystemic collateral circulation. In this situation, portal blood with high ammonia concentrations is shunted away from the liver into the systemic circulation producing autointoxication (Fig. 4b).

SUMMARY

In the small intestine, amino acids are not merely translocated intact, but are also metabolized to a varying degree. As a paradigm, whole-body glutamine metabolism is greatly influenced by the metabolic cooperation between intestine and liver. The interruption of this cooperation may result in life-threating metabolic derangements such as hyperammonaemia and hepatic encephalopathy. Therefore, it seems justified to view this cooperation of intestine and liver as an extended model of metabolic zonation of splanchnic organs.

References

1. Koster AS, Richter E, Lauterbach F, Hartmann F. Intestinal metabolism of xenobiotics. Progr Pharmacol Clinical Pharmacol. 7/2. Stuttgart: Fischer; 1988.
2. Hartmann F, Bissell DM. Metabolism of heme and bilirubin in rat and human small intestinal mucosa. J Clin Invest. 1982;70:23–9.
3. Kuksis A, Shaikh NA, Hoffman AGD. Lipid absorption and metabolism. Environ Health Perspect. 1979;33:45–55.

4. Ingraham RC, Visscher MB. Further studies on intestinal absorption with the performance of osmotic work. Am J Physiol. 1938;121:771–85.
5. Matthews DM, Wiseman G. Transamination by the small intestine of the rat. J Physiol. 1953;120:55P.
6. Dent CE, Schilling JA. Studies on the absorption of proteins: the amino-acid pattern in the portal blood. Biochem J. 1949;44:318–33.
7. Neame KD, Wiseman G. The transamination of glutamic and aspartic acids during absorption by the small intestine of the dog in vivo. J Physiol. 1957;135:442–50.
8. Neame KD, Wiseman G. The alanine and oxo acid concentrations in mesenteric blood during the absorption of L-glutamic acid by the small intestine of the dog cat and rabbit in vivo. J Physiol. 1958;140:148–55.
9. Nakamura J, Noguchi T, Kido R. Aromatic amino acid transaminase in rat intestine. Biochem J. 1973;135:815–18.
10. Weber FL, Maddrey WC, Walser M. Amino acid metabolism of dog jejunum before and during absorption of keto analogues. Am J Physiol. 1977;232:E263–9.
11. Weber FL, Deak SB, Laine RA. Absorption of keto-analogues of branched-chain amino acids from rat small intestine. Gastroenterology. 1978;76:62–70.
12. Finch LR, Hird FJR. The uptake of amino acids by isolated segments of rat intestine. I. A survey of factors affecting the measurement of uptake. Biochim Biophys Acta. 1960;43:268–77.
13. Neptune EM. Respiration and oxidation of various substrates by ileum in vitro. Am J Physiol. 1965;209:329–33.
14. Windmueller HG, Spaeth AE. Uptake and metabolism of plasma glutamine by the small intestine. J Biol Chem. 1974;249:5070–9.
15. Windmueller HG, Spaeth AE. Intestinal metabolism of glutamine and glutamate from the lumen as compared to glutamine from blood. Arch Biophys Biochem. 1975;71:662–72.
16. Windmueller HG, Spaeth AE. Metabolism of absorbed aspartate, asparagine, and arginine by rat small intestine in vivo. Arch Biochem Biophys. 1976;175:670–6.
17. Windmueller HG, Spaeth AE. Respiratory fuels and nitrogen metabolism in vivo in small intestine of fed rats. Quantitative importance of glutamine, glutamate and aspartate. J Biol Chem. 1980;255:107–12.
18. Windmueller HG, Spaeth AE. Source and fate of circulating citrulline. Am J Physiol. 1981;241:E473–80.
19. Pinkus LM, Windmueller HG. Phosphate-dependent glutaminase of small intestine: localization and role in intestinal glutamine metabolism. Arch Biochem Biophys. 1977;182:506–17.
20. Hartmann F, Raible A, Plauth M, Bauder-Groß D, Vieillard-Baron D. Glutamine-dependence of rat enterocyte functions as assessed in cell cultures. Clin Nutr. 1991;10:125–7.
21. Hoogenraad N, Totino N, Elmer H, Wraight C, Alewood P, Johns RB. Inhibition of intestinal citrullin synthesis causes severe growth retardation in rats. Am J Physiol. 1985;249:G792–9.
22. Wakabayashi Y, Yamada E, Yoshida T, Takahashi H. Arginine becomes an essential amino acid after massive resection of rat small intestine. J Biol Chem. 1994;269:32667–71.
23. Plauth M. Die Bedeutung des intestinalen Glutaminmetabolismus im Intermediärstoffwechsel unter normalen und pathophysiologiechen Bedingungen und seine pharmakologische Beeinflussung. [Habilitationsschrift]. Tübingen: Eberhard-Karls-Universität; 1991.
24. Weber FL, Friedman DW, Fresard KM. Ammonia production from intraluminal amino acids in canine jejunum. Am J Physiol. 1988;254:G264–8.
25. Weber FL, Maddrey WC, Walser M. Amino acid metabolism of dog jejunum before and during absorption of keto analogues. Am J Physiol. 1977;232:E263–9.
26. Weber FL, Deak SB, Laine RA. Absorption of keto-analogues of branched-chain amino acids from rat small intestine. Gastroenterology. 1978;76:62–70.
27. Felig P, Wahren J, Karl I, Cerasi E, Luft R, Kipnis DM. Glutamine and glutamate metabolism in normal and diabetic subjects. Diabetes. 1973;22:573–6.
28. Felig P, Wahren J, Räf L. Evidence of inter-organ amino acid transport by blood cells in humans. Proc Natl Acad Sci USA. 1973;70:1775–9.
29. Owen OE, Reichle FA, Mozzoli MA et al. Hepatic gut and renal substrate flux rates in patients with hepatic cirrhosis. J Clin Invest. 1981;68:240–52.
30. Björkman O, Eriksson LS, Nyberg B, Wahren J. Gut exchange of glucose and lactate in basal state and after oral glucose ingestion in postoperative patients. Diabetes. 1990;39:747–51.

31. McAnena OJ, Moore FA, Moore EE, Jones TN, Parsons P. Selective uptake of glutamine in the gastrointestinal tract: confirmation in a human study. Br J Surg. 1991;78:480–2.
32. Van der Hulst RR, Von Meyenfeldt MF, Deutz NE, Soeters PB. Glutamine extraction by the gut is reduced in patients with depleted gastrointestinal cancer. Ann Surg. 1997;225:112–21.
33. Darmaun D, Messing B, Just B, Rongier M, Desjeux J-H. Glutamine metabolism after small intestinal resection in humans. Metabolism. 1991;40:42–4.
34. Matthews DE, Marano MA, Campbell RG. Splanchnic bed utilization of glutamine and glutamic acid in humans. Am J Physiol. 1993;264:E848–54.
35. Fong Y, Tracey KJ, Hesse DG, Albert JD, Barie PS, Lowry SF. Influence of enterectomy on peripheral tissue glutamine efflux in critically ill patients. Surgery. 1990;107:321–6.
36. Souba WW, Wilmore DW. Postoperative alterations of arteriovenous exchange of amino acids across the gastrointestinal tract. Surgery. 1983;94:342–50.
37. Deutz NEP, Reijven PLM, Athanasas G, Soeters PB. Post-operative changes in hepatic, intestinal, splenic and muscle fluxes of amino acids ammonia in pigs. Clin Sci. 1992;83:607–14.
38. Souba WW. The effects of sepsis on intestinal and pulmonary glutamine metabolism. Clin Nutr. 1990;9:49–50.
39. Plauth M, Raible A, Gregor M, Hartmann F. Modulation by endotoxin of intestinal and hepatic glutamine exchange in single and combined organ perfusion. In: Capocaccia L, Merli M, Riggio O, editors. Advances in hepatic encephalopathy and metabolic nitrogen exchange. Boca Raton: CRC Press; 1995;57–60.
40. Cersosimo E, Williams PE, O'Donovan D, Lacy DB, Abumrad NN. Role of acidosis in regulating hepatic nitrogen metabolism during fasting in conscious dog. Am J Physiol. 1987; 252:E313–19.
41. Phromphetcharat V, Jackson A, Dass PD, Welbourne TC. Ammonia partitioning between glutamine and urea: interorgan participation in metabolic acidosis. Kidney Int. 1981;20:598–605.
42. Häussinger D, Gerok W, Sies H. Hepatic role in pH regulation: role of the intercellular glutamine cycle. Trends Biochem Sci. 1984;9:300–2.
43. Welbourne TC, Phromphetcharat V, Givens G, Joshi S. Regulation of interorganal glutamine flow in metabolic acidosis. Am J Physiol. 1986;250:E457–63.
44. Cersosimo E, Williams P, Geer R, Lairmore T, Ghishan F, Abumrad NN. Importance of ammonium ions in regulating hepatic glutamine synthesis during fasting. Am J Physiol. 1989;257:E514–19.
45. Raible A, Plauth M, Hartmann F. Combined perfusion of isolated rat small intestine and liver using perfluorotributylamine as artificial oxygen carrier – first experiences. In: Bengtsson F, Jeppsson B, Almdal T, Vilstrup H, editors. Progress in hepatic encephalopathy and metabolic nitrogen exchange. Boca Raton: CRC Press; 1991;555–60.
46. Raible A, Plauth M, Vieillard-Baron D, Bauder-Groβ D, Gregor M, Hartmann F. Intestinal glucose absorption modulates hepatic glutamine exchange in isolated gut-liver perfusion. In: Capocaccia L, Merli M, Riggio O, editors. Advances in hepatic encephalopathy and metabolic nitrogen exchange. Boca Raton: CRC Press; 1995:507–10.
47. Stümpel F, Kucera T, Gardemann A, Jungermann K. Acute increase by portal insulin in intestinal glucose absorption via hepatoenteral nerves in the rat. Gastroenterology. 1996;110:1863–9.
48. Plauth M, Raible A, Gregor M, Hartmann F. Inter-organ communication between intestine and liver in vivo and in vitro. Semin Cell Biol. 1993;5:231–7.
49. Nance FC, Batson RC, Kline DG. Ammonia production in germ-free Eck-fistula dogs. Surgery. 1971;70:169–74.
50. Schalm SW, van der Mey T. Hyperammonemic coma after hepatectomy in germ-free rats. Gastroenterology. 1979;77:231–4.
51. Weber FL, Veach GA. The importance of the small intestine in gut ammonium production in the fasting dog. Gastroenterology. 1979;77:235–40.
52. Van Leeuwen PAM, Van Berlo CLH, Soeters PB. New mode of action for lactulose. Lancet. 1988;1:55–6.
53. Plauth M, Raible A, Graser TA, Nöldecke I-L, Fürst P, Dölle W, Hartmann F. Lactulose or paromomycin do not affect ammonia generation in the isolated perfused rat small intestine. Z Gastroenterol. 1994;32:141–5.

54. Sugarbaker SP, Revhaug A, Wilmore DW. The role of the small intestine in ammonia production after gastric blood administration. Ann Surg. 1987;206:5–17.
55. Plauth M, Roske A-E, Roth E *et al.* Post-feeding hyperammonemia in liver cirrhosis is caused by small intestinal ammonia production. Gastoenterology. 1997;112:A1360.
56. Häussinger D. Glutamine metabolism in the liver: overview and current concepts. Metabolism. 1989;38(Suppl.1):14–17.
57. Häussinger D, Stoll B, Stehle T, Gerok W. Hepatocyte heterogeneity in glutamate metabolism and bidirectional transport in perfused rat liver. Eur J Biochem. 1989;185:189–95.

12
Drug metabolism in the intestinal wall

U. KLOTZ

INTRODUCTION

Although the liver plays the major role in drug metabolism by oxidative, cytochrome P450 (CYP)-dependent phase I and conjugation or phase II reactions, there is accumulating evidence that drug-metabolizing enzymes in the intestinal wall can significantly contribute to the overall elimination process[1]. The mucosa of the intestinal wall represents the portal entry of orally ingested xenobiotics including drugs, and could be regarded as a first line of defence against such foreign compounds. Enzymes with metabolic activity are primarily localized in epithelial cells. Furthermore, activity is greatest in the villous tips and decreases progressively towards the crypts. Metabolic activity is generally greater in the duodenum and jejunum than in the ileum and colon[2]. A wide range of enzymes are located in the gastrointestinal tract which can metabolize a variety of drugs (see Table 1) and other xenobiotics. Among the various enzymes the P450 gene superfamily[3] and the UDP-glucuronosyltransferase (UGT) isoenzymes[4] are of prime importance. As most data in humans focus on CYP-P450 enzymes, especially on the most abundant CYP3A subfamily, this chapter will concentrate on clinical studies concerning phase I metabolism where such enzymes are involved.

ASSESSMENT OF DRUG-METABOLIZING ENZYMES

Several different methods can be applied to identify or measure drug-metabolizing enzymes in the gut (see Table 2). The activity of an enzyme can be directly assessed *in vitro* by incubating a substrate (probe drug) and cofactors with tissue samples or cell fractions (e.g. microsomes, cytosol) under defined conditions. If the drug is administered intraduodenally, and its metabolites can be identified and quantified in the portal venous system, intestinal metabolism can be evaluated directly *in vivo*. A second *in-vivo* approach can be accomplished in drug disposition studies in the anhepatic phase during liver transplantation. However

Table 1 Examples of drugs metabolized in the intestinal mucosa

Substrate	Enzyme	Reference (see ref. 1)
Acetylgitoxin	Dealcylase	Haustein et al. (1978)
Aspirin (acetylsalicylic acid)	Esterases	Inoue et al. (1980)
		Rowland et al. (1987)
Alcohol (ethanol)	Alcohol dehydrogenase	Inoue et al. (1980)
		Julkunen (1985)
Aminosalicylic acid	Acetyltransferase	Jenne (1963)
Clofibrate	Esterases	Inoue et al. (1980)
Desipramine	N-Sulphotransferase	Romiti et al. (1992)
Ethinyloestradiol	Cytochrome P450	Back et al. (1981)
	Sulphotransferase	Rogers et al. (1987)
Flurazepam	Cytochrome P450	Mahon et al. (1977)
Isoniazid	Acetyltransferase	Jenne (1963)
Isoprenaline (isoproterenol)	Sulphotransferase	Conolly et al. (1972)
Mesalazine (5-ASA)	Acetyltransferase	Allgayer et al. (1989)
Morphine	Glucuronosyltransferase	Mazoit et al. (1990)
Oxodipine	CYP3A4	Flinois et al. (1992)
Paracetamol (acetaminophen)	Sulphotransferase	Rogers et al. (1987)
Phenacetin	Cytochrome P450	Inaba et al. (1979)
Pivampicillin	Esterases	Lund et al. (1976)
Procaine	Deacylase	Haustein et al. (1978)
Sulphonamides	Acetyltransferase	Jenne (1963)
Testosterone	Glucuronosyltransferase	Dahm and Breuer (1966)

Table 2 Methodological approaches to characterize drug metabolism in the intestinal wall

1. Indirect methods ('gene expression')
   Immunohistochemistry
   Immunoblotting of microsomal proteins (e.g. Western blots)
   mRNA isolation/hybridization (Northern blot analysis)
   Characterization of RT-PCR products (e.g. by cloning and nucleotide sequencing)
   In-situ hybridization techniques

2. Pharmacokinetic studies (i.v. versus p.o. or intraduodenal)
   including 'specific' inducers/inhibitors

3. Direct methods ('functional assays')
   In-vitro function tests with subcellular fractions or cultures of enterocytes
   Intraduodenal application and measurements in portal vein

it is not possible to define exactly the extrahepatic site of potential drug metabolism. Pharmacokinetic analysis following intravenous (i.v.) and oral (p.o.) application of a drug dosage (D) in the same subject allows us to calculate, besides bioavailability (F), systemic and oral clearances (CL), also the metabolic extraction (E) by the liver and gastrointestinal tract (see Fig. 1), if a normal hepatic blood flow (Q_H) of 1500 ml/min or 21.6 ml/min per kg is assumed. For the in-vitro and in-vivo studies different probe drugs are used, which are regarded as specific substrates of a particular enzyme[5,6].

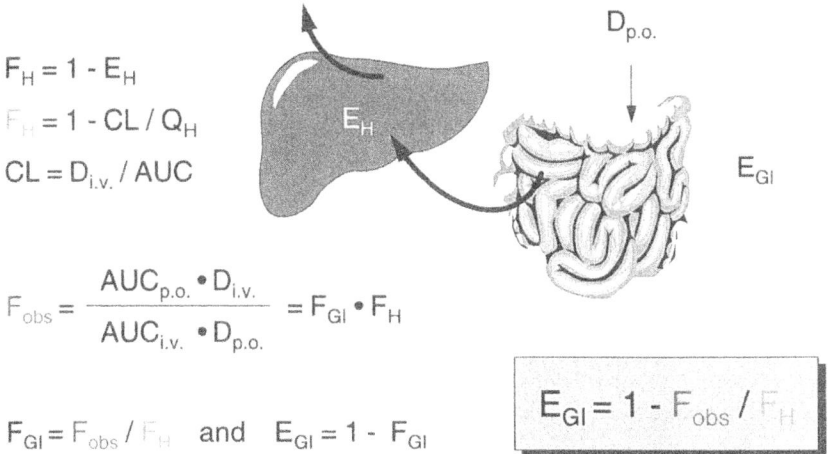

$$F_H = 1 - E_H$$

$$F_H = 1 - CL / Q_H$$

$$CL = D_{i.v.} / AUC$$

$$F_{obs} = \frac{AUC_{p.o.} \cdot D_{i.v.}}{AUC_{i.v.} \cdot D_{p.o.}} = F_{GI} \cdot F_H$$

$$F_{GI} = F_{obs} / F_H \quad \text{and} \quad E_{GI} = 1 - F_{GI}$$

$$E_{GI} = 1 - F_{obs} / F_H$$

Figure 1 Schematic diagram for the calculation of oral bioavailability (F) and sites of presystemic elimination by gastrointestinal (E_{GI}) and hepatic (E_H) extraction. AUC represents the area under the curve following the administration of an intravenous (i.v.) or oral (p.o.) dose (D) in the same individual. A hepatic blood flow (Q_H) of 1500 ml (21.6 ml/min per kg) is assumed

In the past few years various indirect methods – mainly based on molecular biological techniques – have been employed to characterize the location and expression of enzymes in the intestinal wall. However, those methods are not able to quantify the specific activity or function with respect to certain substrates.

Dependent on the specificity of the applied polyclonal or monoclonal antibodies drug-metabolizing enzymes can be identified by immunohistochemical staining in tissue slices of biopsies[7]. Likewise, immunoblot analysis can be used to characterize, in isolated microsomes of different origin, P450 isoenzymes (see Fig. 3) and other drug-metabolizing enzymes[8]. Isolation of mRNA, its hybridization with labelled oligonucleotides specific for certain sequences of drug-metabolizing enzymes or characterization of RT-PCR products and *in-situ* hybridization techniques represent other modern methods, all of which can describe the gene expression of enzymes involved in intestinal drug metabolism[9,10].

PHASE II ENZYMES

The most important phase II reactions are conjugation with glucuronic acid[11] and with glutathione[2,12,13]. In general, these enzyme activities are lower in the gastrointestinal tract if compared to the liver[1,2,8,13]. In a 18-year-old victim of a traffic accident (kidney donor) who was on parenteral nutrition for 4 days before he died, and apparently suffering from Gilbert's syndrome, the longitudinal distribution of UGT activities and glutathione *S*-transferase were measured[12]. In the proximal small intestine two isoforms of UGT and glutathione *S*-transferase declined from duodenum to ileum. Activity of 4-nitrophenol- and 4-methylumbelliferone UGT increased or remained constant, respectively. However, as it is known that Gilbert's syndrome and nutrition can affect xenobiotic metabolizing enzyme activities[14] it remains questionable whether the data of this single patient[12] can be regarded as representative.

CYP-P450 ENZYMES

Immunohistochemistry using a monoclonal antibody closely related to CYP3A identified strong immunoreactivity in hepatocytes, columnar absorptive epithelial cells of the small intestine and polymorphonuclear leucocytes. The immunostaining showed a distinct crypt to villous gradient[7]. More recently, using a specific reverse transcriptase (RT)-polymerase chain reaction (PCR) method, the two subfamily members CYP3A4 and CYP3A5 (but not CYP3A7) could be found in the duodenum of 18 out of 19 patients studied during routine endoscopy for different gastrointestinal diseases[15]. Besides CYP3A4 – the dominant member (70% of total intestinal CYP content) of the CYP3A subfamily – other CYPs (e.g. CYP2C8-10, CYP2D6) could be detected in much lower amounts, but CYP2E1 and CYP1A2 were not identified in the small intestine by immunoblot analysis[8] (see also Fig. 2). On the levels of mRNA and proteins a 'zonal' expression of CYP3A3/3A4 could be shown in human small intestine, with grain density highest in cells within the non-proliferative compartments. In some individuals two CYP3A mRNAs (CYP3A3/3A4 and CYP3A5) were detected in colon samples. It was concluded that there is considerable heterogeneity in the expression of the CYP3A subfamily in human gastrointestinal tissues[10].

A large inter-patient heterogeneity in the expression of CYP3A4 and CYP3A5 in the upper small bowel was seen in terms of CYP3A4 protein

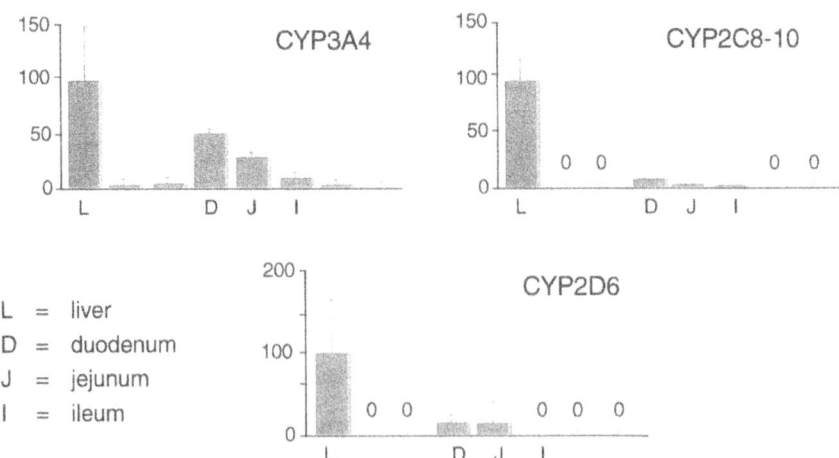

Figure 2 Immunoquantification of P450 enzymes in human liver and intestinal microsomes (data from de Waziers et al.[8])

content (11-fold variation) and CYP3A4 mRNA content (8-fold variation) of intestinal biopsies[16]. There was an excellent correlation between intestinal CYP3A4 protein level and catalytic activity measured *in vitro* with microsomes and the CYP3A4 probe midazolam (see Fig. 3). However, neither parameter significantly correlated with hepatic CYP3A4 activity as measured *in vivo* in the same individuals by the erythromycin breath test (ERMBT). It was concluded that hepatic and intestinal CYP3A4 activities do not correlate well within individuals (probably both sites are regulated differently). The marked inter-patient heterogeneity in the intestinal expression is likely to contribute significantly to the large inter-individual variability in the oral bioavailability of drugs metabolized by the CYP3A subfamily.

PHARMACOKINETIC STUDIES

As already briefly mentioned, besides erythromycin the short-acting benzodiazepine midazolam represents an accepted and validated probe for measuring CYP3A4 activity *in vitro* or *in vivo*. Based on i.v./p.o. crossover studies in healthy volunteers the relative roles of intestinal and hepatic metabolism in the presystemic elimination of a CYP3A substrate can be calculated (see Fig. 1). According to the results of two studies[17,18] in which different doses of midazolam were administered (see Table 3) it is obvious that metabolism by the liver and gastrointestinal tract – expressed as the corresponding extraction ratios (E_H and E_{GI}) – both contribute to a very similar extent to the presystemic elimination, and subsequently to the low oral bioavailability, of 30% (2 mg) or 44% (15 mg) for midazolam. The indirectly calculated and dose-dependent E_{GI}

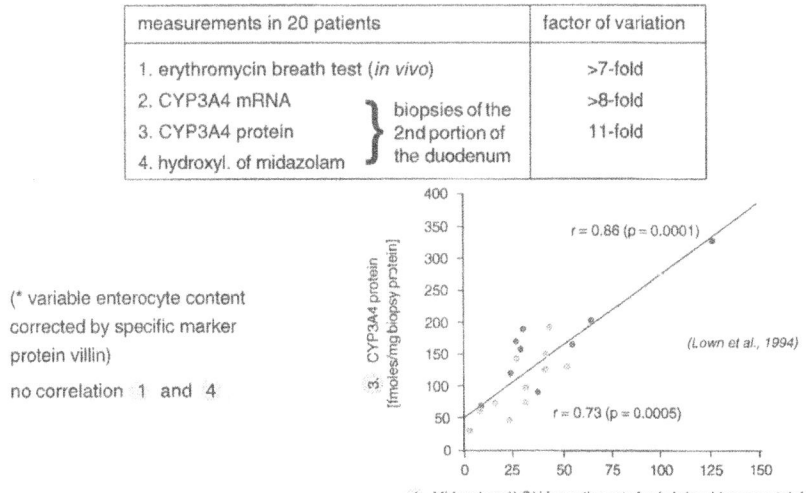

Figure 3 Inter-patient variability of intestinal expression and functional activity of CYP3A4 in duodenal biopsy samples of patients whose CYP3A4 activity was also assessed *in vivo* by the erythromycin breath test (data from Lown *et al.*[16])

Table 3 Example – midazolam

Mean (± SD)	Thummel et al.[18]: oral dose 2 mg (n = 20)	Own data: oral dose 15 mg (n = 6)
F_{obs}	0.30 (± 0.10)	0.44 (± 0.17)
F_H*	0.56 (± 0.14)	0.66 (± 0.06)
E_H	0.44 (± 0.14)	0.34 (± 0.06)
E_{GI}	0.43 (± 0.24)	0.33 (± 0.09)

* Predicted from $1 - CL/Q_H$ with $CL = D_{i.v.}/AUC$ and assuming a liver blood flow of 1500 ml/min.

values of 0.33 ± 0.09[17] and 0.43 ± 0.24[18] were recently confirmed by direct and simultaneous measurement of midazolam and its major metabolite 1'-OH-midazolam in arterial and hepatic portal venous blood samples in liver transplant recipients during the anhepatic phase following i.v. (1 mg) and intraduodenal (2 mg) administration of midazolam. A mass balance approach was used to quantitate intestinal extraction. The mean fraction of the absorbed midazolam dose that was metabolized on transit through the intestinal mucosa averaged 0.43 (± 0.18)[19].

Cyclosporin represents another CYP3A substrate with a low oral bioavailability of about 22% (see Table 4), which is mainly due to presystemic elimination, as an average of 86% of the drug is absorbed intact. With the approach outlined in Fig. 1 a gut extraction ratio between 0.43 and 0.66 was calculated from literature data[20]. When cyclosporin was instilled into the small bowel of two patients during the anhepatic phase of liver transplantation, cyclosporin metabolites (e.g. M1 and 21) were readily detected in considerable amounts in portal venous blood[21]. In addition, when intestinal mucosal microsomes were incubated with cyclosporin (5 μmol/L) for 2 h at 37°C the metabolites M1/M17 could be identified by radiochromatography. Intestinal metabolism was most extensive in duodenum (15% conversion to M1/M17), less in ileum (3–8%) and not detectable in colon[22].

Table 4 Inhibition of intestinal drug metabolism

Probe drug: cyclosporin A, 7.5 mg/kg p.o.; 2.5 mg/kg i.v.
Inhibitor: 250 ml grapefruit juice (–2 h; 0 h)

	Water	Grapefruit juice
F	22%	36% ($p < 0.05$)
E_H	20%	19%
E_{GI}	72%	59% ($p < 0.05$)[24]

	Control	Ketoconazole (200 mg/day)
F	22.4%	56.4% ($p < 0.05$)
F_H	75.2%	86.3% ($p < 0.05$)
F_{GI}	30.2%	65.1% ($p < 0.05$)[23]

INHIBITION OF CYP-P450-MEDIATED INTESTINAL DRUG METABOLISM

As enzymes of the CYP3A subfamily are involved in the metabolism of many drugs[6] it is of clinical importance to test whether the intestinal biotransformation can be inhibited or induced. Some examples will illustrate that such drug interactions exist, both at the site of hepatic and intestinal metabolism. When the CYP3A probe drug cyclosporin was administered orally to subjects pretreated with ketoconazole or erythromycin – known inhibitors of hepatic CYP3A4 – it was suggested that inhibition of enzymes is more effective in the gut than in the liver. Based on 86% absorption of cyclosporin the calculated gut extraction ratio declined from 0.66 to 0.36 (under ketoconazole) or from 0.43 to 0.23 (under erythromycin)[20]. Consequently oral bioavailability was elevated from 22.4% to 56.4% by ketoconazole (see Table 4)[23]. Similarly, when grapefruit juice (250 ml) was ingested immediately before an oral dose of cyclosporin (7.5 mg/kg) its low bioavailability (22%) was increased to 36% by the grapefruit juice. As there were no changes in the systemic clearance after i.v. cyclosporin (2.5 mg/kg infused for 3 h) it was suggested that components of grapefruit juice reduce the gut wall metabolism of cyclosporin[24].

Terfenadine represents a cardiotoxic prodrug, which is metabolized by CYP3A to the active antihistaminic (and not cardiotoxic) agent terfenadine carboxylate. Inhibition of CYP3A by ketoconazole or itraconazole increased the systemic concentration of unchanged terfenadine, resulting in prolongation of the QT interval and increased risk of torsade de points[25]. The same pharmacokinetic interaction with pharmacodynamic consequences can be observed when grapefruit juice is simultaneously ingested with terfenadine. It was suggested that grapefruit juice predominantly may inhibit biotransformation of terfenadine by CYP3A4 in the gut wall[26,27]. Whereas initially naringin and naringenin were claimed as the inhibitory agents, more recently 6′,7′-dihydroxybergamottin was identified as the inhibiting component of grapefruit juice[28,29].

INDUCTION OF CYP-P450-MEDIATED INTESTINAL DRUG METABOLISM

To determine if CYP3A is also inducible in enterocytes, biopsies of small bowel mucosa were obtained from five volunteers before and after they received treatment with rifampin (300 mg b.i.d. for 7 days). Rifampin increased 5–8-fold the mRNA for CYP3A4, intensified staining of CYP3A4 immunoreactive protein and induced, in the one subject tested, the catalytic activity (erythromycin N-demethylase activity) about 10-fold[30]. Therefore it was not surprising that in-vivo rifampin coadministration markedly decreased oral bioavailability of cyclosporin from 27% to 10% because of its significant metabolism in the gut[20].

In the metabolism of verapamil mainly CYP3A4 is involved, and CYP1A2 contributes to the formation of one metabolite (D-617)[31]. In a novel study design before and during treatment with rifampin (600 mg/day for 12 days) racemic verapamil was administered once simultaneously by the i.v. route (10 mg in deuterated form) and p.o. route (120 mg b.i.d. in unlabelled form) using stable isotope technology to exclude intraindividual day-to-day variability in the disposition of this high-clearance drug[32]. Rifampin elevated the systemic clearance of the more cardioactive S-verapamil by 30%, but oral clearance increased 32-fold and consequently bioavailability dropped from 15.6% to 0.7%. This was mainly due to the increase of the gastrointestinal extraction ratio from 0.57 to 0.92, whereas the hepatic extraction ratio increased only moderately from 0.62 to 0.82. Quantitatively very similar results were reported for the less cardioactive R-enantiomer (see Fig. 4). Concomitantly the verapamil-induced maximum PR-interval prolongation was measured as an assessment of the action of verapamil. Following the i.v. dose no significant difference in the changes of this pharmacodynamic parameter could be seen before (19.5%), during (16.8%) or after (20.0%) coadministration of rifampin. However, following oral dosage the maximum PR interval prolongation was significantly less pronounced during rifampin treatment (2.6%) than before (9.0%) and after (6.7%) stopping the inducing agent. These data clearly indicate that gut wall metabolism is preferentially induced by rifampin, and thereby the pharmacological effects of oral verapamil are attenuated[32]. Recently we have finished an identical study in eight elderly subjects to test whether induction by rifampin is age-dependent. Again, during coadministration of rifampin, oral bioavailability of S-verapamil decreased from 14.2% to 0.6% ($p < 0.001$). Effects of orally administered verapamil on AV conduction were nearly abolished (14.4 versus 2.7%; $p < 0.001$). This could be attributed to a considerable increase of prehepatic (intestinal) extraction during treatment with rifampin (E_{GI} of 0.42 versus 0.92; $p < 0.01$) and to a minor extent to induction of heaptic metabolism (E_H of 0.74 versus 0.92; $p < 0.01$; see Table 5). In conclusion, intestinal metabolism and its inducibility is well preserved in the fit elderly[33].

There is increasing evidence that the drug transporter and efflux pump P-glycoprotein (Pgp) is highly expressed in tissues that participate in xenobiotic metabolism. Apparently expression of Pgp and induction of drug metabolism can be affected by the same agents. With a human colon carcinoma cell line a parallel increase in the expression of CYP3A4, CYP3A5 and Pgp by several inducing agents, including rifampin, could be demonstrated[34]. This raises the possibility that the mentioned drug interactions – primarily attributed to intestinal drug metabolism – might be also due (at least in part) to alterations of Pgp-mediated drug transport. The physiological function of Pgp in the gut epithelium

Table 5 Oral bioavailability and inducibility of presystemic extraction of verapamil in the elderly[33]

Mean (± SD) (n = 8)	F (%)	E_{GI} (%)	E_H (%)
S-verapamil			
Before rifampicin	14.2 (± 4.3)	41.7 (± 22.1)	73.7 (± 9.4)
During rifampicin	0.6 (± 0.5)*	91.6 (± 6.6)**	91.6 (± 5.3)**
R-verapamil			
Before rifampicin	38.4 (± 7.3)	29.8 (± 11.2)	45.1 (± 6.4)
During rifampicin	1.0 (± 0.6)*	95.0 (± 4.9)*	78.2 (± 7.6)*

$* p < 0.001$; $** p < 0.01$.

Bioavailability

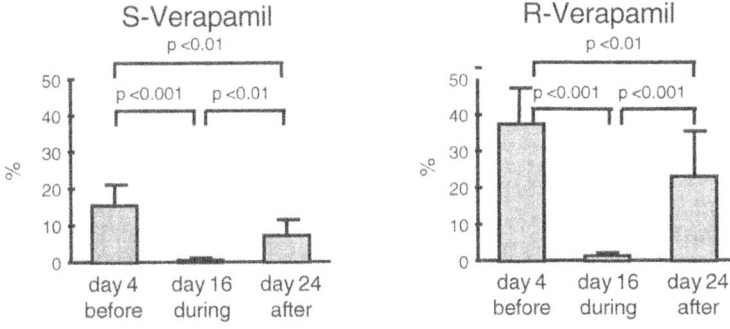

induction by rifampin (600 mg/die; mean ± SD; n = 8)

Hepatic Extraction

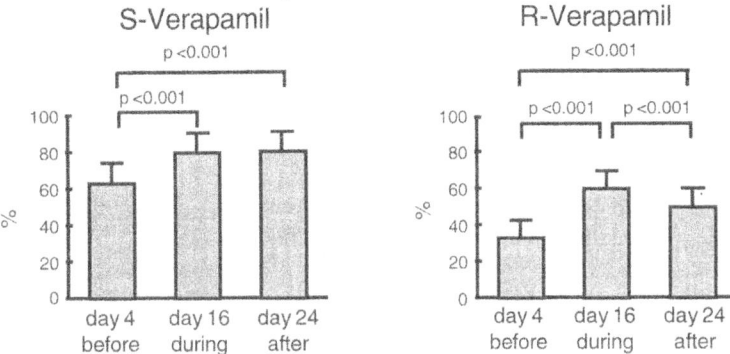

induction by rifampin (600 mg/die; mean ± SD; n = 8)

Gastrointestinal Extraction

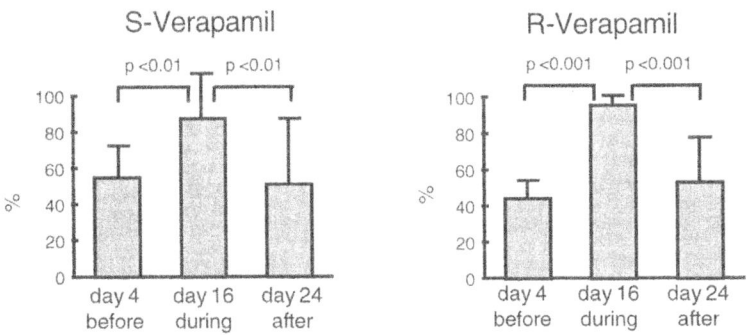

induction by rifampin (600 mg/die; mean ± SD; n = 8)

Figure 4 Rifampin-induced changes (mean ± SD) in the disposition of *S*- and *R*-verapamil in eight healthy volunteers (data from Fromm *et al.*[32])

could be that it protects the body against orally ingested xenotoxins which are substrates of this transport protein. According to the postulated mechanism the oral bioavailability of paclitaxel was elevated from 11.2% to 35.2% in mice with a homozygously disrupted *mdr la gene*, as those animals do not contain functional Pgp in the intestine[35].

Hepatic and/or intestinal drug metabolism is not only responsible for the wide inter-individual variability of drug action in humans, but also plays an important role in toxicology. The dual role of CYP1A1 should be especially remembered, as this enzyme can activate and/or inactivate a broad range of (pro)carcinogens. Therefore the expression and inducibility of the CYP1A subfamily in the gut wall which is exposed to many xenobiotics is of great interest. It was shown that, in endoscopic biopsy specimens obtained from the duodenum of six healthy volunteers, CYP1A1 mRNA and ethoxyresorufin activity were present constitutively in each subject. Omeprazol (20 mg/day for 1 week) induced both parameters in five volunteers. The single 'non-responder' had a marked increase in mRNA and enzymatic activity after receiving 60 mg of omeprazole daily for 1 week (see Fig. 5)[36]. Similarly, 7-ethoxyresorufin O-deethylase (EROD) activity in duodenal biopsy specimens from 10 non-smoking patients receiving omeprazole (20–60 mg/day for at least 1 week) was doubled if compared to 21 non-smoking controls. In smokers EROD activity was 4-fold higher than in non-smokers. Immunoblot analysis substantiated that EROD activity was correlated with CYP1A protein. In contrast, UGT activity towards 4-methylumbelliferone was not significantly affected by smoking or omeprazole[37]. The expression of CYP1A and its induction in the upper small bowel by a frequently given drug may have therapeutic and toxicological implications.

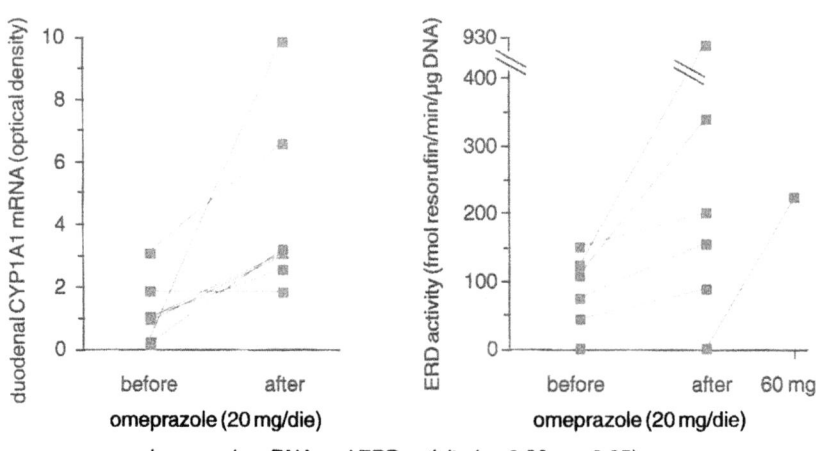

increase in mRNA and ERD activity (r = 0.86; p <0.05)

Figure 5 Quantification of duodenal CYP1A1 mRNA (left) and duodenal ethoxyresorufin deethylase activity (right) before and after treatment with 20 mg omeprazole/day in six individuals ($p < 0.02$). Between the two parameters there was a significant ($r = 0.86$; $p < 0.05$) linear correlation (data from McDonnell *et al.*[36])

XENOBIOTIC METABOLISM AND INTESTINAL DISEASES

According to a recent hypothesis chronic inflammatory bowel disease (IBD), especially ulcerative colitis (UC), might be caused by a reactive xenobiotic metabolite[38]. As cigarette smoking – a known inducer of CYP1A – has a dual effect in IBD (protective in UC, deleterious in Crohn's disease)[39], an association between intestinal xenobiotic metabolism and IBD is more than purely speculative. Previously we could demonstrate that the colon of patients with IBD contained drug-metabolizing activities, e.g. 5-aminosalicylate was N-acetylated[40]. More recently we assessed whether patients with IBD express certain enzymes differently in the gastrointestinal tract than subjects without IBD. Biopsy samples of the terminal ileum and colon were immunohistochemically stained for CYP1A1, CYP2D6, CYP2E1, CYP3A, epoxydehydrolase, α- and π-forms of glutathione transferase, as well as metallothionein. In total, 150 biopsy samples from 21 patients with irritable colon (controls), 37 patients with UC and 25 patients with Crohn's disease (CD) were evaluated. With the exception of CYP1A1 all enzymes were detectable with the same frequency in the three groups (see Table 6). In patients with IBD CYP1A1 staining was more often positive ($p = 0.038$) than in controls, and as CYP1A1 is involved in the activation of toxicologically critical xenobiotics this relationship might offer some new insights into the pathogenesis of IBD[41].

Coeliac disease or gluten-sensitive enteropathy results in small intestinal atrophy which might also affect intestinal drug-metabolizing enzymes. In small bowel biopsy specimens taken from nine patients with active coeliac disease grade 1 CYP3A was hardly expressed, but it was demonstrated that treatment with a gluten-free diet was associated with a significant ($p < 0.05$) increase in CYP3A immunoreactive protein[42]. Thus it is conceivable that enteropathies and alterations in intestinal drug metabolism might in some way be interconnected.

CONCLUSIONS

There is strong and accumulating evidence that the intestinal wall contributes significantly to the metabolism of xenobiotics, especially if they are ingested

Table 6 Expression of drug-metabolizing enzymes in the lower gastrointestinal tract (percentages of samples with positive immunoreactive staining)[41]

Enzyme	Controls (n = 26)	CD (n = 53)	UC (n = 71)
CYP1A1	19.2	**39.6***	**39.0****
CYP2D6	23.1	36.9	29.6
CYP2E1	84.6	77.4	84.5
CYP3A	53.8	58.5	54.9
GST$_\alpha$	19.2	20.8	14.1
GST$_\pi$	19.2	24.1	21.1
Epoxydehydrolase	3.1	1.9	2.8

* $p = 0.057$;   ** $p = 0.050$;   bold figures indicate $p = 0.038$ IBD versus control.

orally. Almost the complete spectrum of phase I and phase II reactions which take place mainly in the liver can also be accomplished by the gut, whose enzymatic capacity can be inhibited and induced, which will have therapeutic and toxicological implications[43]. The variable and low oral bioavailability of CYP3A substrates (e.g. midazolam, cyclosporin, verapamil) – and consequently the action of such drugs – is caused to a considerable extent by the large intra- and inter-individual variation in the expression/activity of the intestinal enzymes. These drug-metabolizing enzymes have a dual function ('friend or foe'?): they can deactivate active drugs or carcinogens to inactive metabolites, but activation of prodrugs or procarcinogens to toxic compounds is possible. Therefore the enterocytes do not necessarily represent a barrier or defence line, but could also be regarded as a type of risk factor, in regard to a variable, potentially ineffective and/or toxic drug response, as well as probably contributing to certain disease states of the gastrointestinal tract. In addition, P-glycoprotein in the gut epithelium may play an important role in the protection of the body against such orally ingested xenotoxins which are substrates of this transport protein.

Acknowledgements

This work was supported by the Robert Bosch Foundation, Stuttgart. The secretarial help of Mrs A. Henker is greatly appreciated.

References

1. Krishna DR, Klotz U. Extrahepatic metabolism of drugs in humans. Clin Pharmacokinet. 1994;26:144–60.
2. Hoensch HP, Hartmann F. The intestinal enzymatic biotransformation system: potential role in protection from colon cancer. Hepato-gastroenterol. 1981;28:221–8.
3. Nelson DR, Koymans L, Kamtaki T et al. P450 superfamily: update on new sequences, gene mapping, accession numbers and nomenclature. Pharmacogenetics. 1996;6:1–42.
4. Burchell B, Brierley CH, Rance D. Specificity of human UDP-glucuronosyltransferases and xenobiotic glucuronidation. Life Sci. 1995;57:1819–31.
5. Kivistö KT, Kroemer HK. Use of probe drugs as predictors of drug metabolism in humans. J Clin Pharmacol. 1997;37:40–8S.
6. Watkins PB. Noninvasive tests of CYP3A enzymes. Pharmacogenetics. 1994;4:171–84.
7. Murray GI, Barnes TS, Sewell HF et al. The immunocytochemical localisation and distribution of cytochrome P-450 in normal human hepatic and extrahepatic tissues with a monoclonal antibody to human cytochrome P-450. Br J Clin Pharmacol. 1988;25:465–75.
8. Waziers de I, Cugnenc PH, Yang CS et al. Cytochrome P450 isoenzymes, epoxide hydrolase and glutathione transferases in rat and human hepatic and extrahepatic tissues. J Pharmacol Exp Ther. 1990;253:387–94.
9. Kolars JC, Lown KS, Schmiedlin-Ren P et al. CYP3A gene expression in human gut epithelium. Pharmacogenetics. 1994;4:247–59.
10. McKinnon RA, Burgess WM, Hall P de la M et al. Characterisation of CYP3A gene subfamily expression in human gastrointestinal tissues. Gut. 1995;36:259–67.
11. Kroemer HK, Klotz U. Glucuronidation of drugs. A re-evaluation of the pharmacological significance of the conjugates and modulating factors. Clin Pharmacokinet. 1992;23:292–310.
12. Peters WHM, Nagengast FM, Tongeren JHM. Glutathione S-transferase, cytochrome P450, and uridine 5'-diphosphate-glucuronosyltransferase in human small intestine and liver. Gastroenterology. 1989;96:783–9.
13. Peters WHM, Jansen PLM. Immunocharacterization of UDP-glucuronyltransferase isoenzymes in human liver, intestine and kidney. Biochem Pharmacol. 1988;37:564–7.

14. Hoensch HP, Steinhardt HJ, Weiss G *et al*. Effects of semisynthetic diets on xenobiotic metabolizing enzyme activity and morphology of small intestinal mucosa in humans. Gastroenterology. 1984;86:1519–30.
15. Kivistö KT, Bookjans G, Fromm MF *et al*. Expression of CYP3A4, CYP3A5 and CYP3A7 in human duodenal tissue. Br J Clin Pharmacol. 1996;42:387–9.
16. Lown KS, Kolars JC, Thummel KE *et al*. Interpatient heterogeneity in expression of CYP3A4 and CYP3A5 in small bowel: lack of prediction by the erythromycin breath test. Drug Metab Dispos. 1994;22:947–55.
17. Allonen H, Ziegler G, Klotz U. Midazolam kinetics. Clin Pharmacol Ther. 1981;30:653–61.
18. Thummel KE, O'Shea D, Paine MF *et al*. Oral first-pass elimination of midazolam involves both gastrointestinal and hepatic CYP3A-mediated metabolism. Clin Pharmacol Ther. 1996;59:491–502.
19. Paine MF, Shen DD, Kunze KL *et al*. First-pass metabolism of midazolam by the human intestine. Clin Pharmacol Ther. 1996;60:14–24.
20. Wu C-Y, Benet LZ, Hebert MF *et al*. Differentiation of absorption and first-pass gut and hepatic metabolism in humans: studies with cyclosporine. Clin Pharmacol Ther. 1995;58:492–7.
21. Kolars JC, Awni WM, Merion RM, Watkins PB. First-pass metabolism of cyclosporin by the gut. Lancet. 1991;338:1488–90.
22. Webber IR, Peters WHM, Back DJ. Cyclosporin metabolism by human gastrointestinal mucosal microsomes. Br J Clin Pharmacol. 1992;33:661–4.
23. Gomez DY, Wacher VJ, Tomlanovich SJ *et al*. The effects of ketoconazole on the intestinal metabolism and bioavailability of cyclosporine. Clin Pharmacol Ther. 1996;58:15–19.
24. Ducharme MP, Warbasse LH, Edwards DJ. Disposition of intravenous and oral cyclosporine after administration with grapefruit juice. Clin Pharmacol Ther. 1995;57:485–91.
25. Kivistö KT, Neuvonen PJ, Klotz U. Inhibition of terfenadine metabolism: pharmacokinetic and pharmacodynamic consequences. Clin Pharmacokinet. 1994;27:1–5.
26. Benton RE, Honig PK, Zamani K *et al*. Grapefruit juice alters terfenadine pharmacokinetics, resulting in prolongation of repolarization on the electrocardiogram. Clin Pharmacol Ther. 1996;59:383–8.
27. Honig PK, Wortham DC, Lazarev A, Cantilena LR. Grapefruit juice alters the systemic bioavailability and cardiac repolarization of terfenadine in poor metabolizers of terfenadine. J Clin Pharmacol. 1996;36:345–51.
28. Edwards DJ, Bernier SM. Naringin and naringenin are not the primary CYP3A inhibitors in grapefruit juice. Life Sci. 1996;59:1025–30.
29. Edwards DJ, Bellevue FH, Woster PM. Identification of 6′, 7′-dihydroxybergamottin, a cytochrome P450 inhibitor, in grapefruit juice. Drug Metab Dispos. 1996;24:1287–90.
30. Kolars JC, Schmiedlin-Ren P, Schuetz JD *et al*. Identification of rifampin-inducible P450 IIIA4 (CYP3A4) in human small bowel enterocytes. J Clin Invest. 1992;90:1871–8.
31. Kroemer HK, Gautier J-C, Beaune Ph *et al*. Identification of P450 enzymes involved in metabolism of verapamil in humans. Naunyn-Schmiedeberg's Arch Pharmacol. 1993; 348:332–7.
32. Fromm MF, Busse D, Kroemer HK, Eichelbaum M. Differential induction of prehepatic and hepatic metabolism of verapamil by rifampin. Hepatology. 1996;24:796–801.
33. Fromm MF, Dilger K, Busse D *et al*. Gut wall metabolism of verapamil in the elderly: effects of rifampin-mediated enzyme induction. Br J Clin Pharmacol. (In press).
34. Schuetz EG, Beck WT, Schuetz JD. Modulators and substrates of P-glycoprotein and cytochrome P4503A coordinately up-regulate these proteins in human colon carcinoma cells. Mol Pharmacol. 1996;49:311–18.
35. Sparreboom A, van Asperen J, Mayer U *et al*. Limited oral bioavailability and active epithelial excretion of paclitaxel (Taxol) caused by glycoprotein in the intestine. Proc Natl Acad Sci USA. 1997;94:2031–5.
36. McDonnell WM, Scheiman JM, Traber PG. Induction of cytochrome P450IA genes (CYP1A) by omeprazole in the human alimentary tract. Gastroenterology. 1992;103:1509–16.
37. Buchthal J, Grund KE, Buchmann A *et al*. Induction of cytochrome P4501A by smoking or omeprazole in comparison with UDP-glucuronosyltransferase in biopsies of human duodenal mucosa. Eur J Clin Pharmacol. 1995;47:431–5.
38. Crotty B. Ulcerative colitis and xenobiotic metabolism. Lancet. 1994;343:35–8.
39. Cope GF, Heatley RV. Cigarette smoking and intestinal defences. Gut. 1992;33:721–3.

40. Allgayer H, Ahnfelt NO, Kruis W *et al.* Colonic *N*-acetylation of 5-aminosalicylic acid in inflammatory bowel disease. Gastroenterology. 1989;97:38–41.
41. Klotz U, Hoensch H, Schütz T *et al.* Expression of intestinal drug metabolizing enzymes in patients with chronic inflammatory bowel disease. Hepato-gastroenterol. (Submitted).
42. Lang CC, Brown RM, Kinirons MT *et al.* Decreased intestinal CYP3A in celiac disease: reversal after successful gluten-free diet: a potential source of interindividual variability in first-pass drug metabolism. Clin Pharmacol Ther. 1996;59:41–6.
43. Park BK, Kitteringham NR, Pirmohamed M, Tucker GT. Relevance of induction of human drug-metabolizing enzymes: pharmacological and toxicological implications. Br J Clin Pharmacol. 1996;41:477–91.

13
The role of gut bacteria in drug metabolism

T. M. BAUER

INTRODUCTION

The role of gut bacteria in drug metabolism has been reviewed regularly over the past 20 years[1-3], but scientific progress has been slow because of the complexity of the issue. However, there is no doubt about the pharmacokinetic relevance of the gastrointestinal microflora and any pathological state it may be affected by.

PRINCIPLES OF BACTERIAL DRUG METABOLISM

The human gastrointestinal tract is inhabited by up to 400 bacterial species. A particular distribution along the axis of the gastrointestinal tract, as well as along the depth of the bowel wall, is maintained by a complex interaction between the host and its microflora. Stomach and proximal small bowel are characterized by low bacterial counts (10^{2-4} CFU/ml), made up primarily of aerobic species such as *Streptococcus* spp. and *Lactobacillus* spp. This relative paucity is contrasted by the abundant flora of distal small bowel and colon, where bacterial counts reach up to approximately 10^7 CFU/ml (terminal ileum) and 10^{12} CFU/g (colon). Anaerobic bacteria such as *Bacteroides* spp. and *Clostridium* spp. outnumber aerobic Enterobacteriaceae and *Streptococcus* spp. by approximately 10^3. The metabolic power of the gut flora is illustrated by a large spectrum of reactions that are potentially relevant for drug metabolism (Table 1).

Research in germ-free or gnotobiotic animals, as well as in healthy humans, has established some basic principles concerning the metabolic activity of the intestinal microflora.

1. There is a group of functional and structural properties of the human gastrointestinal tract that is dependent on the presence of an intact intestinal microflora, designated 'microflora-associated characteristics'[4] (Table 2). Some of those functional properties can be used to monitor the state of the intestinal microflora in health and disease.

Table 1 Biochemical reactions by intestinal bacteria

Hydrolysis	Dehydroxylation	Reduction
Glucuronides	C-hydroxy groups	Double bonds
Glycosides	N-hydroxy groups	Nitro groups, azo groups
Esters	Decarboxylation	Aldehydes
Sulphamates	Demethylation	Alcohols
Amides	Deamination	Acetylation
Nitrates	Dehalogenation	Esterification

Table 2 Microflora-associated characteristics[4]

Breakdown of mucin
Inactivation of tryptic activity
Production of short-chain fatty acids
Formation of coprostanol
Deconjugation of bilirubin
Formation of urobilinogen

2. The metabolic activity of a given bacterial species of human gastrointestinal origin is modified by the presence of other bacterial species, as well as by factors exerted by the human host[5]. Because of this interaction *in vitro* research with isolated bacterial species is of limited value. However, a recently described *in vitro* reactor simulating the human intestinal microbial ecosystem may prove useful for future research[6].

3. Microflora-associated characteristics are subject to a wide inter-individual variability. In terms of intestinal conversion of cholesterol to coprostanol the North American population has been found to fall into two distinct groups, the so-called high converters (comprising approximately three-quarters of the population) and the remaining low converters[7].

ROLE OF BACTERIAL DRUG METABOLISM UNDER PHYSIOLOGICAL CONDITIONS

Given the regional distribution of gut bacteria there is probably little bacterial metabolism in the proximal small intestine, where the majority of nutrients and oral therapeutic agents are absorbed. However, drugs gain access to lower sections of the intestinal tract by two means, i.e. by incomplete absorption after oral administration and by biliary excretion as unabsorbable drug conjugates.

Bacterial metabolism of oral drugs

Bacterial metabolism probably occurs with the majority of incompletely absorbed oral drugs once they are exposed to colonic-type microflora. The effects of this phenomenon on pharmacodynamics and pharmacokinetics are well characterized for a few drugs. Some agents, e.g. sulphasalazine and lactulose, endow their pharmacological activity to prior bacterial transformation[2], whereas other drugs such as digoxin are inactivated[8]. However, the pharmacological relevance of bacterial metabolism remains obscure in many instances: a bacterial reduction product of the antibiotic agent metronidazole, acetamide, is being discussed as a weak human carcinogen, as well as a powerful antibiotic derivative[9].

Role of intestinal microflora in enterohepatic circulation

The role of the intestinal microflora in enterohepatic circulation of endogenous compounds such as bile acids, bilirubin, cholesterol, sex hormones, and vitamin D is well known. These compounds undergo hepatic conjugation with glucuronic acid or sulphate, and are excreted via the bile duct as unabsorbable conjugates. Once they are exposed to colonic-type bacteria such as *Bacteroides* spp., *Veilonella* spp., and *Bifidobacterium* spp. the glycosidic bond is split, resulting in reabsorption of the original compound.

Enterohepatic circulation also occurs with exogenous compounds, including a wide spectrum of orally or parenterally administered drugs. Morphine, rifampin, colchicine, digitoxin, and ethinyloestradiol are agents whose pharmacokinetic properties are influenced by enterohepatic circulation.

EFFECT OF ANTIBIOTICS ON BACTERIAL DRUG METABOLISM

The impact of antibiotics on the intestinal ecosystem is reflected by dramatic effects on various microflora-associated characteristics. Intestinal conversion of cholesterol to coprostanol in healthy volunteers is affected by various antibiotics, and virtually abolished by agents that are particularly active against anaerobes[10]. The administration of antibiotics is therefore likely to have a pharmacokinetic impact in all cases in which gut bacteria are involved in drug metabolism. However, clinical consequences have hitherto only been described for drugs with narrow therapeutic ranges.

Approximately one-third of an oral dose of digoxin remains unabsorbed in the small bowel, and is exposed to drug metabolism by colonic bacteria. Dihydroxydigoxin and other pharmacologically inactive reduction products are formed by anaerobic rods of the genus *Eubacterium* in approximately 10% of the population. The reduction products are absorbed and subsequently excreted by the kidneys. When healthy volunteers on a maintenance dose of digoxin are given antibiotics there is a significant drop in urinary excretion of reduced digoxin metabolites, associated with a two-fold rise in the serum digoxin level[8]. This study is mirrored by several reports on overt digoxin toxicity developing during treatment with various macrolide antibiotics, illustrating the clinical relevance of this drug interaction[11,12].

Another setting in which interference with bacterial drug metabolism can produce therapeutic problems is the patient on oral contraception. Oestrogen compounds of both endogenous and exogenous origin are subject to enterohepatic circulation: their pharmacokinetic properties are therefore dependent on the state of the intestinal microflora. Studies in pregnant women showed that interruption of the enterohepatic circulation by administration of penicillin or ampicillin induces large increases in faecal loss of oestriol, accompanied by reduced urinary oestrogen excretion[13,14]. There are to date no controlled studies indicating that the same applies to ethinyloestradiol, the active oestrogen compound in the contraceptive pill. However, several reports link the co-administration of antibiotics to patients on oral contraception to the occurrence of breakthrough bleeding or unwanted pregnancies[15-17]. It is therefore recommended that women on oral contraception use additional barrier methods during antibiotic treatment.

ROLE OF SMALL INTESTINAL BACTERIAL OVERGROWTH

Small intestinal bacterial overgrowth (SIBO), defined as the presence of more than 10^5 CFU/ml jejunal secretion, has classically been described in patients with structural gastrointestinal tract pathology such as diverticula, fistulas, or blind loops. During the past decade SIBO has been found to be associated with various chronic medical disorders such as diabetes mellitus, chronic renal failure, or cirrhosis of the liver[18]. Malnutrition and vitamin deficiency are known sequelae of SIBO, but its impact on drug resorption and drug metabolism has not yet been investigated systematically. However, the pathogenesis of megaloblastic anaemia in SIBO illustrates what is likely to happen to orally administered drugs. Vitamin B_{12} deficiency in SIBO is due to binding of cobalamin to bacterial cell wall components[19], as well the transformation of exogenous cobalamin to vitamin B_{12} analogues, so-called corrinoids[20], which are inactive and responsible for the development of vitamin B_{12} deficiency. The increasing awareness of the presence of SIBO in various chronic disorders should prompt further research into its pharmacokinetic relevance.

SUMMARY

1. Drug metabolism by intestinal microflora contributes to the pharmacological profile of various drugs. The metabolism of orally administered drugs can result in pharmacodynamic activation or inactivation, and the hydrolysis of biliary drug conjugates is responsible for the enterohepatic circulation of drugs.
2. Interference with bacterial drug metabolism by antibiotics can affect pharmacokinetic properties of various drugs. The administration of antibiotics to patients receiving concurrent drugs can therefore result in treatment failures or unexpected drug toxicity.
3. The impact of small intestinal bacterial overgrowth on drug metabolism and pharmacokinetics is poorly understood and merits systematic studies.

References

1. Goldman P. Therapeutic implications of the intestinal microflora. N Engl J Med. 1973;289:623–8.
2. Goldman P. Biochemical pharmacology of the intestinal flora. Annu Rev Pharmacol Toxicol. 1978;18:523–39.

3. Ilett KF, Tee LBG, Reeves PT, Minchin RF. Metabolism of drugs and other xenobiotics in the gut lumen and wall. Pharmacol Ther. 1990;46:67–93.
4. Midtvedt T, Carlstedt-Duke B, Hoverstadt T et al. Influence of peroral antibiotics upon the biotransformatory activity of the intestinal microflora in healthy subjects. Eur J Clin Invest. 1986;16:11–17.
5. Peppercorn MA, Goldman P. Caffeic acid metabolism by gnotobiotic rats and their intestinal bacteria. Proc Natl Acad Sci USA. 1972;69:1413–15.
6. Molly K, Vande Woestyne M, De Smet I, Verstraete W. Validation of the simulator of the human intestinal microbial ecosystem (SHIME) reactor using microorganism-associated activities. Microbial Ecol Health Dis. 1994;7:191–200.
7. Wilkins TD, Hackman AS. Two patterns of neutral steroid conversion in the feces of normal North Americans. Cancer Res. 1974;34:2250–4.
8. Lindenbaum J, Rund DG, Butler VP, Tse-Eng D, Saha JR. Inactivation of digoxin by the gut flora: reversal by antibiotic therapy. N Engl J Med. 1981;305:789–94.
9. Goldman P, Koch RL, Yeung TC et al. Comparing the reduction of nitro-imidazoles in bacterial and mammalian tissues and relating it to biological activity. Biochem Pharmacol. 1986;35:43–51.
10. Midtvedt T, Lingaas E, Carlstedt-Duike B et al. Intestinal microbial conversion of cholesterol to coprostanol in man. APMIS. 1990;98:839–44.
11. Brown BA, Wallace RJ, Griffith DE, Warden R. Clarithromycin-associated digoxin toxicity in the elderly. Clin Infect Dis. 1997;24:92–3.
12. Friedman HS, Bonventri MV. Erythromycin-induced digoxin toxicity. Chest. 1982;82:202–4.
13. Adlercreutz H, Martin F, Tikkanen MJ, Pulkkinen M. Effect of ampicillin administration on the excretion of twelve oestrogens in pregnancy urine. Acta Endocrinol. 1975;80:551.
14. Pulkkinen M, Willman K. Maternal oestrogen levels during penicillin treatment. Lancet. 1971;i:48.
15. Dossetor J. Drug interactions with oral contraceptives. Lancet. 1975;i:467–8.
16. Reimers D, Jezek A. Rifampicin und andere Antituberkulotika bei gleichzeitiger oraler Kontrazeption. Prax Pneumol. 1971;25:255–62.
17. Sparros MJ. Pregnancies in reliable takers. N Z Med J. 1989;102:575–7.
18. Shindo K, Machida M, Miyakawa K, Fukumura M. A syndrome of cirrhosis, achlorhydria, small intestinal bacterial overgrowth, and fat malabsorption. Am J Gastroenterol. 1993;88:2084–91.
19. Schjonsby H, Peters TJ, Hoffbond AV, Tabaqchali S. The mechanism of vitamin B_{12} malabsorption in the blind loop syndrome. Gut. 1970;11:37.
20. Brandt LJ, Bernstein LH, Wagle A. Production of vitamin B12 analogues in patients with small bowel bacterial overgrowth. Ann Intern Med. 1977;87:546–51.

Section IV
Gut-derived bacterial toxins and liver injury

14
How bacterial toxins affect the intestinal mucosa: molecular mechanism of the action of *Clostridium difficile* toxins

K. AKTORIES

INTRODUCTION

Several enteric bacterial toxins attack the intestinal mucosa by inducing dramatic changes in the physiological function of the intestine, or even severe damage to the gut epithelium. These toxins can be classified in at least two major groups. Whereas one group of enterotoxins increase the net secretion of the intestine without overt histological damage, a second group of enteric toxins are potent cytotoxins that cause major alterations and damage to the mucosa. Well-known 'non-damaging' enterotoxins are cholera toxin and the related *Escherichia coli* heat-labile toxins[1-3]. These toxins act on enterocytes by adenosine diphosphate (ADP) ribosylation of heterotrimeric G proteins (G_s). They increase cAMP production, activate protein kinase A and cause phosphorylation of a major chloride channel (CFTR, cystic fibrosis transmembrane regulator) which results in enhanced Cl^- flux and secretion[4]. Additionally, evidence has been presented for the importance of substances such as prostaglandin E_2 and 5-hydroxytryptamine in cholera toxin-induced secretion[5]. Other members of the group of 'non-damaging' toxins are the heat-stable toxins from *E. coli*, which also affect CFTR by phosphorylation. However, these small polypeptides, that are related to the hormonal factor guanyline, interact with the membrane-bound guanylyl cyclase receptor. They increase cGMP levels, activate the cGMP-dependent protein kinase II and cause CFTR phosphorylation[6-8] (Fig. 1).

Various mechanisms have been described by which 'damaging' enterotoxins attack the mammalian enteric mucosa. One group of cytotoxins alter enterocytes by a *direct* membrane-damaging activity. A typical member of this group is *Clostridium perfringens* enterotoxin (CPE), which is involved in food poisoning but has also been linked to a number of other gastrointestinal illnesses (e.g. antibiotic-associated diarrhoea)[9-11]. Another group of toxins affect *protein*

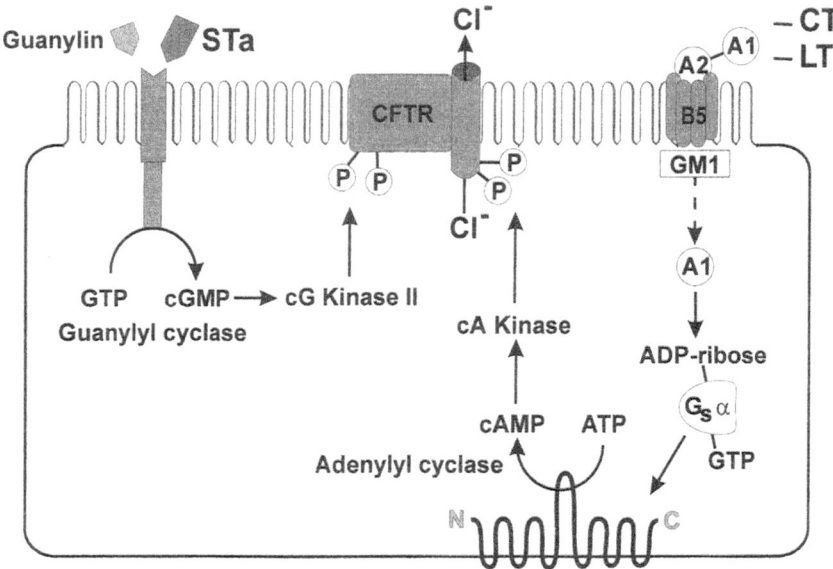

Figure 1   Actions of non-damaging toxins on enterocytes. Cholera toxin (CT) and the related heat-labile enterotoxin from *E. coli* are hexameric AB$_5$ toxins consisting of the biologically active component A (A$_1$–A$_2$) and the binding component (B$_5$). LT and CT bind to their membrane receptor ganglioside G$_{M1}$. Thereafter, the toxins are internalized, followed by translocation of the enzyme component A$_1$ (after nicking of A$_1$–A$_2$) into the cytosol. The enzyme component A$_1$ ADP-ribosylates the α-subunit of the G$_S$ protein involved in adenylyl cyclase activation. Thereby the G protein is persistently active and activates the cyclase. This results in elevated cAMP levels and activation of the cAMP-dependent kinase. The kinase phosphorylates the cystic fibrosis transmembrane regulator (CFTR), a major chloride channel of enterocytes, thereby increasing Cl$^-$ fluxes. The CFTR is also affected by the heat-stable *E. coli* toxins (STa), which are small polypeptides acting on the membrane-bound guanylyl cyclase receptor. This receptor interacts physiologically with guanylin, a hormonal factor. STa binding results in activation of guanylyl cyclase, increase in cGMP formation and activation of G kinase II which phosphorylates and activates CFTR

synthesis of gut cells. Examples of these toxins are *Shiga* toxin and *Shiga*-like toxins which possess RNA-*N*-glycosidase activity and induce the depurination of adenosine at position 4324 of the 28th ribosomal RNA of eukaryotic cells, thereby inhibiting protein synthesis[12,13]. Finally, another large group of intracellularly acting toxins attack the cytoskeleton of cells. One major family of these toxins are the actin-ADP-ribosylating toxins. Members of this family are, for example, *C. perfringens* iota toxin and *C. botulinum* C2 toxin[14–17]. These toxins are binary in structure; they consist of an enzyme component possessing ADP-ribosyltransferase activity and a binding component which is involved in the binding and transport of the enzyme component into the cytosol. In the cytosol the toxins ADP-ribosylate actin at arginine-177, thereby inhibiting actin polymerization[18]. As the actin cytoskeleton is basically involved in the integrity of the epithelial cells, the toxin effects will cause destruction of the epithelial barrier function (Fig. 2).

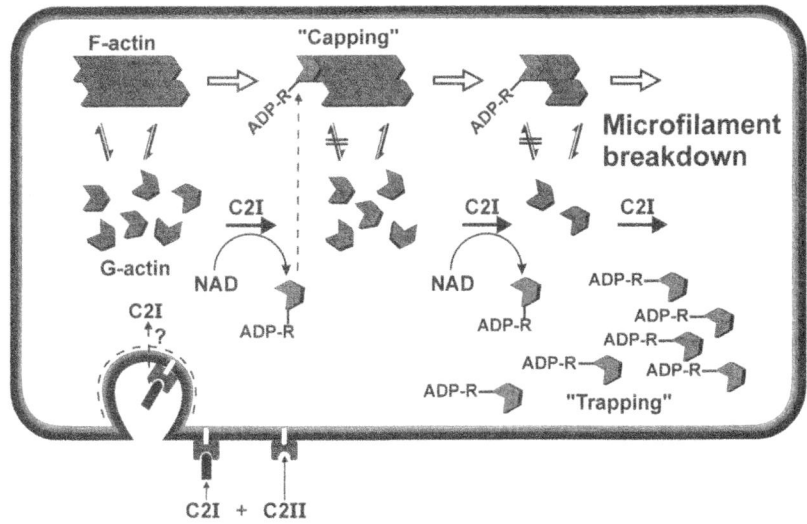

Figure 2   Mechanisms of actin-ADP-ribosylating toxins. Actin-ADP-ribosylating toxins such as C2 toxin from *C. botulinum* and iota toxin from *C. perfringens* are binary in structure: they consist of a binding component (component C2II of C2 toxin) and an enzyme component (component C2I of C2 toxin) which are separated proteins. The components of the toxins meet at the cell surface where component C2II induces a binding site for C2I. After internalization and translocation of C2I into the cytosol monomeric G-actin is ADP-ribosylated. This alters the delicate equilibrium between monomeric G-actin and polymerized F-actin, and induces depolymerization of F-actin. Two major mechanisms are responsible: first, ADP-ribosylated actin is not able to polymerize ('trapping'), second, ADP-ribosylation turns actin into a capping protein that binds to the barbed or fast-growing ends of actin filaments, thereby inhibiting further polymerization of unmodified actin. At the pointed (slow-growing) ends of filaments actin monomers are released which are then modified by the toxins. These events finally result in depolymerization of actin and destruction of the cytoskeleton

Rho PROTEIN-MODIFYING TOXINS

A further group of enteric bacterial cytotoxins are characterized by their indirect action on the cytoskeleton. These are the Rho protein-modifying toxins. Most important members of this group are the large clostridial cytotoxins A and B, which are the major virulence factors of *C. difficile*[19–21]. *C. difficile* is recognized as the cause of about 20% of cases of antibiotic-associated diarrhoea[22], and is suggested as being responsible for most, if not all, cases of antibiotic-induced pseudomembraneous colitis[19,21,23]. The genes encoding these toxins have recently been cloned and sequenced, showing that *C. difficile* toxin A and B consist of 8.130 and 7.089 bp, encoding proteins of 2710 and 2366 amino acids and a molecular mass of about 308 and 270 kDa, respectively[24–27]. The amino acid sequences share 49% identity and 63% similarity. While toxin A induces diarrhoea, inflammation and necrosis, toxin B shows no overt enterotoxicity in animal models[28,29]. However, the cytotoxicity of toxin B is in general 100–1000-fold higher than of toxin A[28,30,31]. Therefore, toxin A is designated as an enterotoxin and toxin B as a cytotoxin. Most likely different cell surface receptors are responsible for these different potencies. Notably, it has been reported recently that in human colonic preparations toxin B is even more toxic than toxin A to induce damage to epithelial cells[32]. Thus, it appears that both toxins may be capable of induction of enterotoxicity, at least in humans.

Although it has been known for some time that *C. difficile* toxins act on the actin cytoskeleton, the precise mechanism was not discovered until recently. It is now clear that these toxins act on the actin cytoskeleton by glucosylating low molecular mass guanosine triphosphate (GTP)-binding proteins of the Rho subfamily (Fig. 3).

Rho GTPases

Rho proteins are members of the superfamily of Ras proteins that act as molecular switches. The Rho subfamily, which consists of at least 10 related small GTPases, is involved in regulation of the actin cytoskeleton and various other signalling processes[33-37]. As known for other GTP-binding proteins, Rho pro-

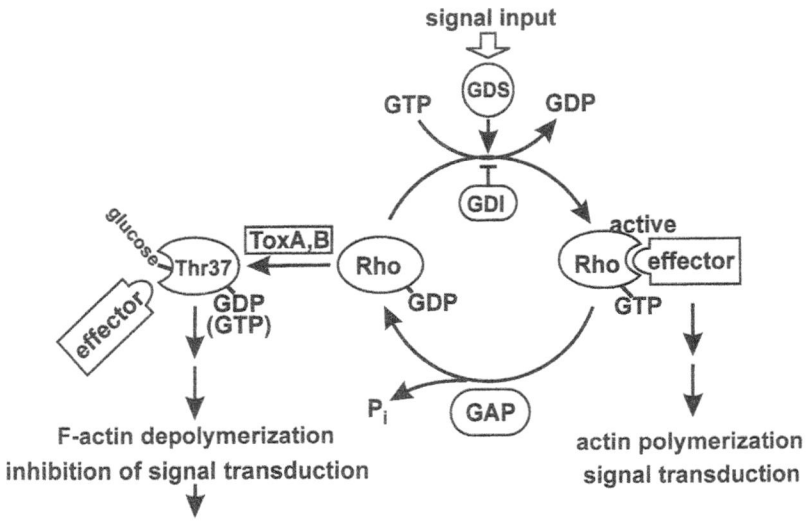

Figure 3 Glucosylation of Rho proteins by *C. difficile* toxins. Rho proteins are small GTPases which regulate the actin cytoskeleton and act as molecular switches in various signal transduction processes. They are involved in the control of integrin signalling, tight junction regulation, wound-healing, cell cycle regulation, cell transformation and apoptosis. Rho proteins are inactive in the GDP-bound form and active after nucleotide exchange, a process that is facilitated by guanine nucleotide dissociation stimulators (GDS). Guanine nucleotide dissociation inhibitors (GDIs) prevent Rho activation. The active GTP-bound form of Rho interacts with its effectors. Hydrolysis of GTP terminates the active state of Rho. This is stimulated by GTPase-activating proteins (GAP). *C. difficile* toxins A and B glucosylate small GTP-binding proteins of the Rho family by using UDP-glucose as a cosubstrate. Modification of Rho occurs at threonine-37, a residue that is crucial for nucleotide-binding, GTPase activity and G-protein-effector coupling. Glucosylation inhibits Rho function, resulting in depolymerization of actin, and inhibition of Rho-dependent signalling

teins are active in the GTP-bound form and inactive when guanosine diphosphate (GDP) is bound. Thus, the active state is terminated by hydrolysis of GTP catalysed by an intrinsic GTPase activity. Because the intrinsic GTPase activity is very low, GTPase-activating proteins that increase the GTPase activity several-fold participate in switching off the active state[38]. Activation of Rho proteins is accomplished by guanine nucleotide dissociation stimulators (GDS). A third group of regulatory proteins, guanine-nucleotide dissociation inhibitors (GDI), block the activation of Rho proteins[39,40]. In the active form, Rho proteins interact with their effector proteins to elicit their specific effects. Several putative effectors of Rho proteins have been described which are protein kinases, lipid kinases, and adaptor proteins.

Best-studied members of the Rho family are Rho (A,B,C), Rac (1 and 2), and Cdc42. Rho GTPases are involved in the control of the actin cytoskeleton, especially in formation of stress fibres and adhesion complexes[41]. In addition, they are also implicated in various signal transduction processes including signalling via phosphoinositide-3-kinase[42], phosphatidylinositol-4-phosphate-5-kinase[43], phospholipase D[44–46], endocytosis[47], transcriptional activation[48–50] and even transformation of cells[51].

Rac proteins (Rac 1 and Rac 2) induce the formation of lamellipodia and of membrane ruffles, and are important for the regulation of the NADPH oxidase and phospholipase A_2[52,53]. Moreover, they are also involved in transcriptional activation[54]. Cdc42 regulates formation of filopodia or microspikes and, in addition to the regulation of the cortical actin filament system, it is also involved in control of transcription[55,56]. Deduced from earlier findings that the Rho and Rac signal pathways converge, it was assumed that the Rho proteins regulate the actin cytoskeleton in a cascade-like manner, starting with Cdc42, which can activate Rac. Activated Rac is then capable of activating Rho. However, recent findings suggest that this regulatory pathway is more complicated, because active Cdc42 is able not only to activate Rac, but also to inhibit stress fibre formation, indicating inhibition of the action of Rho[56–58].

Rho PROTEINS AS TARGETS FOR *C. DIFFICILE* TOXIN

Recently, it has been shown that all Rho proteins are glucosylated by *C. difficile* toxin A and B[59,60]. The toxins use uridine diphosphate (UDP)-glucose as a cosubstrate and transfer the glucose moiety onto Rho proteins. Other small GTPases, e.g. Ras or Rab proteins, are not modified by *C. difficile* toxins. In addition to glucosyltransferase activity, the toxin possesses UDP-glucosyl hydrolase activity, i.e. in the absence of a protein substrate they cleave UDP-glucose into UDP and glucose. This hydrolase activity is much lower than the transferase activity.

Modification of Rho occurs at Thr-37 of Rho, which is equivalent to Thr-35 of Rac and Cdc42. Thr-37 is located in the so-called effector region of the GTPase where coupling with the effector protein takes place. The region adjacent to this crucial amino acid residue undergoes major changes upon activation of Rho. Therefore, this region is called the switch-I region. This amino acid residue is basically involved in coordination of the magnesium ion and of the nucleotide[61–65]. In the active GTP-bound form the hydroxyl group of Thr-37 is directed to the protein and, therefore, not accessible for modification. In contrast, in the GDP-bound form the hydroxyl group is orientated towards the solvent, and available for modification by the toxins. In agreement with this hypothesis it was observed that Rho proteins are poor substrates for glucosylation after loading with GTPγS[59,60]. In order to investigate whether the glucosylation of Rho is sufficient to cause a cytotoxic effect, recombinant Rho A was treated with toxin B in the presence of UDP-glucose. After glucosylation the toxin was removed by membrane filtration and, thereafter, microinjected into culture cells. Only Rho which was previously treated with toxin B and UDP-glucose was capable of induction of cytotoxic effects, indicating that monoglucosylation of Rho is the cause of cytotoxicity[59].

FUNCTIONAL CONSEQUENCES OF Rho GLUCOSYLATION

So far, the precise pathogenetic path which finally results in diarrhoea and/or colitis is not entirely clear. It has been known for some time that C. difficile toxin A increases intestinal permeability and activates chloride secretion[66]. Moreover, in monolayer cells, toxin A induces an increase in tight junction permeability[67]. New studies have recently shown that Rho proteins are involved in tight junction function. When Rho proteins were inhibited by C3, a bacterial toxin that inactivates Rho not by glucosylation but by ADP-ribosylation, depolymerization of the actin cytoskeleton was observed in the vicinity of tight junctions, accompanied by redistribution of the peripheral tight junction protein ZO-1; concomitantly permeability of the epithelial barrier increased dramatically[68]. Previous reports speculated that C. difficile toxins act on the gut mainly by activating neutrophil leucocytes, which then alter the mucosa by release of cytokines and other biologically active agents[19,69]. Although it was demonstrated that C. difficile toxins are able to induce cytokine production (e.g. IL-8[70]), one has to consider that the toxins are potent inhibitors of leucocyte functions. For example, we observed that the activation of leucocytes studied by determination of skeletal rearrangement caused by chemokines is completely blocked by low concentrations of toxin A and B (unpublished observation).

Another Rho function that might be important, in respect to the action of C. difficile, is wound healing. Recently it has been reported that Rho proteins are basically involved in epithelial repair mechanisms[71]. In the course of epithelial damage, enterocytes flatten and start to migrate, to cover the discontinuity of the epithelium caused by the damaging agent. This process appears to be activated by growth factors. Rho proteins play a major role in migration of enterocytes and in the defect-covering process. Thus, inactivation of Rho proteins by C. difficile toxins will block migration of cells and inhibit processes of wound healing. Such processes will definitely support damage of enteric mucosa.

CONCLUSIONS

During recent years much progress has been made in our understanding of the molecular mechanisms of various bacterial toxins acting on the enteric mucosa.

For example, elucidation of the molecular actions of large clostridial cytotoxins which affect the eukaryotic cell by glycosylation of Rho GTPases nicely explains their cytotoxic action on the action cytoskeleton of target cells. However, it should be emphasized that, in spite of this progress at the molecular level, the exact pathogenetic pathways which finally induce the typical features of the respective diseases are still largely unclear. In fact, this is also true for well-known toxins such as cholera toxin, whose action on G-proteins (ADP-ribosylation) has been known for many years. This is, for example, especially the case for *C. difficile* toxins, the causative agents of antibiotic-associated diarrhoea and colitis. Nevertheless, knowledge of the molecular mechanisms of the toxins is an absolute prerequisite to elucidate the pathogenetic steps involved in inducing the secretory misfunction and/or damage to the mucosa. Finally, a better understanding of the molecular mechanism of toxins may be of major importance for the development of novel strategies against these pathogens.

References

1. Spangler BD. Structure and function of cholera toxin and the related *Escherichia coli* heat-labile enterotoxin. Microbiol Rev. 1992;56:622–47.
2. Gill DM. Mechanism of action of cholera toxin. Adv Cyclic Nucleotide Res. 1977;8:85–118.
3. Hol WGJ, Sixma TK, Merritt EA. Structure and function of *E. coli* heat-labile enterotoxin and cholera toxin B pentamer. In: Moss J, Iglewski B, Vaughan M, Tu AT, editors. Bacterial toxins and virulence factors in disease. New York: Marcel Dekker; 1995:185–223.
4. Sears CL, Kaper JB. Enteric bacterial toxins: mechanisms of action and linkage to intestinal secretion. Microbiol Rev. 1996;60:167–215.
5. Zhang G-F, Patton WA, Moss J, Vaughan M. Cholera toxin: mechanism of action and potential use in vaccine development. In: Aktories K, editor. Bacterial toxins – tools in cell biology and pharmacology. Weinheim: Chapman & Hall; 1997:1–13.
6. Cohen MB, Giannelle RA. Enterotoxigenic *Escherichia coli*. In: Blaser MJ, Smith PD, Ravdin JI, Greenberg HB, Guerrant RL, editors. Infections of the gastrointestinal tract. New York: Raven Press; 1995:691–707.
7. Chao AC, de Sauvage FJ, Dong A-J, Wagner JA, Goeddel DV, Gardner P. Activation of intestinal CFTR Cl⁻ channel by heat-stable enterotoxin and guanylin via cAMP-dependent protein kinase. EMBO J. 1994;13:1065–72.
8. Vaandrager AB, Schulz S, de Jonge HR, Garbers DL. Guanylyl cyclase C is an *N*-linked glycoprotein receptor that accounts for multiple heat-stable enterotoxin-binding proteins in the intestine. J Biol Chem. 1993;268:2174–9.
9. Lindsay JA, Dennison JD. Histopathological effect of *Clostridium perfringens* 8–6 enterotoxin on rabbit intestine. Current Microbiol. 1986;13:61–6.
10. McClane BA, Hanna PC, Wnek AP. *Clostridium perfringens* enterotoxin. Microb Pathogen. 1988;4:317–23.
11. Kokai-Kun JF, McClane BA. The *Clostridium perfringens* enterotoxin. In: Rood JI, McClane BA, Songer JG, Titball RW, editors. The clostridia molecular biology and pathogenesis. San Diego: Academic Press; 1997:325–57.
12. Tesh VL, O'Brien AD. The pathogenic mechanisms of *Shiga* toxin and the *Shiga*-like toxins. Mol Microbiol. 1991;5:1817–22.
13. Sandvig K, Van Deurs B. Endocytosis, intracellular transport, and cytotoxic action of *Shiga* toxin and ricin. Physiol Rev. 1996;76:949–66.
14. Aktories K, Sehr P, Just I. Actin-ADP-ribosylating toxins: cytotoxic mechanism of *Clostridium botulinum* C2 toxin and *Clostridium perfringens* iota toxin. In: Aktories K, editor. Bacterial toxins. Weinheim: Champman & Hall; 1997:93–101.
15. Considine RV, Simpson LL. Cellular and molecular actions of binary toxins possessing ADP-ribosyltransferase activity. Toxicon. 1991;29:913–36.
16. Aktories K, Wille M, Just I. Clostridial actin-ADP-ribosylating toxins. Curr Top Microbiol Immunol. 1992;175:97–113.

17. Ohishi, I. Response of mouse intestinal loop to botulinum C2 toxin: enterotoxic activity induced by cooperation of nonlinked protein components. Infect Immun. 1983;40:691–5.
18. Aktories K, Wegner A. Mechanisms of the cytopathic action of actin-ADP-ribosylating toxins. Mol Microbiol. 1992;6:2905–8.
19. Kelly CP, Pothoulakis C, LaMont JT. *Clostridium difficile* colitis. N Engl J Med. 1994;330:257–62.
20. Lyerly DM, Wilkins TD. *Clostridium difficile*. In: Blaser MJ, Smith PD, Ravdin JI, Greenberg HB, Guerrant RL, editors. Infections of the gastrointestinal tract. New York: Raven Press; 1995:867–91.
21. Bartlett JG. *Clostridrium difficile*: history of its role as an enteric pathogen and the current state of knowledge about the organism. Clin Infect Dis. 1994;18:265–72.
22. Bartlett JG. Antibiotic-associated diarrhea. In: Blaser MJ, Smith PD, Ravdin JI, Greenberg HB, Guerrant RL, editors. Infections of the gastrointestinal tract. New York: Raven Press; 1995:893–904.
23. Thielmann NM, Guerrant RL. *Clostridium difficile* and its toxins. In: Moss J, Iglewski B, Vaughan M, Tu AT, editors. Bacterial toxins and virulence factors in disease. New York: Marcel Dekker; 1995:327–66.
24. Dove CH, Wang SZ, Price SB *et al.* Molecular characterization of the *Clostridium difficile* toxin A gene. Infect Immun. 1990;58:480–8.
25. Sauerborn M, Eichel-Streiber C. Nucleotide sequence of *Clostridium difficile* toxin A. Nucl Acids Res. 1990;18:1629–30.
26. Barroso LA, Wang S-Z, Phelps CJ, Johnson JL, Wilkins TD. Nucleotide sequence of *Clostridium difficile* toxin B gene. Nucl Acids Res. 1990;18:4004.
27. Von Eichel-Streiber C, Laufenberg-Feldmann R, Sartingen S, Schulze J, Sauerborn M. Cloning of *Clostridium difficile* toxin B gene and demonstration of high N-terminal homology between toxin A and B. Med Microbiol Immunol. 1990;179:271–9.
28. Lima AAM, Lyerly DM, Wilkins TD, Innes DJ, Guerrant RL. Effects of *Clostridium difficile* toxins A and B in rabbit small and large intestine *in vivo* and on cultured cells *in vitro*. Infect Immun. 1988;56:582–8.
29. Lyerly DM, Saum KE, MacDonald DK, Wilkins TD. Effects of *Clostridium difficile* toxins given intragastrically to animals. Infect Immun. 1985;47:349–52.
30. Rothman SW, Brown JE, Diecidue A, Foret DA. Differential cytotoxic effects of toxin A and B isolated from *Clostridium difficile*. Infect Immun. 1984;46:324–31.
31. Fiorentini C, Arancia G, Paradisi S *et al.* Effects of *Clostridium difficile* toxins A and B on cytoskeleton organization in HEp-2 cells: a comparative morphological study. Toxicon. 1989;27:1209–18.
32. Riegler M, Sedivy R, Pothoulakis C *et al. Clostridium difficile* toxin B is more potent than toxin A in damaging human colonic epithelium in vitro. J Clin Invest. 1995;95:2004–11.
33. Takai A, Sasaki T, Tanaka K, Nakanishi H. Rho as a regulator of the cytoskeleton. Trends Biochem Sci. 1995;20:227–31.
34. Nobes CD, Hall A. Regulation and function of the Rho subfamily of small GTPases. Curr Opin Genet Dev. 1994;4:77–81.
35. Narumiya S. The small GTPase Rho: cellular functions and signal transduction. J Biochem (Tokyo). 1996;120:215–28.
36. Symons M. Rho family GTPases: the cytoskeleton and beyond. Trends Biochem Sci. 1996;21:178–81.
37. Aktories K. Rho proteins: targets for bacterial toxins. Trends Microbiol. 1997;5:282–8.
38. Lamarche N, Hall A. GAPs for rho-related GTPases. Trends Genet. 1994;10:436–40.
39. Ueda T, Takeyama Y, Ohmori T, Ohyanagi H, Saitoh Y, Takai Y. Purification and characterization from rat liver cytosol of a GDP dissociation inhibitor (GDI) for liver24K G, a *ras* p21-like GTP-binding protein, with properties similar to those of *smg* p25A GDI. Biochemistry. 1991;30:909–17.
40. Scherle P, Behrens T, Staudt LM. Ly-GDI, a GDP-dissociation inhibitor of the RhoA GTP-binding protein, is expressed preferentially in lymphocytes. Proc Natl Acad Sci USA. 1993;90:7568–72.
41. Paterson HF, Self AJ, Garrett MD, Just I, Aktories K, Hall A. Microinjection of recombinant p21^{rho} induces rapid changes in cell morphology. J Cell Biol. 1990;111:1001–7.

42. Zheng Y, Bagrodia S, Cerione RA. Activation of phosphoinositide 3-kinase activity by Cdc42Hs binding to p85. J Biol Chem. 1994;269:18727–30.
43. Chong LD, Traynor-Kaplan A, Bokoch GM, Schwartz MA. The small GTP-binding protein Rho regulates a phosphatidylinositol 4-phosphate 5-kinase in mammalian cell. Cell. 1994;79:507–13.
44. Malcolm KC, Ross AH, Qiu R-G, Symons M, Exton JH. Activation of rat liver phospholipase D by the small GTP-binding protein RhoA. J Biol Chem. 1994;269:25951–4.
45. Kuribara H, Tago K, Yokozeki T et al. Synergistic activation of rat brain phospholipase D by ADP-ribosylation factor and rhoA p21, and its inhibition by Clostridium botulinum C3 exoenzyme. J Biol Chem. 1995;270:25667–71.
46. Siddiqi AR, Smith JL, Ross AH, Qiu R-G, Symons M, Exton JH. Regulation of phospholipase D in HL60 cells. J Biol Chem. 1995;270:8466–73.
47. Schmalzing G, Richter HP, Hansen A, Schwarz W, Just I, Aktories K. Involvement of the GTP binding protein Rho in constitutive endocytosis in Xenopus laevis oocytes. J Cell Biol. 1995;130:1319–32.
48. Machesky LM, Hall A. Rho: a connection between membrane receptor signalling and the cytoskeleton. Trends Cell Biol. 1996;6:304–10.
49. Pantaloni D, Carlier M-F. How profilin promotes actin filament assembly in the presence of thymosin β4. Cell. 1993;75:1007–14.
50. Hill CS, Wynne J, Treisman R. The Rho family GTPases RhoA, Rac 1, and CDC42Hs regulate transcriptional activation by SRF. Cell. 1995;81:1159–70.
51. Khosravi-Far R, Solski PA, Clark GJ, Kinch MS, Der CJ. Activation of Rac 1, RhoA, and mitogen-activated protein kinases is required for Ras transformation. Mol Cell Biol. 1995;15:6443–53.
52. Abo A, Pick E, Hall A, Totty N, Teahan CG, Segal AW. Activation of the NADPH oxidase involves the small GTP-binding protein p21rac. Nature. 1991;353:668–70.
53. Bokoch GM. Regulation of the phagocyte respiratory burst by small GTP-binding proteins. Trends Cell Biol. 1995;5:109–13.
54. Minden A, Lin A, Claret F-X, Abo A, Karin M. Selective activation of the JNK signaling cascade and c-Jun transcriptional activity by the small GTPases Rac and Cdc42Hs. Cell. 1995;81:1147–57.
55. Ridley AJ, Paterson HF, Johnston CL, Diekmann D, Hall A. The small GTP-binding protein rac regulates growth factor-induced membrane ruffling. Cell. 1992;70:401–10.
56. Kozma R, Ahmed S, Best A, Lim L. The Ras-related protein Cdc42Hs and bradykinin promote formation of peripheral actin microspikes and filopodia in Swiss 3T3 fibroblasts. Mol Cell Biol. 1995;15:1942–52.
57. Nobes CD, Hall A. Rho, Rac, and Cdc42 GTPases regulate the assembly of multimolecular focal complexes associated with actin stress fibers, lamellipodia, and filopodia. Cell. 1995;81:53–62.
58. Lim L, Manser E, Leung T, Hall C. Regulation of phosphorylation pathways by p21 GTPases – the p21 Ras-related Rho subfamily and its role in phosphorylation signalling pathways. Eur J Biochem. 1996;242:171–85.
59. Just I, Selzer J, Wilm M, Von Eichel-Streiber C, Mann M, Aktories K. Glucosylation of Rho proteins by Clostridium difficile toxin B. Nature. 1995;375:500–3.
60. Just I, Wilm M, Selzer J et al. The enterotoxin from Clostridium difficile (ToxA) monoglucosylates the Rho proteins. J Biol Chem. 1995;270:13932–6.
61. Bourne HR, Sanders DA, McCormick F. The GTPase superfamily: conserved structure and molecular mechanism. Nature. 1991;349:117–27.
62. Bourne HR, Sanders DA, McCormick F. The GTPase superfamily: a conserved switch for diverse cell functions. Nature. 1990;348:125–32.
63. Pai EF, Kabsch W, Krengel U, Holmes KC, John J, Wittinghofer A. Structure of the guanine-nucleotide-binding domain of the Ha-ras oncogene product p21 in the triphosphate conformation. Nature. 1989;341:209–14.
64. Kim S-H, Privé GG, Milburn MV. Conformational switch and structural basis for oncogenic mutations of Ras proteins. In: Dickey BF, Birnbaumer L, editors. GTPases in biology. I. Berlin: Springer-Verlag; 1993:177–94.

65. Wittinghofer A, Pai EF, Goody RS. Structural and mechanistic aspects of the GTPase reaction of H-ras p21. In: Dickey F, Birnbaumer L, editors. GTPases in biology. I. Berlin: Springer-Verlag; 1993:195–211.

66. Moore R, Pothoulakis C, LaMont JT, Carlson S, Madara JL. *C. difficile* toxin A increases intestinal permeability and induces Cl⁻. Am J Physiol. 1990;259:G165–72.

67. Hecht G, Pothoulakis C, LaMont JT, Madara JL. *Clostridium difficile* toxin A perturbs cytoskeletal structure and tight junction permeability of cultured human intestinal epithelial monolayers. J Clin Invest. 1988;82:1516–24.

68. Nusrat A, Giry M, Turner JR *et al.* Rho protein regulates tight junctions and perijunctional actin organization in polarized epithelia. Proc Natl Acad Sci USA. 1995;92:10629–33.

69. Burakoff R, Zhao L, Celifarco AJ *et al.* Effects of purified *Clostridium difficile* toxin A on rabbit distal colon. Gastroenterology. 1995;109:348–54.

70. Mahida YR, Makh S, Hyde S, Gray T, Borriello SP. Effect of *Clostridium difficile* toxin A on human intestinal epithelial cells: induction of interleukin 8 production and apoptosis after cell detachment. Gut. 1996;38:337–47.

71. Santos MF, McCormack SA, Guo Z *et al.* Rho proteins play a critical role in cell migration during the early phase of mucosal restitution. J Clin Invest. 1997;100:216–25.

15
Acute and chronic endotoxaemia: effects on hepatic neutrophil influx and respiratory burst

J. A. SPITZER

INTRODUCTION

Neutrophils (polymorphonuclear leucocytes or PMN) constitute 70% of circulating leucocytes and are considered to be terminally differentiated phagocytic cells. They circulate passively in the blood, ready to be recruited to sites of infection and inflammation, providing the first line of host defence. They can be activated by a variety of stimuli, resulting in increased phagocytic ability and in the generation of reactive oxygen metabolites, nitric oxide and the secretion of several enzymes, e.g. myeloperoxidase and lysozyme, which are located in granules[1,2].

Within minutes of stimulation by a variety of activators and chemotactic factors acting on the neutrophils in the local microvessels, circulating neutrophils attach to the endothelial wall of the blood vessel at the site of infection, migrate out of the vasculature into the tissue and degranulate, releasing defensive antimicrobial products[3]. While the sequestration of activated PMN into tissues provides an important host defence measure, released products of these cells can also cause overall inflammation and massive injury in vital organs[4].

Because of its rich supply of blood sinusoids and direct access to bacteria and their derived components, e.g. endotoxin or lipopolysaccharide (LPS) brought by the portal circulation, as well as the presence of resident macrophages (Kupffer cells) and their derived cytokines (tumour necrosis factor, interleukin-1), the liver is thought to be a target organ for neutrophil influx in the acute phase of the inflammatory response.

Liver injury after LPS exposure is associated with a number of morphological and functional changes, as well as an acute inflammatory response, a prominent feature of which is an early accumulation of PMN at the site of inflammation[5–8]. This early accumulation of PMN in the liver after LPS exposure suggests that these cells might contribute to LPS-induced liver injury, since PMN depletion attenuates liver injury associated with LPS exposure[9]. PMN might cause liver injury by several mechanisms such as the extracellular release of reactive oxygen metabolites, including superoxide anion and hydrogen peroxide[10], as well as proteases and other enzymes from the granules.

HEPATIC PMN INFLUX IN ACUTE AND CHRONIC ENDOTOXAEMIA

We investigated hepatic PMN infiltration in both acute and chronic endotoxaemia. Studies of the cell yield and distribution of liver non-parenchymal cells obtained by elutriation from rats infused with a non-lethal dose of *Escherichia coli* endotoxin for 3 h (acute endotoxaemia) and continuously for 30 h (chronic endotoxaemia) reveal significant changes in total cell yield, as well as a significant influx of PMN at 3 h, which is absent in chronic endotoxaemia[11]. The percentage of PMN in the 45 ml/min elutriation fraction which contains Kupffer cells and elicited PMN is about 55% after 3 h of LPS infusion, whereas in saline-infused animals after 3 h PMN represent only 4–5% of the total cell yield. Upon chronic endotoxaemia PMN have exited or are already destroyed in the liver, because their proportion in the total cell yield is only about 7% (Fig. 1). The significant influx of PMN into the liver in acute endotoxaemia is accompanied by significantly decreased PMN count in the circulating blood. Similar accumulation of PMN is observed in the liver also 3 h after a bolus injection of a comparable dose of *E. coli* LPS[12]. *In-vivo* exposure to LPS for 3 or 30 h primes PMN for enhanced respiratory burst activity upon subsequent stimulation, as shown in Figs 2 and 3[7].

We have documented the recruitment of PMN into the liver of rats infused with non-lethal doses of LPS even earlier than 3 h. By 30 min of infusion of a non-lethal dose of LPS (160 μg/kg total dose delivered), the proportion of neutrophils in the 45 ml/min elutriation fraction was 36% as compared to 8% in the saline-infused animals. By 90 min of infusion the proportion of neutrophils in this fraction was the same as at 3 h of infusion, about 60%. Interestingly, even

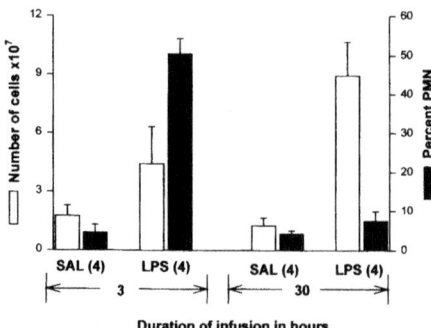

Figure 1 Cell yield and PMN sequestration in the Kupffer cell-enriched (45 ml/min) elutriation fraction of non-parenchymal liver cells from saline- and LPS-infused rats. The percentage of PMN in this fraction after 3 h of LPS infusion is significantly higher than after 3 h of saline infusion. The number of cells in this fraction after 30 h of LPS infusion is significantly higher than after 30 h of saline infusion

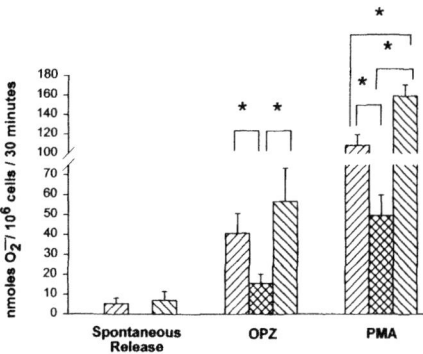

Figure 2 Superoxide O_2^- release spontaneously and upon opsonized zymosan (OPZ, 3500 μg/10^6 cells in 30 min) and PMA (1 nmol/L) stimulation by non-parenchymal liver cells in the 45 ml/min elutriation fraction ⊠, and density gradient separated Kupffer cell ⊠ and PMN ⊠ fractions recovered from rats infused with LPS for 3 h. $^*p < 0.05$. Values are means ± SEM of triplicate determinations of four experiments. (By permission from ref. 7)

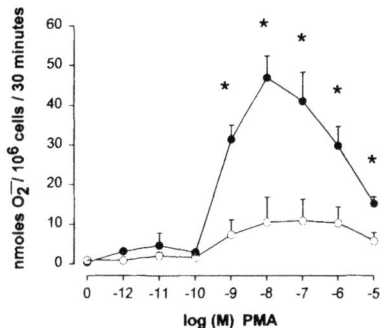

Figure 3 Superoxide release by PMA-stimulated cells of the 45 ml/min elutriation fractions recovered from rats infused with saline (○) or LPS (●) for 30 h. $^*p < 0.05$. Data are expressed as means ± SEM of four independent experiments. (By permission from ref. 7)

though by 30 min of LPS infusion there was a significant influx of PMN into the liver, there was no priming of the non-parenchymal cells for superoxide anion generation in response to *in-vitro* stimulation by phorbol myristate acetate (PMA) or other agents. Likewise, there was no change at this time in the distribution of arachidonic acid metabolites secreted by cells of the 45 ml/min elutriated fraction. However, at 1.5 and 3 h of LPS infusion respiratory burst activity, as shown by superoxide generation, was significantly enhanced, and significant changes were also observed in the arachidonic acid metabolite profile in liver-infiltrated neutrophils[8]. Superoxide generation in the early stages of endotoxaemia was not different in liver-infiltrated PMN from that of circulating PMN of the same LPS-treated rats. However, the respiratory burst activity of PMN from endotoxic animals was higher than in saline control rats[7,8].

FUNCTIONAL DIFFERENCES BETWEEN BLOOD CIRCULATING AND LIVER-RECRUITED PMN OF ENDOTOXIC RATS

The functional states of peripheral blood circulating and liver-recruited PMN of endotoxic animals are different. We have demonstrated significant differences in nitric oxide production, in eicosanoid profile, in CD11b/c expression and in phagocytic activity[13]. Figures 4 and 5 demonstrate significant differences in CD11b/c expression and phagocytic activity between circulating blood and liver-recruited PMN of LPS-infused rats. Studies exploring various signal transduction mechanisms leading to superoxide generation in liver-infiltrated and circulating PMN revealed a significant role of phospholipase A_2 (PLA$_2$) and protein kinase C activity in PMA-stimulated superoxide generation. Because manoalide (MLD), a potent PLA$_2$ inhibitor, inhibited PMA-stimulated superox-

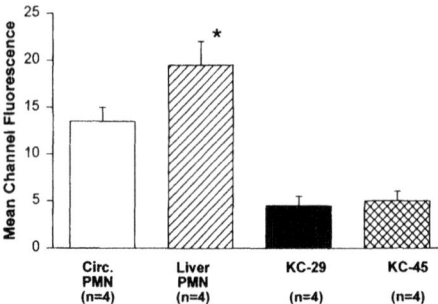

Figure 4 CD11b/expression in liver-sequestered and circulating PMN and in two Kupffer cell fractions of rats infused with LPS for 90 min. Values represent means ± SEM for the number of experiments shown in parentheses. KC-29: Kupffer cells in the 29 ml/min elutriation fraction (small Kupffer cells); KC-45: Kupffer cells in the 45 ml/min elutriation fraction. * = significantly different from Circ. PMN and KC. (By permission from ref. 13)

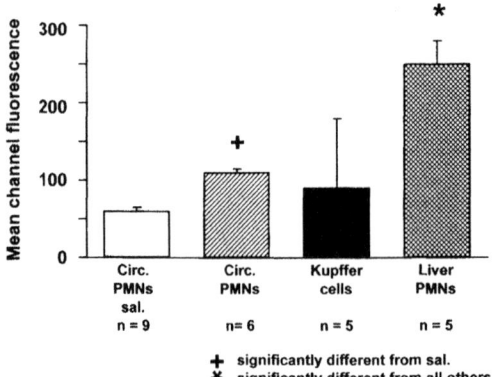

Figure 5 Phagocytic activity (mean channel fluorescence) in circulating PMN, Kupffer cells and liver-sequestered PMN of rats infused with LPS for 90 min. Values are means ± SEM of the number of individual experiments indicated under each bar. (By permission from ref. 13)

198

ide generation, but cyclooxygenase and lipoxygenase inhibitors had no effect, we concluded that PLA_2 activation with a concomitant release of arachidonic acid *per se* were required for PMA-stimulated superoxide generation in both liver-infiltrated and circulating PMN. This contention gained further support from our finding that the inhibitory effect of MLD on PMA-stimulated superoxide generation in the absence of arachidonic acid could be partially reversed in the presence of arachidonic acid[14]. These findings should be helpful in the design of novel therapeutic modalities for the control of superoxide release in the pathogenesis of LPS cytotoxicity.

CYTOKINE-INDUCED NEUTROPHIL CHEMOATTRACTANT (CINC) AND HEPATIC PMN ACCUMULATION

Cytokine-induced neutrophil chemoattractant (CINC) belongs to the CXC chemokine subgroup and is the rat analogue of interleukin-8. CINC is induced in rats by tumour necrosis factor (TNF)-α, interleukin-1 and LPS, and is implicated in neutrophil infiltration in response to inflammatory stimuli. We tested the hypothesis that pretreatment with anti-CINC antibody or by cobra venom factor (CVF) attenuates hepatic neutrophil accumulation induced by a 90-min infusion of *E. coli* endotoxin. Pretreatment with anti-CINC antibody or CVF significantly reduced hepatic neutrophil infiltration (Fig. 6), but did not affect the up-regulation of CD11b/c and CD18 expression on liver-sequestered neutrophils or plasma TNF-α levels. We concluded that attenuation of hepatic neutrophil sequestration by anti-CINC antibody is probably based on blocking the chemotactic activity of CINC, thus diminishing the chemotactic gradient established in the liver[15].

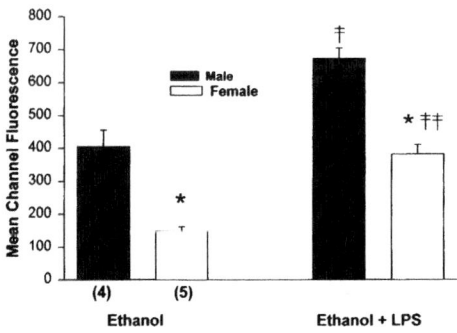

Figure 6   The effect of anti-CINC antibody pretreatment on LPS-induced neutrophil infiltration in the liver. The data represent total cell numbers and percentage of PMN in the 45 ml/min elutriated fractions of rats infused for 90 min with LPS or saline. Anti-CINC antibody treatment consisted of i.v. injections of 1 mg affinity-purified goat anti-CINC IgG 1 h before, and coincident with, the infusion of LPS

GENDER DIFFERENCES IN PMN FUNCTION, CINC GENERATION AND CD11b/c EXPRESSION IN ETHANOL PLUS LPS-TREATED RATS

Several lines of evidence indicate sexual dimorphism in the immune response and in the neuroendocrine–immunological aspects of the acute phase of the inflammatory process. We have demonstrated gender differences in neutrophil function and in CINC generation in endotoxic rats[16]. Subsequently, we have also explored gender differences in the phagocytic response of circulating, and in liver-recruited neutrophils and Kupffer cells, and the generation of CINC in the liver of rats subjected to the dual insult of acute ethanol intoxication and LPS administration. Significant gender differences were noted in neutrophil infiltration into the liver of ethanol plus LPS-treated rats[17] (Fig. 7). Although LPS treatment itself results in hepatic PMN accumulation to the same extent in male and female rats, acute ethanol intoxication in the female exerts a protective effect in that PMN sequestration is significantly reduced compared to that observed in age-matched male animals. Because expression of the adhesion molecule CD11b/c on circulating PMN is a major determinant of the cells' ability to extravasate, we determined CD11b/c expression on circulating PMN in ethanol and ethanol plus LPS-infused rats. CD11b/c expression was significantly reduced in circulating PMN of female rats relative to PMN under the same conditions of ethanol plus LPS treatment in male rats (Fig. 8). Gender differences in phagocytosis were also observed in liver-recruited PMN of acutely ethanol-intoxicated rats with or without LPS treatment (Fig. 9).

Taken together, these studies demonstrate that *in-vivo* exposure of neutrophils to endotoxin primes the cells for enhanced release of reactive oxygen and reac-

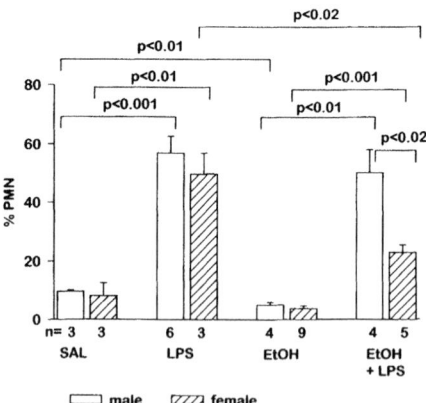

Figure 7 Percentage distribution of PMN in the 45 ml/min elutriation fraction of the non-parenchymal liver cells of saline (SAL), LPS, ethanol (EtOH) and ethanol plus LPS-treated rats. Values are means ± SEM of the number of independent experiments indicated below each bar. Ethanol treatment consisted of a 3 h primed continuous infusion of 20% (v/v) ethanol infusion to a peak blood alcohol level of ~ 180 mg/dl. When LPS was also administered, it was given as an i.v. infusion proceeding through the second 90 min of infusion in a total dose of 167 μg/kg. (By permission from ref. 17)

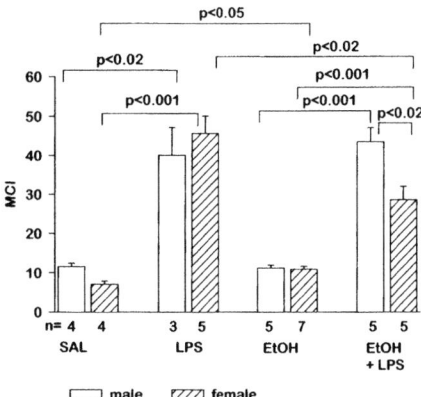

Figure 8 CD11b/c expression (mean channel intensity, MCI) in circulating PMN of saline (SAL), LPS, ethanol (EtOH) and ethanol plus LPS-treated rats. Values are means ± SEM of the number of independent experiments indicated below each bar. (By permission from ref. 17)

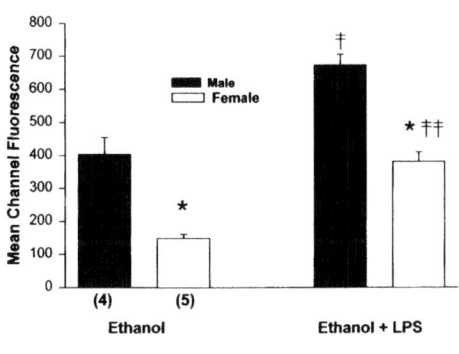

★ p < 0.001 vs Males   ‡ p < 0.01 vs EtOH alone   ‡‡ p < 0.001 vs EtOH alone

Figure 9 Gender differences in phagocytosis by liver-recruited PMN of acutely ethanol-intoxicated rats with or without LPS treatment. Values are means ± SEM of four independent experiments with male rats and five independent experiments with female rats

tive nitrogen intermediates upon subsequent stimulation, and also up-regulates β_2 integrin expression and phagocytosis. Priming may increase host defence to infection, yet predisposes the host to increased tissue damage during inflammation. Several functional attributes of liver-infiltrated neutrophils in the acute endotoxic model are significantly different from those in circulating blood. This is probably a result of the broad construct of endotoxin-induced cytokine networks and interactions of various cell types in the liver. The significant roles played by PLA_2 activity with the resulting availability of arachidonic acid, as well as PKC activity in mediating superoxide generation in acute endotoxaemia, may have relevance in helping to design rational therapeutic approaches to the treatment of cytotoxicity associated with endotoxic injury. Gender differences in hepatic neutrophil influx and several aspects of neutrophil function suggest that, in addition to PMN recruitment-associated liver damage, other factors such as interactions between parenchymal and non-parenchymal cells, differences in the cytokine networks and the interactions of the adrenal and gonadal axes also impact on this aspect of the immune response.

Acknowledgements

The experimental work reported from the author's own laboratory was supported by NIH Grants GM 32654 and AA 09803, and ONR Grant N00014-89-J-1916.

References

1. Korchak HM, Vienne K, Rutherford LE, Weissman G. Neutrophil stimulation: receptor, membrane, and metabolic events. Fed Proc. 1984;43:2749–54.
2. Ignarro LJ. Biosynthesis and metabolism of endothelium-derived nitric oxide. Annu Rev Pharmacol Toxicol. 1990;30:535–60.
3. Osborn L. Leukocyte adhesion to endothelium in inflammation. Cell. 1990;62:3–6.
4. Smith JA. Neutrophils, host defense, and inflammation: a double-edged sword. J Leuk Biol. 1994;56:672–86.
5. Levy E, Ruebner BH. Hepatic changes produced by a single dose of endotoxin in the mouse. Am J Pathol. 1967;51:269–85.
6. Hirata K, Kaneko A. Katsuhiro O et al. Effect of endotoxin on rat liver. Analysis of acid phosphatase isozymes in the liver of normal and endotoxin-treated rats. Lab Invest. 1980;43:165–71.
7. Mayer AMS, Spitzer JA. Continuous infusion of Escherichia coli endotoxin in vivo primes in vitro superoxide anion release in rat polymorphonuclear leukocytes and Kupffer cells in a time-dependent manner. Infect Immun. 1991;59:4590–8.
8. Spitzer JA, Mayer AMS. Hepatic neutrophil influx: eicosanoid and superoxide formation in endotoxemia. J Surg Res. 1993;55:60–7.
9. Hewett JA, Schultze AE, Vancise S et al. Neutrophil depletion protects against liver injury from bacterial endotoxin. Lab Invest. 1992;66:347–61.
10. Fantone JC, Ward PA. Role of oxygen-derived free radicals and metabolites in leukocyte-dependent inflammatory reactions. Am J Pathol. 1982;107:397–418.
11. Rodriguez deTurco EB, Spitzer JA. Eicosanoid production in nonparenchymal liver cells isolated from rats infused with E. coli endotoxin. J Leuk Biol. 1990;48:488–94.
12. Bautista AP, Mészáros K, Bojta J, Spitzer JJ. Superoxide anion generation in the liver during the early stage of endotoxemia in rats. J Leuk Biol. 1990;48:123–8.
13. Spitzer JA, Zhang P, Mayer AMS. Functional characterization of peripheral circulating and liver recruited neutrophils in endotoxic rats. J Leuk Biol. 1994;56:166–73.
14. Mayer AMS, Spitzer JA. Modulation of superoxide anion generation by manoalide, arachidonic acid and staurosporine in liver infiltrated neutrophils in a rat model of endotoxemia. J Pharmacol Exp Ther. 1993;267:400–9.
15. Zhang P, Xie M, Zagorski J, Spitzer JA. Attenuation of hepatic neutrophil sequestration by anti-CINC antibody in endotoxic rats. Shock. 1995;4:262–8.
16. Spitzer JA, Zhang P. Gender differences in neutrophil function and cytokine-induced neutrophil chemoattractant generation in endotoxic rats. Inflammation. 1996;20:485–98.
17. Spitzer JA, Zhang P. Gender differences in phagocytic responses in the blood and liver, and the generation of cytokine-induced neutrophil chemoattractant in the liver of acutely ethanol-intoxicated rats. Alcoholism: Clin Exp Res. 1996;20:914–20.

16
Experimental liver injury: the role of lipopolysaccharides and cytokines

A. WENDEL, M. LEIST, F. GANTNER and G. KÜNSTLE

INTRODUCTION

Overactivation of the host defence

The systemic inflammatory response syndrome (SIRS) is frequently initiated by bacterial infection where cell wall components of germs are recognized by the immune system and cause an overshooting inflammatory response. Shock-like hyperinflammatory conditions may also be elicited in the absence of live microbes by the interaction of their membrane macromolecules with immuno-competent cells. The classical representatives of immunostimulants from Gram-negative bacteria are endotoxins (chemical synonym: lipopolysaccharides, LPS), certain exotoxins as well as superantigens. The toxicity of these substances is indirect, and due to the release of a wide variety of inflammatory mediators in the host. Exposure of the host to such inflammogens frequently results in multi-organ failure as a major clinical complication that affects not only the lungs, kidneys and bowel, but in many cases also the liver[1]. In experimental animals the causal relationship between cytokine release and lethality in different experimental models of sepsis has been firmly established[2-6]. In humans dysregulation and overexpression of various cytokines ('cytokine burst syndrome') has been found to be correlated with these pathological events[7].

Mediators initiated by lipopolysaccharides

Cytokines

LPS from Gram-negative bacteria primarily acts on different populations of macrophages as well as endothelial cells, where the expression and release of various proinflammatory cytokines such as TNF-α, IL-1β, IL-8 and GM-CSF is initiated[8]. It is important to notice that also as counterbalance to overshooting activation, anti-inflammatory factors such as IL-10, TGF-β and the acute-phase cytokine IL-6 are released. LPS also promotes bacterial translocation from the gut, resulting in a further augmentation of endotoxaemia[9]. In addition to activated macrophages, natural killer cells and T lymphocytes release their key proinflammatory cytokine IFN-γ during bacterial infection[10]. The central role of TNF in the pathogenesis of septic shock is addressed in detail in the following sections. Here, we confine ourselves to describing some examples of the forward and feedback interactions that take place within the hyperinflammatory cytokine network.

IL-1 as such shares many activities with TNF, such as the induction of fever and hypotension, as well as the stimulation of IL-6 release and hepatic acute-phase protein production[11]. Evidence for the causal involvement of IL-1 in the pathogenesis of shock is provided by the finding that the blockade of IL-1β actions by IL-1 receptor antagonist protected animals against LPS shock[12]. Moreover, mice deficient in IL-1 converting enzyme (ICE), that have a major defect in the production of mature IL-1β after stimulation with LPS, are resistant to endotoxic shock[13]. IL-6 is released secondary to TNF and IL-1, and is known as a strong inducer of the acute-phase response[14,15], an event that may alleviate the course of endotoxaemia in some cases. IFN-γ, in contrast, contributes considerably to the aggravation of a septic insult. IFN-γ enhances the LPS-induced release of TNF and IL-1 by macrophages[16,17] and mediates the increased sensitivity of mice pretreated with *Propionibacterium acnes* to LPS toxicity[18]. Furthermore, treatment of animals with anti-IFN-γ antibodies[19,20] or disruption of the IFN-γ receptor gene[21] confers protection against endotoxic shock.

Eicosanoids

Secondary to the release of TNF, arachidonic acid release, and its metabolism to prostaglandins, thromboxane and leukotrienes, is initiated[22]. Increased levels of thromboxane A_2 and prostacyclin are found in the circulation of sheep, rodents, and dogs injected with LPS[23-25]. Furthermore, leukotrienes were detected in the bile of rodents and monkeys after administration of LPS[26,27]. Leukotrienes were also described as acting as mediators of septic shock and LPS-induced liver injury[28-30]. The exacerbating effects of leukotrienes in septic shock were attributed either to the increased chemotaxis, broncho- and vasoconstriction, and capillary leakage[28], or to a transient ischaemia/reperfusion caused by the potent vasoconstrictor leukotriene D_4[30].

Nitric oxide (NO)

The pronounced fall in blood during septic shock is largely due to the release of the potent vasodilator NO in response to LPS. NO production is induced by a variety of cytokines and in various cell types, e.g. endothelial cells, macrophages and also hepatocytes and Ito cells[31]. However, endogenous and exogenous NO reduce organ injury or mortality in various models of septic organ failure and shock, including endotoxin-induced liver damage[32,33]. NO produced by constitutive NO synthase (NOS) in endothelial cells inhibits platelet aggregation and improves blood flow in the microcirculation. The net effect of NO in endotoxaemia is accounted for by the actual amount of NO released into the circulation. Whereas high concentrations of NO due to expression of inducible NO synthases result in refractory hypotension, a small amount of NO seems to be indispensable for the maintenance of microcirculation and organ integrity.

The particular role of TNF

The examples discussed so far may suffice to illustrate that endpoint organ destruction, as a consequence of septic shock, cannot be attributed to the actions of a single mediator. Rather, a steadily growing number of agents released from different cellular sources in different organs interacts in a complex network that regulates itself in a way that becomes ever less comprehensible. Therefore, the scheme illustrated in Fig. 1 concentrates only on those processess related to the title of this chapter.

In a variety of different murine models resulting in the release of TNF-α, such as endotoxic shock[34], shock induced by plasmodial antigens[35], or shock induced by T-cell stimulatory superantigens[36–39], a sensitization of up to 10 000-fold towards the initial stimulus by the amino sugar D-galactosamine (GalN) has been observed. Since, in all cases, hepatic injury was the most prominent pathological observation, a rationale for this organotropy has still to be found. Figure 1 might help to clarify why, in spite of the complexity of the cytokine cocktail released during endotoxaemia, it is only TNF-α that acts as a proximal as well as a distal mediator of the sepsis cascade.

1. Administration of small amounts of LPS to healthy volunteers results in enhanced plasma levels of TNF, causing a transient sepsis-like syndrome[40]. The bolus injection of a high dose of LPS to experimental animals causes cardiovascular changes and death, both of which are completely prevented by neutralizing anti-TNF antibodies[41,42]. During the early phase of sepsis, TNF promotes the release of other cytokines such as IL-1, IL-6, IL-8, IL-10, soluble TNF receptors and IL-1 receptor antagonist[43–45].
2. Mice lacking the TNF receptor-1 (TNF-R1) are resistant to endotoxic shock[46,47]. TNF alone elicits all of the pathophysiological alterations observed in endotoxic shock[48–50].

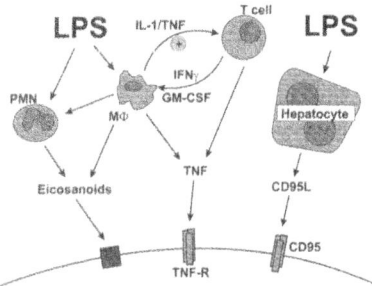

Figure 1 Major proinflammatory factors released from endotoxin (LPS)-activated effector cells to act on the hepatocyte

Sensitizers of experimental liver injury

Since rodents are about three orders of magnitude less sensitive towards LPS than are humans, they are often sensitized by pretreatment with various agents. Bacterial, e.g. *P. acnes* or *Bacillus Calmette-Guerin* (BCG), or viral infection are known to increase the susceptibility of mammals to endotoxin exposure. Among the experimentally used inhibitors of transcription, the aminosugar D-galactosamine (GalN) is the classical example that was initially used to induce an inflammatory liver injury in the rat when administered as such ('GalN hepatitis')[51,52].

GalN is metabolized in rodents exclusively in the liver[53]. For this particular reason it causes a selective depletion of uridine nucleotides in this organ, and thus leads indirectly to a hepatic transcriptional block[54–57]. However, protein synthesis inhibition alone does not sufficiently explain GalN-induced hepatic failure[58]. As candidates that sensitize the liver towards stimuli other than GalN alone, intestinal endotoxins[59] were discussed. The basis for this concept are data showing that GalN induced portal endotoxaemia[60], that GalN hepatitis was prevented either by colectomy[61], or by neutralization of endotoxin with polymyxin B[62] or by anti-LPS antibodies[63], or by induction of tolerance in rats to endotoxin[64].

In spite of the dramatic sensitization by GalN towards the lethal effects of endotoxin it is barely toxic when given to mice alone[65]. By cell transfer experiments between mouse strains of different LPS sensitivity it was demonstrated that macrophages mediate the lethal and hepatotoxic effect of LPS in GalN-sensitized mice[66–68]. Inhibition experiments or direct injection demonstrated that TNF-α was sufficient to mediate lethality and hepatic failure in mice pretreated with GalN[69–72]. In line with this view, in various other murine models resulting in the release of TNF-α, such as endotoxic shock[65], shock induced by plasmodial antigens[73], or shock induced by T-cell stimulatory superantigens[74–77], a sensitization of up to 10 000-fold towards the initial stimulus by GalN has been observed.

Apoptosis in the liver

A large body of histological and biochemical data accumulated during the early 1970s on GalN hepatotoxicity in rats. Retrospectively, it seems that hepatic apoptosis was a key feature of this model, since chromatin condensation and apoptotic bodies (which were then called acidophilic bodies, shrinkage necrosis or Councilman bodies[78–80]) were repeatedly described[81–83]. The molecular mechanisms of hepatic damage, and the cause of lethality, have still not been resolved in the GalN model at the level of the ultimate target cell.

The apoptotic cell death had been originally classified as an own morphological entity with distinct conceptual implications, by Kerr *et al.*[84]. Its defining features are: shrinkage of the cell, detachment from neighbouring cells, preservation of the morphological structure of intracellular organelles, packaging and specific fragmentation of the chromatin, and specific cell membrane alterations indicating a readiness to be phagocytosed. Apoptosis is an inconspicuous type of cell death, allowing rapid removal of the dying cell to prevent tissue damage and inflammation, and favouring rapid reorganization of the tissue to the original structure. For instance, patients may recover from massive (apoptotic?) hepatocyte loss during fulminant viral hepatitis without scarring[85]. In cell cultures, or in pathological situations associated with an extremely high rate of synchronized apoptosis, cells cannot be taken up by phagocytosis, and they eventually lyse. This process of secondary lysis is often confusingly called *secondary necrosis* or *apoptotic necrosis*. However, this post-mortem event does not seem to be related to necrotic/lytic/oncotic cell demise (which describes the transition of living to dead cells). Recent observations suggest that apoptosis and necrosis present only the two extremes of a continuum of different modes of cell death. It is firmly established that the same stimulus may induce either apoptosis or necrosis, depending on the metabolic situation or the intensity of the insult.

HEPATIC APOPTOSIS INDUCED BY ENDOTOXIN

The liver harbours the largest pool of macrophages in the body, and thus is a potent TNF-producing organ[86]. Kupffer cells within the liver may produce TNF after direct stimulation, e.g. with LPS or after interaction with activated lymphocytes in a more complicated immunological setting[87].

Accordingly, LPS injection into GalN-sensitized mice causes TNF release[88,89], and the typical sequence of selective hepatocyte apoptosis followed by widespread necrosis and enzyme release from the liver[90]. Passive immunization of mice against TNF prevented apoptosis[90], as well as transaminase release as a late sign of liver damage[90,91]. When 1000-fold higher doses of LPS were injected into non-sensitized mice the pathological situation was different[92]. We also observed a strictly TNF-dependent liver damage associated with DNA fragmentation. However, the incidence of apoptosis was very low, liver cell types different from hepatocytes were affected, and organ damage was widespread and far from being selective for the liver. Under such excessive intensities of insult the selective triggering of an apoptotic programme may be overridden by many other processes, such as complement activation, neutrophil immigration and activation, ROS generation and many more. In addition, a possibly initiated apoptotic process may not be fully terminated to the stage of chromatin condensation, due to energy failure[93].

Hepatic apoptosis was also observed in GalN-pretreated mice when T-cells were polyclonally activated by stimulation of the T-cell receptor with an anti-CD3 antibody or the superantigen *Staphylococcus aureus* enterotoxin B[94]. Both stimuli strongly increased the serum-TNF concentrations of mice, and passive immunization against TNF prevented this rise, as well as apoptosis and other signs of liver damage. Finally, liver damage associated with hepatocyte apoptosis was induced by the polyclonal T-cell stimulator concanavalin A (ConA)[95]. Again the rise of serum TNF, of apoptosis, and other signs of damage were not present in mice immunized against TNF. Notably, in this model additional sensitization of mice was not required.

HEPATIC APOPTOSIS ELICITED BY CYTOKINES

Growth inhibition by TGF-β

TGF-β acts in the liver; it acts as a negative regulator of hepatocyte growth[96] and mediates collagen deposition by Ito cells and fibrosis[97]. TGF-β was identified as the first defined mediator, eliciting hepatocyte apoptosis[98,99]. It seems to be involved in the normal growth regulation of the liver, rather than in inflammatory or infectious hepatocyte apoptosis. Overexpression of TGF-β in transgenic mice leads to multiple tissue lesions, including hepatocyte apoptosis[100]. The acute toxicity of TGF-β is relatively low[98,101]. Its effects after prolonged exposure seem to depend on the metabolic situation of the liver, e.g. TGF-β-induced apoptosis is greatly enhanced *in vivo* and *in vitro* by tumour promoters, cyproterone acetate treatment or conditions of liver size regression[99,101,102]. A specific characteristic of TGF-β is the arrest of apoptotic DNA fragmentation at the level of 50 kbp fragments in rat liver[103]. This observation demonstrated clearly that oligonucleosomal DNA fragmentation is not required for the apoptotic process.

TNF-α-induced hepatic apoptosis

TNF is an extremely pleiotropic mediator inducing hepatic acute-phase response, hepatic regeneration and growth, stimulation of immune cells, upregulation of adhesion molecules, shock-like conditions, lipolysis, cachexia, tissue destruction and apoptotic or necrotic cell death in various cell types[104,105]. Its cellular effects are mediated by two receptors, i.e. the 55 kDa TNF-RI and the 75 kDa TNF-RII. Its signal transduction involves trimerization and subsequent binding of intracellular proteins[106] to the cytoplasmic tail of the receptor. The coupling of TNF-RI by various adaptor proteins to distinct downstream signalling pathways has been characterized recently: one pathway ends with the activation of caspases, a second involves the generation of ceramide by neutral sphingomyelinase, a third involves jun kinase activation and a further one leads to the activation of the apoptosis-preventing transcription factor NF-κB[107,108]. It is likely that the balance of these pathways determines the cellular fate.

Studies in hepatocyte cultures

The study of TNF-induced apoptosis in isolated hepatocytes has been complicated by the fact that, under standard culture conditions, TNF alone induces no or only a very low percentage of hepatocyte death[109-113]. Cell death was observed only if TNF was present in excessively high concentrations in combination with IFN-γ[114,115]. This difficulty in studying TNF toxicity in hepatocyte cultures is due to the fact that TNF transmits simultaneously possibly cytotoxic signals, and induces various cytoprotective mechanisms, such as the activation of NF-κB[104,105,107]. When these effects are eliminated by blocking transcription, hepatocytes become extremely sensitive towards TNF[109]. Under these conditions 80% of all cells in culture were killed within 16 h, as evidenced by enzyme leakage and loss of the ability to reduce tetrazolium salts. The typical features of cell death were chromatin condensation, budding of the cells, formation of crescent-shaped chromatin lumps and break-up of the chromatin in several apoptotic bodies. These structural changes occurred within hepatocytes which maintained their membrane integrity. In parallel to the structural changes, and well before membrane lysis, the DNA started to fragment and a typical oligonucleosomal pattern of cleavage was observed. All these observations are characteristic for apoptotic cell death. Similar results, i.e. TNF-induced apoptotic cell death under the condition of transcriptional sensitization by ActD (Fig. 1), GalN or α-amanitin, were obtained in cultures of HepG2 human hepatoma cells. Examination of the signal transduction showed that neither reactive oxygen species (ROS) nor NO, nor any of various other well-known signal transduction cascades, played a significant role as mediator of apoptotic death[109].

In vivo studies in mice

TNF has been shown to be hepatotoxic in humans and mice[116,117]. Mice can be dramatically sensitized by viral or bacterial infection, or chemicals such as GalN, which increased the lethality[118] and hepatotoxicity[119] of TNF in mice up to 10 000-fold. The amino sugar GalN selectively depletes uridine in hepatocytes[120,121]. We showed that GalN causes a selective transcriptional inhibition in murine liver. The mechanism of sensitization towards TNF by this substance is due to the selective facilitation of hepatocyte apoptosis caused by such a transcriptional block[90]. Accordingly, selective hepatocyte apoptosis in mice was still observed when GalN was substituted by the general and non-organ-specific transcriptional inhibitor ActD[90,109]. Hepatocyte apoptosis in vivo developed analogously to that observed in vitro. Condensation, margination and fragmentation of the chromatin, associated with oligonucleosomal DNA fragmentation, preceded the loss of intracellular enzymes or a drop in total glutathione levels as parameters for membrane lysis or oxidative stress, respectively[90,109]. Histological examination of the late phases of TNF-induced liver damage in mice sensitized either by GalN or ActD showed widespread necrosis, inflammation and haemorrhage. Thus there is a sequence of events characterized by initially pure hepatocyte apoptosis that is followed by the simultaneous occurrence of apoptosis and necrosis as the liver damage proceeds to virtually complete destruction of the organ. Due to the complexity of the in-vivo approach, it is difficult to decide at this point: (a) whether the occurrence of necrosis was due to secondary actions of TNF, possibly involving other cell types[122]; (b) whether this was due to an inherent, but direct, necrosis-inducing activity of TNF; or (c) whether this was due to an incompletely terminated apoptotic programme in an overstressed or energy-depleted tissue. There is some evidence for each of these possibilities. The last possibility is backed by findings that a variety of insults induce apoptosis at low intensities and cause necrosis, if the intensity or duration of stress is increased[101,123–130]. In addition, we found that typically apoptotic stimuli cause necrosis of T cells, if their ATP levels are reduced[93].

The large-scale induction of hepatocyte apoptosis in vivo and in vitro suggests that a very effective endogenous death programme is present in hepatocytes. This can be very easily triggered under certain metabolic conditions, whereas it is efficiently repressed in others. When activated appropriately such a programme may provide a means to control viral infection and tumour growth in the organ that is most heavily exposed to toxins. If activated inappropriately it may cause rapid destruction of the organ.

Apoptosis via the CD95 (fas/APO-1) system

CD95[131,132] is the nomenclature name for a cell surface receptor homologous to TNF-RI, that was initially identified under the names APO-1[133] and fas[134]. It shares with TNF a short intracellular domain called the 'death domain'. Upon ligand binding and trimerization of the receptor a death-inducing signalling complex (DISC) is formed by association of several molecules to the death domain[106] and initiation of a protease cascade by one of these molecules[135,136]. The CD95 system seems to be less pleiotropic than the TNF/TNF-R system, and cell death mediated by CD95 has always been described as apoptosis.

Studies in hepatocyte cultures

It was shown that injection of an agonistic monoclonal antibody against CD95 (Jo-2) into mice was lethal and associated with fulminant haemorrhagic hepatic failure[137]. Histological examination of these livers showed apoptotic hepatocytes. We were interested in whether these effects of Jo-2 were mediated directly or via other cell types and/or mediators. Therefore, we examined the action of this antibody on primary murine hepatocytes[138]. Analogous to the TNF model a typical sequence of apoptotic events was observed with chromatin and DNA changes preceding the loss of membrane integrity and mitochondrial function. Similar results were obtained in primary human hepatocytes[139]. Notably, murine hepatocyte apoptosis induced by CD95 stimulation did not require any sensitization of the cells. HepG2 human hepatoma cells, however, required sensitization by ActD[140]. These studies suggest that hepatocytes express a second receptor that can directly trigger programmed cell death.

In vivo studies in mice

RNAse protection assays showed that CD95 is highly expressed in murine livers starting at embryonic stages, whereas RNA for the CD95L was not detectable in untreated mice[141]. There are situations in which CD95L can be up-regulated in the liver, e.g. after transformation to hepatocellular carcinoma[142]. Up-regulation may also occur during infection/inflammation in viral or alcoholic liver disease[139], or possibly near the central vein – a region that is thought to be specialized for elimination of aged hepatocytes. In fact, the apoptotic index in the centrilobular region of the liver is increased[143]. Correspondingly, mice with a CD95 null mutation show liver hyperplasia, due to a lack of this death pathway[144].

CD95 expressed in the liver is functional as an apoptosis-triggering receptor, since the liver is the major target organ affected by systemic injection of Jo-2[137]. Subsequently it was shown that apoptotic liver damage also occurred after injection of the CD95 ligand (CD95L) itself[145]. We examined the time-course of various cell death parameters, and whether the liver could be sensitized to CD95-triggered apoptosis by GalN. Analogous to the in-vitro situation, we found only a minor sensitizing effect of GalN towards CD95-mediated liver damage, but the sequence of events (chromatin changes, oligonucleosomal DNA fragmentation and subsequent enzyme release) was similar to that seen with GalN *plus* TNF[138].

RAMIFICATIONS OF THE CD95/CD95L AND THE TNF-R/TNF SYSTEM

Due to the structural homology of CD95 with TNF-RI and CD95L with TNF, and because of the functional redundancy, there were early suggestions that these systems would not act independently. We investigated this question by using mice or hepatocytes from mice that lacked either functional CD95 (lpr) or TNF-RI (tnf-1°) or TNF-RII (tnf-R2°)[138].

1. Hepatocytes from lpr mice were equally sensitive to TNF as were wild-type (wt) mice, but were insensitive towards CD95 stimulation. Similar results were obtained *in vivo*: lpr mice reacted normally towards exogenously injected TNF, or after endogenous TNF induction due to ConA injection, whereas they were insensitive towards CD95 stimulation.
2. In complementary experiments we used hepatocytes from tnf-r1° mice[111,138]. They were completely insensitive towards TNF, but normally susceptible to CD95 stimulation. Similar results were obtained *in vivo*.
3. In a third line of experiments we tested the role of TNF-RII. Hepatocytes from tnf-r2° mice were normally sensitive towards CD95 stimulation and exposure to TNF, *in vivo* or *in vitro*. That is, TNF-RII does not seem to play a major role in the induction of apoptosis by TNF. The transmission of the TNF death signal in hepatocytes by TNF-RI alone is further suggested by the fact that human TNF (which binds to the murine TNF-RI, but not to the murine TNF-RII) induces murine hepatocyte apoptosis *in vivo* and *in vitro*[111].

These studies strongly suggest that two fully independent receptor–ligand systems control hepatocyte apoptosis (Fig. 2, upper part). Additional evidence is provided by the observations that TNF apoptosis is modulated by GalN or variable ambient oxygen tensions, whereas that induced by CD95 stimulation is not[138]. Furthermore the inhibition profile upon immunological, pharmacological or genetic intervention differs between the two stimuli.

MODULATION OF HEPATIC APOPTOSIS

Modulation of hepatic apoptosis is desirable in disease control. Conversely, important mechanistic information can be derived from genetic, pharmacological and immunological intervention studies in disease models.

Pharmacological intervention against apoptosis

Since the signal transduction of CD95 and TNF-RI has been identified only during the past 2 years, earlier intervention strategies could not follow a rational

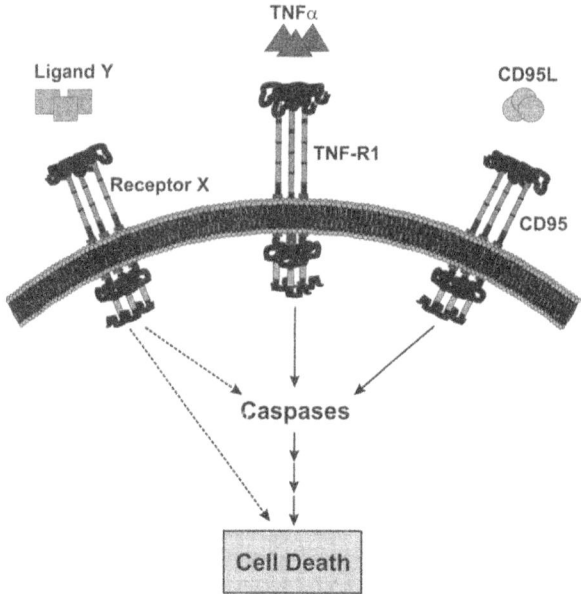

Figure 2 Apoptosis-inducing receptor/ligand systems in the liver

approach. A selective and potent reduction of TNF-induced apoptosis, but not of that induced by CD95, was obtained with fructose treatment. Liver damage due to CD95 activation was prevented by linomide, a substance possibly preventing the intracellular signalling of CD95 via the sphingomyelinase pathway[146].

An early pharmacological approach was based on the assumption that components of the death programme may require *de-novo* protein synthesis. ActD-sensitized hepatocyte cultures were indeed protected by various inhibitors of protein synthesis from TNF-induced apoptosis. Concentration-dependent protection was observed with cycloheximide, puromycin, ricin and tunicamycin[109,147]. Since these substances are chemically and mechanistically unrelated, and only share their inhibitory action on (glyco)protein synthesis, *de-novo* synthesis of some (glyco)protein seems to be required. Protein synthesis inhibitors alone had only a small sensitizing effect towards TNF. Notably, these observations may be specific for TNF-challenged murine hepatocytes. When human hepatoma cells were used, they could be sensitized towards TNF by cycloheximide or ActD. Protein synthesis inhibitors did not protect from apoptosis elicited by CD95 stimulation, but rather had a sensitizing effect[148].

A rise in intracellular cAMP is known to result in suppression of monocyte- or macrophage-derived TNF production. Therefore, a possible pharmacological approach can take advantage of inhibiting the enzymes of the phosphodiesterase (PDE) family, thus arresting the turnover of cyclic nucleotides. In LPS-challenged GalN-sensitized mice, various PDE inhibitors protected from liver injury and lethality[149], and macrophages from these animals were deficient in TNF production when stimulated with LPS. Recently, we extended our previous studies to T-cell-mediated murine liver failure models. Animals pretreated with PDE inhibitors of different isoenzyme selectivity dose-dependently protected against liver injury brought about by overactivation of the lymphocytic cytokine response by the T-cell mitogen ConA, or by the superantigen staphylococcal enterotoxin B[150]. These experiments show that this kind of intervention has a wide potential in preventing hyperinflammatory reactions, independent of the cellular source and the mode of activation.

On a similar background we also checked the pharmacological properties of various methylxanthines in experimental inflammatory liver injury. From a wide variety of analogues the compound A802715 ((5-hydroxy-5-methyl)hexyl-3-methyl-7-propylxanthine) exhibited a special pharmacodynamic profile. In the isolated perfused mouse liver it reversibly abrogated the LPS-stimulated release of TNF-α via regulation of intrahepatic cAMP[151]. Surprisingly, the compound protected *in vivo* not only against LPS, but also (at a higher dose) against TNF-α. We found that pretreatment of mice with A802715 up-regulated the expression and systemic release of the major physiological TNF-α antagonist, i.e. the cytokine IL-10. Moreover, in the presence of the drug an increased shedding of the soluble TNF receptors occurred in the circulation, thus creating a TNF-binding and neutralizing capacity[152]. These experiments not only show a novel principle of pharmacological anti-LPS and anti-TNF strategy via early activation of endogenous counterregulation, but also demonstrate that 'cutting off the tip' of the overshooting TNF production is sufficient for maintenance of organ function and survival.

A completely different mode of prophylactic intervention against endotoxic injury is based on the finding that granulocyte colony-stimulating factor (G-CSF) pretreatment of mice protects the animals[153]. Again, the systemic release of TNF was attenuated under these conditions, and was concluded to be responsible for this protection. However, such an influence of G-CSF on TNF secretion was observed only *in vivo* in mice or rats and *ex vivo* in various macrophage populations, but not *in vitro*. We then examined, in blood taken from volunteers treated with G-CSF, whether similar conditions apply to humans. The release capacity of LPS-stimulated whole blood from G-CSF-treated subjects was decreased for TNF-α and IFN-γ, while the release of anti-inflammatory factors soluble TNF receptors and IL-1 receptor antagonist was strongly increased[154]. It therefore appears that G-CSF treatment had shifted the non-specific host defence towards a lower activation by LPS, i.e. a pharmacological property that is characteristic for a biological response modifier. On the basis of these data there are good reasons to believe that G-CSF can be clinically used for the prophylaxis of sepsis risks to be anticipated before elective major surgery.

In 1995 the intracellular pathway leading from TNF-R stimulation to apoptosis was shown in various cell types to involve the action of caspases[155–157], a new class of proteases structurally related to the *ced-3* cell death gene of *Caenorhabditis elegans*[158]. We and others tested whether inhibition of these proteases may be a useful pharmacological approach to stop pathological processes involving hepatocyte apoptosis[140,159,160]. The result showed unanimously that both TNF- and CD95-mediated hepatic apoptosis in mice was completely prevented when caspase activities were blocked. In addition, liver damage could even be stopped after its initiation, by curative application of caspase inhibitors.

The *in-vitro* use of caspase inhibitors specific for different subclasses allowed us to define a yama/caspase-3 related enzyme as key mediator. In agreement with this, caspase activity measurements *in vivo* showed that this enzyme was particularly activated in the liver by CD95 stimulation. Finally, caspase inhibitors were shown not only to delay hepatotoxicity or to shift the toxicity to another organ; rather, a single dose was sufficient to shift 100% mortality induced via CD95 activation to complete long-term survival. Although the inhibitors used are still at an experimental stage, a novel pharmacological approach to apoptosis-related liver disease may be anticipated. Our current view of individuality of receptors of known function, i.e. CD95 and TNF-RI, and of newly discovered members of this family such as WSL-1/Apo-3[161,162] and TRAMP[163], is shown in Fig. 2.

Immunological and genetic modulation of apoptosis

TNF-induced murine hepatic apoptosis *in vivo* can be inhibited by immune modulators. For example, it has been shown that injection of the NO-donor sodium nitroprusside or IL-1 completely prevented liver damage[90,164]. Conversely, inhibition of endogenous NO formation significantly enhanced TNF-dependent liver damage[92,164], so that NO seems to act as an endogenous protective substance in the liver. The effect of IL-1 is specific for TNF-induced toxicity, since liver damage due to CD95 stimulation is not reduced by this cytokine[138]. Whether NO or IL-1 has an intracellular or extracellular action is not clear, since the protective effect is not seen in hepatocyte cultures.

Molecules modifying the CD95 apoptosis signal inside the cell have been examined by the generation of transgenic mice. In an elegant approach *bcl-2*, a gene controlling apoptosis upstream of the caspase cascade, was overexpressed selectively in murine livers[165]. Such transgenic mice were resistant against CD95-induced apoptosis and also lethality. This approach shows very clearly that fas-induced lethality in mice is exclusively due to stimulation of apoptosis in hepatocytes and the subsequent liver failure.

In another approach a non-transforming mutant of SV40 T antigen was overexpressed in mice. This molecule does not transform cells, but is able to inactivate the putatively proapoptotic protein p53[166]. Hepatocytes from such mice were protected from CD95-mediated apoptosis, but not from TNF. Thus, again, a variation of the two signal transduction pathways of TNF-RI and CD95 is suggested, although both have caspase activation in common. Possible involvement of p53 in CD95 killing, but not in TNF-triggered apoptosis, suggests that alternatives in differentiated modulation of hepatic apoptosis exist.

References

1. Bone RC, Balk RA, Cerra FB *et al*. Definitions for sepsis and organ failure and guidelines for the use of innovative therapies in sepsis. Chest. 1992;101:1644–55.
2. Beutler B, Grau GE. Tumor necrosis factor in the pathogenesis of infectious diseases. Crit Care Med. 1993;21:S423–35.
3. Tracey KJ, Cerami A. Tumor necrosis factor: an updated review of its biology. Crit Care Med. 1993;21:S415–21.
4. Gantner F, Leist M, Lohse AW, Germann PG, Tiegs G. Concanavalin A-induced T cell-mediated hepatic injury in mice: the role of tumor necrosis factor. Hepatology. 1995;21:190–8.

5. Vassalli P. The pathophysiology of tumor necrosis factors. Annu Rev Immunol. 1992; 10:411–52.
6. Tracey KJ, Beutler B, Lowry SF *et al.* Shock and tissue injury induced by recombinant human cachectin. Science. 1986;234:470–4.
7. Waage A. Presence and involvement of TNF in septic shock. In: Beutler B, editor. Tumor necrosis factors: the molecules and their emerging role in medicine. New York: Raven Press; 1993:275–83.
8. Bone RC. Toward a theory regarding the pathogenesis of the systemic inflammatory response syndrome: what we do and do not know about cytokine regulation. Crit Care Med. 1996;24:163–72.
9. Deitch EA, Berg RD. Endotoxin but not malnutrition promotes bacterial translocation of the gut flora in burned mice. J Trauma. 1987;27:161–6.
10. Freudenberg MA, Kumazawa Y, Meding S, Langhorne J, Galanos C. Gamma interferon production in endotoxin-responder and -nonresponder mice during infection. Infect Immun. 1991;59:3484–91.
11. Fischer E, Marano MA, Barber AE *et al.* Comparison between effects of interleukin-1 alpha administration and sublethal endotoxemia in rabbits. Am J Physiol. 1991;261:R442–52.
12. Aiura K, Gelfand JA, Burke JF, Thompson RC, Dinarello CA. Interleukin-1 (IL-1) receptor antagonist prevents *Staphylococcus epidermidis*-induced hypotension and reduces circulating levels of tumor necrosis factor and IL-1 beta in rabbits. Infect Immun. 1993;61:3342–50.
13. Li P, Allen H, Banerjee S *et al.* Mice deficient in IL-1 beta-converting enzyme are defective in production of mature IL-1 beta and resistant to endotoxic shock. Cell. 1995;80:401–11.
14. Heinrich PC, Castell JV, Andus T. Interleukin-6 and the acute phase response. Biochem J. 1990;265:621–35.
15. Kopf M, Baumann H, Freer G *et al.* Impaired immune and acute-phase responses in interleukin-6-deficient mice. Nature. 1994;368:339–42.
16. Collart MA, Belin D, Vassalli J-D, de Kossodo S, Vassalli P. γ Interferon enhances macrophage transcription of the tumor necrosis factor/cachectin, interleukin 1, and urokinase genes, which are controlled by short-lived repressors. J Exp Med. 1986; 164:2113–18.
17. Beutler B, Tkacenko V, Milsark I, Krochin N, Cerami A. Effect of γ interferon on cachectin expression by mononuclear phagocytes. Reversal of the lpsd (endotoxin resistance) phenotype. J Exp Med. 1986;164:1791–6.
18. Katschinski T, Galanos C, Coumbos A, Freudenberg M. Gamma interferon mediates *Propionibacterium acnes*-induced hypersensitivity to lipopolysaccharide in mice. Infect Immun. 1992;60:1994–2001.
19. Heinzel FP. The role of IFN-γ in the pathology of experimental endotoxemia. J Immunol. 1990;145:2920–4.
20. Doherty GM, Lange JR, Langstein HN, Alexander HR, Buresh CM. Evidence for IFN-γ as a mediator of the lethality of endotoxin and tumor necrosis factor-α. J Immunol. 1992; 149:1666–70.
21. Car BD, Eng VM, Schnyder B *et al.* Interferon γ receptor deficient mice are resistant to endotoxic shock. J Exp Med. 1994;179:1437–44.
22. Petrark RA, Balk RA, Bone RC. Prostaglandins, cyclo-oxygenase inhibitors, and thromboxane synthetase inhibitors in the pathogenesis of multiple organ systems failure. Crit Care Clin. 1989;5:303–14.
23. Cook JA, Wise WC, Halushka PV. Elevated thromboxane levels in the rat during endotoxic shock. J Clin Invest. 1980;65:227–30.
24. Demling RH, Smith M, Gunther R, Flynn JT, Gee MH. Pulmonary injury and prostaglandin production during endotoxaemia in conscious sheep. Am J Physiol. 1981;240:H348–53.
25. Yellin SA, Nguyen D, Quinn JV, Buchard KW, Crowley JP, Slotman GJ. Prostacyclin and thromboxane A_2 in septic shock: species differences. Circ Shock. 1986;20:291–7.
26. Hagmann W, Denzlinger C, Keppler D. Production of peptido leukotrienes in endotoxin shock. FEBS Lett. 1985;180:309–13.
27. Denzlinger C, Guhlmann A, Scheuber DH, Wilker D, Hammer DK, Keppler D. Metabolism and analysis of cysteinyl leukotrienes in the monkey. J Biol Chem. 1986;261:15601–6.
28. Lefer AM. Leukotrienes as mediators of ischemia and shock. Biochem Pharmacol. 1986;35:123–7.

29. Keppler D, Hagmann W, Rapp S, Denzlinger C, Koch HK. The relation of leukotrienes to liver injury. Hepatology. 1985;5:883–91.
30. Tiegs G, Wendel A. Leukotriene-mediated liver injury. Biochem Pharmacol. 1988; 37:2569–73.
31. Helyar L, Bundschuh DS, Laskin JD, Laskin DL. Induction of hepatic Ito cell nitric oxide production after acute endotoxemia. Hepatology. 1994;20:1509–15.
32. Bohlinger I, Leist M, Barsig J, Uhlig S, Tiegs G, Wendel A. Interleukin-1 and nitric oxide protect against tumor necrosis factor-α-induced liver injury through distinct pathways. Hepatology. 1995;22:1829–37.
33. Harbrecht BG, Billiar TR, Stadler AJ et al. Nitric oxide synthesis serves to reduce hepatic damage during acute murine endotoxemia. Crit Care Med. 1992;20:1568–74.
34. Galanos C, Freudenberg MA, Reutter WR. Galactosamine-induced sensitization to the lethal effects of endotoxin. Proc Natl Acad Sci USA. 1979;76:5939–43.
35. Bate CA, Taverne J, Playfair JH. Soluble malarial antigens are toxic and induce the production of tumor necrosis factor in vivo. Immunology. 1989;66:600–5.
36. Miethke T, Wahl C, Heeg K, Echtenacher B, Krammer PH, Wagner H. T cell-mediated lethal shock triggered in mice by the superantigen staphylococcal enterotoxin B: critical role of tumor necrosis factor. J Exp Med. 1992;175:91–8.
37. Nagaki M, Muto Y, Ohnishi H et al. Hepatic injury and lethal shock in galactosamine-sensitized mice induced by the superantigen staphylococcal enterotoxin B. Gastroenterology. 1994;106:450–8.
38. Miethke T, Duschek K, Wahl C, Heeg K, Wagner H. Pathogenesis of the toxic shock syndrome: T cell mediated lethal shock caused by the superantigen TSST-1. Eur J Immunol. 1993;23:1494–500.
39. Pfeffer K, Matsuyama T, Kündig TM et al. Mice deficient for the 55 kd tumor necrosis factor receptor are resistant to endotoxic shock, yet succumb to L. monocytogenes infection. Cell. 1993;73:457–67.
40. van Deventer SJH, Buller HR, ten Cate JW, Aarden LA, Hack CE, Sturk A. Experimental endotoxemia in humans: analysis of cytokine release and coagulation, fibrinolytic, and complement pathways. Blood. 1990;76:2520–6.
41. Tracey KJ, Fong Y, Hesse DG et al. Anti-cachectin/TNF monoclonal antibodies prevent septic shock during lethal bacteraemia. Nature. 1987;330:662–4.
42. Beutler B, Milsark IW, Cerami AC. Passive immunization against cachectin/tumor necrosis factor protects mice from lethal effect of endotoxin. Science. 1985;229:869–71.
43. Fong Y, Tracey KJ, Moldawer LL et al. Antibodies to cachectin/tumor necrosis factor reduce interleukin 1β and interleukin 6 appearing during lethal bacteremia. J Exp Med. 1989;170:1627–33.
44. Brouckaert P, Spriggs DR, Demetri G, Kufe DW, Fiers W. Circulating interleukin-6 during a continuous infusion of tumor necrosis factor and interferon-γ. J Exp Med. 1989;169:2257–62.
45. Dinarello CA, Cannon JG, Wolff SM et al. Tumor necrosis factor (cachectin) is an endogenous pyrogen and induces production of interleukin 1. J Exp Med. 1986;163:1433–50.
46. Rothe J, Lesslauer W, Loetscher H et al. Mice lacking the tumor necrosis factor receptor 1 are resistant to TNF-mediated toxicity but highly susceptible to infection by Listeria monocytogenes. Nature. 1993;364:798–800.
47. Pfeffer K, Matsuyama TM, Kündig A et al. Mice deficient for the 55 kD tumor necrosis factor receptor are resistant to endotoxic shock yet succumb to L. monocytogenes infection. Cell. 1993;73:457–67.
48. Mathison JC, Wolfson E, Ulevitch RJ. Participation of tumor necrosis factor in the mediation of Gram negative bacterial lipopolysaccharide-induced injury in rabbits. J Clin Invest. 1988;81:1925–37.
49. Kilbourn RG, Gross SS, Jubran A et al. N^G-methyl-L-arginine inhibits tumor necrosis factor-induced hypotension: implications for the involvement of nitric oxide. Proc Natl Acad Sci USA. 1990;87:3629–32.
50. van der Poll T, Lowry SF. Tumor necrosis factor in sepsis: mediator of multiple organ failure or essential part of host defense? Shock. 1995;3:1–12.
51. Redl H, Bahrami S, Schlag G, Traber DL. Clinical detection of LPS and animal models of endotoxemia. Immunobiology. 1993;187:330–45.

52. Wendel A. Biochemical pharmacology of inflammatory liver injury in mice. Meth Enzymol. 1990;186:675–80.
53. Decker K, Keppler D. Galactosamine hepatitis: key role of the nucleotide deficiency period in the pathogenesis of cell injury and cell death. Rev Physiol Biochem Pharmacol. 1974;71:77–100.
54. Anukarahanonta T, Shinozuka H, Farber E. Inhibition of protein synthesis in rat liver by D-galactosamine. Res Commun Chem Pathol Pharmacol. 1973;5:481–91.
55. Shinozuka H, Martin JT, Farber JL. The induction of fibrillar nucleoli in rat liver cells by D-galactosamine and their subsequent re-formation into normal nucleoli. J Ultrastrucure Res. 1973;44:279–92.
56. Shinozuka H, Farber JL, Konishi Y, Anukarahanota T. D-galactosamine and acute liver cell injury. Fed Proc. 1973;32:1516–26.
57. Konishi Y, Shinozuka H, Farber JL. The inhibition of rat liver nuclear ribonucleic acid synthesis by galactosamine and its reversal by uridine. Lab Invest. 1974;30:751–6.
58. Farber E. Response of cells to inhibition of synthesis of DNA, RNA and protein. Biochem Pharmacol. 1971;20:1023–6.
59. Nolan JP. Intestinal endotoxins as mediators of hepatic injury-an idea whose time has come again. Hepatology. 1989;10:887–91.
60. Grün M, Liehr H, Rasenack U. Significance of endotoxemia in experimental 'galactosamine-hepatitis' in the rat. Acta Hepato-Gastroenterol. 1976;23:64–81.
61. Iwaki Y, Noguchi K, Tanikawa K, Tsuda K. Role of endotoxin in the development of galactosamine-induced hepatic injury. In: Wisse E, Knook DL, Decker K, editors. Cells of the hepatic sinusoid. Rijswijk, Netherlands: Kupffer Cell Foundation; 1989;351–2.
62. Mihas AA, Ceballos R, Mihas TA, Hirshowitz BI. Modification of the hepatotoxicity of D-galactosamine in the rat by an anti-endotoxin. J Med. 1990;21:301–11.
63. Czaja MJ, Xu J, Ju Y, Alt E, Schmiedeberg P. Lipopolysaccharide-neutralizing antibody reduces hepatocyte injury from acute hepatotoxin administration. Hepatology. 1994; 19:1282–98.
64. Grün M, Liehr H, Rasenack U. Significance of endotoxaemia in experimental 'galactosamine-hepatitis' in the rat. Acta Hepato-Gastroenterol. 1976;23:64–81.
65. Galanos C, Freudenberg MA, Reutter WR. Galactosamine-induced sensitisation to the lethal effects of endotoxin. Proc Natl Acad Sci USA. 1979;76:5939–43.
66. Shiratori Y, Tanaka M, Hai K, Kawase T, Shiina S, Sugimoto T. Role of endotoxin-responsive macrophages in hepatic injury. Hepatology. 1990;11:183–92.
67. Chojkier M, Fierer J. D-galactosamine hepatotoxicity is associated with endotoxin sensitivity and mediated by lymphoreticular cells in mice. Gastroenterology. 1985;88:115–21.
68. Freudenberg MA, Keppler D, Galanos C. Requirement for lipopolysaccharide-responsive macrophages in galactosamine-induced sensitization to endotoxin. Infect Immun. 1986;51:891–5.
69. Lehmann V, Freudenberg MA, Galanos C. Lethal toxicity of lipopolysaccharide and tumor necrosis factor in normal and D-galactosamine-treated mice. J Exp Med. 1987;165:657–63.
70. Wendel A, Tiegs G. Pharmacological intervention studies against lipopolysaccharides or TNF-alpha toxicity in mice. In: Fiers W, Buurman WA, editors. Tumor necrosis factor: molecular and cellular biology and clinical relevance. Basel: Karger; 1993:120–5.
71. Tiegs G, Niehörster M, Wendel A. Leukocyte alterations do not account for hepatitis induced by endotoxin or TNF-alpha in galactosamine-sensitized mice. Biochem Pharmacol. 1990;40:1317–22.
72. Tiegs G, Wolter M, Wendel A. Tumor necrosis factor is a terminal mediator in D-galactosamine/endotoxin-induced hepatitis in mice. Biochem Pharmacol. 1989;38:627–31.
73. Bate CA, Taverne J, Playfair JH. Soluble malarial antigens are toxic and induce the production of tumor necrosis factor in vivo. Immunology. 1989;66:600–5.
74. Miethke T, Wahl C, Heeg K, Echtenacher B, Krammer PH, Wagner H. T cell-mediated lethal shock triggered in mice by the superantigen staphylococcal enterotoxin B: critical role of tumor necrosis factor. J Exp Med. 1992;175:91–8.
75. Nagaki M, Muto Y, Ohnishi H et al. Hepatic injury and lethal shock in galactosamine-sensitized mice induced by the superantigen staphylococcal enterotoxin B. Gastroenterology. 1994;106:450–8.

76. Miethke T, Duschek K, Wahl C, Heeg K, Wagner H. Pathogenesis of the toxic shock syndrome. T cell mediated lethal shock caused by the superantigen TSST-1. Eur J Immunol. 1993;23:1494–500.

77. Pfeffer K, Matsuyama T, Kündig TM *et al.* Mice deficient for the 55 kd tumor necrosis factor receptor are resistant to endotoxic shock, yet succumb to *L. monocytogenes* infection. Cell. 1993;73:457–67.

78. Kerr JF, Wyllie AH, Currie AR. Apoptosis: a basic biological phenomenon with wide ranging implications in tissue kinetics. Br J Cancer. 1972;26:239–47.

79. Kerr JFR. Shrinkage necrosis: a distinct mode of cellular death. J Pathol. 1971;105:13–22.

80. Klion FM, Schaffner F. The ultrastructure of acidophilic 'councilman-like' bodies in the liver. Am J Pathol. 1966;48:755–65.

81. Medline A, Schaffner F, Popper H. Ultrastructural features in galactosamine-induced hepatits. Exp Mol Pathol. 1970;12:201–12.

82. Reutter W, Bauer CH, Lesch R. On the mechanism of action of galactosamine: different response to D-galactosamine of rat liver during development. Naturwissenschaften. 1970;57:674–5.

83. Reutter W, Lesch R, Keppler D, Decker K. Galactosamine-hepatitis. Naturwissenschaften. 1968;55:497.

84. Kerr JF, Wyllie AH, Currie AR. Apoptosis: a basic biological phenomenon with wide ranging implications in tissue kinetics. Br J Cancer. 1972;26:239–47.

85. Karvountzis GG, Redeker AG, Peters RL. Long-term follow-up studies of patients surviving fulminant viral hepatitis. Gastroenterology. 1974;67:870–7.

86. Leist M, Auer-Barth S, Wendel A. Tumor necrosis factor production in the perfused mouse liver and its pharmacological modulation by methylxanthines. J Pharmacol Exp Ther. 1996;276:968–76.

87. Gantner F, Leist M, Küsters S, Vogt K, Volk D, Tiegs G. T cell stimulus-induced crosstalk between lymphocytes and liver macrophages results in augmented cytokine release. Exp Cell Res. 1996;229:137–46.

88. Wendel A. Biochemical pharmacology of inflammatory liver injury in mice. Meth Enzymol. 1990;186:675–80.

89. Jilg S, Barsig J, Leist M, Küsters S, Volk H-D, Wendel A. Enhanced release of interleukin-10 and soluble tumor necrosis factor receptors as novel principles of methylxanthine action in murine models of endotoxic shock. J Pharmacol Exp Ther. 1996;278:421–31.

90. Leist M, Gantner F, Bohlinger I, Tiegs G, Germann PG, Wendel A. Tumor necrosis factor-induced hepatocyte apoptosis precedes liver failure in experimental murine shock models. Am J Pathol. 1995;146:1220–34.

91. Tiegs G, Niehörster M, Wendel A. Leukocyte alterations do not account for hepatitis induced by endotoxin or TNF-alpha in galactosamine-sensitized mice. Biochem Pharmacol. 1990;40:1317–22.

92. Bohlinger I, Leist M, Gantner F, Angermüller S, Tiegs G, Wendel A. DNA-fragmentation in mouse organs during endotoxic shock. Am J Pathol. 1996;149:1381–93.

93. Leist M, Single B, Castoldi AF, Kühnle S, Nicotera P. Intracellular ATP concentration: a switch determining the shape of cell death. J Exp Med. 1997;185:1481–6.

94. Gantner F, Leist M, Jilg S, German PG, Freudenberg MA, Tiegs G. Tumor necrosis factor-induced hepatic DNA fragmentation as an early marker of T cell-dependent liver injury in mice. Gastroenterology. 1995;109:166–76.

95. Gantner F, Leist M, Lohse AW, Germann PG, Tiegs G. Concanavalin A-induced T cell-mediated hepatic injury in mice: the role of tumor necrosis factor. Hepatology. 1995; 21:190–8.

96. Bursch W, Oberhammer F, Schulte-Hermann R. Cell death by apoptosis and its protective role against disease. Trends Pharmacol Sci. 1992;13:245–51.

97. Weiner FR, Giambrone M, Czaja MJ *et al.* Ito-Cell gene expression and collagen regulation. Hepatology. 1990;11:111–20.

98. Oberhammer FA, Pavelka M, Sharma S *et al.* Induction of apoptosis in cultured hepatocytes and in regressing liver by transforming growth factor $\beta 1$. Proc Natl Acad Sci USA. 1992;89:5408–12.

99. Oberhammer F, Bursch W, Tiefenbacher R *et al.* Apoptosis is induced by transforming growth factor-beta1 within 5 hours in regressing liver without significant fragmentation of the DNA. Hepatology. 1993;18:1238–46.

100. Sanderson M, Factor V, Nagy P *et al.* Hepatic expression of mature transforming growth factor beta1 in transgenic mice results in multiple tissue lesions. Proc Natl Acad Sci USA. 1995; 92:2572–6.

101. Oberhammer F, Nagy P, Tiefenbacher R *et al.* The antiandrogen cyproterone acetate induces synthesis of transforming factor beta-1 in the parenchymal cells of the liver accompanied by an enhanced sensitivity to undergo apoptosis and necrosis without inflammation. Hepatology. 1996;23:329–37.

102. Oberhammer FA, Qin H. Effect of three tumor promoters on the stability of hepatocyte cultures and apoptosis after transforming growth factor-beta1. Carcinogenesis. 1995;16:1363–71.

103. Oberhammer F, Wilson JW, Dive C *et al.* Apoptotic death in epithelial cells: cleavage of DNA to 300 and/or 50 kb fragments prior to or in the absence of internucleosomal fragmentation. EMBO J. 1993;12:3679–84.

104. Beutler B, editor. Tumor necrosis factors. The molecules and their emerging role in medicine. New York: Raven Press;1992.

105. Aggarwall BB, Vilcek J, editors. Tumor necrosis factors. Structure, function and mechanisms of action. New York: Marcel Dekker; 1992.

106. Peter ME, Kischkel FC, Hellbardt S, Chinnaiyan AM, Krammer PH, Dixit VM. CD95(APO-1/Fas)-associating signalling proteins. Cell Death Diff. 1996; 3:161–70.

107. Zheng-gang L, Hsu H, Goeddel DV, Karin M. Dissection of TNF receptor 1 effector functions: JNK activation is not linked to apoptosis while NF-kB activation prevents cell death. Cell. 1996;87:565–76.

108. Adam-Klages S, Adam D, Wiegmann K *et al.* FAN, a novel WD-repeat protein, couples the p55 TNF-receptor to neutral sphingomyelinase. Cell. 1996;86:937–47.

109. Leist M, Ganter F, Bohlinger I, German PG, Tiegs G, Wendel A. Murine hepatocyte apoptosis induced *in vitro* and *in vivo* by TNF-alpha requires transcriptional arrest. J Immunol. 1994;153:1778–87.

110. Guilhot S, Miller T, Cornman G, Isom HC. Apoptosis induced by tumor necrosis factor-alpha in rat hepatocyte cell lines expressing hepatitis B virus. Am J Pathol. 1996; 148:801–14.

111. Leist M, Gantner F, Jilg S, Wendel A. Activation of the 55 kDa TNF-receptor is necessary and sufficient for TNF-induced liver failure, hepatocyte apoptosis and nitrite release. J Immunol. 1995;154:1307–16.

112. Stadler J, Bentz BG, Harbrecht BG *et al.* Tumor necrosis factor alpha inhibits hepatocyte mitochondrial respiration. Ann Surg. 1992;216:539–46.

113. Shinagawa T, Yoshioka K, Kakumu S *et al.* Apoptosis in cultured rat hepatocytes: the effect of tumour necrosis factor alpha and interferon gamma. J Pathol. 1991;165:247–53.

114. Adamson GM, Billings RE. Cytokine toxicity and induction of NO synthase activity in cultured mouse hepatocytes. Toxicol Appl Pharmacol. 1993;119:100–7.

115. Adamson GM, Billings RE. Tumor necrosis factor induced oxidative stress in isolated mouse hepatocytes. Arch Biochem Biophys. 1992;294:223–9.

116. Jones AL, Selby P. Tumor necrosis factor: clinical relevance. Cancer Surv. 1989; 8:817–36.

117. Talmadge JE, Bowersox O, Tribble H, Lee SH, Shepard M, Liggitt D. Toxicity of tumor necrosis factor is synergistic with gamma-interferon and can be reduced with cyclooxygenase inhibitors. Am J Pathol. 1987;128:410–25.

118. Lehmann V, Freudenberg MA, Galanos C. Lethal toxicity of lipopolysaccharide and tumor necrosis factor in normal and d-galactosamine-treated mice. J Exp Med. 1987; 165:657–63.

119. Tiegs G, Wolter M, Wendel A. Tumor necrosis factor is a terminal mediator in galactosamine/endotoxin-induced hepatitis in mice. Biochem Pharmacol. 1989;38:627–31.

120. Keppler D, Lesch R, Reutter W, Decker K. Experimental hepatitis induced by D-galactosamine. Exp Mol Pathol. 1968;9:279–90.

121. Decker K, Keppler D. Galactosamine hepatitis: key role of the nucleotide deficiency period in the pathogenesis of cell injury and cell death. Rev Physiol Biochem Pharmacol. 1974;71:77–100.

122. Sauer A, Hartung T, Aigner J, Wendel A. Endotoxin-inducible granulocyte-mediated hepatotoxicity requires adhesion and serine protease release. J Leukocyte Biol. 1996; 60:633–43.

123. Dypbukt JM, Ankarcrona M, Burkitt M *et al.* Different prooxidant levels stimulate growth, trigger apoptosis, or produce necrosis of insulin-secreting RINm5F cells. J Biol Chem. 1994;269:30533–6.

124. Ankarcrona M, Dypbukt JM, Bonfoco E *et al*. Glutamate-induced neuronal death: a succession of necrosis or apoptosis depending on mitochondrial function. Neuron. 1995;15:961–73.
125. Bonfoco E, Krainc D, Ankarcrona M, Nicotera P, Lipton SA. Apoptosis and necrosis: two distinct events induced respectively by mild and intense insults with NMDA or nitric oxide/superoxide in cortical cell cultures. Proc Natl Acad Sci USA. 1995; 92:72162–6.
126. Shimizu S, Eguchi Y, Kamiike W *et al*. Induction of apoptosis as well as necrosis by hypoxia and predominant prevention of apoptosis by Bcl-2 and Bcl-XL. Cancer Res. 1996;56:2161–6.
127. Hartley A, Stone JM, Heron C, Cooper JM, Schapira AHV. Complex I inhibitors induce dose-dependent apoptosis in PC12 cells: relevance to Parkinson's disease. J Neurochem. 1994;63:1987–90.
128. Lennon SV, Martin SJ, Cotter TG. Dose-dependent induction of apoptosis in human tumor cell lines by widely diverging stimuli. Cell Prolif. 1991;24:203–14.
129. Jensen JC, Pogrebniak HW, Pass HI *et al*. Role of tumor necrosis factor in oxygen toxicity. J Appl Physiol. 1992;5:1902–7.
130. Corcoran GB, Ray SD, Contemporary issues in toxicology. The role of the nucleus and other compartments in toxic cell death produced by alkylating hepatotoxicants. Toxicol Appl Pharmacol. 1992;113:167–83.
131. Nagata S, Golstein P. The Fas death factor. Science. 1995;267:1449–55.
132. Stanger BZ. Looking beneath the surface: the cell death pathway of Fas/APO-1 (CD95). Mol Med. 1996;2:7–20.
133. Oehm A, Behrmann I, Kalk W *et al*. Purification and molecular cloning of the APO-1 cell surface antigen, a member of the tumour necrosis factor/nerve growth factor receptor family. J Biol Chem. 1992;267:10709–15.
134. Yonehara S, Ishii A, Yonehara M. A cell-killing monoclonal antibody (anti-Fas) to a cell surface antigen co-downregulated with the receptor of tumor necrosis factor. J Exp Med. 1989;169:1747–56.
135. Boldin MP, Goncharov TM, Goltsev YV, Wallach D. Involvement of MACH, a novel MORT1/FADD-interacting protease, in Fas/APO-1- and TNF receptor-induced cell death. Cell. 1996;85:803–15.
136. Muzio M, Chinnaiyan AM, Kischkel FC *et al*. FLICE, a novel FADD-homologous ICE/CED-3-like protease, is recruited to the CD95 (Fas/APO-1) death-inducing signaling complex. Cell. 1996;85:817–27.
137. Ogasawara J, Watanabe-Fukunaga R, Adachi M *et al*. Lethal effect of the anti-fas antibody in mice. Nature. 1993; 364:806–9.
138. Leist M, Gantner F, Künstle G *et al*. The 55 kD tumor necrosis factor receptor and CD95 independently signal murine hepatocyte apoptosis and subsequent liver failure. Mol Med. 1996;2:109–24.
139. Galle PR, Hofmann WJ, Walczak H *et al*. Involvement of the CD95 (APO-1/Fas) receptor and ligand in liver damage. J Exp Med. 1995;182:1223–30.
140. Künstle G, Leist M, Uhlig S *et al*. ICE-protease inhibitors block murine liver injury and apoptosis caused by CD95 or TNF-alpha. Immunol Lett. 1996;55:5–10.
141. French LE, Hahne M, Viard I *et al*. Fas and Fas ligand in embryos and adult mice: ligand expression in several immunoprivileged tissues and coexpression in adult tissues charackterized by apoptotic cell turnover. J Cell Biol. 1996;133:335–43.
142. Strand S, Hofmann WJ, Hug H *et al*. Lymphocyte apoptosis induced by CD95 (APO-1/Fas) ligand expressing tumor cells – a mechanism of immune evasion? Nature Med. 1996; 2:1361–6.
143. Benedetti A, Jezequel AM, Orlandi F. A quantitative evaluation of apoptotic bodies in rat liver. Liver. 1988;8:172–7.
144. Adachi M, Suematsu S, Kondo T *et al*. Targeted mutation in the Fas gene causes hyperplasia in peripheral lymphoid organs and liver. Nature Genet. 1995;11:294–300.
145. Rensing-Ehl A, Frei K, Flury R *et al*. Local Fas/APO-1 (CD95) ligand-mediated tumor cell killing *in vivo*. Eur J Immunol. 1995;25:2253–8.
146. Redondo C, Flores I, Gonzalez A *et al*. Linomide prevents the lethal effect of anti-Fas antibody and reduces Fas-mediated ceramide production in mouse hepatocytes. J Clin Invest. 1996;98:1245–52.
147. Leist M, Wendel A. Tunicamycin potently inhibits tumor necrosis factor-induced hepatocyte apoptosis. Eur J Immunol. 1995;292:201–4.

148. Ni R, Tomita Y, Matsuda K *et al.* Fas-mediated apoptosis in primary cultured mouse hepatocytes. Exp Cell Res. 1994;215:332–7.
149. Fischer W, Schudt C, Wendel A. Protection by phosphodiesterase inhibitors against endotoxin-induced liver injury in galactosamine-sensitized mice. Biochem Pharmacol. 1993;45:2399–404.
150. Gantner F, Küsters S, Wendel A, Hatzelmann A, Schudt C, Tiegs G. Protection from T cell-mediated murine liver failure by phosphodiesterase inhibitors. J Pharmacol Exp Ther. 1997;280:53–60.
151. Leist M, Auer-Barth S, Wendel A. Tumor necrosis factor production in the perfused mouse liver and its pharmacological modulation by methylxanthines, J Pharmacol Exp Ther. 1996;276:968–76.
152. Jilg S, Barsig J, Leist M, Küsters S, Volk H-D, Wendel A. Enhanced release of interleukin-10 and soluble tumor necrosis factor receptors as novel principles of methylxanthine action in murine models of endotoxic shock. J Pharmacol Exp Ther. 1996;278:421–31.
153. Görgen I, Hartung T, Leist M *et al.* Granulocyte colony-stimulating factor treatment protects rodents against lipopolysaccharide-induced toxicity via suppression of systemic tumor necrosis factor-α. J Immunol. 1992;149:918–24.
154. Hartung T, Doecke W-D, Gantner F *et al.* Effect of granulocyte colony-stimulating factor treatment on *ex-vivo* blood cytokine response in human volunteers. Blood. 1995;85:2482–9.
155. Los M, van de Craen M, Penning LC *et al.* Requirement of an ICE/CED-3 protease for Fas/APO-1-mediated apoptosis. Nature. 1995;375:81–3.
156. Tewari M, Dixit VM. Fas- and tumor necrosis factor-induced apoptosis is inhibited by the poxvirus crmA gene product. J Biol Chem. 1995;270:3255–60.
157. Enari M, Hug H, Nagata S. Involvement of an ICE-like protease in fas-mediated apoptosis. Nature. 1995;375:78–81.
158. Kumar S, Lavin MF. The ICE family of cysteine proteases as effectors of cell death. Cell Death Diff. 1996;3:255–67.
159. Rouquet N, Pagès J-C, Molina T, Briand P, Joulin V. ICE inhibitor YVADcmk is a potent therapeutic agent against *in vivo* liver apoptosis. Curr Biol. 1996;6:1192–5.
160. Rodriguez I, Matsuura K, Ody C, Nagata S, Vassalli P. Systemic injection of a tripeptide inhibits the intracellular activation of CPP32-like proteases *in vivo* and fully protects mice against fas-mediated fulminant liver destruction and death. J Exp Med. 1996; 184:2067–72.
161. Kitson J, Raven T, Jiang Y-P *et al.* A death-domain-containing receptor that mediates apoptosis. Nature. 1996; 484:372–5.
162. Marsters SA, Sheridan JP, Donahue CJ *et al.* Apo-3, a new member of the tumor necrosis factor receptor family, contains a death domain and activates NF-κB. Curr Biol. 1996;6:1669–76.
163. Bodmer JL, Burns K, Schneider HK *et al.* TRAMP, a novel apoptosis-mediating receptor with sequence homology to tumor necrosis factor receptor 1 and Fas(Apo-1/CO95). Immunity. 1997;6:79–88.
164. Bohlinger I, Leist M, Barsig J, Uhlig S, Tiegs G, Wendel A. Interleukin-1 and nitric oxide protect against tumor necrosis-factor alpha-induced liver injury through distinct pathways. Hepatology. 1995;22:1829–37.
165. Lacronique V, Mignin A, Fabre M *et al.* Bcl-2 protects from lethal hepatic apoptosis induced by an anti-Fas antibody in mice. Nature Med. 1996;2:80–5.
166. Rouquet N, Allemand I, Grimber G, Molina T, Briand P, Joulin V. Protection of hepatocytes from Fas-mediated apoptosis by a non-transforming SV40 T-antigen mutant. Cell Death Diff. 1996;3:91–6.

17
Endotoxin, Kupffer cells and alcoholic liver injury

R. G. THURMAN, B. U. BRADFORD, K. T. KNECHT, Y. IIMURO,
G. E. ARTEEL, M. YIN, H. D. CONNOR, C. WALL,
J. A. RALEIGH, M. v. FRANKENBERG, Y. ADACHI,
D. T. FORMAN, D. BRENNER, M. KADIISKA and
R. P. MASON

INTRODUCTION

The hepatotoxic effects of alcohol have been described in detail[1], but factors responsible for its hepatotoxicity have been only partially characterized. It is known that chronic ethanol ingestion produces increased hepatic oxygen consumption, fatty liver, hepatomegaly, alcoholic hepatitis, fibrosis, and cirrhosis. It now appears that Kupffer cells participate in several aspects of this pathology.

Interest in the effect of alcohol on the reticuloendothelial system (RES) has mainly been in the context of the known predisposition of alcoholics to infection[2]. After consumption of alcohol, significant changes occur in host defence mechanisms, including altered reticuloendothelial function as well as modified immune, lymphocyte, granulocyte and platelet functions[3,4]. Recently, attention has been directed towards the effect of ethanol on Kupffer cell function, which is stimulated by gut endotoxin (LPS), and its possible relationship to alcohol-induced liver injury[5]. In contrast, most studies on the effects of alcohol on liver function have focused chiefly on the hepatocyte.

The ability of Kupffer cells to remove and detoxify various exogenous and endogenous substances, such as endotoxin, is an important physiological regulatory pathway. Recent work has shown that Kupffer cell function modulates alcohol metabolism in experimental animals[6], supporting the hypothesis that Kupffer cells produce mediators (e.g. prostaglandins or cytokines) that are required for oxidation of alcohol[7].

It has been proposed that the cascade of events leading to alcohol toxicity is initiated by increasing delivery of endotoxin to the liver. We hypothesize that endotoxin initially activates Kupffer cells, a critical step in producing a hypermetabolic state (e.g. the swift increase in alcohol metabolism; SIAM) in parenchymal cells (see Fig. 1). This leads to hypoxia in pericentral regions of the liver lobule, where toxic free radicals are formed upon reintroduction of oxygen, causing cell death. Here we will review new evidence for the proposal that Kupffer cells play a pivotal role in hepatotoxicity following alcohol exposure, focusing predominantly on new information obtained with an enteral alcohol delivery system (Tsukamoto–French model).

IS THE GUT INVOLVED IN ALCOHOL-INDUCED LIVER INJURY?

Considerable evidence suggests that the gut and endotoxin are involved in alcoholic liver injury. Specifically elevated levels of circulating endotoxin delivered to the liver via portal blood could be a cause of hepatic tissue injury (Fig. 1). One hypothesis is that alcohol alters gut microflora, leading to more Gram-negative bacteria, which are the source of gut-derived endotoxin. Alternatively, alcohol could increase gut permeability to macromolecules, increasing the release of endotoxin from the gut into the portal circulation. What evidence supports these ideas?

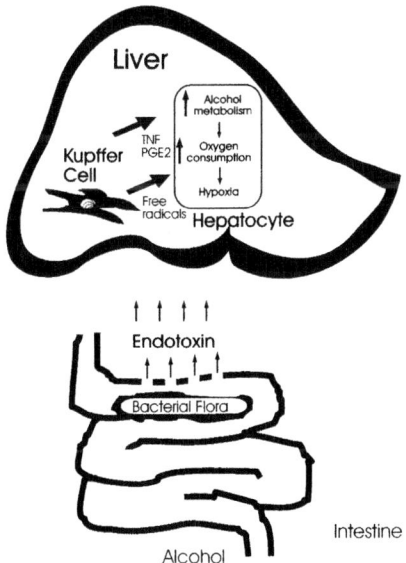

Figure 1 Scheme depicting the involvement of Kupffer cells, endotoxin, hypoxia, and free radicals in the mechanism of alcohol-induced liver injury. Alcohol consumption alters gut permeability and an increase in blood endotoxin occurs. Endotoxin activates Kupffer cells, which release many chemicals including cytokines and eicosanoids. We hypothesize that these substances stimulate hepatocyte metabolism of oxygen and alcohol, leading to hypoxic conditions, free radical generation and ultimately liver injury

DOES DIET OR ALCOHOL ALTER THE GUT FLORA?

The effect of diet and alcohol on the gut flora is a very important consideration, since malnutrition is a common complication in alcoholism[8,9]. French showed that a diet rich in unsaturated fatty acids (linoleic or linolenic) was an absolute requirement for alcohol-induced liver injury in an enteral alcohol delivery model[9]. Rats fed a beef tallow diet showed minimal liver injury after chronic alcohol exposure[9,10] and had normal gut bacterial flora[11]. On the other hand, several studies demonstrated that the gut microflora was relatively insensitive to diet[12]. In spite of these reports, jejunal microflora was increased in alcoholics, and the rise was principally in Gram-negative species, a major source of endotoxin[13]. An important variable in the latter study appeared to be gut pH. A shift of the pH in gastric juice to higher values observed in alcoholics may explain the increase of bacteria in the jejunum[14]. Equally important, when Gram-negative gut microflora was reduced after *Lactobacillus* or antibiotic administration in an enteral alcohol feeding model (Tsukamoto–French), alcohol-induced liver injury was diminished[15]. *Lactobacillus* can suppress the growth of a broad spectrum of Gram-negative bacteria due to the production of low molecular weight substances. Collectively, these studies show that the gut microflora could become more virulent (i.e. produce and/or release more endotoxin) when exposed to alcohol, but by itself does not prove a causal relation to the disease process.

DOES ALCOHOL ALTER GUT PERMEABILITY TO MACROMOLECULES SUCH AS ENDOTOXIN?

Under normal conditions the gut mucosal layer is an imperfect barrier, and small amounts of antigens and other macromolecules pass through the intestinal wall into the blood. It has been shown that gut permeability to macromolecules is increased by exposure to alcohol[16]. Both acute and chronic contact with alcohol increased gut permeability to haemoglobin, horseradish peroxidase and polyvinyl pyrolidone macromolecules[16]. Furthermore, it has been shown that acute *in-vitro* exposure to ethanol increases the permeability of the isolated small intestine to labelled endotoxin in a dose-dependent manner[17]. In alcoholics, permeability to labelled ethylenediaminetetra-acetic acid (EDTA) was elevated about 2-fold compared to healthy controls, and the site of altered permeability was shown to be the intestine[18]. Physical–chemical studies using electron-spin resonance (ESR) of interactions of lipids with membranes have shown that alcohol increases membrane fluidity due to changes in the lipid and lipoprotein composition of the cell membrane[19]. This change in membrane fluidity due to ethanol may result in increased transport and absorption of macromolecules. Data on changes in membrane fluidity by alcohol were known almost 20 years prior to significant experiments using the Tsukamoto–French model, which demonstrated an involvement of a dietary component in toxicity due to alcohol. At this point it is not clear whether dietary effects that prevent liver injury can be explained at the level of gut mucosal barrier.

WHAT IS THE EFFECT OF ENDOTOXIN ON KUPFFER AND PARENCHYMAL CELLS?

Acute exposure to endotoxin causes liver injury, and it has been reported that Kupffer cells play a major role in this mechanism, since they are the principal site for the removal of circulating endotoxin from blood[20]. Endotoxin activates Kupffer cells and triggers the release of a number of potent effectors and cytokines. Most of the biological effects of endotoxin are probably mediated by these chemical factors, including chemoattractants (leukotrienes and tumour necrosis factor), procoagulants, cytotoxic factors (reactive oxygen free radicals, lysosomal enzymes), and vasoactive eicosanoids (leukotrienes, prostaglandins). Furthermore, 90% of endotoxin injected intravenously is scavenged in the liver by Kupffer cells[21]. Possibly the production of mediators from activated Kupffer cells leads directly to parenchymal cell injury[22,23]. Two cytokines which have the ability to produce a shock-like state induced by endotoxin treatment are tumour necrosis factor (TNF) and platelet-activating factor (PAF)[24,25]. TNF can induce the release of PAF, and perhaps both are involved in a cytokine cascade that precipitates the toxic response of LPS. Indeed, it was recently demonstrated that the simple amino acid glycine, which prevents mortality due to LPS[26], decreased TNF release by 80%.

There have been several studies on the direct effect of LPS on hepatocytes[27-29]. Hepatocytes have membrane receptors for both endotoxin and the lipid A component of LPS. Since it has been demonstrated that LPS impairs the uptake and excretion of dyes into the bile[28,29], a direct effect of LPS on hepatocytes could result in liver injury. On the other hand, the fact that LPS causes glycogenolysis in hepatocytes by stimulating Kupffer cells to release prostaglandins[30] suggests an indirect regulatory effect of Kupffer cells on hepatocytes. Thus, Kupffer cells are not only the main site of removal of LPS, but the cell type responsible for mediating the metabolic effects of LPS. Although it is well known that endotoxin stimulates neutrophils and induces their accumulation in the liver very rapidly, inactivation of Kupffer cells by gadolinium chloride ($GdCl_3$) treatment decreases this effect. These results indicate that Kupffer cells may contribute to the mechanism of neutrophil-mediated liver injury, most likely via production of chemoattractants.

Little has been reported on pathological changes or tissue injury induced by chronic treatment with LPS. However, a series of studies indicated a toxic effect of chronic endotoxin exposure. In rats given a choline-deficient diet for a year, cirrhosis developed in 70% of the animals examined; but when neomycin was given in the drinking water, fibrosis was averted[31]. However, if purified *Escherichia coli* LPS was added with neomycin, the protective effect of the antibiotics on the development of pathology was not observed[32]. These results lead to the conclusion that LPS is an important factor in the development of cirrhosis due to choline deficiency.

Carbon tetrachloride (CCl_4) also potentiated the toxic effects of LPS. When CCl_4 was given in small doses, the LD_{50} for endotoxin decreased 600-fold[33], and treatment with antibiotics reduced the intestinal microflora and prevented the toxicity due to CCl_4[34]. Similar results in various experimental animal models of toxic liver injury demonstrated an amelioration of the toxic effects of CCl_4 by limiting the intestinal production of endotoxin.

D-Galactosamine causes liver injury by inhibiting the synthesis of uracil nucleotides; however, when LPS production was blocked by colectomy, no injury occurred even when the hepatocyte was unable to synthesize protein[35]. Recently we have demonstrated that glycine and $GdCl_3$, which act on the Kupffer cell, block D-galactosamine toxicity in the rat[36]. Interestingly, in all of these studies, LPS produced midzonal and pericentral necrosis, lesions similar to those observed in chronic alcohol-induced liver disease.

DOES ALCOHOL AGGRAVATE THE EFFECT OF ENDOTOXIN?

It has been reported previously that blood endotoxin is often elevated in alcoholic subjects[37,38]. In critical experiments in which endotoxin was measured in the Tsukamoto–French model, blood endotoxin began to rise after approximately 2 weeks of continuous intragastric administration of ethanol in the diet[39]. Values increased in the systemic circulation nearly 5-fold, and endotoxin levels in the portal circulation were most likely even higher. Interestingly, a good correlation ($r = 0.84$) between blood endotoxin and pathology (necrosis, infiltration, steatosis, etc.) was observed[39]. The Bodes[16,37] as well as Herbert Remmer[40], have long been proponents of the theory that endotoxaemia participates in alcoholic liver injury.

Recently, it was demonstrated that rats maintained on the Tsukamoto–French model of alcohol-induced liver injury were protected by administration of antibiotics[41]. In this study, rats received diet supplemented with polymixin B and neomycin (150 mg/kg per day and 450 mg/kg per day, respectively) and alcohol. Serum transaminase (AST) levels were significantly decreased about 50% by antibiotics (Fig. 2). Furthermore, the pathology score, which quantitates necrosis, steatosis and inflammation, was decreased from 4.5 to 1 by destruction of endotoxin-producing bacteria. These data are consistent with the hypothesis that elimination of endotoxin from the gut is protective against alcohol-induced liver injury.

Acute exposure to alcohol activates Kupffer cells[42,43]. Carbon uptake by the perfused liver due to phagocytosis of carbon particles by Kupffer cells increased about 25% during acute exposure to ethanol[43]. Further, carbon uptake in the perfused liver was also elevated significantly about 35% following treatment with 5.0 g/kg ethanol 2.5 h prior to perfusion. Similar results have been obtained *in vivo*[44].

Until recently there have been few data linking Kupffer cell function to chronic ethanol exposure[45]. In a recent study it was demonstrated that oxygen radical production by Kupffer cells was increased following chronic ethanol treatment[45]. Others reported that TNF release and the mRNA of TNF expression was increased by alcohol[46], supporting findings that TNF increases in alcoholics[47]. However, one unanswered question is that there are a number of studies showing that alcohol suppresses Kupffer cell function[43,48]. Reasons for these discrepancies remain unclear.

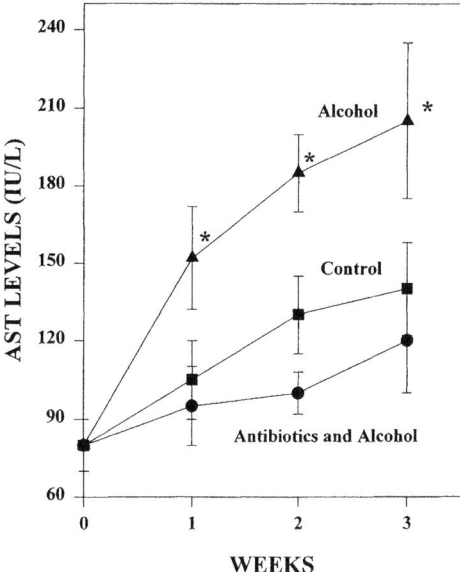

Figure 2 Effect of ethanol and antibiotic treatment on serum AST levels in the rat. Blood was collected from the tail vein weekly and AST was determined spectrophotometrically. Control rats were fed a high-fat corn oil-based liquid diet. Results are expressed as mean ± SEM; $n = 5–10$. $^{*} p = 0.05$ compared with other values

WHAT ARE THE POSSIBLE INTERACTIONS BETWEEN THE KUPFFER CELL AND SIAM?

Israel and his colleagues[49] were the first to describe a hypermetabolic state due to alcohol exposure, and Yuki and Thurman, using the perfused liver, showed that oxygen and ethanol uptake nearly doubled 2.5 h after treatment of rats with a large dose of ethanol[50]. We later demonstrated that hormone-mediated depletion of hepatic carbohydrate reserves accounts for part of this process[51], and we named this phenomenon the 'swift increase in alcohol metabolism' (SIAM).

As stated above, ethanol metabolism is elevated in concert with a decrease in both glycolysis and glycogen reserves during SIAM[50]. Recently, the involvement of Kupffer cells in carbohydrate metabolism has been demonstrated[52]. Specifically, Kupffer cells produce prostaglandins, primarily PGD_2 and PGE_2, which stimulate glucose production from endogenous hepatic glycogen by elevating phosphorylase-*a* activity[52]. Therefore, the role of Kupffer cells in SIAM was studied in the perfused liver using a selective Kupffer cell toxicant, gadolinium chloride. As expected, basal rates of oxygen uptake were nearly doubled, and ethanol metabolism was stimulated following ethanol treatment (Table 1)[6]. This increase was not observed, however, following treatment with ethanol and $GdCl_3$. Thus increases in respiration and ethanol metabolism seen following ethanol treatment were blocked by inactivation of Kupffer cells.

Table 1 Effect of gadolinium chloride treatment on oxygen uptake and ethanol metabolism by the perfused rat liver (μmol/g per hour)

Treatment in vivo	Ethanol uptake	Oxygen uptake
None	76 ± 6	107 ± 12
GdCl$_3$ + ethanol	43 ± 6**	68 ± 14*
Ethanol	95 ± 5*	182 ± 8***

Ethanol (5.0 g/kg i.g. 2.5 h prior to perfusion) or GdCl$_3$ (10 mg/kg i.v. 24 h prior to perfusion) plus ethanol was administered to rats. Oxygen uptake was calculated at 24 min of perfusion from an average of four to eight livers per treatment group. Ethanol (2.0 mmol/L) was infused over a 20-min period and samples of effluent perfusate were collected. Ethanol was measured enzymatically and rates of metabolism were calculated from the change in concentration per unit time. Mean ± SEM. Statistical comparisons used Student's t-test. * $p < 0.05$; ** $p < 0.01$; *** $p < 0.001$ for comparison with appropriate control.

DOES SIAM CAUSE HYPOXIA IN PARENCHYMAL CELLS?

In addition to hypermetabolism, it was shown that high doses of ethanol impair hepatic microcirculation[53] by producing endothelin-1[54]. Furthermore, pathological changes in the Tsukamoto–French model have been demonstrated to be increased by hypoxia[55]. Thus, the background for the idea that hypoxia contributes to alcohol-induced liver injury is substantial. Since alcohol also causes a compensatory increase in hepatic blood flow, which elevates hepatic oxygen concentration, it has been argued that this negates any effect of hypoxia due to hypermetabolism or microcirculatory disturbances[56]. To address this question the hypoxia marker, pimonidazole, was employed[57]. Pimonidazole is reductively activated by nitroreductases, and binds to thiol residues on proteins and macromolecules in the cell in the absence of oxygen. Marker adducts can be detected immunochemically (e.g. ELISA) or immunohistochemically. The results of this study[6] confirmed that downstream (i.e. pericentral) hypoxia occurs after SIAM treatment, which is blocked when Kupffer cells are destroyed with GdCl$_3$. Furthermore, we recently demonstrated that chronic ethanol using the Tsukamoto–French protocol also causes hypoxia[58]. These data provide clear evidence that ethanol *in vivo* increases hypoxia reflected by pimonidazole binding[59].

Studies using miniature oxygen electrodes and microfibre optics have shown that oxygen uptake by the liver is dependent on local oxygen tension[60]. When livers were perfused in the retrograde direction, oxygen uptake was switched predominantly from periportal to pericentral regions of the liver lobule[61]. This was the first suggestion that an oxygen-sensing system was present in the liver. The importance of oxygen is exemplified by the fact that rapid metabolic functions of the liver, such as urea and glucose synthesis, follow the oxygen concentration gradient, whereas very slow processes, such as cytochrome P450-dependent metabolism of drugs, predominate in pericentral areas irrespective of the local oxygen tension[61]. Hypermetabolism associated with a local elevation of the calcium-sensitive enzyme, phosphorylase-a[62], and the effect of oxygen on oxygen uptake, was blocked by W-7, an inhibitor of calcium-calmodulin[63]. It is well known that ethanol activates polyphosphoinositide-specific phospholipase-C in hepatocytes[63]. Thus, calcium is probably involved in oxygen-dependent metabolism, but its precise role remains unclear. It was recently demonstrated that the increase in oxygen uptake due to brief exposure to alcohol in the perfused liver was blocked when Kupffer cells were inactivated[6].

ARE KUPFFER CELLS INVOLVED IN ALCOHOL-INDUCED LIVER INJURY *IN VIVO*?

Several observations support the hypothesis that Kupffer cells are involved in liver injury caused by alcohol. First, alcohol has been reported to affect Kupffer cell functions such as phagocytosis, bactericidal activity and cytokine production[45,47]. Second, increased serum TNF concentrations in alcoholics, reported by Stahnke *et al.*[64], are consistent with the idea that Kupffer cells of patients with alcoholic liver disease are activated, because TNF is produced exclusively by the monocyte–macrophage lineage, and the major population of this lineage is Kupffer cells[65]. Third, Kupffer cells, which contain Ca^{2+} channels[66], are activated by Ca^{2+} (ref. 67), and chronic ethanol treatment makes activation of Ca^{2+} channels in Kupffer cells easier[68]. It has recently been demonstrated that the calcium channel-blocker, nimodipine, reduced alcohol-induced liver in the Tsukamoto–French model, suggesting that calcium channels play an important role in Kupffer cell activation[69]. Collectively, these observations support the hypothesis that chronic exposure to alcohol leads to stimulation of Kupffer cells.

Studies on the mechanism of alcohol-induced liver injury have, until recently, suffered because of the lack of appropriate animal models. The introduction of the *in-vivo* rat model of continuous intragastric alcohol administration, by Tsukamoto and French, represents a major advancement[70,71]. In addition to steatosis present in other models, this model exhibits important characteristics of human alcoholic liver disease, including inflammation, pericentral necrosis, and ultimately fibrosis[72].

Kupffer cells were inactivated in rats during the Tsukamoto–French protocol by twice-weekly treatment with $GdCl_3$, and serum enzyme levels were decreased significantly. Fatty changes, inflammation and necrosis were also all reduced by $GdCl_3$ treatment[73]. The average hepatic pathological score of rats treated with ethanol for 4 weeks of 4.3 ± 0.6 was reduced significantly in ethanol- and $GdCl_3$-treated rats to 1.8 ± 0.5 (see Fig. 4). Additionally, oxygen tension on the surface of the liver was not different from controls when rats were treated with $GdCl_3$ and ethanol. From these results it is concluded that inactivation of Kupffer cells by $GdCl_3$ treatment prevents early injury to the liver. It follows from this conclusion that Kupffer cells play a pivotal role in the early changes that lead ultimately to liver disease.

Oxygen tension on the surface of livers from Tsukamoto–French rats was measured with oxygen electrodes. This methodology takes advantage of the fact that the terminal portal venule stops about 200 μm from the liver surface. Thus, lower values reflect relative hypoxia irrespective of its mechanisms (e.g. hypermetabolism or microcirculatory disturbances). Using this technique, surface hepatic oxygen tension was diminished over 30% by alcohol treatment[41].

Moreover, hypoxia was blocked when Kupffer cells were inactivated with GdCl₃. Furthermore, using the hypoxia marker, pimonidazole, hypoxia could be quantitated in Tsukamoto–French rats following 4 weeks of ethanol feeding. Ethanol treatment for 1 or 4 weeks caused an increase in pimonidazole binding from 18% (control) to 32–35% (ethanol) in the liver using image analysis techniques (Fig. 3)[74]. Thus, direct evidence has now been obtained demonstrating that hypoxia due to ethanol treatment occurs downstream in the clinically relevant Tsukamoto–French model.

HOW DO KUPFFER CELLS, ACTIVATED BY ETHANOL TREATMENT, PARTICIPATE IN LIVER INJURY?

A possible mechanism of alcohol-induced liver injury involves hypoxia as described previously. Israel *et al.* demonstrated that chronic treatment with ethanol increased oxygen uptake by the liver[75,76], and Ji *et al.* reported that the increased tissue respiration induced by chronic ethanol treatment accentuated the intralobular oxygen gradient[77]. This increase in oxygen uptake is due to an alcohol-induced hypermetabolic state[50]. Consequent centrilobular hypoxia may be responsible for pericentral liver injury induced by ethanol, and inactivation of Kupffer cells with GdCl₃ treatment prevented elevated oxygen uptake[6]. In the Tsukamoto–French model, rates of ethanol elimination, which require oxygen, were elevated 2–3-fold in rats exposed to ethanol for 2–4 weeks. However, when Kupffer cells were inactivated by GdCl₃, the elevation in ethanol elimination was blocked. Indeed, centrilobular pathological changes observed in this study are compatible with a mechanism involving hypoxia. Injury in this model

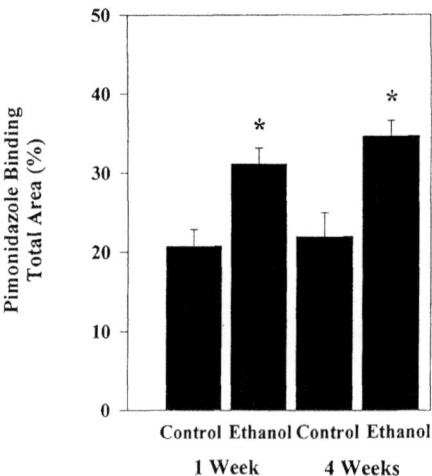

Figure 3 Effect of ethanol on pimonidazole binding quantitated by immunohistochemistry. Controls received a high-fat enteral diet for 7 days or 4 weeks, as indicated. Image analysis was performed to determine the percentage of cells stained in pericentral regions. Results are means ± SEM; $n = 4$. * $p < 0.05$ compared with controls using one-way ANOVA

was increased when O_2 tension in the liver was diminished[55,78]. Importantly, conditioned medium from isolated Kupffer cells of ethanol-treated rats or prostaglandin E_2 stimulated parenchymal cell oxygen consumption. It was further shown[79] that this medium contained elevated levels of prostaglandin E_2.

An alternative explanation for Kupffer cell involvement in liver injury is that activated Kupffer cells release mediators which are directly toxic to liver cells, or serve as chemoattractants for cytotoxic neutrophils which invade the liver. Various toxic mediators including TNF, interleukins, prostaglandins and oxygen radicals are known to be released from activated Kupffer cells[47]. Monden *et al.* reported that TNF, interleukin-1 and superoxide inhibited protein synthesis in cultured rat hepatocytes, and that this effect could be observed in the supernatant of activated Kupffer cell cultures[22]. TNF and interleukin-1 have been demonstrated to be directly cytotoxic to a variety of cell types; thus it is possible that they may be direct mediators of hepatocyte injury. In a recent study, rats treated enterally with alcohol and injected with antibody to TNF were protected from alcohol-induced liver injury[80]. Moreover, TNF and interleukin-1 stimulate neutrophil migration and activation, as well as inducing protease and oxygen radical release[81]. Cellular infiltration of activated neutrophils, which produce oxygen radicals and secrete other toxic mediators, may amplify the inflammatory response and lead to cell injury and death. The inflammatory cell infiltration due to ethanol was blocked by $GdCl_3$ treatment (see Fig. 4). Microcirculatory

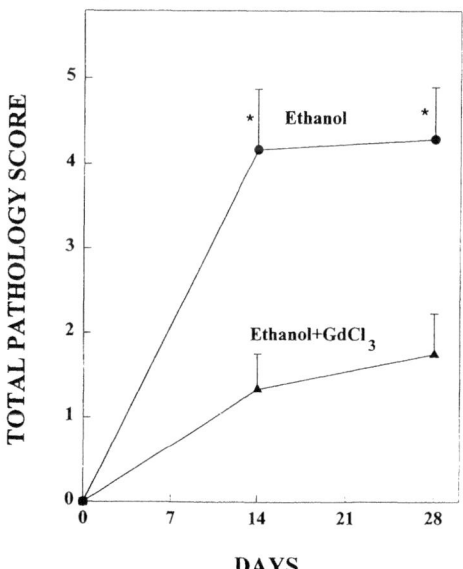

DAYS

Figure 4 Effect of ethanol and $GdCl_3$ on pathology of livers from rats treated chronically with alcohol using the Tsukamoto–French model. Liver pathology was scored as described by Nanji *et al.*[10] as follows: steatosis (the percentage liver cells containing fat): < 25% = 1 +; < 50% = 2 +; < 75% = 3 +; > 75% = 4 +; inflammation and necrosis: 1 focus per low-power field = 1 +; 2 or more = 2 +. One point was given for each grade of severity of histological abnormality as described, and a total score was calculated for each liver. * $p < 0.05$ vs. control value; n = 4–6, mean ± SEM

disturbances due to vasoconstrictive mediators released from Kupffer cells and neutrophils could potentiate hypoxia and lead to a vicious cycle of pathophysiology.

ROLE OF GENDER

It has recently been established that alcohol causes more hepatic injury in female than male rats, using the Tsukamoto–French model of enteral alcohol feeding[82]. In this study, parameters including serum AST, pathological score, levels of circulating endotoxin, neutrophil infiltration and intracellular adhesion molecule-1 expression were all increased significantly more in females than males. The most impressive histological change was the overall deposition of fat in female livers at 2 and 4 weeks of alcohol feeding. The distribution of fat was panlobular in females while it was pericentral in livers from male rats. Plasma endotoxin was significantly higher in female rats after 4 weeks of alcohol (Fig. 5). Furthermore, infiltration of inflammatory cells was not different comparing males and females (Fig. 6); however, significant elevations were produced after 4 weeks of ethanol in both genders, and a 2-fold greater increase was observed in the female liver (Fig. 6). These data collectively demonstrate that the female is more susceptible to alcohol-induced liver injury, and the mechanism of this phenomenon needs to be studied in more detail.

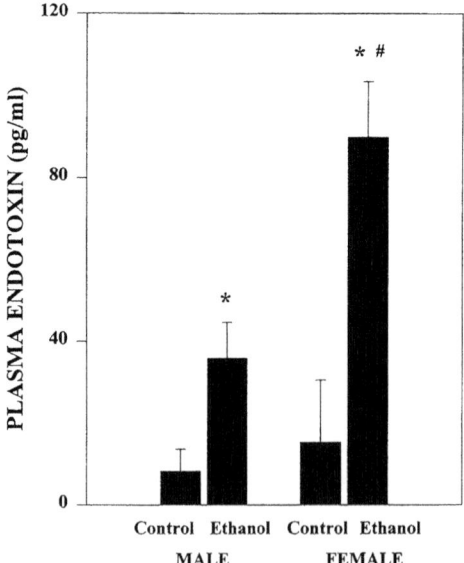

Figure 5 Effect of ethanol on endotoxin levels in plasma. Plasma endotoxin levels in control and ethanol-fed male and female rats was determined with the Limulus amoebocyte lysate assay. Data represent mean ± SEM, $n = 4$–7. * $p < 0.05$ compared with control rats. # $p < 0.05$ compared with male ethanol-fed rats by ANOVA

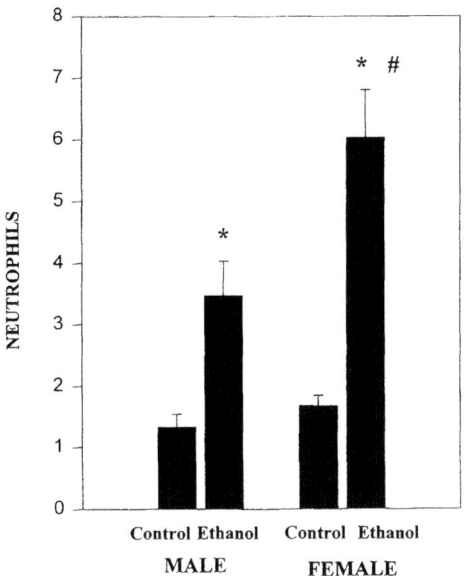

Figure 6   Effect of ethanol treatment on the number of inflammatory cells in the liver. Numbers of inflammatory cells observed in haematoxylin and eosin sections of the liver in control and ethanol-fed rats are depicted. Values were determined by counting polymorphonuclear cells in five high-power fields ($\times$ 400) per slide. The number of hepatocytes was also counted in each field, and the number of inflammatory cells was expressed per 100 hepatocytes. Data represent mean + SEM, $n = 5$–6. * $p < 0.05$ compared with control rats. # $p < 0.05$ compared with male ethanol-fed rats by ANOVA

ARE FREE RADICALS INVOLVED IN THE MECHANISM OF ALCOHOL-INDUCED LIVER INJURY?

Free radical production by ethanol has been suggested to be a factor in its hepatotoxicity. Although evidence of lipid radical formation due to ethanol treatment *in vivo* has been reported, free radicals from ethanol itself have only recently been detected in living animals[83]. By applying the electron spin resonance (ESR) technique of spin trapping to the study of ethanol-treated alcohol dehydrogenase-deficient deermice (*Peromyscus maniculatus*), we detected the α-(4-pyridyl-1-oxide)-*N-t*-butylnitrone (POBN)/α-hydroxyethyl radical adduct in bile from animals given [$^{1-13}$C]ethanol and the spin trap POBN[83]. Spin trapping is a technique in which a diamagnetic molecule reacts with a free radical to produce a more stable species called a radical adduct, which is readily detectable by ESR. Radical adducts are substituted nitroxide free radicals, which tend to be relatively long-lived compared to most free radicals, which are very transient. Nitroxides produced by other biological radicals are sufficiently stable to survive extraction into an organic solvent. Thus, with spin trapping techniques, a very short-lived free radical is replaced by the comparatively long-lived radical adduct.

Placement of a solution containing the free radical adduct in a typical ESR spectrometer's magnetic field will result in unpaired electrons occupying one of two energy states. These states are due to the interaction of the unpaired electron's spin angular momentum with the magnetic field, and they exist only when the sample experiences a magnetic field. The detection of an electron resonance spectrum involves increasing the magnetic field while simultaneously subjecting the sample to microwave radiation. Absorption of the microwave energy, causing electrons in the lower energy state to be excited to higher energy states, occurs only when the energy difference between the two states exactly matches the microwave frequency. The absorption of microwave energy at that particular magnetic field strength is rectified and detected by a microwave diode, and is recorded as the first derivative of the absorption peak. POBN radical adducts characteristically exhibit a six-line ESR spectrum (Fig. 7). ^{13}C substitution on the α-carbon of a spin-trapped species creates an additional hyperfine coupling due to the magnetic interaction of the ^{13}C nucleus with the free electron. The subsequent production of a 12-line spectrum confirms that the trapped radical arises from the labelled parent compound. The use of [^{13}C]ethanol and computer simulation of spectra proves that the subsequent 12-line signal arises from the POBN/α-hydroxyethyl radical adduct[83]. Thus, the radical detected is derived from ethanol, and the unpaired electron density is centred at the α-carbon of ethanol.

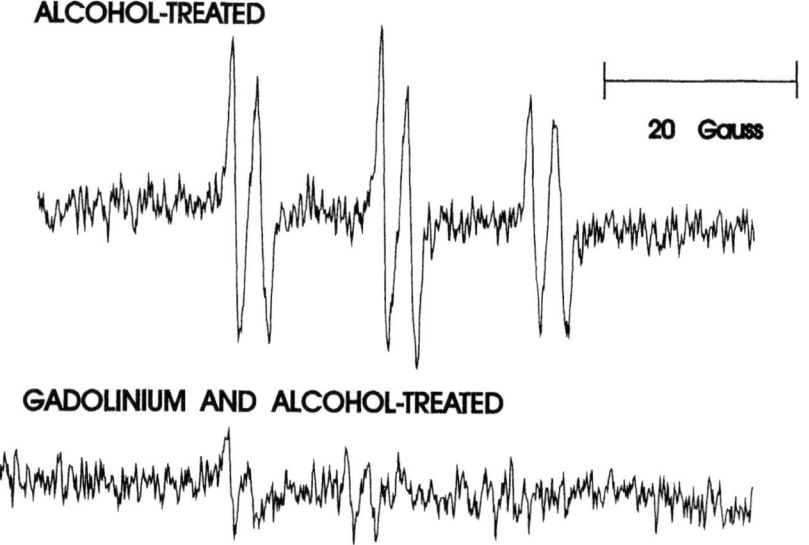

ALCOHOL-TREATED

20 Gauss

GADOLINIUM AND ALCOHOL-TREATED

Figure 7 Enteral alcohol produces free radicals in the liver. Representative ESR spectra of radical adducts in bile from rats treated for at least 2 weeks with continuous intragastric infusion of diet. *Top*, ethanol-containing, high-fat diet; *bottom*, GdCl$_3$-treated ethanol-fed. Bile ducts were cannulated under nembutal anaesthesia and 100 mg/kg of the spin trap POBN was administered i.p. Bile samples were collected into vials containing 50 mmol/L Desferal to prevent *ex-vivo* free radical formation for 3–4 h, frozen on dry ice, and analysed for free radical adducts using ESR spectroscopy

At higher POBN concentrations an additional six-line spectrum was also detected[83]. This radical is most likely derived from an endogenous source such as lipids, based on extraction characteristics and the association between ethanol administration and lipid peroxidation[84]. The six-line species was detectable even in the presence of minimal levels of ethanol, although the signal was stronger when a bolus dose of ethanol was administered. Further, the coupling constants for the radical adduct are similar to those reported in the literature for lipid-derived, carbon-centred radical adducts of POBN[85,86]. Others have also detected free radicals similar to the lipid radical we detected in rats exposed to ethanol[87,88].

Free radical formation probably participates in the progression of early events in alcoholic liver disease. Importantly, we have recently detected a free radical in the bile from rats exposed to ethanol on the Tsukamoto–French model (Fig. 7[73]). This free radical signal was reduced by over 50% when Kupffer cells were eliminated after treatment with $GdCl_3$. A six-line radical adduct spectrum was also detected from the bile of Tsukamoto–French rats treated with an ethanol-containing, high-fat diet, but not in bile from chow-fed animals. Bile from animals fed the control corn oil diet also contained low concentrations of radical adducts. The free radical was identified as α-hydroxyethyl based on a 12-line spectrum obtained when [^{13}C]ethanol was used[89]. Thus, ethanol-derived free radical formation can be detected in the bile of Tsukamoto–French rats treated intragastrically with a high-fat and ethanol-containing diet. Antioxidant-insensitive free radicals have also been obtained from livers of alcohol-treated rats after transplantation[90]. Exact pathways responsible for formation of free radicals in alcohol-treated rats remain unclear; however, since the ESR signal was reduced with $GdCl_3$ treatment, a likely candidate is oxygen radical production by the NADPH oxidase system in resident Kupffer cells and neutrophils. On the other hand, a reperfusion injury involving hypoxia and free radical formation via the xanthine–xanthine oxidase system cannot be ruled out, especially since radicals in bile would be expected to arise from parenchymal cells.

In a recently developed model of pancreatitis using the Tsukamoto–French model of enteral alcohol delivery, radical adducts were measured in pancreatic secretions[89] (Fig. 8). In rats fed control diet, only an ascorbate semiquinone signal was detected in pancreatic secretions (Fig. 8A) while a robust six-line signal was observed in samples collected from ethanol-fed rats (Fig. 8B). This signal was indicative of a carbon-centred radical adduct. Thus, this study demonstrated that early oxidative stress occurs in the pancreas during alcohol exposure, and understanding the source of these radicals could lead to understanding of clinical pathology in patients and tissue using ESR spectroscopy.

CONCLUSIONS

It is likely that alcohol either favours production of Gram-negative bacteria, thereby increasing endotoxin production, or increases membrane permeability of the gut to endotoxin (Fig. 1). Elevated levels of endotoxin activate Kupffer cells to release substances such as eicosanoids, TNF, cytokines, prostaglandins and

Control

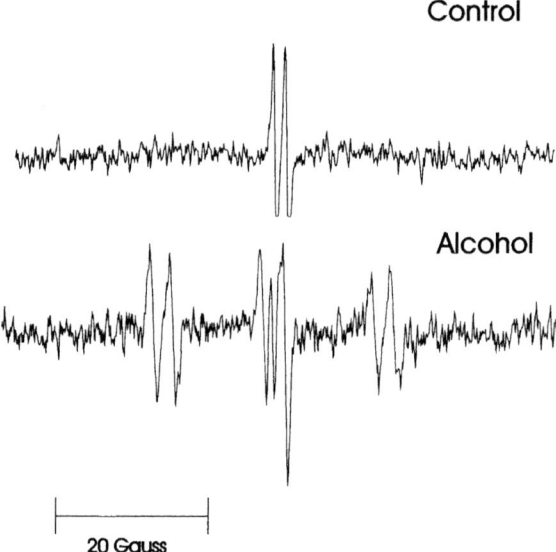

Alcohol

20 Gauss

Figure 8   Radical adducts in pancreatic secretions. Rats were maintained on continuous enteral feeding of control (*top*) or ethanol containing (*bottom*) diet for 4 weeks. Pancreatic secretions were collected by cannulation of the common bile duct after ligation of the bile duct near the liver, and at the end of the duct near the sphincter of Oddi. Samples were collected and analysed by ESR. Representative experiments were repeated three times

free radicals. Prostaglandins increase oxygen uptake and most likely participate in a hypermetabolic state. The increase in oxygen demand leads to hypoxia in the liver and, on reperfusion, free radicals are formed, which lead to tissue damage in pericentral regions of the liver lobule.

Acknowledgements

The authors thank NIAAA for partial support of this work (AA-09156 and AA-03626).

References

1. Lieber CS. Hepatic metabolic and toxic effects of ethanol: 1991 update. Alcohol Clin Exp Res. 1991;15:573–92.
2. Adams HG, Jordan C. Infections in the alcoholic. Med Clin N Am. 1984;68:179–200.
3. McCuskey RS. *In vivo* microscopy of the effects of ethanol on the liver. In: Watson RR, editor. Liver pathology and alcohol. Totowa, NJ: Humana Press; 1991:563–70.
4. Tabakoff B, Hoffman PL, Lee JM, Saito T, Willard B, Leon-Jones FD. Differences in platelet enzyme activity between alcoholics and nonalcoholics. N Engl J Med: 1988;318:134–9.
5. Nolan JP, Leibowitz A, Vladatin AL. Influence of alcohol on Kupffer cell function and possible significance in liver injury. In: Liehr H, Green M, editors. The reticuloendothelial system and pathogenesis of liver disease. Amsterdam: Elsevier; 1980:125–36.
6. Bradford BU, Misra UK, Thurman RG. Kupffer cells are required for the swift increase in alcohol metabolism. Res Commun Subst Abuse. 1993;14:1–6.
7. McCuskey RD, McCuskey PA, Urbaschek R, Urbaschek B. Kupffer cell function in host defense. Rev Infect Dis. 1987;9(Suppl. 5):s616–19.

8. Rao GA, Larkin EC, Derr RF. Inadequate nutrition in the model for alcoholic liver damage using an ethanol + 4-methylpyrazole liquid diet. Biochem Arch. 1987;3:325–30.
9. French SW. Nutrition in the pathogenesis of alcoholic liver disease. Alcohol Alcoholism. 1993; 28:97–109.
10. Nanji AA, Mendenhall CL, French SW. Beef fat prevents alcoholic liver disease in the rat. Alcohol Clin Exp Res. 1989;13:15–19.
11. Hentges DA, Maier BR, Burton GC, Flynn MA, Tsutakawa RK. Effect of a high-beef diet on the fecal bacterial flora of humans. Cancer Res. 1977;37:568–71.
12. Rowland IR, Mallett AK, Wise A. The effect of diet on the mammalian gut flora and its meta-bolic activities. Crit Rev Toxicol. 1985;16:31–103.
13. Bode JC, Bode C, Heidelbach R, Durr H-K, Martini GA. Jejunal microflora in patients with chronic alcohol abuse. Hepatogastroenterology 1984;31:30–4.
14. Ruddell WS, Axon ATR, Findlay JM. Effect of cimetidine on the gastric bacterial flora. Lancet. 1980;1:672–4.
15. Nanji AA, Khettry U, Sadrzadeh SMH. *Lactobacillus* feeding reduces endotoxemia and severity of experimental alcoholic liver disease. Proc Soc Exp Biol Med. 1994;205:243–7.
16. Bode JC. Alcohol and the gastrointestinal tract. In: Frick HP, Harnack GA, Martini GA, Prader A, editors. Advances in internal medicine and pediatrics. Heidelberg: Springer-Verlag; 1980:1–75.
17. Arai M. Effect of ethanol on the intestinal uptake of endotoxin. Nippon Shokakibyo Gakkai Zasshi. 1986;83:1060.
18. Bjarnason I, Ward K, Peters TJ. The leaky gut of alcoholism: possible route of entry for toxic compounds. Lancet. 1984;1:179–82.
19. Chin JH, Goldstein DB. Effects of low concentration of ethanol on the fluidity of spin-labeled erythrocyte and brain membranes. Mol Pharmacol. 1977;13:435–41.
20. Nolan JP, Camara DS. Intestinal endotoxins and macrophages as mediators of liver injury. Trans Am Clin Climatol Assoc. 1988;100:115–25.
21. Arii S, Monden K, Itai S, Sasaoki T, Shibagaki M, Tobe T. The three different phases of reticu-loendothelial system phagocytic function in rats with liver injury. J Surg Res. 1988;45: 314–19.
22. Monden K, Arii S, Itai S, et al. Enhancement and hepatocyte-modulating effect of chemical mediators and monokines produced by hepatic macrophages in rats with induced sepsis. Res Exp Med. 1991;191:177–87.
23. Monden K, Arii S, Itai S. et al. Enhancement of hepatic macrophages in septic rats and their inhibitory effect on hepatocyte function. J Surg Res. 1991; 50:72–6.
24. Tracy K, Beutler B, Lowry S. Shock and tissue injury induced by recombinant human cachectin. Science. 1986;234:470–2.
25. Wallace JL, Steel G, Whittle BJ. Evidence for platelet-activating factor as a mediator of endo-toxin-induced gastrointestinal damage in the rat: effects of three platelet-activating factor antag-onists. Gastroenterology. 1987;93:765–73.
26. Ikejima K, Iimuro Y. Forman DT, Thurman RG. A diet containing glycine improves survival in endotoxin shock in the rat. Am J Physiol. 1996;271:G97–103.
27. Ramadori G, Hopf F, Galanos C. *In vitro* and *in vivo* reactivity of lipopolysaccharides and lipid A with parenchymal and non-parenchymal liver cells in mice. In: Leihr H, Grun M, editors. The reticuloendothelial system and the pathogenesis of liver disease. Amsterdam: Elsevier–North-Holland; 1990:285–90.
28. DePalma RG, Harano Y and Robinson AV. Stucture and function of hepatic mitochondria in hemorrage and endotoxemia. Surg Forum. 1970;21:3–10.
29. Utili R, Abernathy CO, Zimmerman HJ. Hepatic excretory function in the endotoxin tolerant rat. Proc Soc Exp Biol Med. 1979;161:554–60.
30. Kuiper J, Casteleyn E, van Berkel TJ. The role of prostaglandins in endotoxin-stimulated glycogenolysis in the liver. Agents Actions. 1989;26:201–2.
31. Rutenburg AM, Sonnenblick E, Koven I, Aprahamian HA, Reiner L, Fine J. The role of intesti-nal bacteria in the development of dietary cirrhosis in rats. J Exp Med. 1957;106:1–14.
32. Broitman SA, Gottlieb LS, Zamcheck N. Influence of neomycin and ingested endotoxin in the pathogenesis of choline deficiency cirrhosis in the adult rat. J Exp Med. 1964;119:633–47.
33. Formal SB, Noyes HE, Schneider H. Experimental shigella infections. III. Sensitivity of normal, starved, and carbon tetrachloride treated guinea pigs to endotoxin. Proc Soc Exp Biol Med. 1960;103:415–18.

34. Leach BE, Forbes JC. Sulfonamide drugs as protective agents against carbon tetrachloride poisoning. Proc Soc Exp Biol Med. 1941;48:361.
35. Liehr H, Grun M, Seeling H. On the pathogenesis of galactosamine hepatitis. Virchows Arch B Cell Pathol. 1978;26:331–5.
36. Stachlewitz RF, Thurman RG. Dietary glycine prevents acute D-galactosamine hepatotoxicity. Fund Appl Toxicol. 1997;36:229.
37. Bode C, Kugler V. Bode JC. Endotoxemia in patients with alcoholic and non-alcoholic cirrhosis and in subjects with no evidence of chronic liver disease following acute alcohol excess. J Hepatol. 1987;4:8–14.
38. Fukui H, Brauner B, Bode JC, Bode C. Plasma endotoxin concentrations in patients with alcoholic and non-alcoholic liver disease: reevaluation with an improved chromogenic assay. J Hepatol. 1991;12:162–9.
39. Nanji AA, Khettry U, Sadrzadeh SM, Yamanaka T. Severity of liver injury in experimental alcoholic liver disease. Correlation with plasma endotoxin, prostaglandin E_2, leukotriene B_4, and thromboxane B_2. Am J Pathol. 1993;142:367–73.
40. Remmer H. Die Wirkungen des Alkohols. Alkoholwirkungen. 1981;17:1–11.
41. Adachi Y, Moore LE, Bradford BU, Gao W, Thurman RG. Antibiotics prevent liver injury in rats following long-term exposure to ethanol. Gastroenterology. 1995;108:218–24.
42. D'Souza NB, Baustista AP, Lang CH, Spitzer JJ. Acute ethanol intoxication prevents lipopolysaccharide-induced down regulation of protein kinase C in rat Kupffer cells. Alcohol Clin Exp Res. 1992;16:64–7.
43. D'Souza NB, Bagby GJ, Lang CH, Deaciuc IV, Spitzer JJ. Ethanol alters the metabolic response of isolated, perfused rat liver to a phagocytic stimulus. Alcohol Clin Exp Res. 1993;17:147–54.
44. Earnest DL, Sim WW, Smith TL, Eskelson CD. Ethanol, acetaldehyde and Kupffer cell function: potential role for Kupffer cells in alcohol induced liver injury. Prog Clin Biol Res. 1990;325:255–65.
45. Yamada S, Mochida S, Ohno A, et al. Evidence for enhanced secretory function of hepatic macrophages after long-term ethanol feeding in rats. Liver. 1991;11:220–4.
46. Earnest DL., Abril ER, Jolley CS, Martinez F. Ethanol and diet-induced alterations in Kupffer cell function. Alcohol Alcoholism. 1993;28:73–83.
47. Martinez F, Abril ER, Earnest DL, Watson RR. Ethanol and cytokine secretion. Alcohol. 1992;9:455–8.
48. Nelson S, Bagby GJ, Bainton BG, Summer WR. The effects of acute and chronic alcoholism on tumor necrosis factor and the inflammatory response. J Infect Dis. 1989;160:422–9.
49. Israel Y, Videla L, Bernstein J. Liver hypermetabolic state after chronic ethanol consumption: hormonal interrelations and pathogenic implications. Fed Proc. 1975;34:2052–9.
50. Yuki T, Thurman RG. The swift increase in alcohol metabolism: time course for the increase in hepatic oxygen uptake and the involvement of glycolysis. Biochem J. 1980;186:119–26.
51. Yuki T, Bradford BU, Thurman RG. Role of hormones in the mechanism of the swift increase in alcohol metabolism in the rat. Pharmacol Biochem Behav. 1980;13:67–71.
52. Casteleijn E, Kuiper J, Van Rooij HCJ et al. Hormonal control of glycogenolysis in parenchymal liver cells by Kupffer and endothelial liver cells. J Biol Chem. 1988;263:2699–703.
53. Hijioka T, Sato N, Matsumura T et al. Ethanol-induced disturbance of hepatic microcirculation and hepatic hypoxia. Biochem Pharmacol. 1991;11:1551–7.
54. Oshita M, Takei Y, Kawano S et al. Roles of endothelin-1 and nitric oxide in the mechanism for ethanol-induced vasoconstriction in rat liver. J Clin Invest. 1993;91:1337–42.
55. French SW, Benson NC, Sun PS. Centrilobular liver necrosis induced by hypoxia in chronic ethanol-fed rats. Hepatology. 1984;4:912–17.
56. Shaw S, Heller EA, Friedman HS, Lieber CS. Increased hepatic oxygenation following ethanol administration in the baboon. Proc Soc Exp Biol Med. 1977;156:509–13.
57. Arteel GE, Thurman RG, Yates JM, Raleigh JA. Evidence that hypoxia markers detect oxygen gradients in liver: Pimonidazole and retrograde perfusion of rat liver. Br J Cancer. 1995;72:889–95.
58. Adachi Y, Bradford BU, Gao W, Thurman RG. Mechanisms of alcohol-induced liver injury: hypoxia and role of Kupffer cells. Toxicologist. 1994;14:369.
59. Arteel GE, Raleigh JA, Bradford BU, Thurman RG. Acute alcohol produces hypoxia directly in rat liver tissue in vivo: role of Kupffer cells. Am J Physiol. 1996;271:G494–500.

60. Matsumura T, Thurman RG. Measuring rates of O_2 uptake in periportal and pericentral regions of liver lobule: stop-flow experiments with perfused liver. Am J Physiol. 1983;244:G656–9.
61. Thurman RG, Kauffman FC. SCOPE: metabolic fluxes in periportal and pericentral regions of the liver lobule. Hepatology. 1985;5:144–51.
62. Matsumura T, Yoshihara H, Jeffs R et al. Hormones increase oxygen uptake in periportal and pericentral regions of the liver lobule. Am J Physiol. 1992;262:G645–50.
63. Hoek JB, Rubin E. Alcohol and membrane-associated signal transduction. Alcohol Alcoholism. 1990;25:143–56.
64. Stahnke LL, Hill DB, Allen JI. TNFα and IL-6 in alcoholic liver disease. In: Wisse E, Knook DL, McCluskey RS, editors. Cells of the hepatic sinusoid. Leiden: Kupffer Cell Foundation; 1991:472–5.
65. Decker T, Lohmann-Matthes ML, Karck U, Peters T, Decker K. Comparative study of cytotoxicity, tumor necrosis factor, and prostaglandin release after stimulation of rat Kupffer cells, murine Kupffer cells, and murine inflammatory liver macrophages. J Leukocyte Biol. 1989;45:139–46.
66. Hijioka T, Rosenberg RL, Lemasters JJ, Thurman RG. Kupffer cells contain voltage-dependent calcium channels. Mol Pharmacol. 1992;41:435–40.
67. Decker K. Biologically active products of stimulated liver macrophages (Kupffer cells). Eur J Biochem. 1990;192:245–61.
68. Goto M, Lemasters JJ, Thurman RG. Activation of voltage-dependent calcium channels in Kupffer cells by chronic treatment with alcohol in the rat. J Pharmacol Exp Ther. 1994;267:1264–8.
69. Iimuro Y, Ikejima K, Rose ML, Bradford BU, Thurman RG. Nimodipine, a dihydropyridine-type calcium channel blocker, prevents alcoholic hepatitis due to chronic intragastric ethanol exposure in the rat. Hepatology. 1996;24:391–7.
70. Tsukamoto H, Reiderberger RD, French SW, and Largman C. Long-term cannulation model for blood sampling and intragastric infusion in the rat. Am J Physiol. 1984;247:R595–9.
71. Tsukamoto H, French SW, Reidelberger RD, and Largman C. Cyclical pattern of blood alcohol levels during continuous intragastric ethanol infusion in rats. Alcohol Clin Exp Res. 1985;9:31–7.
72. French SW, Miyamoto K, Tsukamoto H. Ethanol-induced hepatic fibrosis in the rat: role of the amount of dietary fat. Alcohol Clin Exp Res. 1986;10:13–19S.
73. Adachi Y, Bradford BU, Gao W, Bojes HK, Thurman RG. Inactivation of Kupffer cells prevents early alcohol-induced liver injury. Hepatology. 1994;20:453–60.
74. Arteel GE, Iimuro Y, Yin M, Raleigh JA, Thurman RG. Chronic enteral ethanol treatment causes hypoxia in rat liver tissue in vivo. Hepatology. 1997;25:920–6.
75. Videla L, Bernstein J, Israel Y. Metabolic alteration produced in the liver by chronic alcohol administration. Increased oxidative capacity. Biochem J. 1973;134:507–14.
76. Bernstein J, Videla L, Israel Y. Metabolic alterations produced in the liver by chronic ethanol administration. Changes related to energetic parameters of the cell. Biochem J. 1973;134:515–21.
77. Ji S, Lemasters JJ, Thurman RG. Intralobular hepatic pyridine nucleotide fluorescence: evaluation of the hypothesis that chronic treatment with ethanol produces pericentral hypoxia. Proc Natl Acad Sci USA. 1982;80:5415–19.
78. Tsukamoto H, Xi XP. Incomplete compensation of enhanced hepatic oxygen consumption in rats with alcoholic centrilobular liver necrosis. Hepatology. 1989;9:302–6.
79. Qu W, Zhong Z, Goto M, Thurman RG. Kupffer cell prostaglandin E_2 stimulates parenchymal cell O_2 consumption: effect of alcohol treatment on cell-cell communication. Am J Physiol. 1996;270:G574–80.
80. Thurman RG, Iimuro Y, Gallucci RM, Luster MI. Anti-TNFα antibody prevents liver injury due to chronic intragastric ethanol exposure in the rat. FASEB J. 1996;10:4612.
81. Thiele DL. Tumor necrosis factor, the acute phase response and the pathogenesis of alcoholic liver disease. Hepatology. 1989;9:497–9.
82. Iimuro Y, Frankenberg M, v. Arteel GE, Bradford BU, Wall CA, Thurman RG. Female rats exhibit greater susceptibility to early alcohol-induced injury than males. Am J Physiol. 1997;272:G1186–94.
83. Knecht KT, Bradford BU, Mason RP, Thurman RG. In vivo formation of a free radical metabolite of ethanol. Mol Pharmacol. 1990;38:26–30.

84. Di Luzio NR. Prevention of the acute ethanol-induced fatty liver by the simultaneous adminis-tration of antioxidants. Life Sci. 1964;3:113–18.
85. McPhail DB, Nicol F, Arthur JR, Goodman BA. The influence of dietary history on the produc-tion of free radicals in rat liver microsomes. Free Radic Res Commun. 1988;4:337–42.
86. Connor HD, Fischer V, Mason RP. A search for oxygen-centered free radicals in the lipoxygenase/linoleic acid system. Biochem Biophys Res Commun. 1986;141:614–21.
87. Tomasi A, Albano E, Biasi F, Slater TF, Vannini V, Dianzani MU. Activation of chloroform and related trihalomethanes to free radical intermediates in isolated hepatocytes and in the rat *in vivo* as detected by the ESR-spin trapping technique. Chem Biol Interact. 1985;55:303–16.
88. Reinke LA, Lai EK, DuBose CM, McCay PB. Reactive free radical generation in the heart and liver of ethanol-fed rats: correlation with *in vitro* radical formation. Proc Natl Acad Sci USA. 1987;84:9223–7.
89. Knecht KT, Adachi Y, Bradford BU, *et al.* Free radical adducts in the bile of rats treated chroni-cally with intragastric alcohol: inhibition by destruction of Kupffer cells. Mol Pharmacol. 1995;47:1028–34.
90. Gao W, Connor HD, Lemasters JJ, Mason RP, Thurman RG. Primary nonfunction of fatty livers produced by alcohol is associated with a new, antioxidant-insensitive free radical species. Transplantation. 1995;59:674–9.

18
Hepatic injury and biliary tract diseases associated with small intestinal bacterial overgrowth

R. B. SARTOR and S. N. LICHTMAN

INTRODUCTION

Hepatobiliary inflammation is associated with a number of clinical and experimental intestinal disorders (Table 1), with the common thread being increased mucosal permeability and exposure to luminal bacteria[1]. To examine mechanisms by which resident luminal bacteria stimulate hepatobiliary inflammation in genetically susceptible hosts, Lichtman and colleagues employed the well-established jejunal self-filling blind loop (SFBL) model in rats[2]. An overgrowth of predominantly anaerobic bacteria (10^9/ml) occurs within 1 week of creation of a SFBL (Fig. 1). The surgical control is a jejunal self-emptying blind loop (SEBL) (Fig. 1), which contains approximately 5×10^5 luminal bacteria/ml, compared with normal jejunal levels[3] of 5×10^3 bacteria/ml. A series of studies have shown that genetically susceptible rats develop progressive hepatobiliary inflammation and fibrosis, resembling to some extent sclerosing cholangitis, in response to cell wall polymers of anaerobic bacteria, especially *Bacteroides* spp., mediated in part by tumour necrosis factor alpha (TNF-α) from activated Kupffer cells.

Table 1 Intestinal inflammation or bacterial overgrowth associated with hepatobiliary disease

Clinical	Animal models
Ulcerative colitis	Intravenous injection of non-viable *Escherichia coli*
Crohn's disease (colitis)	Repeated systemic injection of TNF-α
Jejunoileal bypass	Colitis in IL-2 knockout mice
Whipple's disease	Colitis in cottontop tamarins
Coeliac disease	Small intestinal bacterial overgrowth in susceptible rats.
	Indomethacin-induced enteritis in Lewis rats

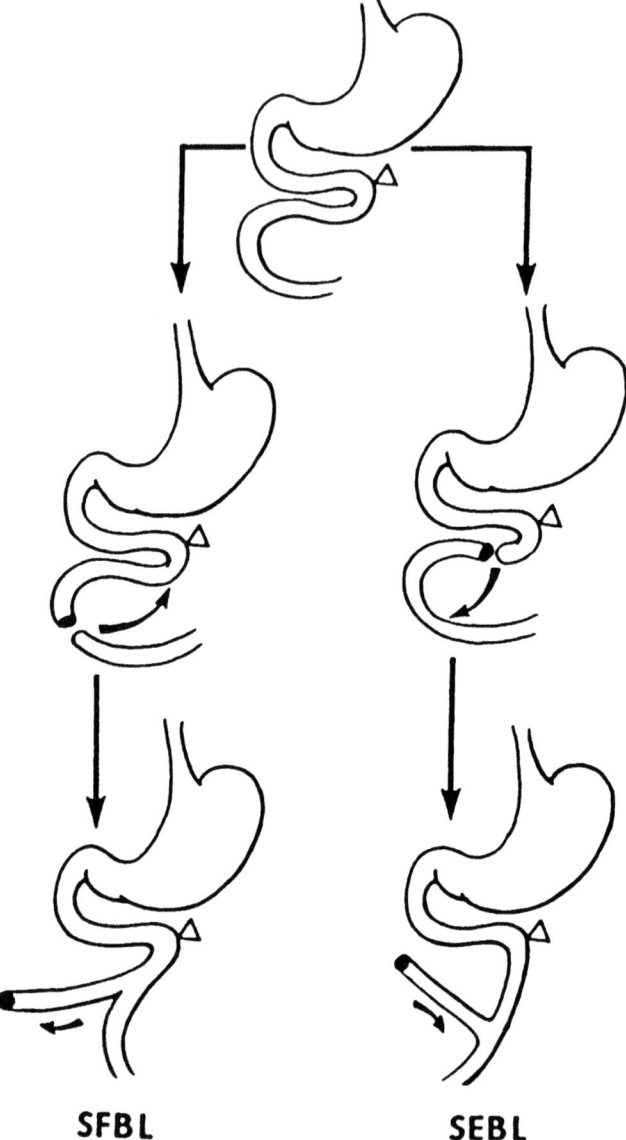

SFBL   **SEBL**

Figure 1 Surgical construction of self-filling (SFBL) and self-emptying (SEBL) blind loops in the jejunum of rats

HEPATOBILIARY INFLAMMATION IN GENETICALLY SUSCEPTIBLE RATS

Susceptible rats develop progressive hepatomegaly, hepatobiliary inflammation, elevated plasma transaminase values and increased mortality in response to jejunal bacterial overgrowth[3]. Inflammation is centred around the bile ducts, with an infiltrate of predominatly mononuclear cells in the portal tract, marked bile duct proliferation, and biliary epithelial injury (Fig. 2). Kupffer cells are increased in number and engorged with PAS-positive, diastase-resistant material. In later stages prominent fibrosis occurs. The extrahepatic bile duct becomes enlarged with an increased diameter and hyperplasia of the wall (wall area 249 ± 95 μm^2 SFBL vs 87 ± 20 μm^2 sham-operated control, $p < 0.001$)[4]. Cholangiograms of rats with SFBL show widening of the extrahepatic duct with ectasia, irregular stenosis and pruning of the intrahepatic bile ducts, in contrast to smoothly tapered bile ducts in rats with SEBL (Fig. 3). Of considerable relevance to the relatively low instance of sclerosing cholangitis in patients with inflammatory bowel disease (IBD), genetic susceptibility strongly influences the incidence and aggressiveness of hepatobiliary injury following experimental small bowel bacterial overgrowth (SBBO) in inbred strains[3]. As demonstrated in

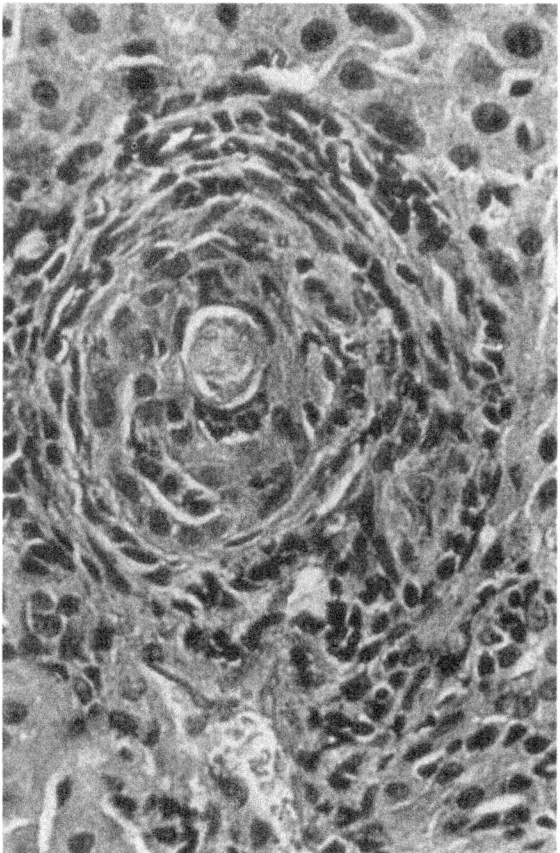

Figure 2 Photomicrograph of an inflamed portal tract with biliary duct injury in a Wistar rat 12 weeks after creation of an SFBL. An 'onion-skin' lesion is present with lymphocytes, macrophages and occasional neutrophils concentrically surrounding an injured mid sized bile duct ($\times$ 400 magnification). (From ref. 2, with permission)

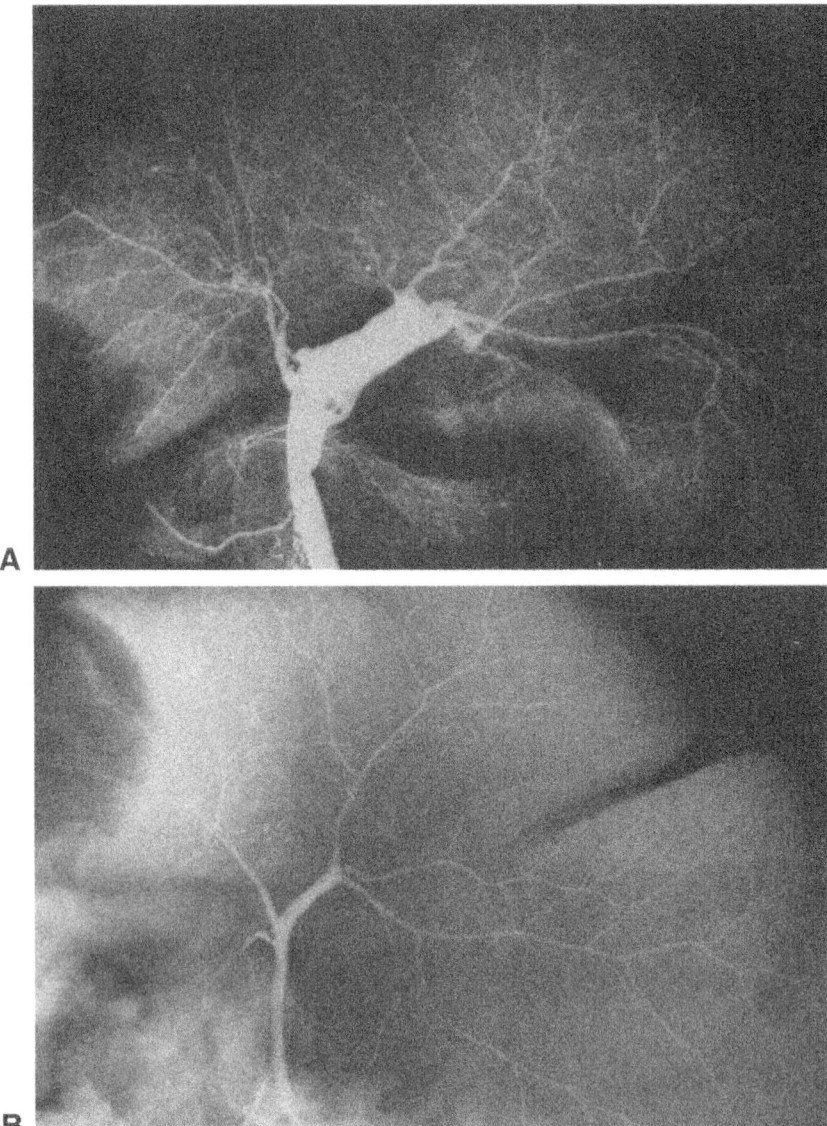

Figure 3 Cholangiograms of rats with SFBL (**A**) and surgical control (**B**). Intrahepatic bile ducts in the inflamed liver (**A**) are ectatic and pruned, with dilatation of the extrahepatic duct

Fig. 4, Lewis rats exhibited significantly increased histological and biochemical evidence of hepatobiliary injury within 2–4 weeks of the SFBL, Wistar rats developed inflammation by 12 weeks and Buffalo rats failed to develop inflammation even when followed up to 24 weeks, despite almost identical levels of anaerobic bacteria in the SFBL of all rats (9.1 ± 1.2 vs 8.7 ± 0.9 $\log_{10}$ bacteria/ml luminal contents).

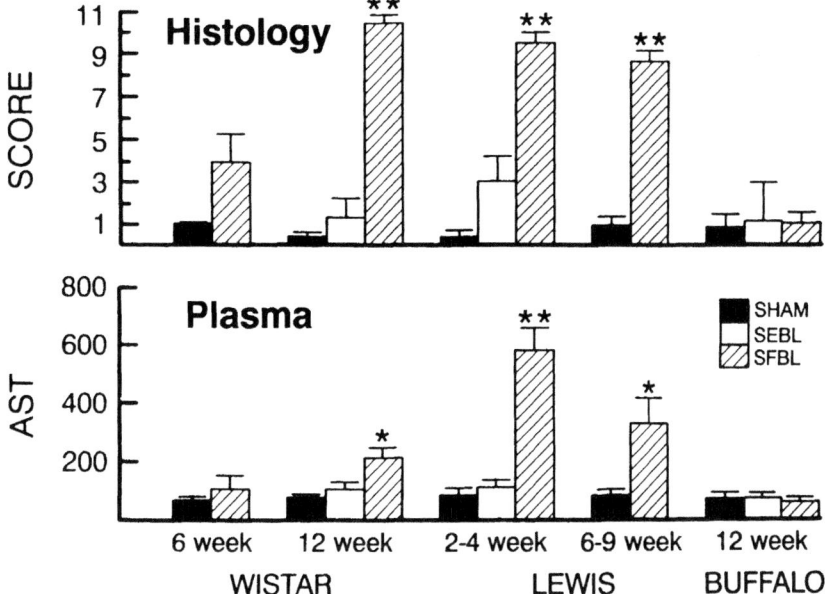

Figure 4 Differential susceptibility of inbred rat strains to hepatobiliary injury with experimental small bowel bacterial overgrowth. Blinded histological scores and plasma ALT values were obtained at various periods after self-filling blind loop (SFBL), self-emptying blind loop (SEBL) or sham operations

INFLUENCE OF LUMINAL ANAEROBIC BACTERIA AND THEIR CELL WALL POLYMERS ON HEPATOBILIARY INJURY

As mentioned above, anaerobic bacteria rapidly proliferate in the SFBL to a much greater extent than in the SEBL, which is not associated with liver damage. Furthermore, bacteria could be cultured from the mesenteric lymph nodes of 66–80% of rats with SFBL vs 25–33% of sham-operated controls and 23% of rats with SEBL[3]. However, cultures of livers, bile and blood from rats with SFBL were reproducibly sterile[3]. To determine which bacterial subset had the greatest influence on this inflammatory response, we treated rats with antibiotics having variable activities against luminal bacteria (Fig. 5). Metronidazole and tetracycline, but not gentamicin or polymyxin B (oral or intraperitoneal), prevented the hepatobiliary inflammation[5]. The protective antibiotics (metronidazole and tetracycline) eliminated *Bacteroides* spp. from the blind loop but had minimal effects on total anaerobic bacterial concentrations, suggesting that *Bacteroides* have a preferential ability to induce hepatobiliary inflammation, similar to the ability of *Bacteroides vulgatus* to induce colitis in HLA-B$_{27}$ transgenic rats[6] and carrageenan-fed guinea pigs[7].

Because the liver and bile of inflamed rats were sterile, we then examined whether non-viable bacterial products could cause inflammation. The lack of efficacy of polymyxin B, which binds LPS, in this model[5] suggests that endotoxin was not involved. Brand *et al.*[8] demonstrated that endotoxaemia is present

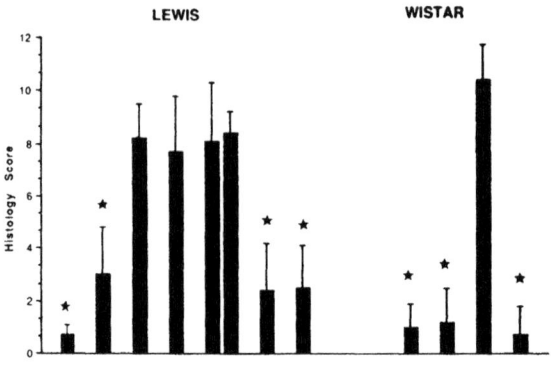

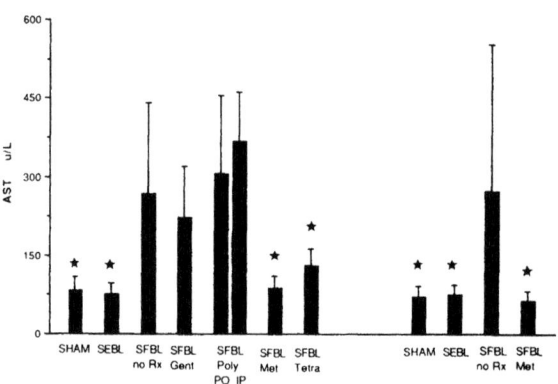

Figure 5 Blinded histological scores and plasma AST values in Lewis and Wistar rats with SFBL after treatment with various antibiotics

following SFBL, but did not correlate with the presence of hepatic injury. We found no detectable biliary FMLP during hepatobiliary inflammation (Lichtman and Chadwick, unpublished observations), in contrast to observations in patients with sclerosing cholangitis[9]. However, we have demonstrated compelling evidence that peptidoglycan–polysaccharide (PG-PS) polymers from the luminal bacteria induced inflammation. Rats with SFBL have increased plasma and luminal anti-PG-PS antibodies and enhanced mucosal absorption, hepatic concentrations and biliary excretion of PG-PS[10]. PG-PS is concentrated in Kupffer cells, where it remains for at least 3 months after intraperitoneal injection[11]. These results suggests that the cell wall polymers undergo an enterohepatic circulation similar to that described for FMLP[12].

The most compelling evidence incriminating PG-PS in the pathogenesis of hepatobiliary information in this model is the observation that degradation of PG-PS prevents and treats inflammation[13]. Mutanolysin, a muralytic enzyme derived from a *Streptomyces globisporus*, degrades PG-PS by splitting the B_{1-4}

linkage of N-acetylmuramyl-N-acetylglucosamine in the glycan backbone of the polymer[14], similar to the activity of lysozyme. This linkage is highly conserved among bacterial species. Systemically administered mutanolysin beginning immediately before creation of the SFBL, and continuing for 4 or 8 weeks, prevented mortality and significantly attenuated biochemical and histological evidence of hepatobiliary inflammation (Table 2) with no change in luminal total bacterial or *Bacteroides* spp. concentrations[13]. Furthermore, delayed administration of mutanolysin (16–21 days after SFBL) partially reversed established inflammation, although it had little effect if treatment was delayed for over 1 month after the creation of the SBFL (Table 2). Mutanolysin prevented elevation of plasma anti-PG antibodies and circulating TNF-α, although it had no effect on mucosal permeability. These results strongly suggests that systemic uptake of PG-PS derived from resident enteric bacteria contributes to hepatobiliary inflammation induced by SBBO in susceptible rats.

IMMUNE MECHANISMS OF HEPATOBILIARY INJURY

Potential mechanisms by which biologically active PG-PS polymers could induce hepatobiliary injury include direct toxic effect of PG-PS on the biliary epithelium as they undergo enterohepatic circulation, immune complex formation, and stimulation of immune cells. Our studies in the SFBL model suggest that TNF-α secreted by activated Kupffer cells mediate this inflammation. PG-PS polymers stimulate TNF-α, IL-Iβ and TGF-β secretion by isolated Kupffer cells and *in-vitro* digestion of PG-PS inhibits TNF-α production by Kupffer cells[13,15,16]. Plasma TNF levels are increased in Lewis rats with experimental SBBO, with maximal levels occurring 18–28 days after creation of the SFBL,

Table 2 *In-vivo* protective effect of degrading endogenous PG-PS by the muralytic enzyme mutanolysin

I.   Prevention (beginning 1 day before SFBL creation)

Rx group	Mortality	AST	Histology score
Sham	0	75 ± 12	1.6 ± 0.9
SFBL-buffer	44%	240 ± 142	7.5 ± 0.8
SFBL-mutanolysin (200 μg 3 $\times$ week)	0*	$111 \pm 32*$	$2.9 \pm 1.7**$
SFBL-mutanolysin (heat-inactive)	63%	183 ± 67	7.7 ± 1.2

II. Treatment (delayed onset of mutanolysin therapy)

Rx	Onset Rx after SFBL	Mortality (%)	AST pre-Rx	AST post-Rx	Histology score
Buffer	16–21 days	45	108 ± 52	247 ± 142	7.1 ± 2.4
Mutanolysin	16–21 days	9*	142 ± 80	$103 \pm 24*$	$2.6 \pm 2.0**$
Mutanolysin	33–53 days	50	219 ± 40	172 ± 102	6.5 ± 17

* $p < 0.05$ vs buffer;   ** $p < 0.001$.

which coincides with onset of liver injury[13]. In addition, plasma TNF-α levels do not increase in mutanolysin-treated rats. Prevention of hepatobiliary damage with pentoxifylline, which inhibits TNF-α production, and palmitate, which inhibits Kupffer cell phagocytosis, further implicates this pathway of tissue damage[17]. Surprisingly, there is no consistent clinical response to ursodeoxycholic acid, methotrexate or cyclosporin A in this model[13], diminishing the likelihood of toxic bile acids and T lymphocytes as major aetiological factors.

SUMMARY AND CONCLUSION

These results demonstrate that hepatobiliary inflammation associated with experimental SBBO is caused by PG-PS polymers from luminal anaerobic bacteria (possibly *Bacteroides* spp.) which activate Kupffer cells to secrete TNF-α (Fig. 6). Aggressiveness of the inflammatory response is strongly influenced by host genetic susceptibility, with inbred Lewis rats more responsive than Wistar rats, whereas inbred Buffalo and Fischer F_{344} rats are totally resistant. These observations are relevant to the pathogenesis of sclerosing cholangitis, hepatic inflammation associated with jejunal ileal bypass for morbid obesity, and non-specific liver injury associated with intestinal inflammation or infection (Table 1). Only a minority of patients with ulcerative colitis, Crohn's disease, or

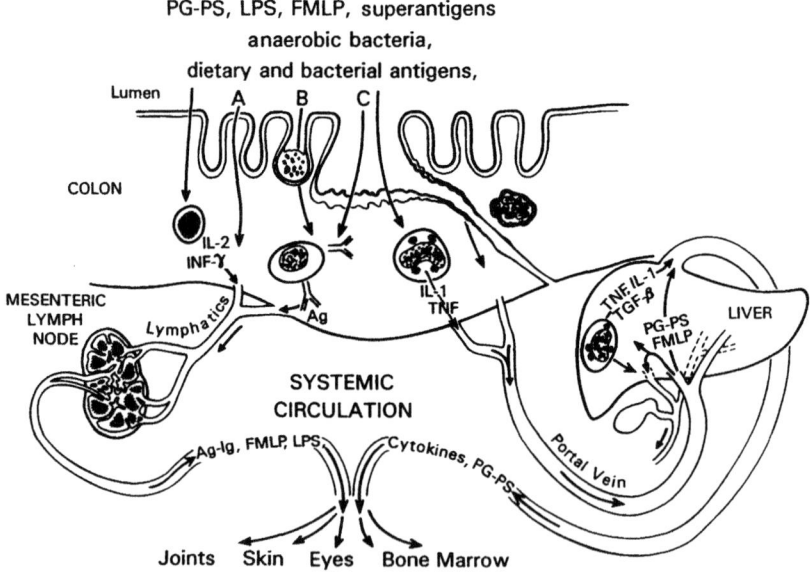

Figure 6 Uptake of luminal peptidoglycan–polysaccharide polymers (PG-PS) produced by resident bacteria through the inflamed or ulcerated intestinal mucosa, with transport to the liver via the portal vein. PG-PS and FMLP undergo biliary secretion and activate resident Kupffer cells to secrete proinflammatory cytokines, including TNF-α, IL-1β and transforming growth factor-β (TGF-β). (Adapted from ref. 1, used with permission)

jejunal bypass develop clinically evident hepatobiliary injury[1], possibly due to as-yet-unrecognized genetic susceptibility factors. Although metronidazole and tetracycline effectively treat systemic manifestations of jejunoileal bypass, no trials have been conducted in sclerosing cholangitis. Our data in this experimental model suggest that diminishing anaerobic bacteria with antibiotics, degrading PG-PS polymers with muralytic enzymes, and inhibiting TNF-α production by Kupffer cells would be fruitful areas for clinical therapeutic trials in sclerosing cholangitis.

Acknowledgements

The authors thank Kim Harrison and Susie May for their secretarial assistance, John Keku for technical support and John H. Schwab, PhD, for his intellectual input into these studies. Original data were supported by the Crohn's and Colitis Foundation of America and NIH grants DK 40249, DK 34987 and DK 44233.

References

1. Sartor RB, Lichtman SN. Mechanisms of systemic inflammation associated with intestinal injury. In: Targan SR, Shanahan F, editors. Inflammatory bowel disease: from bench to bedside. Baltimore, MD: Williams & Wilkins; 1993:210–22.
2. Sherman P, Wesley A, Forstner GG. Sequential disaccharidase loss in rat intestinal blind loops: impact of malnutrition. Am J Physiol. 1985;248:G626–32.
3. Lichtman SN, Sartor RB, Keku J, Schwab JH. Hepatic injury due to small bowel bacterial overgrowth in rats. Gastroenterology. 1990;98:414–23.
4. Lichtman SN, Keku J, Clark RL, Schwab JH, Sartor RB. Biliary tract disease in rats with experimental small bowel bacterial overgrowth. Hepatology. 1991;13:766–72.
5. Lichtman SN, Keku J, Schwab JH, Sartor RB. Hepatic injury associated with small bowel bacterial overgrowth is prevented by metronidazole and tetracycline. Gastroenterology. 1991;100:513–19.
6. Rath HC, Herfarth HH, Ikeda JS et al. Normal luminal bacteria, especially Bacteroides species, mediate chronic colitis, gastritis, and arthritis in HLA-B27/human β2 microglobulin transgenic rats. J Clin Invest. 1996;98:945–53.
7. Onderdonk AB, Franklin ML, Cisneros RL. Production of experimental ulcerative colitis in gnotobiotic guinea pigs with simplified microflora. Infect Immun. 1981;32:225–31.
8. Brand HS, Maas MA, Bosma A, Van Ketel RJ, Speelman P, Chamuleau RA. Experimental colitis in rats induces low-grade endotoxinemia without hepatobiliary abnormalities. Dig Dis Sci. 1994;39:1210–15.
9. Anderson RP, Friend GM, Ferry DM, Chadwick VS. Formyl peptidemia in patients with inflammatory bowel disease and primary sclerosing cholangitis. Gastroenterology. 1991;100:A557.
10. Lichtman SN, Keku J, Schwab JH, Sartor RB. Evidence for peptidoglycan absorption in rats with experimental small bowel bacterial overgrowth. Infect Immun. 1991;59:555–62.
11. Dalldorf FG, Cromartie WJ, Anderle SK, Clark RL, Schwab JH. The relation of experimental arthritis to the distribution of streptococcal cell wall fragments. Am J Pathol. 1980;100:383–402.
12. Hobson CH, Butt TJ, Ferry PM et al. Enterohepatic circulation of bacterial chemotactic peptide in rats with experimental colitis. Gastroenterology. 1988;94:1006–13.
13. Lichtman SN, Okoruwa EE, Keku J, Schwab JH, Sartor RB. Degradation of endogenous bacterial cell wall polymers by the muralytic enzyme mutanolysin prevents hepatobiliary injury in genetically susceptible rats with experimental intestinal bacterial overgrowth. J Clin Invest. 1992;90:1313–22.
14. Janusz MJ, Esser RE, Schwab JH. In vivo degradation of bacterial cell wall by the muralytic enzyme mutanolysin. Infect Immun. 1986;52:459–67.

15. Lichtman SN, Wang J, Schwab JH, Lemasters JJ. Comparison of peptidoglycan–polysaccharide and lipopolysaccharide stimulation of Kupffer cells to produce TNFα and IL-1. Hepatology. 1994;19:1013–22.
16. Manthey CL, Kossmann T, Allen JB, Corcoran ML, Brandes ME, Wahl, SM. Role of Kupffer cells in developing streptococcal cell wall granulomas. Streptococcal cell wall induction of inflammatory cytokines and mediators. Am J Pathol. 1992;140:1205–14.
17. Lichtman SN, Wang J, Reinstein JL, Currin R, Lemasters JJ. Role of tumor necrosis factor in causing hepatobiliary injury in rats with experimental small bowel bacterial overgrowth. Sixth International Symposium on Cells of the Hepatic Sinusoid, 1993;Vol.4:141–4.

19
Endotoxaemia in chronic hepatitis and cirrhosis: Epiphenomenon or of pathological relevance?

H. FUKUI, S. TSUJITA, M. MATSUMOTO, H. KITANO,
K. HOPPOU, M. MORIMURA, A. TAKAYA, S. OKAMOTO,
T. TSUJII, Ch. BODE and J. Ch. BODE

INTRODUCTION

Much interest has focused on the roles of endotoxin in the pathophysiology of liver diseases, either as a cause of hepatic injury or as a possible mediator of the clinical manifestations in patients with liver disease[1]. Until recently, gelation of the test medium has been used for detection of plasma endotoxin. However, non-specific gelation has been reported, and interpretation of the results has often caused confusion[2]. In 1978 Iwanaga et al.[3] developed a quantitative endotoxin assay using a synthetic chromogenic peptide as a substrate for the endotoxin-sensitive Limulus enzyme. This assay has been shown to give reliable results for minute amounts of endotoxin in water[3]. However, measurements of endotoxin in blood still present difficulties.

Major problems in plasma endotoxin assay are: (a) disagreement about the best way of preparing standard curves[4-6], (b) lack of an optimal method for eliminating plasma inhibitors for endotoxin assay[7], and (c) necessity of endotoxin-specific chromogenic substrate[8].

We have insisted that a standard curve should be prepared for each individual plasma sample in the endotoxin determination, because ideal 100% recovery of endotoxin could not be validated in any trial of plasma pretreatment[7]. The internal standard is especially necessary in the perchloric acid treatment, in which strict adjustment of pH in samples is difficult before the chromogenic assay[9]. Our study demonstrated a hidden extra portion of endotoxin in the plasma of patients with chronic liver diseases, using new methods of plasma pretreatment, either using Tween 80 in the dilution and heating method or using triethylamine in the perchloric acid method[10].

The chromogenic substrate widely used throughout the world is considered to react not only to endotoxin but also to other substances such as

(1,3)-β-D-glucan, a component of the cell wall of fungus[8]. The endotoxin-specific chromogenic substrate Endospecy was produced by removing the G-factor from the lysate[8]. In this study we measured plasma endotoxin using our improved perchloric acid method[9] and this endotoxin-specific chromogenic substrate in patients with chronic hepatitis and liver cirrhosis, and showed that endotoxaemia observed in these patients has a pathophysiological meaning.

SUBJECTS AND METHODS

Subjects and blood sampling

Blood was sampled from eight healthy subjects, 11 patients with chronic hepatitis (all hepatitis C-associated) and 90 patients with liver cirrhosis (11 alcoholic, 26 hepatitis B-associated, 53 hepatitis C-associated). Fifteen patients were classified to Child's grade A, 39 patients to grade B and 36 patients to grade C. Ascites, hepatocellular carcinoma and oesophageal varices were noted in 51, 59 and 74 patients, respectively. In patients with bleeding from oesophagocardial varices, blood was sampled repeatedly after the bleeding. Ten millilitres of blood was drawn from a peripheral antecubital vein using an aseptic technique. All blood specimens were mixed with endotoxin-free heparin (Midorijuji Co., Tokyo, Japan), producing a final concentration of 15 units heparin per millilitre of blood, placed on ice and transported immediately to the laboratory. Platelet-rich plasma was prepared by centrifugation at 150 g for 20 min at 0°C. The separated plasma was stored at −80°C in pyrogen-free polyethylene tubes (Eppendorf, Hamburg, Germany). The diagnosis of chronic hepatitis was based on liver biopsy. The diagnosis of liver cirrhosis was based on clinical symptoms, clinical chemical findings, ultrasonography, computerized tomography and, if possible, liver biopsy. This research was approved by the Human Studies Committee in the Nara Medical University Hospital.

Measurement of plasma endotoxin

Two-hundred microlitres of plasma samples were mixed with 400 μl of 0.32 mol/L perchloric acid as described by Obayashi et al.[11]. The mixture was incubated for 20 min at 37°C and centrifuged at 1000 g for 10 min at 0°C. Each supernatant fraction was neutralized by adding an equal amount of 0.18 mol/L NaOH solution, and each precipitate fraction was neutralized and dissolved in 400 μl pyrogen-free water by adding 30–60 μl of the 10% triethylamine as described elsewhere[5]. The final pH of the sample was always adjusted to 7 by careful titration of triethylamine. To each neutralized sample from supernatant and precipitate pyrogen-free water or endotoxin standard were added to final exogenous endotoxin concentrations of 0, 12.5 and 25 pg/μl. The endotoxin activity of each sample was measured by a chromogenic substrate assay using the endotoxin-specific substrate Endospecy (Seikagaku Kogyo Co., Tokyo, Japan) with kinetic analysis. The absorbance was measured at 37°C every 5 min until 40 min by a microprocessor-controlled reader (MTP-32, Corona Electrics Co., Katsuta, Japan). The linear part of the kinetic curve was read, and endogenous plasma endotoxin concentrations were calculated from the standard curve obtained.

Analysis of plasma endotoxin-inactivating rate and endotoxin binding of proteins

Fifty-four samples from 90 patients with liver cirrhosis and eight healthy subjects were used. The aetiology of cirrhosis was alcoholic in five patients, hepatitis C virus-associated in 37 and hepatitis B virus-associated in 12. Sixteen patients were classified to Child's grade A, 26 patients to grade B and 13 patients to grade C. Ascites, hepatocellular carcinoma and oesophageal varices were noted in 17, 31 and 43 patients, respectively. None of the patients had evidence of recent gastrointestinal bleeding or hepatic coma.

Measurement of endotoxin-inactivating rate of plasma

Endotoxin from *Escherichia coli* 0111:B4 was added to each sample plasma to a final concentration of 250 pg/ml. The endotoxin activities of the mixtures, either with or without an incubation (37°C for 1 h), were measured by the endotoxin-specific substrate Endospecy after pretreatment by an improved perchloric acid method described by Inada *et al.*[12]. The endotoxin-inactivating rate was calculated as follows[13]:

$$\text{Endotoxin inactivating rate } (\%) = (B - A)/B \times 100$$

where: A = Endotoxin activity measured after preincubaion (37°C, 1 h)
B = Endotoxin activity measured without preincubaion

Endotoxin-binding capacity of albumin, high-density lipoprotein and transferrin

[3H]-labelled endotoxin was prepared from *Salmonella anatum* A_1 *epi* using ethylenediaminetetraacetic acid (EDTA, Nacalai Tesque, Inc., Kyoto, Japan) extraction[13]. Briefly the culture medium was centrifuged at 10 000 r.p.m for 10 min at 0°C and the precipitate was suspended in 1 ml of 0.01 mol/L EDTA-Na_2, 0.015 mol/L trishydroxymethylaminomethane (pH 8). Then the supernatant, after centrifugation at 10 000 r.p.m. for 10 min, was dialysed and stored. *S. anatum* A_1 *epi* was supplied by Professor S. Kanegasaki (Institute of Medical Science, University of Tokyo, Japan). [3H]-labelled endotoxin was added to each plasma sample at a final concentration of 300 pg/ml (1.5×10^4 dpm/ml).

Endotoxin bound to albumin was counted by liquid scintilation counter after affinity chromatography using Blue Sepharose CL-6B (Pharmacia LKB, Uppsala, Sweden). Briefly 50 μl of sample plasma containing labelled endotoxin was applied to a Blue Sepharose column. Albumin, once adsorbed to Blue Sepharose, was eluted by 0.05 mol/L Tris buffer containing 1.5 mol/L KCl.

Endotoxin bound to HDL and transferrin in 100 μl sample plasma was counted by liquid scintilation counter after immunoprecipitation. As primary antibodies, 1 : 10 diluted anti-human apolipoprotein A1 (Boehringer, Mannheim, Germany) and anti-human transferrin sheep serum (Binding Site, Ltd, Birmingham, UK) were used, and as secondary antibody anti-sheep γ-globulin rabbit serum (Organon Teknika, Co., PA, USA) was used. Non-specific binding was blocked by treatment of each sample by 1 : 10 diluted anti-bovine albumin rabbit serum (ICN Biomedicals, Co., Tokyo, Japan) before the immunoprecipitation. The endotoxin-binding capacity of each protein was expressed as picogram endotoxin per millilitre of sample plasma.

Statistical analyses

Statistical differences were analysed by using one-way analysis of variance and Student's t-test. All data are presented as means ± SD.

RESULTS

Plasma endotoxin concentration

There was an increase of plasma endotoxin with the progression of chronic liver disease (healthy subjects 6.1 ± 3.0 pg/ml; chronic hepatitis 22.8 ± 18.3 pg/ml; liver cirrhosis 89.0 ± 109.9 pg/ml). In patients with chronic hepatitis, endotoxin in the precipitate fraction after perchloric acid treatment increased somewhat (healthy subjects 3.1 ± 2.1 pg/ml vs chronic hepatitis 22.6 ± 18.4 pg/ml). In cirrhotics, a marked increase of endotoxin, both in the supernatant and precipitate fraction, was noted (supernatant 37.5 ± 65.6 pg/ml, precipitate 52.3 ± 69.1 pg/ml).

Further, the total endotoxin level increased as the progression of Child–Pugh grades. Endotoxin in the precipitate fraction showed a tendency to increase, initially. This was followed by an increase in endotoxin in the supernatant fraction (Fig. 1).

In patients bleeding from oesophageal varices, plasma endotoxin increased for 3 days after the bleeding, and thereafter decreased. Endotoxin in the supernatant fraction increased immediately after bleeding; then the endotoxin in the precipitate fraction also increased (Fig. 2).

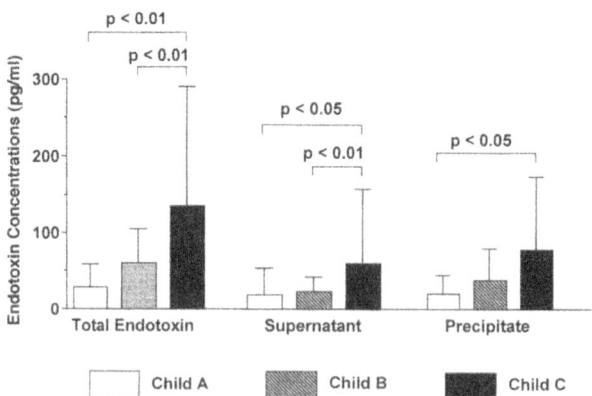

Figure 1 Relationship between plasma endotoxin concentrations and Child–Pugh classification in cirrhotics

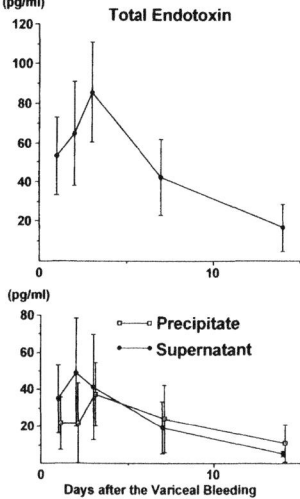

Figure 2 Changes in plasma endotoxin concentrations after rupture of oesophageal varices in patients with liver cirrhosis

Relationships of plasma endotoxin to liver function tests and clinical course in cirrhotics

The endotoxin concentrations revealed significant negative correlations with prothrombin time and hepaplastin test (Fig. 3).

In cirrhotics with hepatocellular carcinoma, those with multiple or large carcinoma showed higher endotoxin levels than those with less-advanced carcinoma

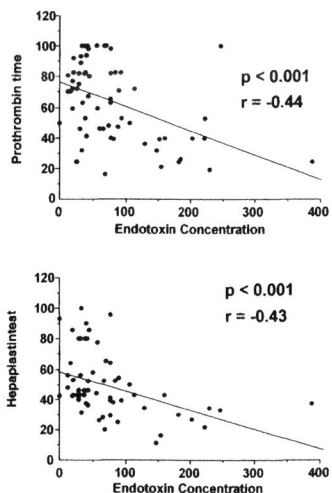

Figure 3 Relationship of plasma endotoxin concentrations to prothrombin time and hepaplastin test in cirrhotics

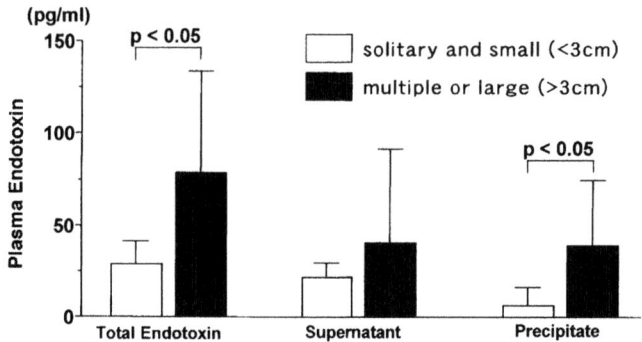

Figure 4   Plasma endotoxin concentrations in cirrhotic patients with hepatocellular carcinoma

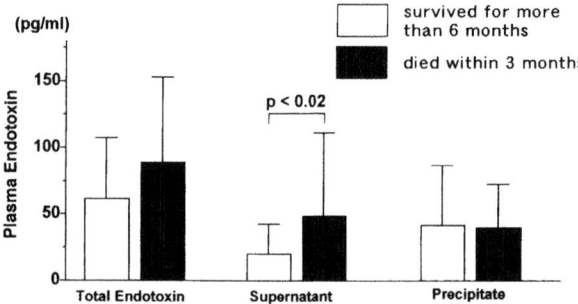

Figure 5   Relationship between plasma endotoxin concentrations and prognosis of cirrhotics

(Fig. 4). Cirrhotics who died within 3 months showed higher endotoxin levels than those who survived more than 6 months (Fig. 5).

There is a weak positive relationship of endotoxin in the precipitate to body temperature and serum C-reactive protein in cirrhotics as a whole ($r = 0.36$, $p < 0.0025$; $r = 0.56$, $p < 0.001$). On the other hand, there is a positive relationship of endotoxin in the supernatant fraction to plasma tumour necrosis factor-α and interleukin-6 in cirrhotics with ascites ($r = 0.86$, $p < 0.0002$; $r = 0.83$, $p < 0.0005$).

Endotoxin binding of plasma proteins and endotoxin-inactivating rate

Serum levels of albumin, HDL-cholesterol and transferrin decreased as the liver cirrhosis progressed (Table 1). The endotoxin-binding capacity of albumin was decreased in severe cirrhosis. On the contrary, the endotoxin-binding capacity of HDL and transferrin was preserved even in these cases (Fig. 6).

The plasma endotoxin-inactivating rate was decreased in Child C cirrhotics (Fig. 7). The plasma endotoxin-inactivating rate was positively correlated to the endotoxin-binding capacity of albumin (Fig. 8) and serum HDL-cholesterol levels.

Table 1 Serum albumin, high-density lipoprotein–cholesterol and transferrin levels in liver cirrhotic Child classification

	Albumin (g/dl)			HDL-cholesterol (mg/dl)			Transferrin (mg/dl)		
Child A	3.58 ± 0.39 ⌉		⌉	40.6 ± 13.9 ⌉		⌉	282.7 ± 75.5 ⌉		⌉
		*			****			****	
Child B	3.12 ± 0.47 ⌋	*		31.9 ± 9.1 ⌋		*	241.8 ± 67.0 ⌋		*
		****			**			****	
Child C	2.93 ± 0.34 ⌋		⌋	17.6 ± 15.2 ⌋		⌋	180.2 ± 22.3 ⌋		⌋

HDL = high-density lipoprotein.
$* p < 0.001$; $** p < 0.005$; $*** p < 0.01$; $**** p < 0.05$.

Serum albumin was negatively correlated to plasma interleukin-1b ($r = -0.31$, $p < 0.05$), interleukin-6 ($r = -0.33$, $p < 0.05$) and tumour necrosis factor-α level ($r = -0.37$, $p < 0.02$) in cirrhotics. High plasma cytokine levels are found only in cirrhotics with decreased endotoxin-binding capacity of albumin (Fig. 9). Further, the endotoxin-binding capacity of albumin was negatively correlated to serum C-reactive protein levels ($r = -0.47$, $p < 0.01$).

DISCUSSION

Iwanaga *et al.*[3] developed a quantitative endotoxin assay using a synthetic chromogenic substrate for the endotoxin-sensitive *Limulus* enzyme. This assay provides reliable results for minute amounts of endotoxin in water. However, the major problem with the plasma endotoxin assay by this method is that an optimal method for eliminating plasma inhibitors has not yet been established[7]. In order to improve the recovery of endotoxin in the dilution and heating method, we added a detergent (Tween 80) after heating the plasma[14]. Using this method we found a marked elevation of plasma endotoxin in chronic alcoholics and in cirrhotics with upper gastrointestinal bleeding, including those with oesophageal varices[14]. However, the chromogenic substrate S-2423, which we used then, was known to react not only to endotoxin but also to other substances such as (1,3)-β-D-glucan. In this study we improved the recovery of endotoxin in the perchloric acid method by using triethylamine, and measured plasma endotoxin by an endotoxin-specific substrate, Endospecy[8]. As a result we confirmed that plasma endotoxin was elevated in patients with chronic liver diseases, especially in those with liver cirrhosis. Moreover, the total endotoxin level, which was determined by this new acid method and Endospecy, was increased with the progression of Child–Pugh grades in patients with liver cirrhosis. This correlated well to prothrombin time and hepaplastin test. The elevation of plasma endotoxin was prominent in cirrhotics with poor prognosis, variceal bleeding and advanced hepatoma.

As we reported previously, a large amount of endotoxin is lost from the assay system if we do not measure the precipitate fraction in addition to the supernatant fraction using the perchloric acid method[7]. The precipitate fraction was

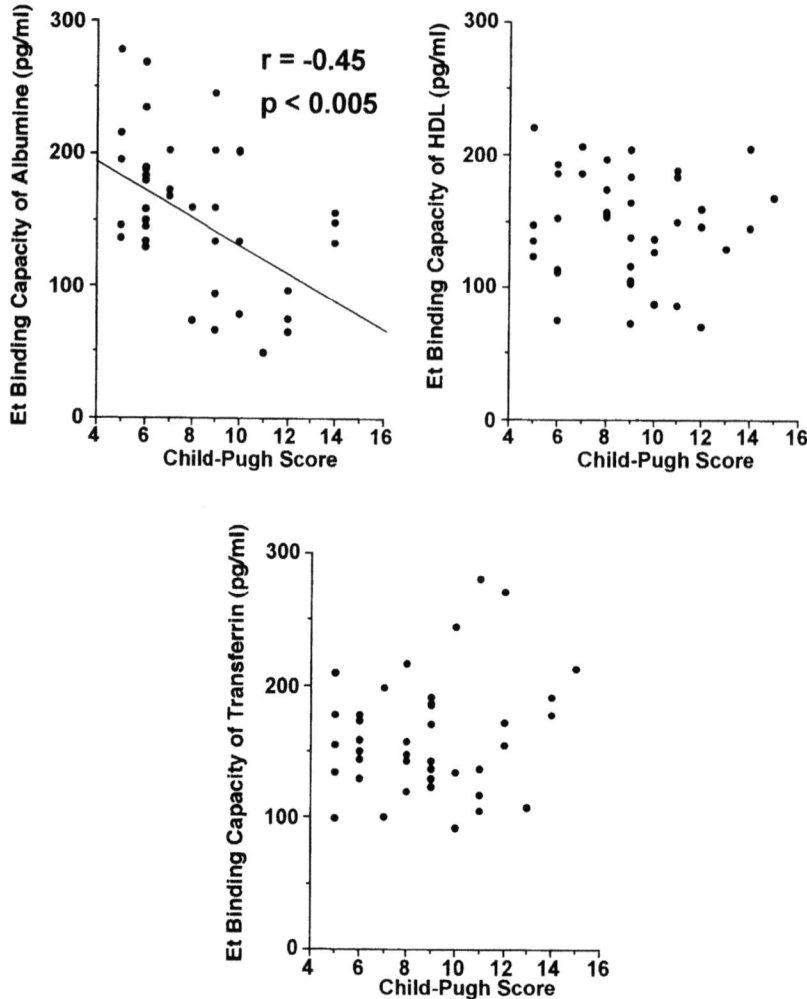

Figure 6 Correlations between Child–Pugh score and endotoxin-binding capacities of plasma albumin, high-density lipoprotein (HDL) and transferrin in cirrhotics

dissolved and neutralized by adding triethylamine. This procedure enabled us to detect all endotoxin in the plasma sample using the perchloric acid method. In the present study endotoxin in the supernatant fraction increased first, after bleeding from oesophageal varices; thereafter that in the precipitate fraction increased. On the contrary, the increase of endotoxin in the precipitate fraction preceded that in the supernatant fraction with the progression of chronic liver diseases. Correlation to body temperature or C-reactive protein was confined to endotoxin in the precipitate fraction, while correlation to plasma tumour necrosis factor α or interleukin-6 was confined to endotoxin in the supernatant fraction. The meaning of these endotoxin activities in the supernatant and in the precipitate fractions after perchloric acid treatment is still unclear. However, a differ-

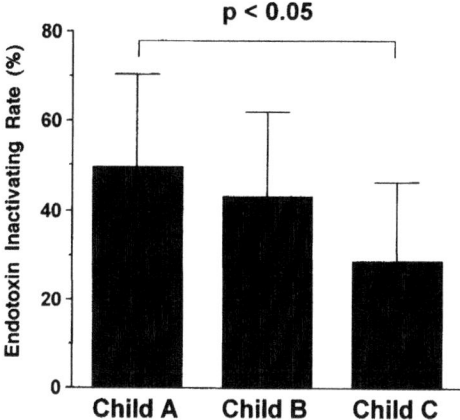

Figure 7 Correlations between Child–Pugh grade and plasma endotoxin-inactivating rate in cirrhotics

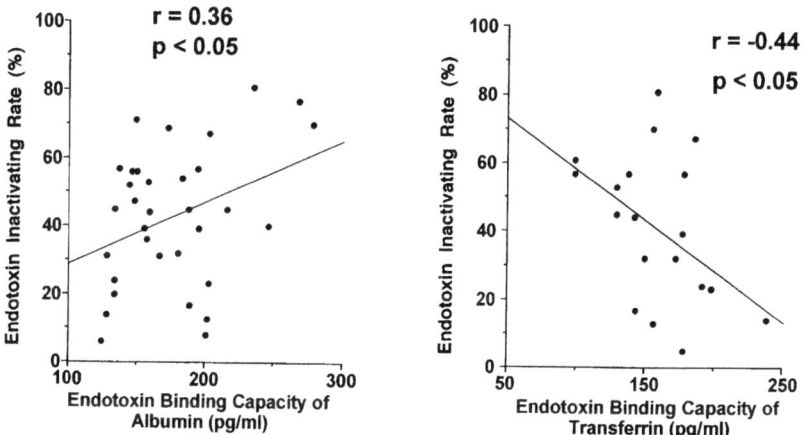

Figure 8 Relationships of endotoxin-binding capacities of plasma albumin and transferrin to plasma endotoxin-inactivating rate in cirrhotics

ence in the binding state of endotoxin to proteins, or the structure of endotoxin itself, is thought to lead to this separation.

As an alternative method to recover all endotoxin after perchloric acid treatment, Inada et al.[12] added NaOH to the sample plasma before perchloric acid (PCA) treatment. Using this new PCA method, plasma total endotoxin can be measured in one fraction, because an addition of NaOH to the sample plasma inhibited the formation of precipitate after PCA treatment[12]. Total plasma endotoxin was supposed to be measurable as sodium-binding state. In this study we measured plasma endotoxin using our improved PCA method, using triethylamine. However, for determination of endotoxin-inactivating rate we used the new PCA method by Inada et al.[12] because of its simplicity. Loss of endotoxin

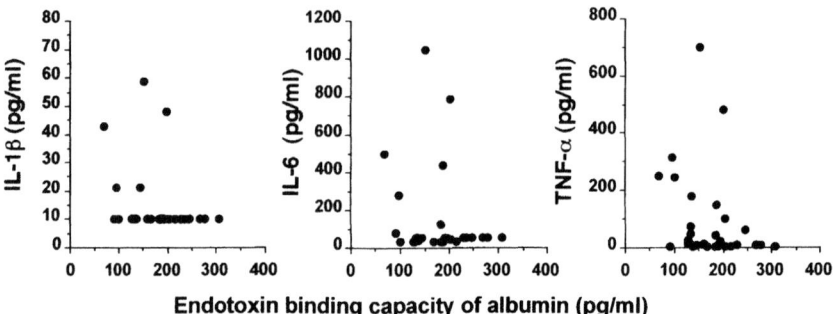

Figure 9 Relationships of endotoxin-binding capacity of serum albumin to plasma interleukin (IL)-1β, IL-6 and tumour necrosis factor (TNF)-α levels in cirrhotics

activity by incubation with plasma in this method seems to be related to the structural and functional change of endotoxin with binding to plasma protein.

As discussed above, patients with liver cirrhosis frequently have elevated levels of plasma endotoxin. However, it is true that the endotoxin level does not necessarily correlate to the severity of liver disease. Endotoxin was generally cleared and detoxified by the reticuloendothelial system. The fact that the toxicity of endotoxin does not appear, in spite of its high plasma level, led us to hypothesize that there is some endotoxin-inactivating mechanism in the blood. HDL[15], transferrin[16] and lipopolysaccharide-binding protein (LBP)[17] have been reported to show endotoxin-binding activity and considered as transporting proteins of endotoxin in the blood. However, it is undetermined whether they can really inactivate endotoxin by their binding. Mathison *et al.*[18] provided evidence that binding to HDL retards the clearance of endotoxin in rabbits. Freudenberg *et al.*[19] further demonstrated that uptake of free endotoxin by mouse macrophage was much greater than that of HDL-bound endotoxin. However, Abdelnoor *et al.*[20] showed the inability of HDL to neutralize endotoxin *in vivo*. LBP has been reported to enhance both endotoxin uptake and tumour necrosis factor secretion by macrophage[17]. It is not clear what protein is chiefly responsible for binding and inactivating endotoxin in the blood.

At present we cannot differentiate free 'active' endotoxin from protein-bound 'inactive' endotoxin by the chromogenic substrate assay. Fractionation of minute endogenous endotoxin to free form and protein-bound forms without contamination is at present difficult. On the basis of these limitations in the study we added radiolabelled endotoxin to sample plasma and measured the protein-bound fraction by affinity chromatography and immunoprecipitation.

Until now the endotoxin-binding and inactivating capacity of albumin have been disregarded. In a trial of stabilizing standard endotoxin by an addition of albumin, we happened to notice that albumin inhibited endotoxin activity in the chromogenic assay system[21]. This observation led us to hypothesize that albumin may act as a protective protein against endotoxaemia. In our preliminary study we first noted that 250 pg/ml endotoxin lost most activity in the presence of albumin at physiological concentrations (unpublished data). Another interesting result was that albumin inhibits LPS-stimulated interleukin-1 secretion in the macrophage culture system (unpublished data). The present result of affinity chromatography supports the concept that albumin can bind and inactivate endotoxin in the blood of cirrhotics. We further noted that the capacity of albumin to bind exogenous [^{3}H]-labelled endotoxin decreased in the plasma of cirrhotics. Although serum levels of HDL and transferrin decreased in patients with advanced liver cirrhosis, in our study the endotoxin-binding capacity of HDL and transferrin did not decrease with the progression of liver disturbance. Albumin has a protective effect against encephalopathy in advanced cirrhosis[22]. Substances which require albumin binding – such as bilirubin, free fatty acids and organic anions[23] – markedly increase in the blood in this situation. The increase of these substances may limit the endotoxin-binding capacity of albumin. In Child C cirrhotics, in whom albumin showed very low endotoxin-binding capacity, endotoxin increased in the supernatant fraction rather than in the precipitate fraction using the perchloric acid method. To delineate an albumin–endotoxin complex in the blood we should perform a saturation study. Future research will focus on the molecular structure and dynamics in association with this binding.

In conclusion, endotoxaemia is closely related to the pathophysiology of chronic liver disease. Endotoxaemia, together with a failure to inactivate endotoxin in the blood, may aggravate the clinical course of patients with chronic liver diseases.

Acknowledgements

This study was supported by the Ministry of Education, Science and Culture, Japan; Grant 06670578. The authors thank Professor S. Kanegasaki and Dr S. Kobayashi in the Institute of Medical Science, University of Tokyo, for instruction on the preparation of [^{3}H]endotoxin, and for their valuable advice.

References

1. Lumsden A, Henderson J, Kutner M. Endotoxin levels measured by a chromogenic assay in portal, hepatic and peripheral venous blood in patients with cirrhosis. Hepatology. 1988;8:232–6.
2. Scully M. Measurement of endotoxemia by the limulus test. Int Care Med. 1984;10:1–2.
3. Iwanaga S, Morita T, Harada T. Chromogenic substances for horseshoe crab clotting enzyme, its application for the assay of bacterial endotoxin. Hemostasis 1978;7:183–188.
4. Sturk A, Joop K, ten Cate JW, Thomas LLM. Optimalization of a chromogenic assay for endotoxin in blood. In: ten Cate JW, Buller HR, Sturk A, Levin J, editors. Bacterial endotoxins: structure, biomedical significance and detection with *Limulus* amebocyte lysate test. New York: A. R. Liss; 1985:117–36.
5. Friberger, P. The design of a reliable endotoxin test. In: ten Cate JW, Buller HR, Sturk A, Levin J, editors. Bacterial endotoxins: structure, biomedical significance and detection with *Limulus* amebocyte lysate test. New York: A. R. Liss; 1985:139–49.
6. Sturk A, Janssen ME, Muylaert FR, Joop K, Thomas LLM, ten Cate JW. Endotoxin testing in blood. Progr Clin Biol Res. 1987;231,371–85.
7. Fukui H, Brauner B, Bode JC, Bode C. Chromogenic endotoxin assay in plasma – selection of plasma pretreatment and production of standard curves. J Clin Chem Biochem. 1989;27:941–6.
8. Obayashi T, Tamura H, Tanaka S. A new chromogenic endotoxin-specific assay using recombined *Limulus* coagulation enzymes and its clinical applications. Clin Chim Acta. 1985;149:55–65.

9. Fukui H, Matsumoto M, Tsujita S et al. Plasma endotoxin concentration and endotoxin binding capacity of plasma acute phase proteins in cirrhotics with variceal bleeding: an analysis by new method. J Gasroenterol Hepatol. 1994;9:582–6.

10. Bode C, Fukui H, Bode JC. 'Hidden' endotoxin in plasma of patients with alcoholic liver disease. Eur J Gastroenterol Hepatol. 1993;5:257–62.

11. Obayashi T. Addition of perchloric acid to blood samples for colorimetric Limulus test using chromogenic substrate: comparison with conventional procedures and clinical application. J Lab Clin Med. 1984;104:321–30.

12. Inada K, Endo S, Takahashi K et al. Establishment of a new perchloric acid treatment method to allow determination of the total endotoxin content in human plasma by the Limulus test and clinical application. Microbiol Immunol. 1991;35:303–14.

13. Fukui H, Tsujita S, Matsumoto M et al. Endotoxin inactivating action of plasma in patients with liver cirrhosis. Liver. 1995;15:104–9.

14. Fukui H, Matsumoto M, Bode C, Bode JC, Tsujita S, Tsujii T. Endotoxemia in patients with liver cirrhosis and upper gastrointestinal bleeding: detection by the chromogenic assay with plasma Tween 80 pretreatment. J Gasroenterol Hepatol. 1993;8:577–81.

15. Ulevitch RJ, Johnston AR, Weinstein DB. New function for high density lipoproteins: their participation in intravascular reactions of bacterial lipopolysaccharides. J Clin Invest. 1979;64:1516–24.

16. Berger D, Beger HG. Evidence for endotoxin binding capacity of human Gc-globulin and transferrin. Clin Chim Acta. 1987;163:289–99.

17. Schumann RR, Leong SR, Flaggs GW et al. Structure and function of lipopolysaccharide binding protein. Science. 1990;249:1429–31.

18. Mathison J, Ulevitch R. The clearance, tissue distribution, and cellular localization of intravenously injected lipopolysaccharide in rabbits. J Immunol. 1979;123:2133–43.

19. Freudenberg MCG. The metabolic fate of endotoxin. In: Levin J, Buller H, ten Cate J, van Deventer SJH, Sturk A, editors. Bacterial endotoxins: pathophysiological effects, clinical significance, and pharmacological control. New York: Alan R Liss; 1988:63–75.

20. Abdelnoor A, Harvie N, Johnson A. Neutralization of bacteria- and endotoxin-induced hypotension by lipoprotein-free human serum. Infect Immun. 1982;38:157–61.

21. Fukui H, Brauner B, Bode JC. Plasma endotoxin concentrations in patients with alcoholic and non-alcoholic liver disease: reevaluation with an improved chromogenic assay. J Hepatol. 1991;12:162–9.

22. Zieve L. Hepatic encephalopathy: summary of present knowledge with an elaboration on recent developments. In: Popper, Schaffner F, editor. Progress in liver diseases, Vol. VI. New York: Grune & Stratton; 1979:327–41.

23. Sorrentino D, Potter B, Berk P. From albumin to the cytoplasm: the hepatic uptake of organic anions. In: Popper, Schaffner F, editor. Progress in liver diseases, Vol. IX. New York: Grune & Stratton; 1990:203–35.

20
Endotoxaemia and disseminated intravascular coagulation in cirrhosis

F. VIOLI, S. BASILI and D. FERRO

INTRODUCTION

The clinical history of chronic liver disease is often complicated by haemorrhagic episodes occurring prevalently in the gastrointestinal tube. This bleeding complication is partly dependent on the important functional relationship between liver cells and the clotting system. All the procoagulant factors, except von Willebrand factor, are synthesized by liver cells[1–4]; furthermore, the hepatic cell is an important regulator of the clotting system, since it also synthesizes clotting inhibitors, i.e. antithrombin (AT) III, protein C and S, heparin cofactor II[5–9] and important components of the fibrinolytic system, i.e. plasminogen and plasmin inhibitors such as α_2-antiplasmin and α_2-macroglobulin[10,11]; in addition, cultured human hepatocytes were demonstrated to synthesize the inhibitor of tissue plasminogen activator (PAI)[12,13]. Finally, the reticuloendothelial liver cells play an important role in the clearance of activated clotting factors and plasminogen activators[14–18]. One of the most common abnormalities found in patients with liver cirrhosis (LC) is the reduced activity of almost all the components of the clotting and fibrinolytic system, due to diminished hepatocellular protein synthesis[19]. Other alterations can also be detected, including changes in primary haemostasis and in the activation of the fibrinolytic system[20–23] (Table 1). Among these clotting changes, hyperfibrinolysis has been shown to be an important risk factor, since cirrhotic patients with hyperfibrinolysis are at

Table 1 Clotting and platelet abnormalities in liver cirrhosis

Decreased synthesis of clotting factors	Thrombocytopenia
Dysfibrinogenaemia	Thrombocytopathia
Hyperfibrinolytic syndrome	

higher risk of bleeding. This overview deals with the relationship between hyperfibrinolysis and bleeding, and the mechanism(s) accounting for it.

HYPERFIBRINOLYSIS AND BLEEDING COMPLICATION IN CIRRHOTIC PATIENTS

The prognosis of patients with liver cirrhosis after gastrointestinal bleeding is poor, since only 50% survive 6 weeks after the first episode, and about 10–20% are still alive after 4 years[24–26]. Therefore, the identification of risk factors of first bleeding may be of potential clinical relevance for the future management of cirrhotic patients. The rupture of oesophageal varices is the most important cause of gastrointestinal bleeding[27,28]; therefore, many trials with drugs that reduce portal hypertension, such as β-blockers, have been performed to prevent gastrointestinal bleeding[29–31]. Liver failure is another important factor that increases the risk of variceal bleeding[32]. Even if the mechanism underlying such association is yet to be defined, clotting changes observed in patients with severe liver failure could play a role. Thus, it has been shown that hyperfibrinolysis is often detected in patients with severe liver failure, and is a good predictor of gastrointestinal bleeding[22,33,34]. These studies, however, have been performed in relatively small cohorts of cirrhotic patients with advanced cirrhosis, and excluded patients with compensated cirrhosis[35]. Furthermore, it has not been investigated whether hyperfibrinolysis increases the risk of gastrointestinal bleeding in cirrhotic patients without a clinical history of bleeding. Finally, the methodological approach used to detect hyperfibrinolysis, i.e. the measurement of fibrin(ogen) degradation products (FDP), is a semiquantitative assay which may give false-positive results[36,37].

Following a more adequate procedure for the diagnosis of hyperfibrinolysis it has recently been demonstrated that cirrhotic patients have high values of tissue-plasminogen activator (t-PA) activity and D-dimer[38,39], a marker of thrombin and plasmin activation[36,40]; furthermore, we found a close association between high values of t-PA and D-dimer, so providing clear-cut support to the suggestion that hyperfibrinolysis complicates the clinical course of cirrhosis[35].

In a recent study[41] we analysed whether hyperfibrinolysis increases the risk of bleeding, in an unselected cohort of cirrhotic patients with low-to-severe liver failure who had not experienced gastrointestinal bleeding before entry into the study; furthermore, we examined the association of hyperfibrinolysis with clinical variables, such as the degree of liver failure, classified by Child–Pugh criteria[42], ascites and variceal size, which have previously been reported to be independent predictors of gastrointestinal bleeding[25,43].

From October 1990 to July 1994 all patients who were seen at any of the participating institutions with diagnosis of cirrhosis of the liver underwent routine upper gastrointestinal endoscopy. All patients with oesophageal varices, but no history of bleeding from varices or any other source in the upper gastrointestinal tract, were eligible for the study. Oesophageal varices were classified as small, moderate-sized, large and varices with red signs[24,43]. After baseline evaluation of clinical and laboratory variables, including clotting (prothrombin activity, activated partial thromboplastin time (aPTT), fibrinogen) and fibrinolytic indices

(D-dimer, t-PA activity), patients were examined periodically, normally every 2–4 months, and rehospitalized in case of worsening of liver failure or bleeding. At each visit a study of the coagulation and fibrinolytic system was carried out. Patients were considered to have hyperfibrinolysis if they had high values of both D-dimer (> 216 ng/ml, mean ± 2 SD of controls) and t-PA activity (> 3.6 U/ml, mean ± 2 SD of controls) in two consecutive controls. None of the patients had received drugs that interfered with the coagulation or fibrinolytic system, vitamin K and β-blockers, throughout follow-up. The end-point of the study was bleeding from the gastrointestinal tract. Gastrointestinal bleeding was defined as the presence of haematemesis or melaena (or both), together with a decrease in the haemoglobin level of ≥ 2 g/dl. Emergency endoscopy was able to establish the source of bleeding in 25 patients. The endoscopic diagnoses were bleeding varices in 23 patients (92%) and acute gastric erosions in two (8%). In the remaining nine patients the source of bleeding was not verified endoscopically, either because of death before hospital admittance ($n = 3$) or because endoscopic findings were inconclusive ($n = 6$). Fatal bleeding was defined as occurring when a patient died within 6 weeks of a bleeding episode[43]. One hundred and twelve patients (67 males, 45 females; age 30–84 years, 61 ± 10; class A ($n = 26$), B ($n = 52$), and C ($n = 34$) according to Child–Pugh criteria) entered the study. Eighty-two (73%) patients had serological markers for hepatitis B virus (HBV) and/or hepatitis C virus (HCV), 21 (19%) had cryptogenic cirrhosis and nine (8%) had a history of alcoholic consumption.

Follow-up

During the follow-up (median, (range): 12 (1–48) months) 13 (12%) patients died and 34 (30%) bled. The cause of death could be attributed to liver disease ($n = 9$) and to fatal gastrointestinal bleeding ($n = 4$). The gastrointestinal tract was the source of bleeding in all 34 patients who bled during follow-up; four bleedings were fatal.

Bleeding patients had more severe liver failure and variceal size, and a higher prevalence of ascites and varices with red signs, than patients who did not bleed; they also had higher serum values of bilirubin, a more prolonged aPTT, lower blood values of albumin, fibrinogen, prothrombin activity and a high prevalence of hyperfibrinolysis. Multivariate analysis (Cox regression model) showed that hyperfibrinolysis was the only predictor of bleeding (regression coefficient: 3.75, standard error: 0.57, hazard ratio: 42.5, 95% confidence limits: 14–129, $p < 0.001$). Similar results were obtained using prothrombin activity, aPTT, serum albumin, plasma fibrinogen and serum bilirubin as continuous variables.

Association among hyperfibrinolysis, clinical variables and bleeding

At entry, 33 (29%) patients were classified as having hyperfibrinolysis. Hyperfibrinolysis was absent in patients of A class, while it was found in 21% of B and 79% of C class patients. It is noteworthy that all patients with hyperfibrinolysis were ascitic; conversely there were 29 (47%) ascitic patients without hyperfibrinolysis. Abnormal values of serum albumin, bilirubin, fibrinogen and prothrombin activity were associated with hyperfibrinolysis.

All patients who had hyperfibrinolysis at entry persistently had high values of D-dimer and t-PA activity throughout follow-up. Conversely, eight patients (six males and two females, one of A, six of B and one of C class) who had no hyperfibrinolysis at entry, showed elevated values of D-dimer and t-PA activity during follow-up. All but one of these patients had no ascites at entry; conversely, all were ascitic when hyperfibrinolysis was detected. Four of these patients experienced gastrointestinal bleeding during follow-up (4–18 months after the hyperfibrinolysis was detected). Since previous studies demonstrated that Child–Pugh classes, ascites and variceal size were significantly associated to bleeding, we analysed the relationship among these clinical variables, hyperfibrinolysis and bleeding.

Kaplan–Meier curves for the whole series of cirrhotic patients (panel A) and for ascitic patients (panel B) with and without hyperfibrinolysis are reported in Fig. 1. This analysis shows that patients with hyperfibrinolysis have a higher probability of suffering from gastrointestinal bleeding.

Figure 2 shows the Kaplan–Meier curves inherent to Child–Pugh classes with and without hyperfibrinolysis. While it is evident that, in patients without hyperfibrinolysis, the occurrence of bleeding is related to the entity of liver failure, the presence of hyperfibrinolysis is associated with early haemorrhage independently of liver failure score. The relationship between hyperfibrinolysis and bleeding was also analysed, taking variceal size into account. Within each subclass group of variceal size the presence of hyperfibrinolysis discriminated patients who bled from those who did not. It is interesting to note that all patients with small varices who bled during follow-up had hyperfibrinolysis.

The mechanism accounting for the association between hyperfibrinolysis and gastrointestinal bleeding in cirrhotic patients needs to be clarified, but the interference of hyperfibrinolysis with clotting activation and platelet function could perhaps account for it. Thus, as a consequence of hyperfibrinolysis, clotting activation may be delayed due to clotting factor consumption and fibrin polymerization inhibition[44]. Hyperfibrinolysis also reduces platelet adhesion and aggregation by degradation of von Willebrand factor and fibrinogen platelet receptors (glycoprotein Ib and IIb/IIIa)[45–47]. Finally, hyperfibrinolysis may provoke clot lysis by inducing platelet disaggregation and haemostatic plug disruption[48].

The interference of hyperfibrinolysis with clotting and platelet activation may cause or simply facilitate the occurrence of bleeding. Several studies support the idea that hyperfibrinolysis favours bleeding in a case of vascular injury[44]. Accordingly, a possible 'scenario' may be that, in a case of rupture of oesophageal varices, the presence of hyperfibrinolysis may delay clotting activation or induce disruption of haemostatic plug, so facilitating the occurrence of bleeding.

The mechanisms which lead to the activation of the fibrinolytic system in liver cirrhosis are currently under investigation. There are at least three mechanisms potentially accounting for: (a) imbalance between tissue-plasminogen activator and its inhibitor (PAI-1), due to reduced clearance of t-PA[49]; (b) reduced levels of α2-antiplasmin, which are due to diminished protein liver synthesis[50,51]; (c) intravascular clotting activation[52]. While the first two

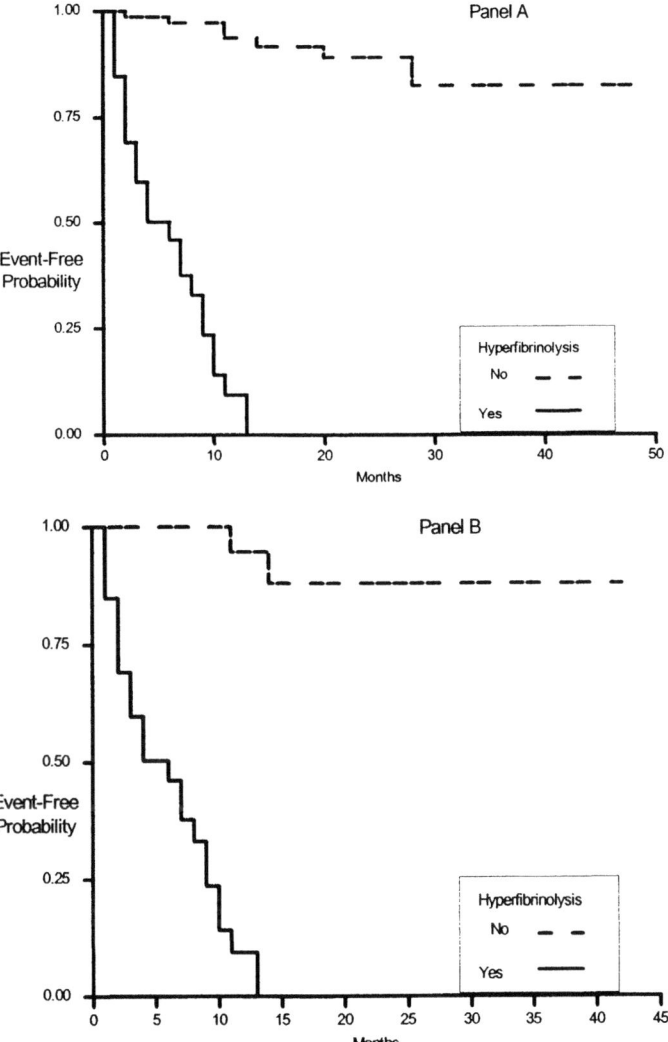

Figure 1 Kaplan–Meier curves for the series of cirrhotic patients (panel A) and ascitic patients (panel B)

mechanisms suggest the presence of primary hyperfibrinolysis, the third hypothesis is in favour of hyperfibrinolysis secondary to clotting activation.

HYPERFIBRINOLYSIS AND CLOTTING ACTIVATION: THE ROLE OF ENDOTOXAEMIA

Even though several studies have attempted to elucidate whether hyperfibrinolysis in LC is primary or secondary to intravascular clotting activation, no

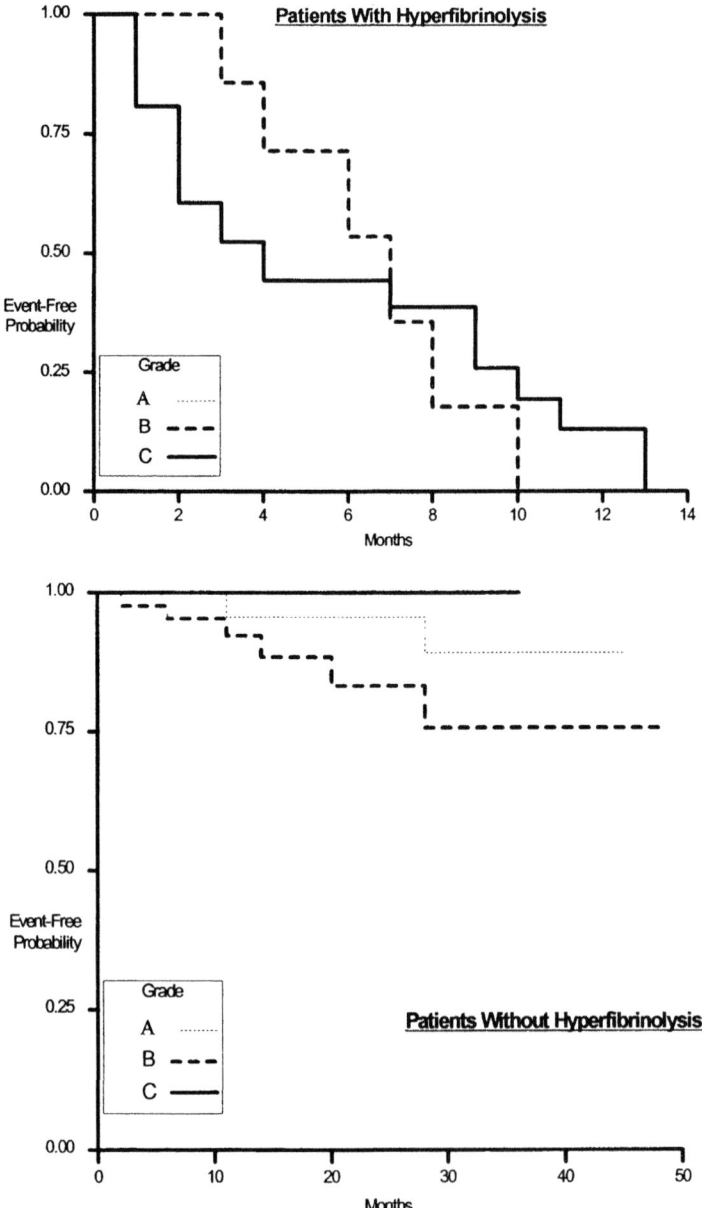

Figure 2 Kaplan–Meier curves inherent to Child–Pugh classes with and without hyperfibrinolysis

conclusive data are available to support the former or the latter hypothesis[51-53]. Primary hyperfibrinolysis is alleged to occur as a result of either an imbalance between tissue-plasminogen activator (t-PA) and its inhibitor (PAI-1), due to impaired hepatic t-PA clearance, or a reduced synthesis by the liver of the plasmin inhibitor α_2-antiplasmin[50,54,55]. None of these studies, however, could clarify if a casual relationship exists between hyperfibrinolysis and intravascular clotting activation. Previous studies demonstrated that LC patients have a reduced half-life of fibrinogen, prothrombin and plasminogen, which are reversed by heparin administration[56,57]. This led us to hypothesize that low-grade disseminated intravascular coagulation (low-grade DIC) complicates the clinical course of cirrhosis. However, the accelerated catabolism was not considered as a possible contributing factor to peritoneal loss of clotting factors[58].

Further studies have investigated the presence of a hypercoagulability state in LC. Two markers of *in-vivo* clotting activation have been measured in LC patients: the fibrinopeptide A (FpA), which is an index of the enzymatic activity of thrombin, and the thrombin–antithrombin III complexes, which represent an index of thrombin generation rate. The results of these assays, however, have been conflicting: the pattern of plasma concentrations shown by the two markers was inconsistent, as both high and normal values have been reported[39,59,60]. Moreover, no evidence has been found that the clotting activation was associated with hyperfibrinolysis and blood coagulation factors consumption, even in those cases in which high values of FpA and thrombin–antithrombin complexes were detected.

Recently a new method has been developed to assess the presence of a hypercoagulability state; namely the measurement of circulating levels of prothrombin fragment F1+2, which is cleaved by factors Xa and Va through prothrombin conversion to thrombin, and is considered a marker of thrombin generation rate[61]. The measurement of F1+2 seems to be a more reliable method to explore clotting activation, since its half-life (90 min) is longer than that reported for FpA (5 min) or thrombin–antithrombin III complexes (15 min). Preliminary studies demonstrated that F1+2 is elevated in LC[62,63] but its prevalence, and the relationship to hyperfibrinolysis, have never been investigated.

Recently we carried out a study[64] to assess if patients with LC have primary hyperfibrinolysis or low-grade DIC, or both. In addition we investigated the behaviour of endotoxaemia, which is elevated in LC[65] and may represent a potential stimulus for clotting pathways[66,67]. We studied 41 consecutive patients (27 males, 14 females; aged 48–79 years; six assigned to A, 25 to B and 10 to C class according to Child–Pugh criteria) affected by liver cirrhosis and 20 healthy volunteers (13 males, seven females, aged 41–72 years). Patients were given no non-absorbable antibiotics during the previous 30 days.

In a first study a cross-sectional comparison of clotting tests and endotoxaemia was performed between patients and controls.

A second study was carried out to explore the relationship between endotoxaemia and clotting system activation. Thirty patients were randomly assigned to standard therapy (spironolactone, furosemide, ethacrinic acid, albumin, and lactulose) or to standard therapy plus non-absorbable antibiotics: (1) colistin 6 000 000 U/day; (2) neomycin 200 000 U/day; (3) bacitracin 20 000 U/day; (4) nystatin 4 000 000 U/day. The two groups had similar age, sex and degree of liver failure data. None of these LC patients had had gastrointestinal bleeding in the previous 4 months, or had been given non-absorbable antibiotic therapy in the previous 30 days. A blood sample to measure endotoxaemia, D-dimer, fibrin(ogen) degradation products (FDP), t-PA, PAI-1, F1+2, fibrinogen, prothrombin activity and serum albumin was taken before and after 7 days of treatment.

Clotting activation and hyperfibrinolysis in different degrees of liver failure

Changes in the clotting and fibrinolytic system were closely related to liver failure. Thus, patients with severe liver failure, i.e. patients of C class, had lowest values of prothrombin activity, fibrinogen and PAI, and highest values of D-dimer and t-PA; the prevalence of patients with FDP > 10 μg/ml was 0% in patients of A class and 44% and 100% in those of B and C class, respectively.

F1+2 plasma levels were significantly higher in LC patients than in controls (1.75 ± 1.05 vs 0.62 ± 0.23 nmol/L, $p = 0.0001$). F1+2 progressively increased from A to C class; patients of B and C classes having F1+2 values higher ($p < 0.01$) than patients of A class and controls (Fig. 3).

Conversely, no difference was observed between A class and controls. F1+2 plasma levels greater than 1 nmol/L (mean ± 2 SD of controls) were observed in no patient of A class, in 17 (68%) patients of B class and in all patients (100%) of C class ($p = 0.0002$). Among patients of B class with F1+2 > ($n = 13$) or ≤ ($n = 7$) 1.0 nmol/L, matched for age and sex, serum albumin (3.2 ± 0.4 vs 3.3 ± 0.5 g/dl, $p > 0.05$) and prothrombin activity (61 ± 9 vs 66 ± 9%, $p > 0.05$) showed no statistical difference, suggesting that F1+2 behaviour was not closely dependent upon liver function.

Nineteen (46%) LC patients were considered to have hyperfibrinolysis, since they had high values of both D-dimer and FDP. High values of F1+2 were closely associated with fibrinolytic system activation. Thus, patients with F1+2 > 1 nmol/L had higher values of D-dimer and t-PA, and higher t-PA/PAI ratio than patients with F1+2 < 1 nmol/L. These differences were also observed in patients matched for degree of liver failure.

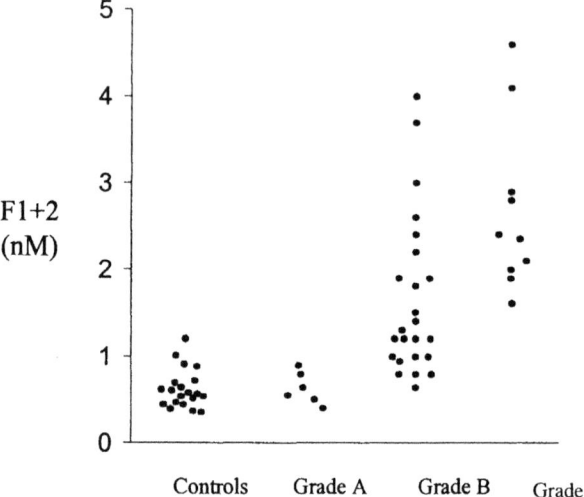

Figure 3 F1+2 plasma levels in healthy subjects and in liver cirrhotic patients with low (A), moderate (B) or severe (C) liver failure

Seventy per cent of patients with F1+2 > 1.0 nmol/L had D-dimer plasma values > 216 ng/ml (mean ± 2 SD of controls); conversely, all patients with normal F1 + 2 had D-dimer < 216 ng/ml.

F1+2 was significantly correlated with D-dimer (rho = 0.67, p = 0.0001) and t-PA (r = 0.79, p = 0.0001). It is noteworthy that t-PA values > 3.6 U/ml (mean ± 2 SD of controls) were observed only in patients with high values of both F1+2 and D-dimer, while they were in the normal range in patients with normal F1+2 or high F1+2 but normal D-dimer.

All 19 patients with D-dimer > 216 ng/ml had F1+2 > 1 nmol/L. In comparison to patients with D-dimer < 216 ng/ml (n = 22) they showed lower α_2-antiplasmin, higher values of t-PA and higher values of t-PA/PAI antigen ratio. They also had significantly lower values of fibrinogen by clotting and radial immunodiffusion assays. Similar results were obtained in a homogeneous group of cirrhotic patients, i.e. 20 patients of B class with high (n = 7) or normal (n = 13) D-dimer (data not shown), indicating that hyperfibrinolysis, but not liver failure, was responsible for the findings reported above.

In comparison to patients with F1+2 > 1 nmol/L but normal D-dimer (n = 8), patients with D-dimer > 216 ng/ml (n = 19) had significantly lower values of ATIII (38.7 ± 11.6 vs 62.9 ± 15.1%; p = 0.0001).

Among the 41 patients examined 17 (41%) had a clinical history of gastro-intestinal bleeding. Patients who had previously bled had significantly higher values of F1+2 (2.6 ± 1.1 vs 1.2 ± 0.5 nmol/L, p = 0.0001) and D-dimer – median (range): 1156 (113–2206) vs 86 (38–1611) ng/ml, p = 0.0001 – than patients who did not. Fifteen out the 17 bleeding patients had values of D-dimer higher than 216 ng/ml.

Relationship among endotoxaemia, clotting activation and hyperfibrinolysis

Endotoxaemia was significantly higher in LC patients than in controls – median (range): 13.6 (0–188.9) vs 4.3 (0–9.6) pg/ml, p = 0.003 – and progressively increased from A to C class (p = 0.003) (Fig. 4). Similar findings were obtained after exclusion of patients with a clinical history of alcoholism.

In order to assess the variability of endotoxaemia it was measured 1 month apart in 15 patients (10 males and five females, aged 42–70 years, 12 of B and three of C class), four with and 11 without systemic signs of hyperfibrinolysis. Throughout this period the patients, whose clinical characteristics and liver failure score remained stable, did not show significant changes of endotoxaemia: 19.2 (0–41.5) vs 19.7 (0–59.0) pg/ml.

Endotoxaemia was closely associated with clotting and fibrinolytic system activation. Thus, we found a strong correlation between endotoxaemia and F1+2 (Fig. 5).

Patients with D-dimer > 216 ng/ml also had significantly higher endotoxaemia than patients with D-dimer < 216 ng/ml.

Comparison of baseline laboratory characteristics between patients assigned to standard therapy or standard therapy plus non-absorbable antibiotics disclosed no significant differences. In patients given standard therapy liver failure score and laboratory indices did not change significantly. In the patients given

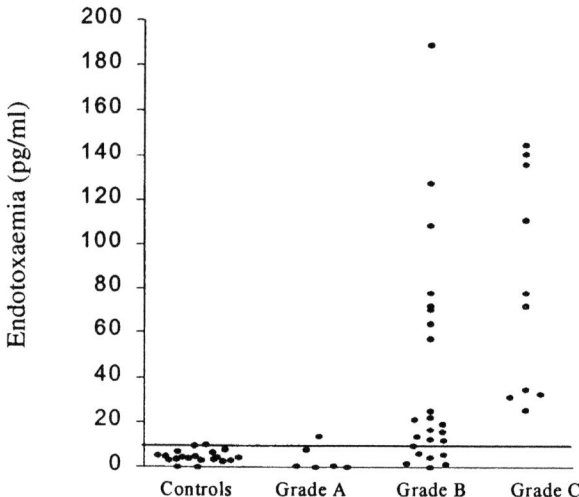

Figure 4 Endotoxaemia in healthy subjects and in liver cirrhotic patients with low (A), moderate (B) or severe (C) liver failure

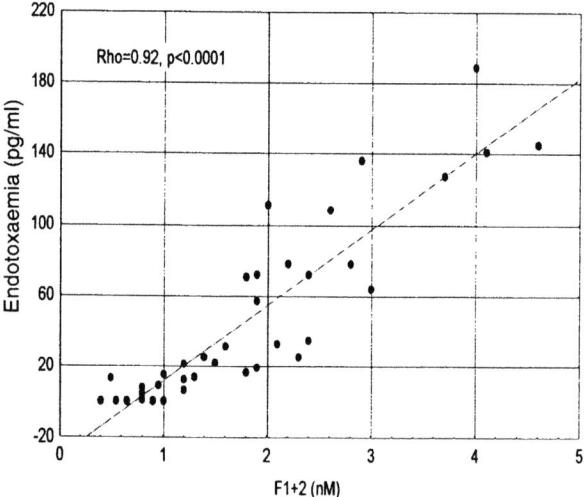

Figure 5 Correlation between endotoxaemia and plasma levels of F1+2 in patients with liver cirrhosis

standard therapy plus non-absorbable antibiotics a significant decrease of endotoxaemia ($p = 0.0125$, Fig. 6, panel A), F1+2 plasma levels ($p = 0.002$, Fig. 6, panel B), D-dimer, t-PA antigen and activity and a significant increase of fibrinogen plasma levels were observed. Child–Pugh score, PAI-1, prothrombin activity, and albumin serum levels did not change significantly. A reduction of endotoxaemia more than 11%, which is the day-to-day variability of the assay

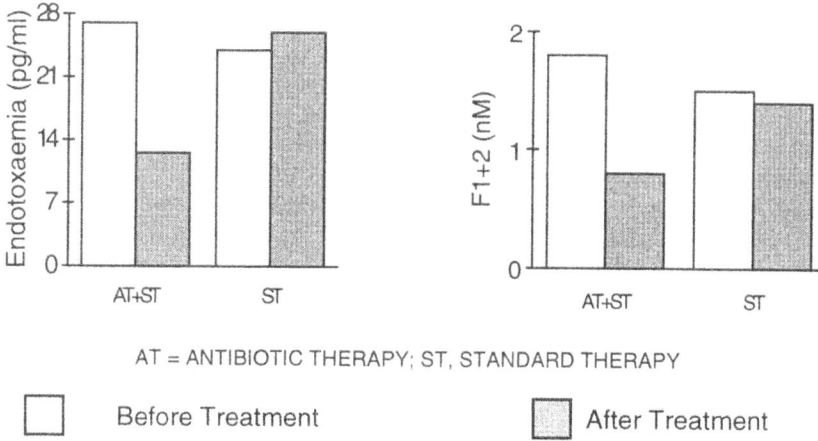

AT = ANTIBIOTIC THERAPY; ST, STANDARD THERAPY

☐ Before Treatment   ▦ After Treatment

Figure 6 Endotoxaemia and F1+2 plasma levels in liver cirrhotic patients treated for 7 days with standard therapy or standard therapy plus non-absorbable antibiotics

method, was observed in all but four patients. In these latter endotoxaemia [75 (15–78) vs 78 (15–92) pg/ml], as well as F1+2 [1.4 (1.0–2.8) vs 2.0 (1.0–2.6) nmol/L], D-dimer [1016 (50–1821) vs 806 (80–1640) ng/ml], t-PA [9.5 (1.3–12.6) vs 9.2 (1.4–11.0) U/ml], and fibrinogen [126 (101–208) vs 162 (60–305) mg/dl], did not change significantly. In the whole series of patients given non-absorbable antibiotics a statistically significant correlation between percentage changes of endotoxaemia and F1+2 was observed (rho = 0.85, $p = 0.0015$).

Taken together these data strongly suggest that in LC fibrinolysis is not primary, but is the result of a hypercoagulability state. However, our study did not fully elucidate the mechanism which favours the occurrence of low-grade DIC in patients with high F1+2 values. It is possible that ATIII levels, which are lower in patients with low-grade DIC, may have a role, but we cannot exclude the possibility that ATIII behaviour is a mere consequence of low-grade DIC. In order to investigate the mechanism of intravascular clotting activation, we measured endotoxaemia, which could represent a plausible explanation of the high rate of thrombin generation. Endotoxin induces an increase in tissue factor expression on the surface of macrophages and endothelial cells, and promotes the macrophage synthesis of tumour necrosis factor which, in turn, activates extrinsic clotting pathway[66,68–70]. The procoagulant activity of endotoxin has been well documented in clinical trials showing that a bolus injection increases the plasma levels of prothrombin fragment F1+2 and thrombin–antithrombin III complexes[71].

Endotoxin, a constituent of the cell wall of Gram-negative bacilli, can be absorbed, under normal circumstances, from the gastrointestinal tract into the portal circulation, and then undergoes clearance by the hepatic reticuloendothelial system[72,73]. In patients with acute and chronic liver disease an impairment of the reticuloendothelial system and/or the presence of portosystemic shunts may lead, in the absence of sepsis, to the presence of endotoxin in the systemic circulation[74]. Gastrointestinal bleeding, hypotension and alcohol consumption can increase endotoxin absorption[75,76]. Previous studies reported a great variability of endotoxaemia in LC patients, probably due to the poor sensitivity and reproducibility of the *Limulus* lysate test[77]. Recently, using a new sensitive chromogenic assay, it has been shown that cirrhotic patients have significantly higher endotoxaemia than healthy subjects[65]; this study demonstrated that the presence of endotoxaemia is closely related to liver failure, since only patients with moderate–severe hepatic insufficiency have high values. In patients in whom endotoxaemia was measured 1 month apart, a very small variation was observed, indicating a highly reproducible measurement for this laboratory index and, overall, that endotoxaemia may be persistently elevated for a long time.

Our study provides evidence for a direct relationship between clotting activation and endotoxaemia. The hypothesis is supported on the one hand by the strong association between endotoxaemia and high plasma levels of F1+2 and D-dimer, and on the other hand by the decrease of clotting and fibrinolytic activation following the reduction of endotoxaemia. Further evidence for this suggestion was provided by the strong correlation between percentage changes of F1+2 and endotoxaemia observed after non-absorbable antibiotic therapy. These data indicate that endotoxaemia plays a role in the activation of clotting and fibrinolytic pathways, but they do not clarify the mechanism accounting for this effect. Further study is therefore necessary to explain how endotoxaemia induces clotting activation in cirrhosis.

CLOTTING ACTIVATION IN THE PORTAL VEIN: THE ROLE OF ENDOTOXAEMIA

Thrombosis may also occur in cirrhosis, prevalently in the portal blood, as shown by anatomopathological study, angiography and enhanced computerized tomography[78–80]; about 15% of cirrhotic patients may experience thrombosis of the portal vein[79]. The mechanism accounting for thrombosis is unclear even if certain factors such as antiphospholipid antibodies and hepatitis C virus may have a role[81,82]. Endotoxin, which is elevated in cirrhosis[64,83], particularly in the portal circulation[84], may represent an important trigger as it stimulates the clotting system[85], but to date there is no study aimed at evaluating the relationship between endotoxaemia and clotting activation in the portal circulation of cirrhotic patients.

In a recent study[86] we analysed the behaviour of the clotting system and endotoxaemia in the portal vein and peripheral circulation of cirrhotic patients undergoing transjugular portosystemic shunt (TIPS). We studied 11 patients (seven males and four females; age 55 ± 16, range 26–78 years; five of A, five of B and one of C class according to Child–Pugh criteria) affected by liver cirrhosis, diagnosed by needle liver biopsy. TIPS was indicated for the presence of recurrence of variceal bleeding ($n = 8$) or refractory ascites ($n = 3$). No patient was treated by TIPS on an emergency basis.

Insertion of TIPS

The TIPS procedure (Fig. 7) was performed following the usual method previously described[87,88]. With the patients under heavy sedation, or under general anaesthesia, the right jugular vein was punctured and a catheter needle assembly was advanced through the right atrium and the hepatic vein into a portal branch. At this moment blood samples were taken to study endotoxaemia and the clotting system. After blood sampling the procedure was continued by measuring the pressure gradient between the right atrium and the portal, and by deploying a metallic stent between the hepatic vein and the portal system to establish direct communication. The stents we used were either Wallstents (Schneider, Bulach, Switzerland), or Nitinol-Strecker stents (Ultraflex Biliary Stent system–Meditech, Boston Scientific Co., Natick, MA, USA).

Design of the study

In all patients a blood sample was taken both in the peripheral circulation and portal vein to study the clotting system (prothrombin activity, fibrinogen, prothrombin fragment F1+2, D-dimer), and to measure endotoxaemia. Blood samples were taken on the same day using a 19 G needle for the peripheral blood and a puncture needle, advanced transjugularly in a catheter (Cooks), for the portal vein.

In separate experiments blood samples were taken from the antecubital vein of volunteers with a 19 G needle, as well as with the catheter used for portal vein puncture, in order to assess if the use of the catheter might cause *per se* artifactual assay. Clotting variables obtained with these two techniques showed no significant differences.

In the peripheral circulation cirrhotic patients had significantly higher values of F1+2 [1.1 (0.6–2.1) vs 0.57 (0.3–1.2) nmol/L, $p = 0.0005$], D-dimer [192 (64–813) vs 66.5 (32–270) ng/ml, $p = 0.0009$], endotoxaemia [13.7 (7.5–23.5) vs 4.34 (0–9.6) pg/ml, $p = 0.0008$] and lower fibrinogen [134 (75–244) vs 235 (150–361) mg/dl, $p = 0.0008$] than controls. In particular five patients had F1+2 > 1.2 nmoL (upper limit of control values), five had D-dimer > 216 ng/ml

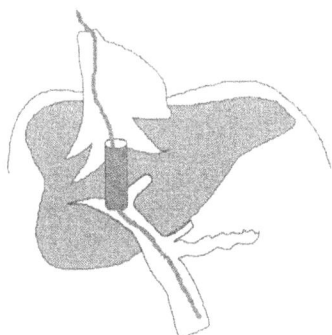

Figure 7   Insertion of TIPS

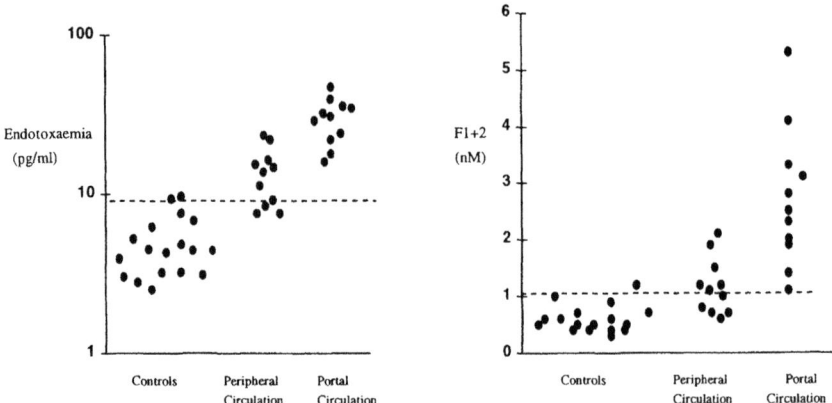

Figure 8 Endotoxaemia and F1+2 in peripheral circulation of controls and in peripheral and portal circulation of cirrhotic patients. Dashed line represents the upper limit of control values

(mean ± 2 SD of controls), and seven had endotoxaemia > 9.6 pg/ml (upper limit of control values) (Fig. 8).

Samples taken from the portal vein had significantly higher values of F1+2 [2.5 (1.1–5.3) nmol/L, $p < 0.01$], D-dimer [765 (184–1713) ng/ml, $p < 0.01$] and endotoxaemia [31 (16–47.2) pg/ml, $p < 0.01$] than those found in the peripheral circulation; fibrinogen values were lower in the portal vein but the difference was not significant [85 (58–195) mg/dl, $p > 0.05$] (Fig. 7). In the portal vein all but one sample had F1+2 > 1.2 nmol/L, all but one had D-dimer > 216 mgdl and 100% had values of endotoxaemia > 9.6 pg/ml. Portal blood showed no difference in F1+2 ($p = 0.27$) and D-dimer ($p = 0.20$) in patients with low ($n = 5$) or moderate-severe ($n = 6$) liver failure.

In the portal vein endotoxaemia was significantly correlated with F1+2 (rho = 0.92 $p = 0.006$) and D-dimer (rho = 0.93, $p = 0.005$); in peripheral circulation we obtained similar findings, since endotoxaemia was significantly correlated with F1+2 (rho = 0.91, $p = 0.004$) and D-dimer (rho = 85, $p = 0.007$). A strong significant correlation between F1+2 and D-dimer was found in portal (rho = 0.99, $p = 0.0017$) and in peripheral (rho = 0.83, $p = 0.0084$) circulation.

These data have potential clinical relevance, since they give insights into the mechanism leading to thrombotic complication in the portal circulation of cirrhotic patients. Indeed, the ongoing prothrombotic state found in the portal vein is similar to other clinical settings characterized by elevated values of F1+2 and thrombotic recurrence in the systemic circulation[89]. As clotting activation was present in almost all portal samples, future studies on larger cohorts should be performed to identify the relationship between clotting changes and the risk of portal thrombosis.

CONCLUSION

These data provide evidence that clotting activation occurs in both peripheral and portal circulation of cirrhotic patients, and might explain the concomitant presence of thrombosis and bleeding in this clinical setting. In both peripheral and portal circulation endotoxaemia was closely related to *in-vitro* thrombin generation, suggesting a role for endotoxaemia in activating the clotting system. Further study is in progress to evaluate the mechanism allowing endotoxaemia to activate the clotting system in cirrhosis.

References

1. Roberts HR, Cederbaum AI. The liver and blood coagulation: physiology and pathology. Gastroenterology. 1972;63:297–320.
2. Brozovic M. Acquired disorders of coagulation. In: Bloom AL, Thomas DP, editors: Hemostasis and thrombosis. Edinburgh: Churchill Livingstone; 1987:519–34.
3. Joist JH. Hemostatic abnormalities in liver disease. In: Colman RW, Hirsh J, Marder VJ *et al.* editors. Hemostasis and thrombosis: basic principles and clinical practice, 2nd edn. Philadelphia: Lippincott; 1987:861–72.
4. Wion KL, Kelly D, Summerfield JA, Tuddenham EGD, Lawn RM. Distribution of factor VIII mRNA and antigen in human liver and other tissues. Nature. 1985;317:726–9.
5. Leon M, Aiach M, Coezy E, Guennec JY, Fiessinger JN. Antithrombin III synthesis in rat liver parenchymal cells. Thromb Res. 1983;30:369–75.
6. Esmon CT, Esmon NL. Protein C. Semin Thromb Hemost. 1984; 10:122–30.
7. Strickland DK, Kessler CM. Biochemical and functional properties of protein C and protein S. Clin Chim Acta. 1987;170:1–23.
8. Jaffer EA, Armellino D, Tollefsen DM. Biosynthesis of functionally active heparin cofactor II by a human hepatoma-derived cell liver. Biochem Res Commun. 1985;132:368–74.
9. Tran TH, Lammle B, Zbinden B, Duckert F. Heparin cofactor II: purification and antibody production. Thromb Haemost. 1986;55:19–23.
10. Collen D, Verstraete M. Molecular biology of human plasminogen. II. Metabolism in physiological and some pathological conditions in man. Thromb Diath Haemorrh. 1975;34:403–8.
11. Saito H, Goodnough LT, Knowles BB, Aden TP. Synthesis and secretion of alpha-2-plasmin inhibitor by endothelial human liver cell lines. Proc Natl Acad Sci USA. 1982;79:5684–7.
12. Sprengers ED, Princen HMG, Koistra T, Van Hinsberg VWM. Inhibition of plasminogen activators by conditioned medium of human hepatocytes and hepatoma cell line hep. G2. J Lab Clin Med. 1985;105:751–8.
13. Sprengers ED, Kluft C. Plasminogen activator inhibitors. Blood. 1987;69:381–7.
14. Spaet TH, Horowitz HI, Franklin DZ, Cintron J, Biezensi JJ. Reticuloendothelial clearance of blood thromboplastin in rats. Blood. 1961;17:196–205.
15. Gans H, Lowman JT. The uptake of fibrin and fibrin degradation products by isolated perfused rat liver. Blood. 1967;29:526–9.
16. Deykin D, Cochios F, De Camp G. Hepatic removal of activated factor X by the perfused rat liver. Am J Physiol. 1968;214:414–19.
17. Korninger C, Stassen JM, Collen D. Turnover of human exstrinsic (tissue-type) plasminogen activator in rabbits. Thromb Hemost. 1981;46:658–61.
18. Emers JJ, Van Den Hooger CM, Jensen D. Hepatic clearance of tissue-type plasminogen activator in rats. Thromb Hemost. 1985;54:661–4.
19. Ratnoff OD. Disordered hemostasis in hepatic disease. In: Schiff L, Schiff R, editors. Disease of the liver. New York: Lippincott; 1987:187–207.
20. Ingeberg S, Jacobsen P, Fisher E, Bentsen KD. Platelet aggregation and release of ATP in patients with hepatic cirrhosis. Scand J Gastroenterol. 1985;20:285–8.
21. Marongiu F, Mamusa AM, Mameli G *et al.* Thrombocytopenia and liver cirrhosis. Evidence for relationship between platelet count, spleen size and hepatic synthetic activity. Thromb Res. 1987;45:275–8.
22. Francis RB Jr, Feinstein DI. Clinical significance of accelerated fibrinolysis in liver cirrhosis. Haemostasis. 1984;14:460–5.
23. VandeWater I, Carr JM, Aronson D, Mc Donagh J. Analysis of elevated fibrin(ogen) degradation products levels in patients with liver disease. Blood. 1986;67:1468–73.
24. Graham DY, Smith JL. The course of patients after variceal hemorrhage. Gastroenterology. 1981;80:800–9.

25. The North Italian Endoscopic Club for the Study and Treatment of Oesophageal Varices. Prediction of the first variceal hemorrhage in patients with cirrhosis of the liver and oesophageal varices. N Engl J Med. 1988;319:983–9.
26. Pinto C, Abrantes A, Esteves AV, Almeida M, Pinto Correia J. Long-term prognosis of patients with cirrhosis of the liver and upper gastrointestinal bleeding. Am J Gastroenterol. 1989;84:1234–43.
27. Lebrec D, De Fleury P, Rueff B, Nahum M, Benhamou JP. Portal hypertension, size of oesophageal varices and risk of gastrointestinal bleeding in alcoholic cirrhosis. Gastroenterology. 1980;79:1139–44.
28. Kleber G, Sauerbruch T, Ansari M, Paumgartner G. Prediction of variceal hemorrhage in cirrhosis: a prospective follow-up study. Gastroenterology. 1991;100:1332–7.
29. Lebrec D, Poynard T, Hillon P, Benhamou JP. Propranolol for prevention of recurrent gastrointestinal bleeding in patients with cirrhosis. A controlled study. N Engl J Med. 1981;305:1371–4.
30. Pascal JP, Cales P. and the Multicenter Study Group. Propranolol in the prevention of first upper gastrointestinal tract hemorrhage in patients with cirrhosis of the liver and oesophageal varices. N Engl J Med. 1987;317:856–61.
31. The Italian Multicenter Project for Propranolol in Prevention of Bleeding. Propranolol prevents first gastrointestinal bleeding in non-ascitic cirrhotic patients. Final report of a multicenter randomized trial. J Hepatol. 1989;9:75–83.
32. Heresbach D, Bretagne JF, Raoul JL et al. Pronostic et fecteurs pronostiques de l'hemorragie par rupture de varice chez le cirrhotique a l'ere de la sclerosendoscopique. Gastroenterol Clin Biol. 1991;15:838–44.
33. Bertaglia E, Belmonte P, Vertolli V, Azzurro M, Martines D. Bleeding in cirrhotic patients: a precipitating factor due to intravascular coagulation or to hepatic failure? Hemostasis. 1983;13:328–34.
34. Boks AL, Brommer EJP, Schalm SW, Van Vliet HHDM. Hemostasis and fibrinolysis in severe liver failure and their relation to hemorrhage. Hepatology. 1986;6:79–86.
35. Violi F, Ferro D, Basili S et al. Hyperfibrinolysis increases the risk of gastrointestinal hemorrhage in patients with advanced cirrhosis. Hepatology. 1992;15:672–6.
36. Carr JM. Disseminated intravascular coagulation in cirrhosis. Hepatology. 1989;10:103–10.
37. van De Water L, Carr JM, Aronson D, McDonagh J. Analysis of elevated fibrin(ogen) degradation product levels in patients with liver disease. Blood. 1986;67:1468–73.
38. Huber K, Kircheimer JC, Korninger C, Binder BR. Hepatic synthesis and clearance of components of the fibrinolytic system in healthy volunteers and in patients with different stages of liver cirrhosis. Thromb Res. 1991;62:491–500.
39. Bakker CM, Knot EAR, Stibbe J, Wilson JHP. Disseminated intravascular coagulation in liver cirrhosis. J Hepatol. 1992;15:330–5.
40. Violi F, Ferro D, Quintarelli C, Saliola M, Cordova C, Balsano F. Clotting abnormalities in chronic liver disease. Dig Dis. 1992;10:167–72.
41. Violi F, Basili S, Ferro D, Quintarelli C, Alessandri C, Cordova C, CALC group. Association between high values of D-dimer and tissue-plasminogen activator activity and first gastrointestinal bleeding in cirrhotic patients. Thromb Haemost. 1996;76:177–83.
42. Pugh RNH, Murray-Lyon IM, Dawson JL, Petroni MC, Williams R. Transection of oesophagus for bleeding oesophagus varices. Br J Surg. 1973;60:646–9.
43. Poynard T, Cales P, Pasta L et al. and the Franco-Italian Multicenter Study Group. Beta-adrenergic-antagonist drugs in the prevention of gastrointestinal bleeding in patients with cirrhosis and esophageal varices. N Engl J Med. 1991;324:1532–8.
44. Marder VJ, Sherry S. Thrombolytic therapy: current status. N Engl J Med. 1988;318:1585–95.
45. Stricker RB, Wong D, Shin DT, Reyes PT, Shiman MA. Activation of plasminogen by tissue plasminogen activator on normal and thromboasthenic platelets: effects on surface proteins and platelet aggregation. Blood. 1986;68:275–80.
46. Adelman B, Michelson AD, Greenberg J, Handin RI. Proteolysis of platelet glycoprotein Ib by plasmin is facilitated by plasmin lysine-binding regions. Blood. 1986;68:1280–4.
47. Moake JL, Olson JD, Troll JH, Tang SS, Funicella T, Peterson DM. Binding of radioiodinate human von Willebrand factor to Bernard-Soulier, thromboasthenic and von Willebrand's disease platelets. Thromb Res. 1980;19:21–7.
48. Loscalzo J, Vaughan DE. Tissue plasminogen activator promotes platelet disaggregation in plasma. J Clin Invest. 1987;79:1749–55.

49. Lasierra J, Aza MJ, Vilades E *et al.* Tissue plasminogen activator and plasminogen activator inhibitor in patients with liver cirrhosis. Fibrinolysis. 1991;5:117–20.
50. Leebeek FWG, Kluft C, Knot EAR, De Maat MPM, Wilson JHP. A shift in balance between profibrinolytic and antifibrinolytic factor causes enhanced fibrinolysis in cirrhosis. Gastroenterology. 1991;101:1382–90.
51. Hersch SL, Kunelis T, Francis RB. The pathogenesis of accelerated fibrinolysis in liver cirrhosis: a critical role for tissue plasminogen activator inhibitor. Blood. 1987;69:1315–19.
52. Violi F, Ferro D, Basili S, *et al.* and the C.A.L.C. Group. Hyperfibrinolysis resulting from clotting activation in patients with different degrees of cirrhosis. Hepatology. 1993;17:78–83.
53. Ferro D, Quintarelli C, Saliola M *et al.* Prevalence of hyperfibrinolysis in patients with liver cirrhosis. Fibrinolysis. 1993;7:59–62.
54. Nilsson T, Wallen P, Mellbring G. *In-vivo* metabolism of human tissue type plasminogen activator. Scand J Haematol. 1984;33:49–53.
55. Knot EAR, Drijfhout HR, ten Cate JW *et al.* α2 plasmin inhibitor mechanism in patients with liver cirrhosis. J Lab Clin Med. 1985;105:353–8.
56. Coleman M, Finalyson N, Bettigole RE, Sadula D, Cohn M, Pasmantin M. Fibrinogen survival in cirrhosis: improvement by 'low dose' heparin. Ann Intern Med. 1975;83:79–81.
57. Cordova C, Musca A, Violi F, Alessandri C, Vezza E. Improvement of some blood coagulation factors in cirrhotic patients treated with low doses of heparin. Scand J Haematol. 1982;29:235–40.
58. Ruegg R, Straub PW. Exchange between intravascularly and extravascularly injected radioiodinated fibrinogen and its *in-vivo* derivatives. J Lab Clin Med. 1980;95:842–56.
59. Coccheri S, Mannucci PM, Palareti G, Gervasoni W, Poggi M, Vigano S. Significance of plasma fibrinopeptide A and high molecular weight fibrinogen in patients with liver cirrhosis. Br J Haematol. 1982;52:503–9.
60. Mombelli G, Monotti R, Haeberli A, Straub PW. Relationship between fibrinopeptide A and fibrinogen/fibrin fragment E in thromboembolism, DIC, and various non-thromboembolic diseases. Thromb Haemost. 1987;58:758–63.
61. Teitel JM, Bauer KA, Lau HK, Rosemberg RD. Studies of the prothrombin activation pathway utilizing radioimmunoassay for the F2/F1+2 fragment and thrombin–antithrombin complex. Blood. 1982;59:1086–97.
62. Bruhn HD, Conard J, Mannucci PM *et al.* Multicentric evaluation of a new assay for prothrombin fragment F1+2 determination. Thromb Haemost. 1992;68:413–17.
63. Violi F, Ferro D, Quintarelli C *et al.* Systemic clotting activation in liver cirrhosis patients: the role of endotoxemia. Clin Res. 1994;42:242.
64. Violi F, Ferro D, Basili S *et al.* Association between low-grade disseminated intravascular coagulation and endotoxemia in patients with liver cirrhosis. Gastroenterology. 1995;1099:531–9.
65. Lumsden AB, Henderson JM, Kutner MH. Endotoxin levels measured by a chromogenic assay in portal, hepatic and peripheral venous blood in patients with cirrhosis. Hepatology. 1988;8:232–6.
66. Semeraro N, Biondi A, Lorenzet R, Locati D, Mantovani A, Donati MB. Direct induction of tissue factor synthesis by endotoxin in human macrophages from diverse anatomical sites. Immunology. 1983;50:529–35.
67. Moore KL, Andreoli SP, Esmon NL, Esmon CT, Bang NU. Endotoxin enhances tissue factor and suppresses thrombomodulin expression of human vascular endothelium *in vitro*. J Clin Invest. 1987;79:124–30.
68. Colucci M, Balconi G, Lorenzet R, Pietra A, Locati D. Cultured human endothelial cells generate tissue factor in response to endotoxins. J Clin Invest. 1983;71:1893–6.
69. Michie HR, Manogue KR, Spriggs DR, Roux-Lombard P, J5 Study Group, Lambert PH. Detection of circulating tumor necrosis factor after endotoxin administration. N Engl J Med. 1988;318:1481–6.
70. Van der Poll T, Buller HR, ten Cate H *et al.* Activation of coagulation after administration of tumor necrosis factor to normal subjects. N Engl J Med. 1990;322:1622–7.
71. Van Deventer SJH, Buller HR, ten Cate JW, Aarden LA, Hack CE, Sturk A. Experimental endotoxemia in humans: analysis of cytokine release and coagulation, fibrinolytic, and complement pathways. Blood. 1990;12:2520–6.
72. Ravin HA, Rowey D, Jenkins C, Fine J. On the absorption of bacterial endotoxin from the gastrointestinal tract of the normal and shocked animal. J Exp Med. 1960;112:783–92.

73. Wolter J, Liehr H, Grun M. Hepatic clearance of endotoxins: differences in arterial and portal perfusion. J Reticuloendothel Soc. 1978;3:145–52.
74. Liehr H. Endotoxins and the pathogenesis of hepatic and gastrointestinal diseases. Ergeb Inn Med Kinderheilkd. 1982;48:117–93.
75. Nolan JP. The role of endotoxin in liver injury. Gastroenterology. 1975;69:1346–56.
76. Fukui H, Brauner B, Bode JC, Bode C. Plasma endotoxin concentrations in patients with alcoholic and non-alcoholic liver disease: reevaluation with an improved chromogenic assay. J Hepatol. 1991;12:162–9.
77. Triger DR. Endotoxemia in liver disease – time for re-appraisal? J Hepatol. 1991;12:136–8.
78. Oka K, Tanaka K. Intravascular coagulation in autopsy cases with liver disease. Thromb Haemost. 1979;42:564–70.
79. Belli L, Romani F, Sansalone CV, Aseni P, Rondinara G. Portal thrombosis in cirrhotics. A retrospective analysis. Ann Surg. 1986;203:286–91.
80. Witte CL, Brewer ML, Witte MH, Pond GB. Protean manifestations of pylethrombosis. A review of thirty-four patients. Ann Surg. 1985;202:191–202.
81. Violi F, Ferro D, Basili S et al. Relation between lupus anticoagulant and splanchnic venous thrombosis in cirrhosis of the liver. Br Med J. 1994;309:239–40.
82. Violi F, Ferro D, Basili S, Levrero M, Cordova C. Venous thrombosis in hepatitis C virus liver cirrhosis. J Invest Med. 1996;43:550–4.
83. Guarner C, Soriano C, Tomas A et al. Increased serum nitrite and nitrate levels in patients with cirrhosis: relationship to endotoxemia. Hepatology. 1993;18:1139–43.
84. Lumsden AB, Henderson JM, Kutner MH. Endotoxin levels measured by a chromogenic assay in portal, hepatic and peripheral blood in patients with cirrhosis. Hepatology. 1988;8:232–6.
85. Van Deventer SJH, Buller HR, Ten Cate JW, Aarden LA, Hack Ce, Sturk A. Experimental endotoxemia in human: analysis of cytokine release and coagulation fibrinolytic and complement pathways. Blood. 1990;12:2520–6.
86. Violi F, Ferro D, Basili S et al. Ongoing prothrombotic state in the portal circulation of cirrhotic patients. Thomb Haemost. 1997;77:44–7.
87. Rössle M, Haag K, Ochs A et al. The transjugular intrahepatic portosystemic stent–shunt procedure for variceal bleeding. N Engl J Med. 1994;330:165–71.
88. Ochs A, Rössle M, Haag K et al. The transjugular intrahepatic portosystemic stent–shunt procedure for refractory ascites. N Engl J Med. 1995;332:1192–7.
89. Bauer KA, Rosemberg RD. The pathogenesis of the prethrombotic state in humans: insights from studies using markers of hemostatic system activation. Blood. 1987;70:343–50.

21
The role of gut-derived bacterial toxins (endotoxin) for the development of alcoholic liver disease in man

Ch. BODE, C. SCHÄFER and J. Ch. BODE

GUT-DERIVED BACTERIAL TOXINS AND LIVER INJURY – IMPORTANT EARLIER FINDINGS

Evidence that intestinal bacteria might contribute to acute and chronic experimental hepatic injury was already published four decades ago.

In 1954 it was shown that antibiotic suppression of intestinal flora with neomycin and aureomycin effectively prevented hepatic damage in rats fed a choline-deficient diet[1]. Other authors found that long-term administration of a non-absorbable antibiotic significantly delayed the development of liver fibrosis in rats receiving a cirrhogenic diet[2]. The assumption that endotoxin (= lipopolysaccharide, LPS) of Gram-negative bacteria is of pivotal importance was confirmed in a crucial study by Broitman et al.[3]. These authors demonstrated that the protective effect of oral neomycin administration against the development of dietary cirrhosis in rats is completely abolished by feeding purified LPS (1–4 mg/kg) together with the choline-deficient diet. Furthermore, polymyxin B, which has unique anti-endotoxin properties, was shown[4] to prevent markedly hepatic necrosis in rats treated with sublethal doses of CCl_4.

Details on the rapidly increasing knowledge of functional disturbances and morphological alterations in the liver caused by LPS have been summarized in several extensive reviews[5–7]. Until the late 1970s endotoxemia was detected in the peripheral venous blood of patients with cirrhosis in a number of studies. However, the observed frequency of endotoxaemia in cirrhotics varied greatly, and some authors even questioned its existence. More reliable results were obtained when an endotoxin assay was developed using a synthetic chromogenic peptide as substrate[8]. This assay was more sensitive than the previous gelation assay, and provided quantitative measurement of endotoxin[9,10].

In addition to the experimental studies mentioned above, a number of clinical findings suggest that enhanced uptake of LPS from the gut might play a role in the development and progression of alcohol-induced liver disease. First, marked leucocytosis is frequently observed in patients with alcoholic hepatitis without evidence of bacterial infections. Second, 30–40% of patients with alcoholic hepatitis have fever of otherwise unexplained causes. Third, the histology of alcoholic hepatitis is characterized by an infiltrate of mainly neutrophil polymorphs. Furthermore, in alcoholics who had been drinking shortly before, upper gastrointestinal endoscopy frequently revealed signs of mucosal damage such as erosions and haemorrhage in the stomach and in the upper duodenum, which might facilitate the translocation of LPS and other bacterial toxins from the lumen to the portal blood.

ALCOHOL-INDUCED MUCOSAL INJURY IN THE UPPER GASTROINTESTINAL TRACT

Gastric mucosa

Alcoholic beverages have repeatedly been shown to be an important cause of haemorrhagic erosive gastric lesions in humans[11,12]. No relation seems to exist between the subepithelial haemorrhages in alcoholics and the presence of *Helicobacter pylori*[13]. Administration of alcohol solutions of 20% or more also leads to severe haemorrhage and erosions of gastric mucosa in animal experiments[11]. Several mechanisms may contribute to the development of these mucosal injuries. Alcohol in concentrations of 15% and more disrupts the gastric mucosal barrier in various animal species and in humans, thereby increasing hydrogen, sodium and potassium ion fluxes[14]. The results of a number of studies support the hypothesis that decreased prostaglandin formation might play a role in the mucosal injury induced by alcohol[15,16]. From the results of other studies it was assumed that increased leukotriene production might contribute to the development of alcohol-induced mucosal injury[14,17].

Mucosa in the small intestine

In experimental animals, administration of alcoholic solutions at concentrations corresponding to those of commonly available alcoholic beverages leads to damage of the mucosa of the upper small intestine that extends to pronounced exfoliation of the tips of the villi and haemorrhage[11,18]. The exact pathomechanism of these mucosal injuries has not yet been clarified. The results of earlier studies led to the assumption that alcohol has a direct toxic effect on the integrity of the mucosal epithelium[11,19]. On the basis of very elegant studies in dogs, other authors have proposed an indirect effect via alterations in the mucosal microcirculation that leads to enhanced transcapillary fluid infiltration and subsequent rupture of the epithelial lining or a combination of these two events[20]. In subsequent studies the same authors provided evidence supporting the hypothesis that the mechanism of the injury to the intestinal mucosa by alcoholic beverages may be the induction of villous contraction that leads to villous-tip bleb formation, lymphatic obstruction, and finally to exfoliation of the tips of the villi when the blebs rupture[21]. On the basis of additional experiments it was suggested that the initial event in response to alcohol is the release of noxious mediators such as histamine[22] and leukotrienes[23], which cause microvascular injury. The observation that marked duodenal erythema with subepithelial bleeding developed following a single large oral dose of alcohol to volunteers supports the assumption that similar mucosal injury occurs in humans[24].

INCREASED GUT PERMEABILITY TO MACROMOLECULES

The mucosal barrier in normal mammals is incomplete so that small amounts of macromolecules may pass through the mucosa of the small intestine[25]. For example, the escape of minute amounts of LPS from the luminal side across the normal mucosa into the portal vein and intestinal lymphatics has been shown to occur in animal experiments[6].

In experimental animals acute and chronic administration of alcohol results in an increased intestinal permeability to macromolecules, such as haemoglobin, horseradish peroxidase, polyvinyl pyrolidone[11], polyethylene glycol (PEG) 1.5 kDa[26] and ^{51}Cr-labelled EDTA[27]. Increased intestinal permeability to macromolecules has also been observed in alcoholic patients without liver cirrhosis when ^{51}Cr-labelled EDTA was used as the permeability probe[28]. This increased intestinal permeability in alcoholics without cirrhosis was recently confirmed for larger molecules, such as PEG 4 kDa and 10 kDa[29]. No significant changes of intestinal permeability in chronic alcoholics were observed when smaller molecules, such as lactulose and mannitol[30] or PEG 0.4 kDa[29] were used.

The enhanced permeability of the intestinal mucosa to macromolecules following acute or chronic alcohol ingestion could result in the absorption of toxic compounds such as endotoxin and other bacterial toxins which would not normally be absorbed, and which might play a role in the development of alcohol-related damage to the liver and other organs. This assumption is supported by the observation of endotoxaemia in patients with early forms of alcohol-related liver damage, such as fatty liver[31], or the transient endotoxaemia observed following acute alcohol consumption in subjects with no evidence of alcoholic liver disease[32].

BACTERIAL OVERGROWTH IN ALCOHOLICS

Marked qualitative and quantitative changes have been observed in the microflora in the jejunum of recently imbibing chronic alcoholics[33]. The most significant finding was the increase in the number of facultative and obligate anaerobic bacteria and the total number of bacteria per unit volume of jejunal juice (Table 1). Similar changes in the bacterial flora have recently been reported in samples of duodenal juice of alcoholics[34]. Evidence of an increased incidence of bacterial overgrowth in alcoholics also stems from studies using the H_2-breath test after ingestion of lactulose[35] or glucose[36]. Bacterial overgrowth in the small intestine might lead to an increased production of endotoxin and other bacterial

Table 1 Incidence of low numbers ($< 10^2$/ml) and markedly enhanced numbers of colony-forming units (CFU) in jejunal juice obtained from patients with alcoholic liver disease (ALD) and controls under anaerobic and aerobic conditions (data from ref. 33) (percentages)

Type of bacteria	No. of CFU/ml				p
	Controls (n = 13)		Alcoholics (n = 25)		
	$< 10^2$	$> 10^5$	$< 10^2$	$> 10^5$	
Anaerobes	46.2	7.6	0	48.1	< 0.001
Aerobes	46.2	23	11.1	40.8	< 0.025

toxins, which can more readily pass through the mucosa as a result of the alcohol-induced mucosal damage.

ENDOTOXAEMIA IN PATENTS WITH ALCOHOLIC LIVER DISEASE

Endotoxaemia in patients with alcoholic and non-alcoholic cirrhosis

Using a qualitative *Limulus* gelation test, endotoxaemia was detected in the peripheral venous blood of patients with cirrhosis in a number of studies, irrespective of the aetiology of the underlying liver disease[5,6,31]. However, the observed frequency of endotoxaemia in these patients varied distinctly. When an endotoxin assay using a synthetic chromogenic peptide as substrate was developed, LPS determination in plasma became more sensitive, and the test provided quantitative measurement of LPS[8–10]. However, even in studies in which this new test was used to determine LPS concentrations in the plasma of patients with cirrhosis, the results obtained varied considerably[36,37,38]. In the latter studies the results were evaluated with no consideration given to the aetiology of cirrhosis. When the aetiology of the liver disease was taken into account, endotoxaemia was found in a significantly higher percentage of patients with alcoholic cirrhosis than in patients with non-alcoholic cirrhosis[32]. In a study with an improved chromogenic substrate assay using individual standard curves for each plasma sample[10], the mean LPS concentration was significantly higher in patients with alcoholic cirrhosis than in patients with non-alcoholic cirrhosis[31].

Endotoxaemia in alcoholics without advanced liver disease

Endotoxaemia in patients with liver cirrhosis is assumed to mainly reflect impairment of hepatic clearance of LPS caused by intra- and extrahepatic portosystemic shunts and functional defects in the phagocytic capacity of the hepatic reticuloendothelial system (RES) due to the advanced stage of the liver disease[5,7]. The endotoxaemia is more a consequence of the advanced chronic liver disease than a causative factor. Regarding the potential role of LPS for the development and progression of alcoholic liver disease, the occurrence of endotoxaemia in the initial stages might be of more relevance.

When LPS concentration was determined with an improved chromogenic substrate assay, markedly elevated LPS concentrations were already seen in patients

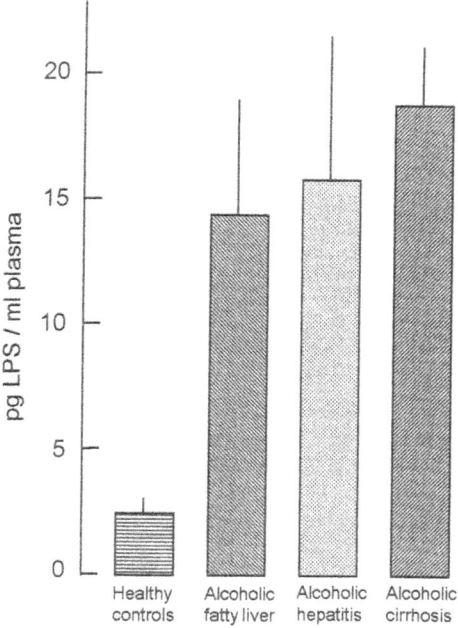

Figure 1 Plasma endotoxin concentrations in patients with early stages of alcoholic liver disease and alcoholic cirrhosis compared to those obtained in healthy controls. Mean values ± SEM. (From ref. 30, with permission of the publisher)

with fatty liver who had had a high consumption of alcohol right up to the time of admission (Fig. 1)[31]. Similar results were obtained in patients with mild forms of alcoholic hepatitis (Fig. 1). Endotoxaemia was reversible in the majority of the patients with alcoholic fatty liver within 6–8 days following cessation of alcohol intake[31]. In addition, transient endotoxaemia was found in non-alcoholic subjects following acute alcohol intoxication[32]. Since in the latter subjects, and in patients with alcoholic fatty liver, portosystemic shunting is unlikely to be involved in the occurrence of endotoxaemia, the transient increase in LPS concentration might be the result of an enhanced uptake of LPS from the intestinal tract and/or of an inhibition of the RES.

Binding of LPS to plasma factors and LPS inactivation

Endotoxin clearance by Kupffer cells

The Kupffer cells form the main protective barrier between the portal blood and the systemic circulation by removing LPS from the blood[6,39]. The uptake of LPS by Kupffer cells is assumed to occur by absorptive pinocytosis[40]. After internalisation of LPS into Kupffer cells LPS is modified in such a way that detoxification occurs[41]. Alcohol ingestion has been shown to lead to depression in Kupffer cell clearance of gut-derived LPS[6]. Impairment of phagocytic activity of Kupffer cells has also been demonstrated in chronic alcoholics[40,42].

LPS binding by plasma factors and blood cells

In addition to the uptake of LPS by Kupffer cells and other macrophages, the body has a further effective system for the neutralization of LPS, by binding of LPS to various plasma proteins which are rapidly produced in increased amounts during the 'acute-phase response' to endotoxaemia. Proteins assumed to be of importance for the binding of LPS are high-density lipoprotein (HDL) cholesterol, albumin and transferrin[43]. The assumption that plasma contains a considerable portion of 'bound' LPS was confirmed by a study on plasma LPS in patients with alcoholic liver disease and healthy subjects[43]. When plasma samples of patients with various stages of alcoholic liver disease were studied after treatment with a detergent (Tween 80) or with a solvent for LPS (tri-ethanolamine), the 'hidden' LPS concentrations were shown to be about 2–4-fold higher than the LPS concentrations found by the standard LPS assay (Fig. 2)[43]. Of special interest is the finding that, even in patients with early stages of alcoholic liver disease (ALD), such as fatty liver and mild alcoholic hepatitis, the concentration of 'hidden' LPS was 6–10-fold higher than in healthy controls (Fig. 2). When using these methods the LPS concentrations in patients with alcoholic liver disease revealed a significant negative correlation with the con-

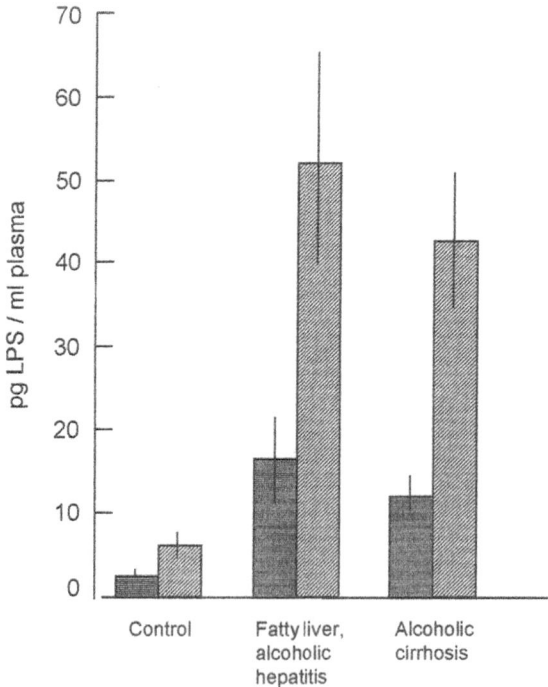

Figure 2 Plasma endotoxin concentrations in healthy controls and in patients with different stages of alcoholic liver disease. Comparison of the results obtained using a standard method (⊟) and a method using acid precipation and dissolution with triethanolamine (= 'hidden' endotoxin; ☒). Mean values ± SEM. (Slightly modified from ref. 42, with permission of the publisher)

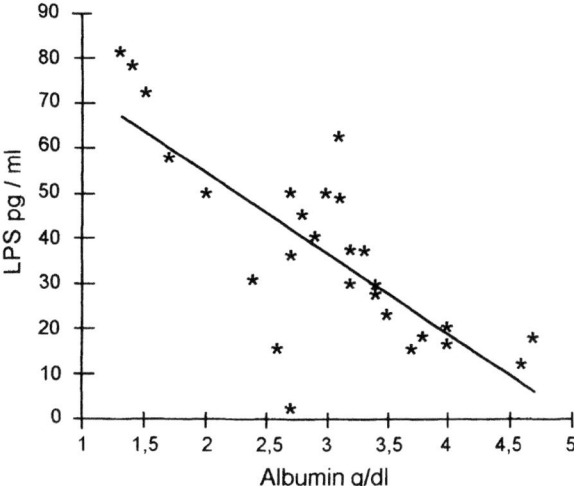

Figure 3 Negative correlation between plasma endotoxin concentrations and concentrations of albumin in patients with alcoholic liver disease, $r = -0.76$, $p < 0.01$. (From ref. 42, with permission of the publisher)

centrations for HDL cholesterol, transferrin and albumin (Fig. 3)[43]. In a more recent study the overall LPS binding capacity of whole blood was markedly diminished not only in patients with alcoholic cirrhosis, but also in patients with alcoholic hepatitis without cirrhosis[44]. From these findings it was suggested that reduced LPS binding capacity may enhance the adverse effects of endotoxaemia.

Gut-derived endotoxin in experimental alcohol-induced liver injury

More direct evidence supporting the hypothesis that gut-derived bacterial toxins are involved in the pathomechanism of alcohol-induced liver injury stems from animal experiments. In a study using the animal model established by Tsukamoto and French[45], plasma levels of LPS increased in rats fed alcohol, and the levels correlated well with the pathology scores of liver injury[17]. The hypothesis that endotoxaemia is a major cause of alcoholic liver injury was further supported by a study in which blocking LPS production by intestinal sterilization using antibiotics prevented alcohol-induced liver injury in rats on the Tsukamoto–French protocol[46].

BINDING OF LPS TO MONOCYTES/MACROPHAGES

A key event regarding the biological actions of LPS is its binding to the cell membrane. The most important receptor shown to bind LPS, and to be involved in LPS-induced cell activation, is CD14[47]. CD14 has been shown to exist in two forms. The first is extracellular, membrane-associated CD14 (mCD14) which is anchored in the membrane of myeloid cells as a glycerophosphatidylinositol tailed protein. This 55 kDa glycoprotein is strongly expressed on monocytes and macrophages and weakly on neutrophils[48]. Binding of LPS to mCD14 and activation of cells is strongly facilitated by LPS binding protein (LBP)[49]. The binding of LPS–LBP complex to mCD14 is essential for the activation of myeloid cells by low concentrations of LPS (pg/ml to ng/ml range)[50,51]. The latter concentrations correspond to those which have been found in patients with alcoholic liver disease[31]. The second form of CD14 is soluble CD14 (sCD14). Soluble CD14 might compete with mCD14 for LPS-binding, thereby negatively modulating the activation of monocytes/macrophages by LPS[52]. Soluble CD14 is required for binding of LPS to endothelial (and epithelial) cells and to activate these cells[52]. Again, LBP is important to form LPS–sCD14 complexes which bind on specific LPS–sCD14 receptors on endothelial cells[52]. LBP is a 60 kDa serum glycoprotein which is formed by hepatocytes as an acute-phase reactant[50]. Complexation of LPS with LBP occurs via the lipid A moiety.

In patients with alcoholic liver disease, LBP levels were shown to be markedly elevated[53]. A 2–3-fold increase in serum LBP concentrations was already observed in patients with early forms of alcoholic liver disease without cirrhosis. A significant increase compared to non-alcoholic controls was also observed for sCD14 concentration in plasma of patients who had been drinking shortly before, with alcoholic fatty liver or alcoholic hepatitis[53].

Bactericidal/permeability-increasing protein (BPI) is a protein with strong homology to LBP[50]. BPI binds to LPS with high affinity and was shown to inhibit effects of LPS, such as tumour necrosis factor-alpha (TNF-α) production and LPS-induced priming of neutrophils in *in-vitro* experiments[54]. The concentration of BPI, which also has strong bactericidal capacity[54], was found to be increased in plasma of patients with alcoholic liver disease[53].

ENDOTOXAEMIA AND FACTORS INFLUENCING THE BIOLOGICAL ACTIVITY OF LPS – SUMMARY OF RESULTS IN PATIENTS WITH EARLY STAGES OF ALCOHOLIC LIVER DISEASE

As already outlined in the preceding sections, the occurrence of endotoxaemia in the initial stages of alcoholic liver disease, and its biological effects, are of special interest with respect to the primordial pathomechanism that leads to the onset of alcoholic hepatitis and its progression to fibrosis and cirrhosis. The main findings concerning endotoxaemia, and factors that may influence the biological activity of LPS in patients with early stages of alcoholic liver disease, are summarized in Table 2. Marked endotoxaemia is found in actively drinking alcoholics with fatty liver or mild to moderately severe alcoholic hepatitis. Both the 'free' LPS in plasma and the 'bound' fraction of plasma LPS are distinctly elevated[43]. Endotoxaemia is reversible in most of these patients within 1–2 weeks of abstinence. In addition to a depression in the clearance of gut-derived LPS by macrophages following alcohol ingestion[6,18] (not shown in Table 2) the LPS-binding capacity in the blood is already reduced in patients with alcoholic hepatitis without cirrhosis[44]. In contrast to the decrease in the capacity to eliminate or neutralize LPS, those plasma factors which are essential for activation of macrophages and other cells by LPS, such as LPS-binding protein (LBP) and

Table 2 Endotoxaemia and factors influencing the biological activity of LPS in patients with early stages of alcoholic liver disease. Summary of data presented in the text

Parameter	Alcoholic fatty liver	Alcoholic hepatitis without cirrhosis
LPS concentration in plasma		
'free' LPS	↑↑	↑↑
'bound' (= 'hidden') LPS	↑↑↑↑	↑↑↑↑
Decrease of LPS concentration to control levels within 1 week of abstinence	Most cases	About 50% of cases
LPS binding capacity in whole blood	No change	↓↓
LPS-binding protein (LBP) concentration	↑↑	↑↑
Soluble CD14 (sCD14) concentration	↑	↑

soluble CD14 (sCD14) are significantly enhanced in patients with early stages of alcoholic liver disease[53]. Together with the results obtained in animal experiments[1-6,45-47] the data summarized in Table 2 strongly support the assumption that LPS does play a significant role in the initiation and progression of alcoholic hepatitis in humans.

LPS-INDUCED RELEASE OF CYTOKINES AND OTHER MEDIATORS FROM MACROPHAGES/MONOCYTES IN ALCOHOLIC LIVER DISEASE

In the past decade there has been an explosion of information regarding the direct and indirect effects of LPS on the cells of the specific and unspecific immune system. Macrophages/monocytes are assumed to play a central role in the mediation of the physiological effects of LPS[55,56]. Some of the more important mediators which are produced by these cells in response to LPS are summarized in Fig. 4. Exaggerated production of mediators, such as TNF-α, interleukin-1 (IL-1) and oxygen radicals may cause microvascular injury, disseminated intravascular coagulation and other deleterious manifestations which finally lead to organ injury[7,55]. TNF-α and IL-1 are mediators of the acute-phase response which includes fever, neutropenia followed by leucocytosis with neutrophilia and an increase in acute-phase proteins. In addition to stimulation of mediator release, LPS leads to numerous other events. LPS activates complement through both the alternative pathway and the classical pathway, the proteolytic cascade and coagulation pathways[56]. Furthermore, at the cellular level, LPS affects the function of T lymphocytes, B lymphocytes, polymorphonuclear neutrophils, platelets and endothelial cells[55,56]. Despite the tremendous progress in our knowledge of the physiological, biochemical, cell biological, and molecular biological properties and actions of cytokines and other mediators in recent years, it has to be stressed that our understanding of the pathophysiological relevance of changes in the production or concentrations of single cytokines or other mediators for diseases in humans is incomplete. The manifold, multifunctional cytokines act together as a complex biological regulatory system. The single

289

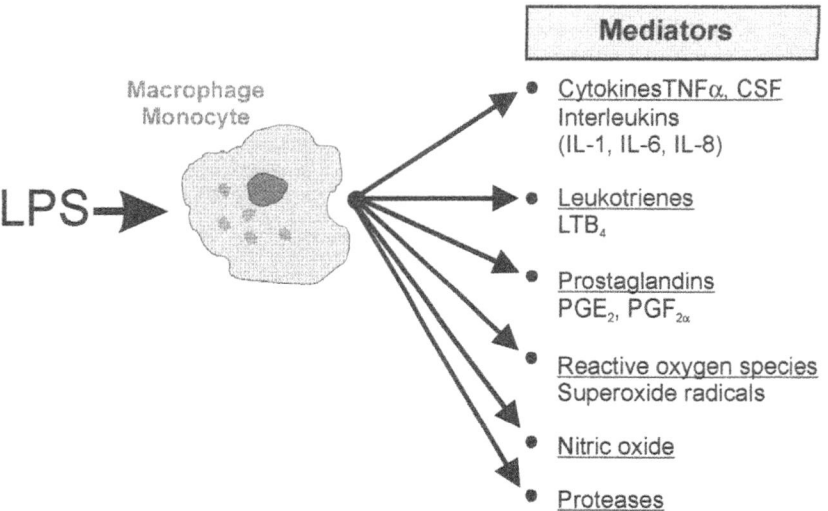

Figure 4 Schematic representation of the effects of LPS on mediator release from monocytes/macrophages

parts of this system can react synergistically or antagonistically, or may be functionally redundant. Some factors which influence the effects of a specific cytokine are summarize in Table 3. They emphasize that the production and the physiological or pathophysiological effects of single cytokines depend on numerous factors of the complicated network of cytokines[57,58]. This fact must be considered when interpreting the results of new studies on the meaning of cytokines for the pathogenesis of alcoholic liver disease reviewed in the following sections. The discussion deals almost exclusively with the results of clinical studies. Further discussion of the numerous studies on this topic, involving experiments with animals, can be found in other chapters of this book and in other works that give a general overview[59,60].

A common drawback in studies in human subjects is the inability to gain access to portal venous blood or sufficient amounts of liver tissue for direct investigation of the intrahepatic cytokine crosstalk between parenchymal and non-parenchymal cells, and its relation to the LPS influx from the intestine. Therefore, information regarding cytokines in patients with alcoholic liver disease stems from an indirect approach by testing peripheral blood monocytes and plasma. Although the implications that can be drawn from studies using this

Table 3 Factors which influence the effects of a specific cytokine

Local concentration of the cytokine affected by formation/release/inactivation
Expression of receptors on the surface of the target cells
Presence of receptor antagonists
Pattern of other cytokines and additional mediators
Differences in coupling to intracellular signal transduction pathways in different cell types

more indirect approach are limited, they may provide some information regarding the role of cytokines, together with endotoxaemia, in the pathogenesis of alcoholic liver disease.

Serum/plasma levels of cytokines

In patients with severe forms of alcoholic hepatitis, with or without cirrhosis, plasma concentrations of *TNF-α, IL-1 and IL-6* were found to be elevated[61,62]. In another study in patients with severe alcoholic hepatitis, increased plasma levels of TNF-α but not increased IL-1 was found to be correlated with decreased long-term survival[63]. However, significantly elevated serum levels of TNF-α, IL-1 and IL-6 were also found in patients with chronic liver disease of other aetiology, such as chronic hepatitis B and C, autoimmune hepatitis, primary biliary cirrhosis and haemochromatosis[64]. The levels of the three cytokines were significantly higher in cirrhotics than in non-cirrhotics. The authors concluded from their results that enhanced serum levels of proinflammatory cytokines represent a consequence of liver dysfunction independent of the aetiology of the underlying chronic liver disease[64]. The significance of elevated plasma levels of TNF-α and IL-1 with respect to a possible role of these cytokines in the pathogenesis of alcoholic liver disease, which has repeatedly been discussed[59,61,62], remains doubtful at least as long as measurements are performed only in patients with advanced stages of alcoholic liver disease. In a recent study in patients with different stages of alcoholic liver disease, plasma TNF-α was found to be elevated only in patients with alcoholic cirrhosis, while the plasma concentration of this cytokine in actively drinking patients with non-cirrhotic liver disease was not significantly increased[65]. It was suggested that elevated *TNF plasma levels* are not associated with the primordial pathomechanism that induces the damaging process at the onset of alcoholic liver disease. However, in a second study in a larger group of alcoholics, significantly elevated plasma levels of TNF-α and IL-6 were also found in patients with fatty liver or alcoholic hepatitis[66]. The increased levels of these cytokines were associated with enhanced plasma LPS concentrations in the same patients.

Recently increased serum concentrations of soluble tumour necrosis factor receptor type I (sTNFR) have been observed in serum of patients with alcoholic cirrhosis[67]. sTNFR has been shown to inhibit or antagonize the function of TNF-α[68]. High levels of sTNFR-I in patients with alcoholic cirrhosis may reflect a response to the enhanced levels of TNF-α in this disease[61,62] and add to the difficulty of assessing the pathophysiological role of increased plasma TNF-α concentrations in this disease.

Interleukin-8 (IL-8)

This neutrophil chemotaxin, secreted by monocytes, macrophages and Kupffer cells[69], has also been incriminated in mediating hepatic neutrophil infiltration and hepatic injury induced by alcohol[70]. Increased plasma IL-8 concentrations in patients with alcoholic hepatitis have recently been demonstrated[70–72]. As opposed to the conflicting findings regarding the plasma levels of TNF-α, IL-1 and IL-6, mentioned above, distinctly increased plasma levels of IL-8 were found in patients with alcoholic hepatitis without cirrhosis, and even in patients with alcoholic fatty liver[72]. Furthermore, the serum IL-8 concentrations were closely correlated with the histological score for alcoholic hepatitis and aspartate transaminase (AST) values[72]. It was suggested that the increased production of IL-8 in alcoholic liver disease is probably mediated by LPS, but LPS plasma levels were not determined in these studies.

Cytokine release of peripheral blood monocytes

Several studies emphasize the pivotal role of macrophages and mediators released from macrophages (e.g. TNF-α, IL-1, IL-6) in multiple types of experimental liver diseases[58,73,74], including the type of alcohol-induced liver injury observed in rats and other animal species[45,58,75]. However, the form of progressive alcoholic liver disease typically observed in humans, especially alcoholic hepatitis[76], cannot be reproduced in experimental animals. The only exception is a model of alcoholic liver disease in the baboon[77].

Because of the manifold shortcomings of all experimental models of alcoholic liver injury in non-primate animals, only limited conclusions can be drawn from results obtained in such animal experiments regarding their relevance for the pathophysiology of alcoholic liver disease in humans. Therefore, it would be important to evaluate whether enhanced release of cytokines and other mediators from macrophages does occur in patients with alcoholic liver disease, especially in early stages of alcoholic hepatitis, and whether this enhanced mediator release is associated with endotoxaemia. The lack of access to sufficient amounts of human liver tissue does not allow a direct approach to the study of this topic. An indirect way of obtaining information about changes in the function of the monocyte/macrophage system is to study the cytokine release in isolated circulating monocytes.

Very little information is available regarding the *spontaneous release* of cytokines from peripheral monocytes in alcoholic liver disease patients. In one study, circulating monocytes obtained from patients with severe alcoholic hepatitis were shown to be more likely to exhibit spontaneous release of TNF-α during *in-vitro* culture than monocytes from controls[78]. The reliability of the results was questioned, since the incubation medium in the latter experiments contained commercial lots of fetal calf serum which has been found to contain varying quantities of LPS[79]. In fact, no release of bioactive TNF-α from isolated monocytes from patients with alcoholic hepatitis or alcoholic cirrhosis was observed when LPS-free fetal calf serum was used in another study[65].

In-vitro investigation of *LPS-stimulated monocytes* from patients with severe alcoholic hepatitis or alcoholic cirrhosis has shown both the elevated[78,80] and depressed[81] release of TNF-α and the depressed release of IL-1[81]. In all three studies very high concentrations of the LPS stimulus, far above the relevant range found in patients with alcoholic hepatitis and cirrhosis[30,65], were used. This, apart from differences in patient selection, may be responsible for the contradictory findings. In a more recent study by our group, using markedly lower LPS concentrations for stimulation, a significantly enhanced release of bioactive TNF-α was observed from monocytes of actively drinking alcoholics with various stages of liver disease[65]. The secretion of TNF-α was dependent on the dose of stimulatory LPS (Fig. 5) and the duration of the stimulation period[65].

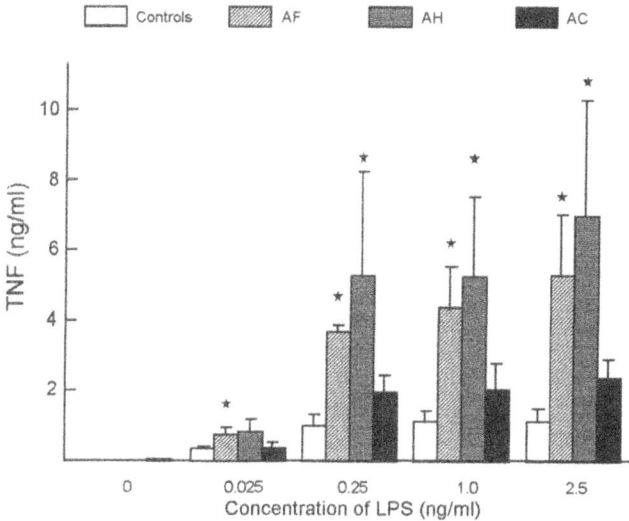

Figure 5   Release of bioactive TNF-α from isolated monocytes stimulated with various amounts of LPS over 3 h. Mean values ± SEM. AF = alcoholic fatty liver, AH = alcoholic hepatitis, AC = alcoholic cirrhosis. * = $p < 0.05$ vs controls. (From ref. 65, with permission of the publisher)

In the groups with alcoholic fatty liver and alcoholic hepatitis the TNF-α response was 3–4 times as high as in the control group. In patients with alcoholic cirrhosis the TNF-α response was less pronounced in up to 3 h of stimulation (Fig. 5) but was similar after prolonged incubation[65]. After 1 week of abstinence from alcohol the TNF-α secretion from monocytes of the same patients decreased by approximately 50–60% in the groups with fatty liver or alcoholic hepatitis, while no decrease was observed in the patients with alcoholic cirrhosis[65]. In the same study a significant increase in IL-6 release was observed in monocytes from patients with alcoholic fatty liver[65]. Increased production of IL-6 has also been reported in monocytes of patients suffering from alcoholic cirrhosis[82]. Taken together these findings seem to indicate the presence in early alcoholic liver disease of some degree of *in-vivo* activation of monocytes in a manner which potentiates the production of cytokines, such as TNF-α and IL-6. In addition to the induction of the changes that have been referred to as the acute-phase response[55], the increased production of TNF-α may contribute to the up-regulation of the CD95 receptor and/or ligand which has been reported in patients with alcoholic liver disease, thereby favouring apoptosis of hepatocytes[83].

CONCLUSIONS

The findings reviewed in the preceding sections lend strong support to the hypothesis which our group proposed for the first time 15 years ago[84]. We stated that alcohol-induced changes in the gut, and their consequences, may play an important role in the pathophysiology of alcoholic liver disease in humans. The main sequence of events is schematically sketched in Fig. 6:

1. Abuse of alcoholic beverages leads to mucosal damage in the upper gastro-intestinal tract extending to erosions in the stomach and duodenum, and to exfoliations of the tips of the villi in the upper jejunum.
2. The mucosal defects favour an increase in the permeability of the mucosa for macromolecules, such as endotoxin and other bacterial toxins.
3. In a high percentage of alcohol abusers bacterial overgrowth in the small intestine with faecal flora increases the production of endotoxin and other toxins.
4. The resulting enhanced translocation of LPS from the gut to the portal blood and/or the lymphatics leads to endotoxaemia. The occurrence of endotox-aemia is favoured by the inhibitory effect of alcohol on the phagocytic function of Kupffer cells and other macrophages.
5. Stimulation of monocytes/macrophages by gut-derived LPS results in an increased release of potentially toxic mediators such as TNF-α, IL-1, IL-6 and reactive oxygen species.
6. The chronic overproduction of such mediators may induce neutrophil activ-ation, endothelial lesions, increased permeability of sinusoids/capillaries, disturbed microcirculation and a multitude of other injurious events which

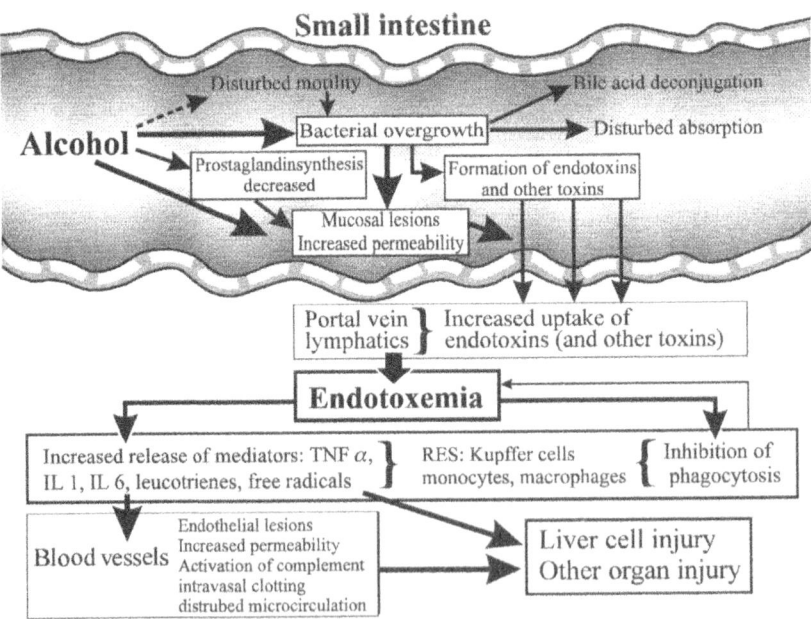

Figure 6 Schematic representation of the possible causes and consequences of changes induced by alcohol abuse in the intestine, the resulting endotoxaemia and the effects of endotoxaemia on mono-cytes/macrophages which may contribute to alcoholic liver disease and other organ injury. (Modified from ref. 14, with permission of the publisher)

lead to cellular damage extending to hepatocyte necrosis, inflammatory infiltrates of neutrophils and deposition of collagen.

Acknowledgements

The original work presented in this article was supported by the Deutsche Forschungs-gemeinschaft (DFG), Grants Scha 530/1-1 and Scha 530/1-3, and by the Robert-Bosch-Stiftung

References

1. György P. Antibiotics and liver injury. Ann NY Acad Sci. 1954;57:925–30.
2. Rutenberg AM, Sonnenblick E, Koven I. The role of intestinal bacteria in the development of dietary cirrhosis in rats. J Exp Med. 1957;106:1–6.
3. Broitman SA, Gottlieb LS, Zamcheck N. Influence of neomycin and ingested endotoxin in the pathogenesis of choline deficiency cirrhosis in the adult rat. J Exp Med. 1964;119:633–40.
4. Nolan JP, Leibowitz AI. Endotoxin and the liver. III. Modification of acute carbon tetrachloride injury by polymyxin b – an antiendotoxin. Gastroenterology. 1978;75:445–9.
5. Liehr H. Endotoxins and the pathogenesis of hepatic and gastrointestinal diseases. Ergeb Inn Med Kinderheilkd. 1982;48:117–93.
6. Nolan JP. Intestinal endotoxins as mediators of hepatic injury – an idea whose time has come again. Hepatology. 1989;10:887–891.
7. Hewett JA, Roth RA. Hepatic and extrahepatic pathobiology of bacterial lipopolysaccharides. Pharmacol Rev. 1993;45:382–411.
8. Iwanaga S, Morita T, Harada T et al. Chromogenic substrates for horseshoe crab clotting enzyme. Its application for the assay of bacterial endotoxins. Haemostasis. 1978;7:183–8.
9. Sturk A, Joop K, ten Cate JW, Thomas LL. Optimalization of a chromogenic assay for endotoxin in blood. Prog Clin Biol Res. 1985;189:117–37.
10. Fukui H, Brauner B, Bode JC, Bode C. Chromogenic endotoxin assay in plasma. Selection of plasma pretreatment and production of standard curves. J Clin Chem Clin Biochem. 1989;27:941–6.
11. Bode JC. Alcohol and the gastrointestinal tract. Ergeb Inn Med Kinderheilkd. 1980;45:1–75.
12. Laine L, Weinstein WM. Histology of alcoholic hemorrhagic 'gastritis': a prospective evaluation. Gastroenterology. 1988;94:1254–62.
13. Laine L, Marin Sorensen M, Weinstein WM. Campylobacter pylori in alcoholic hemorrhagic 'gastritis'. Dig Dis Sci. 1989;34:677–80.
14. Bode JC, Bode C. Alcohol malnutrition and the gastrointestinal tract. In: Watson RR, Watzl B, editors. Nutrition and alcohol. London: CRC Press; 1992:403–28.
15. Bode C, Ito T, Rollenhagen A, Bode JC. Effect of acute and chronic alcohol feeding on prostaglandin E2 biosynthesis in rat stomach. Dig Dis Sci. 1988;33:814–18.
16. Bode C, Maute G, Bode JC. Prostaglandin E2 and prostaglandin F2a biosynthesis in human gastric mucosa: effect of chronic alcohol misuse. Gut. 1996;39:348–52.
17. Nanji AA, Khettry U, Sadrzadeh SM, Yamanaka T. Severity of liver injury in experimental alcoholic liver disease. Correlation with plasma endotoxin, prostaglandin E2, leukotriene B4, and thromboxane B2. Am J Pathol. 1993;142:367–73.
18. Persson J. Alcohol and the small intestine. Scand J Gastroenterol. 1991;26:3–15.
19. Hunter CK, Treanor LL, Gray JP, Halter SA, Hoyumpa AJ, Wilson FA. Effects of ethanol in vitro on rat intestinal brush-border membranes. Biochim Biophys Acta. 1983;732:256–65.
20. Beck IT, Dinda PK. Acute exposure of small intestine to ethanol: effects on morphology and function. Dig Dis Sci. 1981;26:817–38.
21. Ray M, Dinda PK, Beck IT. Mechanism of ethanol-induced jejunal microvascular and morphologic changes in the dog [see comments]. Gastroenterology. 1989;96:345–54.
22. Dinda PK, Leddin DJ, Beck IT. Histamine is involved in ethanol-induced jejunal microvascular injury in rabbits. Gastroenterology. 1988;95:1227–33.
23. Beck IT, Boyd AJ, Dinda PK. Evidence for the involvement of 5-lipoxygenase products in ethanol-induced intestinal plasma protein loss. Am J Physiol. 1988;254:G483–8.

24. Gottfried EB, Korsten MA, Lieber CS. Alcohol-induced gastric and duodenal lesions in man. Am J Gastroenterol. 1978;70:587–92.
25. Chadwick VS, Anderson RP. Inflammatory products of commensal bacteria and gastro-intestinal disorders. Dig Dis. 1990;8:253–68.
26. Bode C, Vollmer E, Hug J, Bode JC. Increased permeability of the gut to polyethylene glycol and dextran in rats fed alcohol. Ann NY Acad Sci. 1989;837–40.
27. Bjarnason I, Marsh MN, Price A, Levi AJ, Peters TJ. Intestinal permeability in patients with coeliac disease and dermatitis herpetiformis. Gut. 1985;26:1214–19.
28. Bjarnason I, Peters TJ, Wise RJ. The leaky gut of alcoholism: possible route of entry for toxic compounds. Lancet. 1984;1:179–82.
29. Parlesak A, Bode JC, Bode C. Parallel determination of gut permeability in man with M(r) 400, M(r) 1500, M(r) 4000 and M(r) 10,000 polyethylene glycol. Eur J Clin Chem Clin Biochem. 1994;32:813–20.
30. Keshavarzian A, Fields JZ, Vaeth J, Holmes EW. The differing effects of acute and chronic alcohol on gastric and intestinal permeability. Am J Gastroenterol. 1994;89:2205–11.
31. Fukui H, Brauner B, Bode JC, Bode C. Plasma endotoxin concentrations in patients with alcoholic and non-alcoholic liver disease: reevaluation with an improved chromogenic assay. J Hepatol. 1991;12:162–9.
32. Bode C, Kugler V, Bode JC. Endotoxemia in patients with alcoholic and non-alcoholic cirrhosis and in subjects with no evidence of chronic liver disease following acute alcohol excess. J Hepatol. 1987;4:8–14.
33. Bode JC, Bode C, Heidelbach R, Durr HK, Martini GA. Jejunal microflora in patients with chronic alcohol abuse. Hepatogastroenterology. 1984;31:30–4.
34. Scherenbacher P, Kullak K, Bode JC, Bode C. Alcohol abuse leads to bacterial overgrowth in the duodenum and to alterations in the faecal flora. Alcohol Clin Exp Res. 1996;20:81.
35. Bode C, Kolepke R, Schäfer K, Bode JC. Breath hydrogen excretion in patients with alcoholic liver disease – evidence of small intestinal bacterial overgrowth. Z Gastroenterol. 1993;31:3–7.
36. Morencos FC, de las Heras Castano G, Martin Ramos L et al. Small bowel bacterial overgrowth in patients with alcoholic cirrhosis. Dig Dis Sci. 1995;40:1252–6.
37. Obayashi T. Addition of perchloric acid to blood samples for colorimetric Limulus test using chromogenic substrate: comparison with conventional procedures and clinical applications. J Lab Clin Med. 1984;104:321–30.
38. Bigatello LM, Broitman SA, Fattori L et al. Endotoxemia, encephalopathy, and mortality in cirrhotic patients. Am J Gastroenterol. 1987;82:11–15.
39. Fox ES, Broitman SA, Thomas P. Bacterial endotoxins and the liver. Lab Invest. 1990;63:733–41.
40. Toth CA, Thomas P. Liver endocytosis and Kupffer cells. Hepatology. 1992;16:255–66.
41. Rietschel ET, Kirikae T, Schade FU et al. Bacterial endotoxin: molecular relationships of structure to activity and function. FASEB J. 1994;8:217–25.
42. Tarao K, So K, Moroi T, Ikeuchi T, Suyama T. Detection of endotoxin in plasma and ascitic fluid of patients with cirrhosis: its clinical significance. Gastroenterology. 1977;73:539–42.
43. Bode C, Fukui H, Bode JC. 'Hidden' endotoxin in plasma of patients with alcoholic liver disease. Eur J Gastroenterol Hepatol. 1993;5:257–62.
44. Schäfer C, Greiner B, Landig J et al. Decreased endotoxin-binding capacity of whole blood in patients with alcoholic liver disease. J Hepatol. 1997;26:567–73.
45. French SW, Miyamoto K, Tsukamoto H. Ethanol-induced hepatic fibrosis in the rat: role of the amount of dietary fat. Alcohol Clin Exp Res. 1986;10:13–19S.
46. Adachi Y, Moore LE, Bradford BU, Gao W, Thurman RG. Antibiotics prevent liver injury in rats following long-term exposure to ethanol. Gastroenterology. 1995;108:218–24.
47. Wright SD, Ramos RA, Tobias PS, Ulevitch RJ, Mathison JC. CD14, a receptor for complexes of lipopolysaccharide (LPS) and LPS binding protein. Science. 1990;249:1431–3.
48. Dentener MA, Von Asmuth EJU, Francot GJM, Buurman WA. Interaction between CD14, lipopolysaccharide-binding protein and bactericidal/permeability increasing protein during lipopolysaccharide-induced cell activation. In: Levin J, van Deventer, SJH, van der Poll T, Sturk A, editors. Bacterial Endotoxins; Progress in Clinical and Biological Research Vol. 388. New York. Brisbane, Toronto, Singapore: Wiley-Liss; 1994:59–70.

49. Heumann D, Gallay P, Barras C et al. Control of lipopolysaccharide (LPS) binding and LPS-induced tumor necrosis factor secretion in human peripheral blood monocytes. J Immunol. 1992;148:3505–12.
50. Tobias PS, Ulevitch RJ. Lipopolysaccharide binding protein and CD14 in LPS dependent macrophage activation. Immunobiology. 1993;187:227–32.
51. Grunwald U, Fan X, Jack RS et al. Monocytes can phagocytose Gram-negative bacteria by a CD14-dependent mechanism. J Immunol. 1996;157:4119–25.
52. Grunwald U, Kruger C, Schutt C. Endotoxin-neutralizing capacity of soluble CD14 is a highly conserved specific function. Circ Shock. 1993;39:220–5.
53. Schäfer C, Parlesak A, Carroll SF, Bode JC, Bode C. Endotoxin plasma levels and endotoxin binding factors in patients with alcoholic liver disease. Alcohol Clin Exp Res. 1996;20:127.
54. Elsbach P, Weiss J. The bactericidal/permeability-increasing protein (BPI), a potent element in host defense against gram-negative bacteria and lipopolysaccharide. Immunobiology. 1993;187:417–29.
55. Cybulsky MI, Chan MK, Movat HZ. Acute inflammation and microthrombosis induced by endotoxin, interleukin-1, and tumor necrosis factor and their implication in gram-negative infection. Lab Invest. 1988;58:365–78.
56. Chaby R, Girard R. Interaction of lipopolysaccharides with cells of immunological interest. Eur Cytokine Netw. 1993;4:399–414.
57. Grell M, Scheurich P, Meager A, Pfizenmaier K. TR60 and TR80 tumor necrosis factor (TNF)-receptors can independently mediate cytolysis. Lymphokine Cytokine Res. 1993;12:143–8.
58. Tilg H. The role of cytokines in the pathophysiology of chronic liver diseases. Int J Clin Lab Res. 1993;23:179–85.
59. Watson RR, Borgs P, Witte M et al. Alcohol, immunomodulation, and disease. Alcohol Alcoholism. 1994;29:131–9.
60. McClain C, Hill D, Schmidt J, Diehl AM. Cytokines and alcoholic liver disease. Semin Liver Dis. 1993;13:170–82.
61. Khoruts A, Stahnke L, McClain CJ, Logan G, Allen JI. Circulating tumor necrosis factor, interleukin-1 and interleukin-6 concentrations in chronic alcoholic patients. Hepatology. 1991;13:267–76.
62. Bird GL, Sheron N, Goka AK, Alexander GJ, Williams RS. Increased plasma tumor necrosis factor in severe alcoholic hepatitis. Ann Intern Med. 1990;112:917–20.
63. Felver ME, Mezey E, McGuire M et al. Plasma tumor necrosis factor alpha predicts decreased long-term survival in severe alcoholic hepatitis. Alcohol Clin Exp Res. 1990;14:255–9.
64. Tilg H, Wilmer A, Vogel W et al. Serum levels of cytokines in chronic liver diseases. Gastroenterology. 1992;103:264–74.
65. Schäfer C, Schips C, Landig J, Bode JC, Bode C. Tumor-necrosis-factor and interleukin-6 response of peripheral blood monocytes to low concentrations of lipopolysaccharide in patients with alcoholic liver disease. Z Gastroenterol. 1995;33:503–8.
66. Bode C, Scherenbacher P, Schäfer C, Landig J, Parlesak A, Bode JC. Bacterial overgrowth in the duodenum of chronic alcoholics is associated with increased plasma levels of endotoxin, tumour necrosis factor alpha, interleukin 6, and enhanced susceptibility of monocytes to endotoxin stimulation. In: Faist E, editor. Proceedings of the 4th International Congress on 'The Immune Consequences of Trauma, Shock and Sepsis – Mechanisms and Therapeutic Approaches'. Bologna: Monduzzi Editore; 1997:247–52.
67. Diez Ruiz A, Tilz GP, Guitierrez Gea F et al. Neopterin and soluble tumor necrosis factor receptor type I in alcohol-induced cirrhosis. Hepatology. 1995;21:976–8.
68. Peetre C, Thysell H, Grubb A, Olsson I. A tumor necrosis factor binding protein is present in human biological fluids. Eur J Haematol. 1988;41:414–19.
69. Thornton AJ, Ham J, Kunkel SL. Kupffer cell-derived cytokines induce the synthesis of a leukocyte chemotactic peptide, interleukin-8, in human hepatoma and primary hepatocyte cultures. Hepatology. 1991;14:1112–22.
70. Sheron N, Bird G, Koskinas J et al. Circulating and tissue levels of the neutrophil chemotaxin interleukin-8 are elevated in severe acute alcoholic hepatitis, and tissue levels correlate with neutrophil infiltration. Hepatology. 1993;18:41–6.
71. Hill DB, Marsano LS, McClain CJ. Increased plasma interleukin-8 concentrations in alcoholic hepatitis. Hepatology. 1993;18:576–80.

72. Huang YS, Chan CY, Wu JC, Pai CH, Chao Y, Lee SD. Serum levels of interleukin-8 in alcoholic liver disease: relationship with disease stage, biochemical parameters and survival. J Hepatol. 1996;24:377–84.
73. Freudenberg MA, Keppler D, Galanos C. Requirement for lipopolysaccharide-responsive macrophages in galactosamine-induced sensitization to endotoxin. Infect Immun. 1986;51:891–5.
74. Cornell RP. Endotoxin-induced hyperinsulinemia and hyperglucagonemia after experimental liver injury. Am J Physiol. 1981;241:E428–35.
75. Bhagwandeen BS, Apte M, Manwarring L, Dickeson J. Endotoxin induced hepatic necrosis in rats on an alcohol diet. J Pathol. 1987;152:47–53.
76. Hall P. Pathological spectrums of alcoholic liver disease. In: Hall P, editor. Alcoholic liver disease, 2nd edn. London: Arnold; 1995:41–70.
77. Lieber CS, Robins SJ, Li J, et al. Phosphatidylcholine protects against fibrosis and cirrhosis in the baboon [see comments]. Gastroenterology. 1994;106:152–9.
78. McClain CJ, Cohen DA. Increased tumor necrosis factor production by monocytes in alcoholic hepatitis. Hepatology. 1989;9:349–51.
79. Wood DD, Cameron PM. The relationship between bacterial endotoxin and human B cell-activating factor. J Immunol. 1978;121:53–60.
80. Deviere J, Content J, Denys C et al. Excessive in vitro bacterial lipopolysaccharide-induced production of monokines in cirrhosis. Hepatology. 1990;11:628–34.
81. Muzes G, Deak G, Lang I Gonzalez Cabello R, Gergely P, Feher J. Depressed monocyte production of interleukin-1 and tumor necrosis factor-alpha in patients with alcoholic liver cirrhosis. Liver. 1989;9:302–6.
82. Muller C, Zielinski CC. Interleukin-6 production by peripheral blood monocytes in patients with chronic liver disease and acute viral hepatitis. J Hepatol. 1992;15:372–7.
83. Galle PR, Hofmann WJ, Walczak H. Involvement of the APO-1/Fas (CD95) receptor and ligand in liver damage. J Exp Med. 1995;182:1223–30.
84. Bode JC, Bode C, Kugler V. Bacterial toxins and liver fibrosis. In: Gerlach U, Pott G, Rauterberg J, Voss B, editors. Connective tissues of the normal and fibrotic human liver. Stuttgart; Thieme; 1982:137–42.

22
Endotoxaemia and cholestasis

E. WALTER

INTRODUCTION

Endotoxins, lipopolysaccharide constituents of the outer membrane of Gram-negative bacteria, are the prime initiators of sepsis and septic shock. Cholestasis is an often-observed complication of sepsis and all severe inflammatory or infectious diseases. Clinically significant portal and systemic endotoxaemia, however, also occurs in the absence of documented sepsis or infections from localized sites. Lipopolysaccharides released in the gut from the lysis of bacteria, as well as from growing intact bacteria, can normally transit the gut wall in small amounts[1-3]. In states of gut inflammation or ischaemia significantly increased amounts of these bacterial products may be absorbed. Patients with alcoholic liver disease have been found to have portal vein and systemic endotoxaemia[4]. Endotoxins play a role in the pathogenesis of total parenteral nutrition-associated jaundice[5]. The focus of this short overview, however, is on the incidence, clinical diagnosis and differential diagnosis of sepsis-associated cholestasis. Important advances in the understanding of the cellular and molecular mechanisms of hepatic inflammation and endotoxaemia-induced hepatocellular dysfunction, including cholestasis, have been made mainly from experimental models. They have been reviewed recently[6-10].

INCIDENCE

The syndrome of cholestasis in the neonatal period with bacterial infection is well known to the paediatrician. In adults septic liver injury often occurs in critically ill patients as part of the progressive multiple-organ dysfunction syndrome, sepsis and septic shock[11,12]. The frequency of sepsis-associated cholestasis is difficult to assess, and the reported frequencies of jaundice as a result of Gram-negative and Gram-positive bacteremia range from 0.6% to 55%[13-15]. The organisms most often identified with hepatic dysfunction in bacteraemia are *Escherichia coli*, *Klebsiella pneumoniae*, *Pseudomonas aeruginosa*, *Haemophilus influenzae*, *Proteus* species, *Bacteroides* species and *Staphylococcus aureus*. The sites of infection include all severe intra-abdominal and pelvic

299

infections (e.g. appendicitis, diverticulitis), urinary tract infections, pneumonia and endocarditis[16]. In one study of 47 consecutive patients with *Staphylococcus aureus* endocarditis 11 patients (23%) were noted to have hyperbilirubinaemia[17].

PATHOGENESIS

Absorption of endotoxins from the gut with portal endotoxaemia is a normal physiological process. The liver is the major site for removal of all gut-derived endotoxins from the circulation. In addition, endotoxins from systemic sites of infection enter the liver. The endotoxins are cleared from the circulation primarily by resident liver macrophages, Kupffer cells, with supplemental uptake by sinusoidal endothelial cells and hepatocytes[18]. The exposure to endotoxins results in a characteristic hepatocellular response, including the activation of Kupffer cells. The production and release of bioactive lipids, reactive species of oxygen, acute-phase proteins and proinflammatory cytokines (TNF-α, IL-6, IL-8), acting independently or in sequence, damage immediately adjacent hepatocytes and sinusoidal endothelial cells[19,20]. A significant amount of TNF-α is also released into the circulation. Inactivation of Kupffer cells prevents endotoxin-induced hepatic damage, demonstrating the central pathogenetic role of Kupffer cells[21,22].

The release of TNF-α and other cytokines causes a profound down-regulation of hepatocellular bile formation[23–25]. Endotoxins have been shown to inhibit hepatocyte bile salt uptake in a TNF-α-dependent manner[23]. Basolateral and canalicular bile acid and organic anion transport are both significantly impaired[26,27]. Sodium-dependent basolateral bile acid transport and ATP-dependent and membrane-potential-dependent canalicular transport of the bile acids are reduced. Rats injected intravenously with endotoxins were shown to exhibit decreased canalicular secretion capacity for organic anions transported by the canalicular multiple organic anion transporter (canalicular multiple-drug resistance protein: MRP 2). Endotoxins and inflammatory cytokines cause a reduction of gene expression of carrier proteins at the basolateral membrane by more than 90%. The exact molecular mechanism of the reduction of the canalicular carrier capacity (at the translational or transcriptional level) still remains unclear[19]. Nitric oxide synthesis is induced in Kupffer cells and hepatocytes by endotoxins, and NO-mediated inhibition of hepatocyte protein synthesis may also regulate hepatocyte transport of bile acids and organic anions[10,28,29]. It appears possible that, in endotoxaemia, the basolateral transport exceeding the canalicular transport (due to the larger surface area of the basolateral surface) may lead to intracellular accumulation of potentially toxic compounds[27].

CLINICAL FEATURES AND DIAGNOSIS

Patients with sepsis-associated cholestasis typically show clinical manifestations and laboratory findings that are sufficiently characteristic to allow a distinction from other causes of cholestasis. In patients with sepsis and septic shock the signs of systemic inflammatory response and the manifestations of multiple-organ dysfunction usually dominate the clinical picture. Liver enzyme abnormalities in critically ill patients are very frequent; in patients with sepsis-associated, 'isolated' cholestasis; however, a pattern of disproportionate and occasionally isolated elevation of direct and total serum bilirubin values compared with values from other liver function tests (e.g. alkaline phosphatase, aspartate aminotransferase, etc.) is characteristic[15]. Jaundice may develop as early as within a few days of onset of bacteraemia, and is typically progressive. Hepatomegaly is common. Coagulopathy, encephalopathy or hypoglycaemia characteristically found in patients with hepatic failure are not associated with sepsis-induced cholestasis[14].

The most prominent histopathological feature of septic liver disease is a centrilobular cholestasis. There is usually little or no hepatocellular necrosis. Hyperplastic Kupffer cells and an increase in inflammatory mononuclear cells in the portal areas, as well as mild fatty infiltration, have been described, but usually portal tracts are not substantially affected by endotoxaemia. After long-standing cholestasis dilated canaliculi filled with bile, and minute stones impacted in the canaliculi and small bile ducts may be observed[8]. As a diagnosis of sepsis-associated cholestasis can be suggested from the pattern of laboratory values and the clinical findings, however, a liver biopsy is only rarely needed.

DIFFERENTIAL DIAGNOSIS AND PROGNOSIS

The differential diagnosis includes all infections directly affecting the liver, such as Weil's disease, toxoplasmosis, brucellosis, malaria, legionnaires' disease or infections with hepatotropic viruses. Usually serum transaminases are substantially increased, as in these cases the primary damage is hepatocellular.

A careful review of all medications received by the patient should be performed, to detect potential hepatotoxic drugs. Liver disease associated with total parenteral nutrition (TPN) is an important differential diagnosis[5]. Approximately 25% of premature infants receiving TPN develop clinical and biochemical evidence of hepatic dysfunction. In children cholestasis is predominant. In adults TPN leads more frequently to steatosis with inflammatory infiltrates and bile duct proliferation, further steatohepatitis and hepatomegaly. On ultrasound all signs of fatty change of the liver can be detected, mild elevation of transaminases and alkaline phosphatase occur typically 1–4 weeks after the start of TPN. The cause of TPN-associated hepatobiliary disease is still unclear. Lipid overload, bacterial endotoxins and overgrowth, and nutrient deficiencies are all possible pathogenetic factors of TPN-induced cholestasis and steatosis.

Biliary sludge formation and cholelithiasis occur frequently in both age groups. Impaired bile flow and the reduced enterohepatic circulation of bile acids appear to predispose to the formation of sludge in the gall bladder in patients receiving TPN[5].

Jaundice resulting from sepsis may portend a poor prognosis. However, the patients do not succumb from hepatic failure but the prognosis is determined from the underlying illness. Patients with liver cirrhosis, who develop sepsis or multiple organ failure, have a very poor prognosis, however[30]. There are only a few recent studies that examine this clinical experience. Pinsky et al. studied cytokine levels in 53 patients with septic shock. As in other studies the range of TNF-α or IL-6 levels was very high, with a high inter-patient and intra-patient variability. Sixty-seven per cent of the patients with cirrhosis developed multi-organ failure and died, whereas the mortality of non-cirrhotic patients was only 33%. All patients showed elevated TNF levels over 48 h, but there was no relationship between peak TNF levels and outcome. However, serum levels of TNF-α and IL-6 did not decrease over time in the cirrhotic patients. The failure to clear cytokines from the blood cells may thus explain the worse outcome in cirrhotic patients with sepsis[31].

There is no proven therapy for sepsis-induced cholestasis. Rapid and specific antibiotic therapy is mandatory, and the recognition of contributing factors.

The increasing knowledge of the molecular mechanisms of sepsis-induced hepatocellular dysfunction and cholestasis will provide possible therapeutic approaches to patients with sepsis-associated cholestasis as well as those with other liver diseases.

References

1. van Deventer SJH, ten Cate JW, Tytgat GNJ. Intestinal endotoxemia – clinical significance. Gastroenterology. 1988;94:825–31.
2. Bird GLA, Sheron N, Goka AKJ, Alexander GJ, Williams RS. Increased plasma tumor necrosis factor in severe alcoholic hepatitis. Ann Intern Med. 1990;112:917–20.
3. Nolan JP. Intestinal endotoxins as mediators of hepatic injury – an idea whose time has come again. Hepatology. 1989;10:887–91.
4. Bode C, Kugler V, Bode JC. Endotoxemia in patients with alcoholic and non-alcoholic cirrhosis and in subjects with no evidence of chronic liver disease following acute alcohol excess. J Hepatol. 1987;4:8–14.
5. Quigley EM, Marsh MN, Shaffer JL, Markin RS. Hepatobiliary complications of total parenteral nutrition. Gastroenterology. 1993;104:286–301.
6. Fox ES, Broitman SA, Thomas P. Biology of disease – bacterial endotoxins and the liver. Lab Invest. 1990;63:733–41.
7. Crawford JM. Cellular and molecular biology of the inflamed liver. Cur Opin Gastroenterol. 1997;13:175–85.
8. Green RM Crawford JM. Hepatocellular cholestasis: pathobiology and histological outcome. Semin Liver Dis. 1995;15:372–89.
9. Meier PJ. Molecular biology of cholestasis. In: Alvaro D, Benedetti A, editors. Vanishing bile duct syndrome. Lancaster: Kluwer; 1997:107–16.
10. Moseley RH. Sepsis-associated cholestasis. Gastroenterology. 1997;112:302–6.
11. Rangel-Frausto MS, Pittet D, Costigan M, Hwang T, Davis CS, Wenzel RP. The natural history of the systemic inflammatory response syndrome (SIRS). J Am Med Assoc. 1995;273:117–23.
12. Wenzel RP, Pinsky MR, Ulevitch RJ, Young L. Current understanding of sepsis. Clin Infect Dis. 1996;22:407–13.
13. Zimmerman HJ, Fang M, Utili R, Seeff LB, Hoofnagle J. Jaundice due to bacterial infection. Gastroenterology. 1979;77:362–74.
14. Herrera JL. Hepatobiliary abnormalities in the critically ill. Cur Opin Crit Care. 1995;1:147–51.
15. Franson TR, Hierholzer Jr, WJ, LaBrecque DR. Frequency and characteristics of hyperbilirubinemia associated with bacteremia. Rev Infect Dis. 1985;7:1–9.
16. Vermillion SE, Gregg JA, Bagenstoss AH, Bartholomew CG. Jaundice associated with bacteremia. Arch Intern Med. 1969;124:611–18.
17. Quale JM, Mandel LJ, Bergasa NV, Straus EW. Clinical significance and pathogenesis of hyperbilirubinemia associated with *Staphylococcus aureus* septicemia. Am J Med. 1988;85:615–18.
18. van Bossuyt H, Wisse E. Cultured Kupffer cells, isolated from human and rat liver biopsies, ingest endotoxin. J Hepatol. 1988;7:45–56.
19. Decker K. Biologically active products of stimulated liver macrophages (Kupffer cells). Eur J Biochem. 1990;192:245–61.

20. Andus T, Bauer J, Gerok W. Effects of cytokines on the liver. Hepatology. 1991;13:364–75.
21. Sarphie TG, D'souza NB, Deaciuc IV. Kupffer cell inactivation prevents lipopolysaccharide-induced structural changes in the rat liver sinusoid: an electron-microscopic study. Hepatology. 1996;23:788–96.
22. Suzuki S, Nakamura S, Serizawa A. *et al.* Role of Kupffer cells and the spleen in modulation of endotoxin-induced liver injury after partial hepatectomy. Hepatology. 1996;24:219–25.
23. Whiting JF, Green RM, Rosenbluth AB, Goll JL. Tumor necrosis factor-alpha decreases hepatocyte bile salt uptake and mediates endotoxin-induced cholestasis. Hepatology. 1995;22:1273–78.
24. Green RM, Beier D, Gollan JL. Regulation of hepatocyte bile salt transporters by endotoxin and inflammatory cytokines in rodents. Gastroenterology. 1996;111:193–8.
25. Moseley RH, Wang W, Takeda H *et al.* Effect of endotoxin on bile acid transport in rat liver: a potential model for sepsis-associated cholestasis. Am J Physiol. 1996;271:G137–46.
26. Utili R, Abernathy C, Zimmerman H. Cholestatic effects of *Escherichia coli* endotoxin on the isolated perfused rat liver. Gastroenterology. 1976;70:248–53.
27. Bolder U, Ton-Nu N-T, Schteingart CD, Frick E, Hofmann AF. Hepatocyte transport of bile acids and organic anions in endotoxemic rats: impaired uptake and secretion. Gastroenterology. 1997;112:214–25.
28. Rockey DC, Chung JJ. Regulation on inducible nitric oxide synthase in hepatic sinusoidal endothelial cells. Am J Physiol. 1996;271:G260–7.
29. Kitade H, Sakitani K, Inoue K *et al.* Interleukin 1β markedly stimulates nitric oxide formation in the absence of other cytokines or lipopolysaccharide in primary cultured rat hepatocytes but not in Kupffer cells. Hepatology. 1996;23:797–802.
30. Moreau R, Hadengue, A, Soupison T *et al.* Septic shock in patients with cirrhosis: hemodynamic and metabolic characteristics and intensive care unit outcome. Crit Care Med. 1992;20:746–50.
31. Pinsky MR, Vincent J-L, Deviere J, Alegre M, Kahn RJ, Dupont E. Serum cytokine levels in human septic shock – relation to multiple-system organ failure and mortality. Chest. 1993;103:565–75.

Section V
Gastrointestinal dysfunction in liver disease

23
Altered gastrointestinal motility in chronic liver disease

R. K. ZETTERMAN

INTRODUCTION

There is often a concurrence of gastrointestinal symptoms in the patient with advanced liver disease. Nausea, vomiting, vague abdominal pain (which is typically right upper quadrant or epigastric in location), and diarrhoea have been noted to occur in up to 30% of chronic liver patients[1,2]. Symptoms of gastro-oesophageal reflux are also frequent, though the cause of reflux in liver patients is unclear[3]. These non-specific symptoms appear to relate to: (a) gastrointestinal functional alterations that develop as a consequence of the underlying liver disease; (b) the associated aetiological factors for the liver disease, such as ethanol; (c) the effects of therapeutic interventions such as sclerotherapy; (d) the simultaneous presence of complicating illnesses such as pancreatitis (e.g. in the alcoholic or sclerosing cholangitis patient); or (e) the result of complications of portal hypertension such as mesenteric venous hypertension or ascites. For many patients, however, the exact cause of the symptoms may not be immediately evident. In this review we will discuss the associated motility disorders that develop in those with chronic liver disease, including what is known regarding their causes.

GASTRIC EMPTYING

The patient with end-stage liver disease frequently develops gastric varices and/or portal hypertensive gastropathy as a consequence of portal hypertension. Other associations with advanced liver disease include acute mucosal diseases such as gastritis and peptic ulcer disease[4]. However, what effect changes of portal hypertension may have on gastric function has been unclear.

Gastric emptying is reported to be enhanced[5], delayed[6-8], or unchanged[9,10] in the presence of portal hypertension. Most recent studies, however, have suggested that gastric emptying is decreased when both liquid- and solid-phase emptying are evaluated[6-8]. The underlying aetiology of liver injury does not seem to play a role. In the past, altered emptying was attributed to displacement of the stomach by ascites, or by an enlarged liver or spleen, assuming that compression or distortion of the stomach would lead to mechanical impairment of emptying. However, this seems unlikely as impaired gastric emptying can occur in the absence of ascites[8] or portal hypertension[7].

The severity of symptoms such as anorexia, nausea, vomiting, and epigastric pain may directly relate to a reduction of gastric emptying[6]. This study also addressed the question of autonomic dysfunction as a cause of symptoms, and no relationship was identified. Though elevated portal pressure (as determined by wedged hepatic venous pressure measurement) does not appear to correlate directly with impairment of gastric emptying, more rapid emptying has been described in those with oesophageal varices, whether or not sclerotherapy had been undertaken[7]. Why emptying should be more rapid in this subset is not clear, and other studies have not confirmed this finding. Some studies have suggested a relationship of reduced gastric function to the severity of associated liver disease as measured by indocyanine green clearance, prothrombin time, and serum albumin[6]. Others, however, have failed to find such a relationship to other markers of disease severity such as a reduction of serum albumin or elevation of serum bilirubin[8]. While portal hypertension or lowered serum albumin might cause worsening portal hypertensive gastropathy, or mucosal oedema of the stomach, no direct correlation of gastropathy to impaired emptying has been observed[7].

It has also been suggested that gastric colonization with *Helicobacter pylori* might contribute to abnormal gastric emptying in those with chronic liver disease. In a study of 50 patients with cirrhosis, however, no correlation between portal hypertensive gastropathy (PHG) and *H. pylori* presence was seen[10]. All patients in this study underwent endoscopy with visual assessment of portal hypertensive gastropathy, and had a stomach mucosal biopsy for determination of *H. pylori* presence by histology and quantitation of gastric secretion. While patients with cirrhosis as a group had reduced basal and stimulated gastric acid secretion, the presence of PHG did not further alter secretion. The presence of *H. pylori*, however, did indicate that acid secretion would be additionally reduced in this subset. However, there was no correlation between *H. pylori* presence and alteration of gastric emptying, presence or absence of varices, or the severity of liver disease in patients with cirrhosis.

One study has suggested that portal hypertension may contribute to altered antral function[11]. Patients with cirrhosis were divided based on the presence or absence of gastric antral vascular ectasia (GAVE) and antral function assessed with ultrasound to determine antral contraction amplitude and frequency and emptying following a solid–liquid meal. Those with GAVE tended to be older and were more likely to have a lower frequency and amplitude of antral contraction. However, no relationship of GAVE to overall emptying was observed.

What contributes to impaired gastric emptying in patients with end-stage liver disease? It does not appear to be a direct consequence of portal hypertension, varices, *H. pylori* infection, or autonomic dysfunction, though further studies will be needed to determine relationships of portal hypertension to antral function through direct measurement of antroduodenal motility. Such measurements are also needed in patients with varying severity of liver injury, in other disorders associated with impaired emptying such as alcohol consumption, and in those with other local factors which may alter motility, such as subclinical pancreatitis and ascites. Whatever the aetiology, there does seem to be a correlation of upper gastrointestinal symptoms with reduced gastric emptying. Could this impairment add to injury, and more severe liver disease be a result? It has been hypothesized that the presence of impaired gastric emptying in the chronic alcoholic could play a further role in macronutrient deficiency, and lead to greater malnutrition[12].

SMALL INTESTINAL TRANSIT

The studies of small bowel transit in patients with chronic liver disease to date have led to equally diverse results. In part this may be a result of the varying techniques utilized to determine small intestinal function. Overall, slowing of transit seems evident in those with cirrhosis[13,14]. In these studies, orocaecal transit was determined through measurement of breath-hydrogen levels following oral ingestion of lactulose. The lactulose, being non-absorbed, passes to the bacteria-filled caecum, where digestion and release of hydrogen occurs to indicate its arrival. Both studies also determined liquid gastric emptying to ensure that its alteration did not add to total orocaecal transit time. Both failed to demonstrate an association of cirrhosis with impaired gastric emptying, indicating that altered small bowel function accounted for prolonged orocaecal transit. It has also been suggested that slow small bowel transit might have a role in hepatic encephalopathy, as transit time improves following treatment with a low-protein diet and oral neomycin[14].

Direct manometric measurement of small bowel motility does indicate that alterations of small bowel motility during fasting occur in the patient with cirrhosis[15]. A prolonged interval between bursts of cyclical motor activity and more frequent clusters of phase 2 activity were more common in those with cirrhosis than in normal controls. These clusters of phase 2 activity tended to occur with a frequency of up to 12 per hour, while less than four clusters per hour were observed in controls. The underlying aetiology of liver disease did not seem to make a difference in the observed motor abnormalities. An effect of portal hypertension on myoelectric activity of the small intestine has been described in a portal vein ligation rat model, suggesting that such alteration may be the cause of impaired small bowel motility[16]. However, in another model, utilizing an isolated jejunal loop in dogs, no alteration of small bowel motility was observed in the presence of mesenteric venous hypertension[17].

Reduction of small bowel motility also does not correlate with Child–Turcotte–Pugh score, with serum albumin level, or with the presence of small intestinal bacterial overgrowth[15]. Furthermore, while tetracycline can shorten the interval between cyclic activity in those with cirrhosis, the difference was not significant. However, in conjunction with other studies which observed that antibiotic therapy will reduce orocaecal transit time[14], it seems likely that bacterial overgrowth might alter small intestinal function in patients with chronic liver disease. Other factors affecting motility should also be considered, as alcohol in the absence of associated liver disease may alter gut transit time[18].

These provocative studies suggest that impaired small bowel motility with attendant effects that prolong transit do occur in some patients with end-stage liver disease. When motility patterns result in a delay of normal migrating motor complex (MMC) activity, an increased risk of bacterial overgrowth of the small intestine and a further decrease in small bowel function may be the result.

BACTERIAL OVERGROWTH

If small intestinal transit is delayed in patients with chronic liver disease, it seems likely that bacterial overgrowth will develop. In a study of 89 patients with alcoholic cirrhosis, 30.3% had evidence of small intestinal bacterial overgrowth as compared to 0% of the normal control population[19]. These patients and controls were studied by breath-hydrogen testing following ingestion of a 50 g glucose load, where an early appearance of hydrogen in the breath of enrollees indicated the presence of bacterial overgrowth. Bacterial overgrowth also correlated with the presence of ascites (37.1% vs 5.3% in those lacking ascites) and with severity of illness (48.3% Child's C vs 13.1% Child's A and 27% Child's B). As 63 of 89 patients were actively consuming ethanol at the time of study, a direct effect of ethanol on motility cannot be excluded, since other studies have indicated that ethanol alone can affect small bowel motility[20]. These effects of ethanol may be due to either ethanol or its proximate metabolite, acetaldehyde, through impairment of contractile proteins in jejunal smooth muscle[21].

Small bowel bacterial overgrowth may also contribute to development of spontaneous bacterial peritonitis (SBP)[20]. In those patients with ascites and coexisting small bowel bacterial overgrowth, 30.7% developed an episode of SBP compared to only 9.1% of those with ascites who lacked bacterial overgrowth. As transudation of bacteria across the bowel wall may be the major cause of SBP, these data are intriguing, and this seems to be corroborated by other studies in which oral antibiotics reduced the risk of SBP in those with ascites and gastrointestinal bleeding, or those with a prior episode of SBP.

EFFECT OF ETHANOL ON MOTILITY

Up to 30% of patients with chronic alcoholism complain of non-specific gastrointestinal symptoms, including epigastric and right upper quadrant abdominal pain, diarrhoea, nausea, and vomiting[22–24]. Some of these effects seem to be a direct consequence of ethanol, as they abate when alcohol consumption is stopped.

Oesophagus

Recent ethanol ingestion reduces lower oesophageal sphincter pressure (LOSP) and increases gastro-oesophageal reflux[25,26]. Besides symptoms, these patients with chronic alcohol consumption also have a greater prevalence of gastro-oesophageal reflux disease (GERD) as manifest by oesophagitis[26–28]. The effects of ethanol appear to be complex, and the results of oesophageal studies in the alcoholic vary, depending on whether patients are studied while actively drinking, undergoing withdrawal, or abstinent.

The administration of intravenous ethanol to normal adults results in the reduction of LOSP, but has a lesser effect when administered to those with chronic alcoholism[29]. This suggests that the lower oesophageal sphincter of the alcoholic may develop tolerance to the effects of alcohol. In those with chronic alcoholism undergoing withdrawal, however, LOSP may be transiently elevated[27,28], returning to normal in most with continued abstinence[28].

High-amplitude oesophageal waves during swallowing are common in the alcoholic[27,28], suggesting that high-amplitude mid-oesophageal pressure waves may identify the presence of alcoholism[28]. Peripheral neuropathy does not correlate with oesophageal dysfunction in the alcoholic[28].

These data are similar to studies in animal models in which an acute effect of ethanol on LOSP[30] and an increase of oesophageal contraction amplitude[31] have been described. These changes also indicate that ethanol may increase the risk of development of GERD in the alcoholic.

Oesophageal transit is also altered in some patients with alcohol-related cirrhosis[32]. Untilizing a radionuclide oesophageal technique in sitting patients, 153 alcoholic cirrhotics were studied, and prolonged oesophageal transit defined as arrival of the bolus in the stomach more than 9 s following initiation of the swallow. Patients with more severe underlying liver disease, as defined by Child–Turcotte–Pugh classification, were more likely to have prolonged oesophageal transit. In those who were Child's C, 61.8% of swallows were prolonged, as compared to only 23.8% of swallows in Child's A patients ($p < 0.01$). The presence of varices also indicated that delayed transit would be present (47.3% of swallows prolonged in the presence of varices vs 29.2% of those without, $p < 0.05$). However, increasing grade of varices did not correlate with greater impairment of transit. When oesophageal transit in patients was assessed within each class (Child–Turcotte–Pugh) based on the presence or absence of varices, there was no difference, though the difference in transit based on severity of underlying liver disease remained significant in those with varices.

Other studies have also suggested that the presence of oesophageal varices will affect oesophageal motility[33]. The role of varices in oesophageal stasis, and in impairment of oesophageal clearance, needs further study. It is tempting to consider that impaired clearance of acid could increase the likelihood of acute mucosal injury, and thereby increase the risk of variceal haemorrhage.

Gastric emptying

Ethanol has been suggested to reduce gastric emptying based on animal studies[34,35] and some[13,36], but not all[37], human studies.

Small bowel motility

The ingestion of ethanol will interrupt the normal migrating motor complex (MMC) pattern of the small intestine, producing a fed pattern[20,38]. Ethanol also reduces phase III activity, clusters, and phasic bursts of the small intestine[20].

Colon

Many patients with chronic alcoholism complain of diarrhoea, which typically abates with cessation of ethanol consumption. In a study of 20 chronic alcoholics undergoing detoxification, colon transit time, as determined utilizing ingested markers, was determined on day 1 and day 10 following alcohol cessation[39]. Transit time was initially shorter, and increased as the interval since the last consumption of alcohol lengthened. These data suggest that colon transit is shorter in those recently consuming alcohol, and coupled with the acceleration of small intestine motility observed by others[13], may explain the frequent occurrence of diarrhoea in the alcoholic. Even modest ethanol consumption may enhance whole-gut transit[18].

EFFECT OF SCLEROTHERAPY ON OESOPHAGEAL MOTILITY

Most patients develop symptoms following sclerotherapy of oesophageal varices, including chest pain, dysphagia, and odynophagia[40,41]. When oesophageal motility is determined before and immediately following sclerotherapy, some[42], but not all[43], have found that relaxation of the lower oesophageal sphincter (LOS) may be initially impaired. With a longer interval following sclerotherapy, however, LOS function is generally found to be normal[43–47]. Two studies have compared the differences in oesophageal motility following either sclerotherapy or banding of oesophageal varices[42,48]. No difference in LOSP compared to controls was noted in either group following treatment.

Motility of the oesophagus is initally altered following sclerotherapy[44–49]. Reduced amplitude[44], simultaneous contractions[46], broad-based or double contraction waves[45,47], and reduced peristalsis in the distal oesophagus[44,49] have been described. These changes may account for the symptoms such as dysphagia that occur post-sclerotherapy. Oesophageal transit is also affected by sclerotherapy[50,51].

Some patients develop gastric emptying disorders and pseudo-obstruction following sclerotherapy of oesophageal varices[52,53], suggesting that vagal nerve integrity may be compromised by sclerotherapy. To assess vagal nerve function, secretion of pancreatic polypeptide (PP) following insulin-induced hypoglycaemia was determined[54]. Reduced PP secretion was initially observed following sclerotherapy, but returned to normal with time, suggesting that transient vagal injury might develop following sclerotherapy, and account for previously observed gastrointestinal complications such as gastric bezoar formation or pseudo-obstruction.

SUMMARY

Non-specific upper gastrointestinal symptoms are common in patients with chronic liver disease. However, varied and sometimes conflicting results of oesophagogastrointestinal function are described. Furthermore, such effects on function may be a consequence of either the underlying causes of liver disease, such as active ethanol consumption, or the therapies of complications of liver disease, such as sclerotherapy. Altered motility may also account for the development of some complications of liver disease, such as the contribution of small intestinal bacterial overgrowth to development of spontaneous bacterial peritonitis. The variation of aetiology, complications, and severity of illness in current studies suggest that more must be done to understand the interrelationship of liver disease and altered motility. Additional studies are clearly needed.

References

1. Galati JS, Monsour HP, Dyer CH, Seagren S, Quigley EMM. A survey of the frequency of gastrointestinal complaints in patients with chronic liver disease. Gastroenterology. 1995;108:A1068.
2. Quigley EMM, Zetterman RK. Gastrointestinal complications of chronic liver disease. In: Rector WE, Jr, editor. Complications of chronic liver disease. Chicago: Mosby; 1992:317–38.
3. Andreica V, Pascu O, Graghici A. Gastroesophageal reflux in patients with liver cirrhosis and ascites. Rom J Gastroenterol. 199;4:133–41.
4. Khodadoost J, Glass JBG. Erosive gastritis and acute gastroduodenal ulcerations as a source of upper gastrointestinal bleeding in liver cirrhosis. Digestion. 1972;7:129–38.
5. Reilly JA, Forst CF, Quigley EMM, Rikkers LF. Gastric emptying of liquids and solids in the portal hypertensive rat. Dig Dis Sci. 1990;35:781–6.
6. Isobe H, Hironori S, Satoh M, Sakamoto S, Hajime N. Delayed gastric emptying in patients with liver cirrhosis. Dig Dis Sci. 1994;39:983–7.
7. Balan KK, Grime S, Sutton R, Phil M, Critchley M, Jenkins SA. Abnormalities of gastric emptying in portal hypertension. Am J Gastroenterol. 1996;91:530–4.
8. Galati JS, Holdeman KP, Dalrymple GV, Harrison KA, Quigley EMM. Delayed gastric emptying of both the liquid and solid components of a meal in chronic liver disease. Am J Gastroenterol. 1994;89:708–11.
9. Galati JS, Holdeman KP, Bottjen PL, Quigley EMM. Gastric emptying and orocecal transit in portal hypertension and end-stage chronic liver disease. Liver Transplant Surg. 1997;3:34–8.
10. Balan KK, Jones AT, Roberts NB, Pearson JP, Critchley M, Jenkins SA. The effects of *Helicobacter pylori* colonization on gastric function and the incidence of portal hypertensive gastropathy in patients with cirrhosis of the liver. Am J Gastroenterol. 1996;91:1400–6.
11. Charneau J, Petit R, Cales P, Dauver A, Boyer J. Antral motility in patients with cirrhosis with or without gastric antral vascular ectasia. Gut. 1995;37:488–92.
12. Sankaran H, Larkin EC, Rao GA. Induction of malnutrition in chronic alcoholism: role of gastric emptying. Med Hypoth. 1994;42:124–8.
13. Wegener M, Schaffstein J, Dilger U, Coenen C, Wedmann B, Schmidt G. Gastrointestinal transit of solid–liquid meal in chronic alcoholics. Dig Dis Sci. 1991;36:917–3.
14. Van Thiel DH, Fagiuoli S, Wright HI, Chien M-C, Gavaler JS. Gastrointestinal transit in cirrhotic patients: effect of hepatic encephalopathy and its treatment. Hepatology. 1994;19:67–71.
15. Chesta J, Defilippi C, Defilippe C. Abnormalities in proximal small bowel motility in patients with cirrhosis. Hepatology. 1993;17:828–32.
16. Stewart JJ, Battarbee HD, Farrar GE, Betzing KW. Intestinal myoelectrical activity and transit time in chronic portal hypertension. Am J Physiol. 1992;263:G474–9.
17. Jacobs DL, Eamonn JL, Quigley EMM, Spanta AD, Rikkers LF. The effect of mesenteric venous hypertension on gut motility and absorption. J Surg Res. 1990;48:562–7.
18. Probert CSJ, Emmett PM, Heaton KW. Some determinants of whole-gut transit time: a population based study. Q J Med. 1995;88:311–15.
19. Morencos FC, Castano GD, Ramos LM, Lopez-Arias MJ, Ledesma F, Romero FP. Small bowel bacterial overgrowth in patients with alcoholic cirrhosis. Dig Dis Sci. 1995;40:1252–6.
20. Charles F, Evans DF, Castillo FD, Wingate DL. Daytime ingestion of alcohol alters nighttime jejunal motility in man. Dig Dis Sci. 1994;39:51–8.
21. Marway JS, Preedy VR. The acute effects of ethanol and acetaldehyde on the synthesis of mixed and contractile proteins of the jejunum. Alcohol Alcoholism. 1995;30:211–17.
22. Levi AJ, Chalmers DM. Recognition of alcoholic liver disease in a district general hospital. Gut. 1978;19:521–5.

23. Wilson FA, Hoyumpa AM. Ethanol and small intestinal transport. Gastroenterology. 1979;76:388–403.
24. Beck IT, Dinda PK. Acute exposure of the small intestine to ethanol. Dig Dis Sci. 1981;26:817–38.
25. Mayer EM, Grabowski CJ, Fisher RS. Effects of graded doses of alcohol upon esophageal motor function. Gastroenterology. 1987;75:1133–6.
26. Arsene D, Bruley des-Varannes GB, Galmiche JP et al. Gastroesophageal reflux and alcoholic cirrhosis. A reappraisal. J Hepatol. 1987;4:250–8.
27. Silver LS, Worner TM, Korsten MA. Esophageal function in chronic alcoholics. Am J Gastroenterol. 1986;81:423–7.
28. Grande L, Monforte R, Ros E et al. High-amplitude contractions in the middle third of the oesophagus: a manometric marker of chronic alcoholism. Gut. 1996;38:655–62.
29. Keshavarzian A, Polepalle C, Iber FL, Durkin M. Esophageal motor disorder in alcoholics: result of alcoholism or withdrawal? Alcohol Clin Exp Res. 1990;14:561–7.
30. Keshavarzian A, Urban G, Sedghi S et al. Effect of acute ethanol on esophageal motility in cat. Alcohol Clin Exp Res. 1991;15:116–21.
31. Keshavarzian A, Rizk G, Urban G, Wilson C. Ethanol-induced esophageal motor disorder: development of an animal model. Alcohol Clin Exp Res. 1990;14:76–81.
32. Ham HR, Urban D. Esophageal transit of liquid in chronic alcoholism in patients with cirrhosis. Influence of esophageal varices. Clin Nucl Med. 1994;19:809–12.
33. Passaretti S, Mazzotti G, de Franchis R, Cipolla M, Testoni PA, Tittobello A. Esophageal motility in cirrhotics with and without esophageal varices. Scand J Gastroenterol. 1989;24:334–8.
34. Knight LC, Maurer AH, Wikander R, Krevsky B, Malmud LS, Fisher RS. Effect of ethyl alcohol on motor function in the canine stomach. Am J Physiol. 1992;262:G223–30.
35. Willson CA, Bushnell DA, Keshavarzian A. The effect of acute and chronic ethanol administration on gastric emptying in cats. Dig Dis Sci. 1990;35:444–8.
36. Jian R, Cortot A, Ducrot F, Jobin G, Chayvialle JA, Modigliani R. Effect of ethanol ingestion on post prandial gastric emptying and secretion, biliopancreatic secretions, and duodenal absorption in man. Dig Dis Sci. 1986;31:604–14.
37. Kaufman SE, Kaye D. Effect of ethanol upon gastric emptying. Gut. 1979;20:688–92.
38. Demol P, Singer MV, Hotz J et al. Action of intragastric ethanol on pancreatic exocrine secretion in relation to the interdigestive gastrointestinal motility in humans. Arch Int Physiol Biochim. 1986;94:251–9.
39. Bouchoucha M, Nalpas B, Berger M, Cugnenc PH, Barbier J-Ph. Recovery from disturbed colonic transit time after alcohol withdrawal. Dis Colon Rectum. 1991;34:111–14.
40. Shoenut JP, Micflikier AB. Retrosternal pain subsequent to sclerotherapy. Gastrointest Endosc. 1986;32:84–7.
41. Schuman BW, Beckman JW, Tedesco FJ, Griffin JW, Assad RT. Complications of endoscopic injection sclerotherapy. A review. Am J Gastroenterol. 1987;82:823–30.
42. Goff JS, Reveille MR, Stiegmann GV. Endoscopic sclerotherapy versus endoscopic variceal ligation: esophageal symptoms, complications, and motility. Am J Gastroenterol. 1988;83:1240–4.
43. Cohen LB, Simon C, Korsten MA et al. Esophageal motility and symptoms after endoscopic injection sclerotherapy. Dig Dis Sci. 1995;30:29–32.
44. Grande L, Planas R, Lacima G et al. Sequential esophageal motility studies after endoscopic injection sclerotherapy: a prospective investigation. Am J Gastroenterol. 1991;86:36–40.
45. Larson GM, Vandertoll DJ, Netscher DT, Polk HC Jr. Esophageal motility: effects of injection sclerotherapy. Surgery. 1984;96:703–9.
46. Snady H, Korsten MA. Esophageal acid-clearance and motility after endoscopic sclerotherapy of esophageal varices. Am J Gastroenterol. 1986;84:419–22.
47. Reilly JJ, Schade RR, Van Thiel DS. Esophageal function after injection sclerotherapy pathogenesis of esophageal stricture. Am J Surg. 1984;147:85–8.
48. Berner JS, Gaing AA, Sharma R, Almenoff PL, Muhlfelder T, Korsten MA. Sequelae after esophageal variceal ligation and sclerotherapy: a prospective randomized study. Am J Gastroenterol. 1994;89:852–8.
49. Soderlund C, Thor K, Wiechel K-L. Oesophageal motility after sclerotherapy for bleeding varices. Acta Chir Scand. 1985;151:249–53.
50. Spence RAJ, Smith JA, Isaacs S, Terblanche J. Disturbed oesophageal motility after eradication of varices by chronic sclerotherapy: a scintigraphic study. S Afr Med J. 1990;77:138–40.

51. Sidhu SS, Bal C, Karak P, Garg PK, Bhargava DK. Effect of endoscopic variceal sclerotherapy on esophageal motor functions and gastroesophageal reflux. J Nucl Med. 1995;36:1363–7.
52. Sabanathan K, Dean S, Carr-Locke D, Phol JEF. Acute gastric dilation after endoscopic injection sclerotherapy. Lancet. 1984;1:1240–1.
53. Rasbridge S, Sheldon G, Hardman SMC, Vicary FR. Intestinal pseudo-obstruction. A new complication of esophageal sclerotherapy. Br Med J. 1986;292:991.
54. Masclee AAM, Lamers CBHW. Effect of endoscopic sclerotherapy of esophageal varices on vagus nerve integrity. J Hepatol. 1994;21:724–9.

24
Portal hypertensive intestinal vasculopathy

T. R. VIGGIANO

INTRODUCTION

Since McCormick *et al.'s* report on 'congestive gastropathy' in 1985[1], we have learned more about the association between portal hypertension and intestinal mucosal changes. Sarfeh and Tarnawski[2] reported that the fundamental structural change is a vasculopathy that can occur in all portions of the intestine. We reviewed the clinical, endoscopic, and histopathological features of intestinal mucosal changes associated with portal hypertension, and proposed the term 'portal hypertensive intestinal vasculopathy'[3] to describe the spectrum of intestinal mucosal changes.

PORTAL HYPERTENSIVE GASTROPATHY

The changes which occur in the stomach mucosa in patients with portal hypertension are the most significant clinically, because they are the most frequent cause of non-variceal bleeding in portal hypertensive patients[4]. Portal hypertensive gastropathy (PHG) has been estimated to occur in 50–80% of cirrhotic patients with portal hypertension, and in approximately 40% of patients with non-cirrhotic portal hypertension[5–8]. PHG has also been observed more frequently in patients who have undergone endoscopic sclerotherapy of oesophageal varices[1,6–10]. There are conflicting reports as to whether the presence of PHG correlates with the presence of oesophageal or gastric varices[5,7,8,11–13], severity of liver disease as assessed by Child–Pugh classification[1,8,11–13], hepatic venous pressure gradient measurements[10,13], or measurements of intravariceal pressure[8,12]. Thus, mechanisms other than portal hypertension alone may be important in the pathogenesis of PHG.

There is some confusion about the endoscopic appearance of PHG[3]. McCormick *et al.*[1] used the classification for gastritis proposed by Taor *et al.*[14]. In September 1992 the New Italian Endoscopic Club Consensus Conference proposed that the endoscopic appearance of PHG be classified into three stages:

(a) non-specific redness, (b) mosaic pattern, (c) red spots[15,16]. The risk of bleeding correlates with the endoscopic finding of hamorrhagic gastritis[3,15,16]. There is some evidence that the risk of bleeding correlates with red spots, but no convincing evidence that significant risk for bleeding correlates with either mosaic pattern or redness[3,15,16].

The role of endoscopic biopsy in the diagnosis of PHG is limited. Dilatation of mucosal vessels without inflammatory changes is consistent with PHG[1,11,13], but several studies have shown no correlation between endoscopic and histological findings[6,7,17,18]. There has been some discussion as to whether the diagnostic yield can be improved by obtaining larger mucosal samples by using large biopsy forceps[11] or diathermy snare biopsy techniques[19]. It has also been proposed that the diagnostic yield may be improved by using special stains, and observing for mucosal vessel wall thickening[3]. Practising endoscopists usually rely on the endoscopic appearance, and the observation that PHG usually involves the proximal stomach, to confirm a clinical diagnosis without obtaining biopsies.

Although the exact mechanisms have not been established, it has been postulated that portal hypertension renders the gastric mucosa more susceptible to injury. In experimental animals it has been shown that the portal hypertensive gastric mucosa is more susceptible than normal gastric mucosa to injury when exposed to aspirin[20], bile salts[21], alcohol[22], and endotoxins[23]. Multiple studies have shown that the portal hypertensive gastric mucosa is not more susceptible to injury from *Helicobacter pylori* infection[7,24–26]. It has been postulated that patients with PHG have impaired mucosal defence mechanisms, and it has been reported that gastric mucus secretion is quantitatively and qualitatively impaired, and that gastric bicarbonate production is decreased in PHG[27,28].

Alterations in gastric mucosal blood flow in patients with PHG have been extensively investigated by several different indirect methods. There have been reports of decreased gastric mucosal blood flow in patients with PHG[29–31] which has been attributed to 'stasis' or passive congestion. There are also reports of increased gastric mucosal blood flow in PHG attributed to 'overflow' or active congestion caused by a hyperdynamic circulation[32–35]. Although this controversy continues to be debated[36,37] at this time it is not possible to form conclusions. It may be that better methods of measuring gastric mucosal blood flow will need to be developed to accurately characterize the haemodynamic alterations of the portal hypertensive gastric mucosa[36].

There is also controversy as to whether or not there is impaired oxygenation of the portal hypertensive gastric mucosa. Sarfeh *et al.*[38] reported reduced gastric mucosal oxygenation with normal gastric serosal oxygenation in portal hypertensive patients, and postulated that the increased susceptibility of the portal hypertensive gastric mucosa to injury is a consequence of impaired mucosal oxygenation. Other investigators have found decreased gastric mucosal oxygenation[39,40], and in one report the impaired mucosal oxygenation resolved after liver transplantation[40]. Panes *et al.*[32] reported increased gastric mucosal haemoglobin concentration with normal gastric mucosal oxygen concentration, consistent with the hyperaemic pattern of the hyperdynamic circulation. Using a new probe that measures oxygen diffusion from the epithelium, Piasecki *et al.*[41] reported gastric mucosal hypoxaemia in patients with PHG. Using tonometry,

Lamarque et al.[42] found no difference in gastric mucosal pH between controls and patients with PHG, and suggested that ischaemia did not play a significant role in PHG.

The search for factors in addition to portal hypertension that could be responsible for the development of either stasis or overflow congestion have largely focused on circulating vasoactive substances that could cause vasodilation or inhibit vasoconstriction. Again there is controversy, because there are conflicting reports about the association of PHG with elevated levels of serum gastrin[11,18], serum glucagon[46,47], and prostaglandins[18,48–50]. Ohta et al.[51] reported higher levels of gastric mucosal 6-keto-PGF$_{1\alpha}$, a stable metabolite of prostacyclin, in patients with PHG, but there was no correlation between plasma and gastric mucosal levels of prostaglandin E$_2$. Recent studies[52,53] strongly suggest that enhanced production of nitric oxide plays an important role in the vasodilatation and vascular hyporeactivity observed in patients with portal hypertension. Increased gastric mucosal nitric oxide synthase activity has been reported in patients with PHG[54]. The role that tumour necrosis factor-alpha plays in the regulation of nitric oxide synthase activity is currently under investigation.

The endoscopic appearance of severe portal hypertensive gastropathy has been confused with gastric antral vascular ectasia (watermelon stomach syndrome), which also occurs in patients with cirrhosis and portal hypertension[55,56]. Although there are some overlapping features in patients with cirrhosis, severe portal hypertensive gastropathy and antral vascular ectasia are distinct entities[3,56]. Gastric antral vascular ectasia usually involves the antrum, while PHG involves the proximal stomach. The watermelon stomach syndrome has distinct pathological findings of capillary dilatation, intravascular fibrin thrombi and fibromuscular hyperplasia of the lamina propria[43,44]. In PHG intravascular fibrin thrombi occur less commonly, and fibromuscular hyperplasia of the lamina propria has not been reported. Most important, watermelon stomach responds well to endoscopic coagulation; however, PHG responds to portal decompression.

The treatment of PHG is portal decompression, which can be accomplished by medical, radiological, and surgical methods. Propranolol has been shown to prevent acute bleeding from PHG[45,57]. Vasopressin[58,59], oestrogen progesterone[60], and Teprenone[61] have been studied, and appear promising. Transjugular intrahepatic portal shunting is effective, but is considered a temporary measure. Surgical portal decompression has prevented both acute and chronic rebleeding, and reverses both the endoscopic and histological manifestations of PHG[3].

PORTAL HYPERTENSIVE ENTEROPATHY

McCormick et al.[25] described endoscopic and histological changes consistent with congestion in the duodenum, jejunum and ileum of patients with portal hypertension and coexisting gastropathy. Thiruvengadam and Gostout[62] described endoscopic changes of erythema and scattered petechia in the stomach, duodenum, and jejunum of three patients who presented with bleeding.

No biopsy specimens were obtained. Nagral *et al.*[63] examined 26 consecutive patients with portal hypertension of different aetiologies, and found endoscopic evidence for portal hypertensive gastropathy in 17 patients (65%) and evidence for 'congestive duodenopathy' in four patients (16%). Review of the endoscopic findings in this study revealed that two patients had mild patchy erythema, one patient had diffuse erythema, and one patient has cherry-red spots. Thus, only one patient (4%) had endoscopic changes consistent with the NIEC criteria for PHG. In our experience the number of patients with small bowel involvement is small, and other than contributing to bleeding in patients with coexisting gastropathy, the clinical significance of portal hypertensive enteropathy is unknown[3].

PORTAL HYPERTENSIVE COLOPATHY

Portal hypertensive intestinal vasculopathy may involve the colon, and presents as rectal varices or portal hypertensive colopathy (PHC). It is important to distinguish between haemorrhoids and rectal varices[64,65]. Haemorrhoids are prolapsed normal anal vascular cushions that do not occur more frequently in portal hypertension. Anorectal varices are portosystemic collaterals that develop in portal hypertension and usually occur 4–5 cm above the anal verge. Two recent reports found a 40–44% prevalence of rectal varices in portal hypertensive patients, which is similar to previously reported prevalence rates[67,68]. Ligation of rectal varices appears to be effective treatment, with minimal morbidity[3].

Kozarek *et al.* reported 20 patients with portal hypertension and evidence for intestinal bleeding[66]. Fourteen of the 20 patients (70%) had vascular-appearing lesions (cherry-red spots, spider telangiectasias and angiodysplasia-like lesions). Four of these 14 patients also had an endoscopic appearance compatible with chronic colitis, and biopsy specimens from all four patients showed inflammation. Histological examination of biopsies from four patients without an endoscopic appearance compatible with colitis endoscopically showed oedema and capillary dilatation with minimal inflammation. Sixty per cent of the patients with PHC had previously undergone variceal sclerotherapy, and 50% of the patients with PHC had coexisting PHG. There was no correlation between the severity of hepatic dysfunction and the presence of vascular-appearing lesions.

Ganguly *et al.*[67] reported endoscopic changes compatible with PHC in 26 (52%) of 50 consecutive patients with portal hypertension. PHC was found to be significantly more common in patients with PHG than in those without PHG (81% versus 31%), and PHC was observed more commonly in patients who had bleeding than in those who did not (52% versus 12.5%). There was no significant difference in the frequency of PHC in patients with cirrhosis, non-cirrhotic portal fibrosis, or extrahepatic portal vein obstruction. PHC did not occur more frequently in patients who had previous sclerotherapy, or in patients with gastric varices, and there was no correlation between the presence of PHC and the severity of liver disease as assessed by Child's classification. PHC and RV coexisted in 15 of 50 (30%) patients.

Misra *et al.*[68] evaluated 70 consecutive cirrhotic patients with portal hypertension and found PHC in 34 patients (48.5%). Diffuse hyperaemia and oedema suggestive of chronic colitis was found in 19 patients (27%), patchy erythema was found in 14 patients (20%), spider-like vascular lesions in four patients (5%), and spontaneous bleeding resembling acute colitis in three patients (4%). Biopsy specimens were obtained in all 70 patients. There was no correlation between the endoscopic and histological appearances, except that all three patients with acute colitis showed congested vessels with superficial haemorrhage. The presence of PHC did not correlate with the severity of liver disease, previous sclerotherapy, or with the presence of PHG. PHC was more common in patients without rectal varices and in patients with large oesophageal varices or gastric varices.

Tam et al.[69] found an 84% prevalence rate of PHC in 75 cirrhotic patients with recent bleeding. Histopathological findings in the patients with telangiectasias or angiodysplastic-like lesions showed dilatation of vessels and oedema of the mucosa. We previously reported that the histopathological findings of dilated mucosal capillaries with thickened basement membranes, and no evidence for mucosal inflammation, are specific for PHC[3]. Thus, endoscopic biopsy may play a more important role in diagnosing PHC than PHG. Munakata[70] recently reported that endoscopic image processing and topological analysis of colonic mucosal veins demonstrated that persistent portal hypertension alters the colonic mucosal venous structure by increasing the calibre of the veins and the number of branches or anastomoses between them.

Although we have learned much about portal hypertensive intestinal vasculopathy (PHIV) over the past decade, there is much yet to be learned. Future research should address why PHIV develops in some patients with portal hypertension but not in others. If we can better understand the pathophysiology of the portal hypertensive circulation, we will be able to develop better methods of treatment.

References

1. McCormack PM, Sims J, Eyre-Brook I et al. Gastric lesions in portal hypertension: inflammatory gastritis or congestive gastropathy? Gut. 1985;26:1226–32.
2. Sarfeh J, Tarnawski. Gastric mucosal vasculopathy in portal hypertension. Gastroenterology. 1987;93:1129–31.
3. Viggiano TR, Gostout CJ. Portal hypertensive intestinal vasculopathy: a review of clinical, endoscopic and histopathological features. Am J Gastroenterol. 1992;87:944–54.
4. D'Amico G, Montalbano L, Traina M et al. Natural history of congestive gastropathy in cirrhosis. Gastroenterology. 1990;99:1558–64.
5. Amarapurkar D, Dhawan P, Chopra K et al. Stomach in portal hypertension. J Assoc Phys India. 1993;10:638–40.
6. Sarin SK, Misra SP, Singal A et al. Evaluation of the incidence and significance of the 'mosaic pattern' in patients with cirrhosis, noncirrhotic portal fibrosis, and extrahepatic obstruction. Am J Gastroenterol. 1988;83:1235–9.
7. Misra SP, Dwivedi M, Misra V et al. Endoscopic and histologic appearance of the gastric mucosa in patients with portal hypertension. Gastrointest Endosc. 1990;36:575–9.
8. Sarin SK, Sreenivas DV, Lahoti D et al. Factors influencing development of portal hypertensive gastropathy in patients with portal hypertension. Gastroenterology. 1992;102:994–9.
9. Papazian A, Braillon A, Dupas JL et al. Portal hypertensive gastric mucosa: an endoscopic study. Gut. 1986;27:1199–203.
10. Lin W, Lee F, Lin H et al. Snake skin pattern gastropathy in cirrhotic patients. J Gastroenterol Hepatol. 1991;6:145–9.
11. Quintero E, Pique JM, Bombi JA et al. Gastric mucosal vascular ectasias causing bleeding in cirrhosis. Gastroenterology. 1987;93:1054–61.

12. Taranto D, Suozzo R, Romano M *et al.* Gastric endoscopic features in patients with liver cirrhosis: correlation with esophageal varices, intra-variceal pressure, and liver dysfunction. Digestion. 1994;55:115–20.
13. Parikh SS, Desai SB, Prabhu SR *et al.* Congestive gastropathy: factors influencing development, endoscopic features, *Helicobacter pylori* infection, and microvessel changes. Am J Gastroenterol. 1994;89:1036–42.
14. Taor RE, Box B, Ware J *et al.* Gastritis – gastroscopic and microscopic. Endoscopy. 1975;7:209–15.
15. GP Spina, R Arcidiacono, J Bosch *et al.* Gastric endoscopic features in portal hypertension: final report of a consensus conference, Milan. Ita J Hepatol. 1994;21:461–7.
16. Hashizume M, Sugimachi K. Classification of gastric lesions associated with portal hypertension. J Gastroenterol Hepatol. 1995;10:339–43.
17. Corbishley CM, Saverymuttu S, Maxwell JD. Use of endoscopic biopsy for diagnosing congestive gastropathy. J Clin Pathol. 1988;41:1187–90.
18. Vigneri S, Termini R, Piraino A *et al.* The stomach and liver appearance of the gastric mucosa in patients with portal hypertension. Gastroenterology. 1991;101:472–8.
19. Saperas E, Pique JM, Perez-Ayuso RP *et al.* Comparison of snare and large forceps biopsies in the histologic diagnosis of gastric vascular ectasia in cirrhosis. Endoscopy. 1989;21:165–7.
20. Sarfeh IJ, Tarnawski A, Hajduczek J *et al.* Does portal hypertension predispose gastric mucosa to aspirin injury? Histologic, ultrastructural and functional analysis. Gastroenterology. 1987;92:1614.
21. Sarfeh J, Tarnawski A, Maeda R *et al.* The gastric mucosa in portal hypertension effects of topical bile acid. Scand J Gastroenterol. 1984;19:189–94.
22. Sarfeh IJ, Tarnawski A, Malki A *et al.* Portal hypertension and gastric mucosal injury in rats: effects of alcohol. Gastroenterology. 1983;84:987–93.
23. Shibayama Y. An experimental study into the cause of acute hemorrhagic gastritis in cirrhosis. J Pathol. 1986;149:307–13.
24. Tarnawski A, Sarfeh IJ, Stachura J *et al.* Microvascular abnormalities of the portal hypertensive gastric mucosa. Hepatology. 1988;8:1488–94.
25. McCormick PA, Sankey EA, Cardin F *et al.* Congestive gastropathy and *Helicobacter pylori*: an endoscopic and morphometric study. Gut. 1991;32:351–4.
26. Bhargava N, Venkateswaran S, Ramakrishna BS *et al.* Colonization by *Helicobacter pylori* and its relationship to histological changes in the gastric mucosa in portal hypertension. J Gastroenterol Hepatol. 1994;9:507–11.
27. Guslandi M, Sorghi M, Foppa L *et al.* Mucosal defensive mechanisms in congestive gastropathy. Gastroenterology. 1992;102:A816.
28. Guslandi M, Sorghi M, Foppa L *et al.* Congestive gastropathy versus chronic gastritis: a comparison of some pathophysiological aspects. Digestion. 1993;54:160–2.
29. Iwao T, Toyonaga A, Ikegami M *et al.* Reduced gastric mucosal blood flow in patients with portal hypertensive gastropathy. Hepatology. 1993;18:36–40.
30. Kotzampassi I, Eleftheriadis E, Aletras H. Gastric mucosal blood flow in portal hypertension patients – a laser Doppler flowmetry study. Hepatogastroenterology. 1992;39:39–42.
31. Sawant P, Bhatia R, Kulhalli P *et al.* Comparison of gastric mucosal blood flow in normal subjects and in patients with portal hypertension using endoscopic laser-Doppler velocimetry. Indian J Gastroenterol. 1995;14:87–90.
32. Panes J, Bordas JM, Pique JM *et al.* Increased gastric mucosal perfusion in cirrhotic patients with portal hypertensive gastropathy. Gastroenterology. 1992;103:1875–82.
33. Pique JM, Pizcueta P, Perez-Ayuso RM *et al.* Effects of propranolol on gastric microcirculation and acid secretion in portal hypertension rates. Hepatology. 1990;12:476–80.
34. Paye JL, Cales P. Modifications gastriques au cours de la cirrhose. Gastroenterol Clin Biol. 1991;15:285–95.
35. Vorobioff J, Bredfeldt JE, Groszmann RJ. Hyperdynamic circulation in portal hypertensive rat model: a primary factor for maintenance of chronic portal hypertension. Am J Physiol. 1983;244:G52–7.
36. Aggarwal R, Naik SR. Portal hypertensive gastropathy and gastric mucosal blood flow. Indian J Gastroenterol. 1995;14:83–6.
37. Guslandi M. Gastric mucosal hemodynamics in portal hypertensive gastropathy: the debate goes on. Hepatology. 1995;22:1002–4.

38. Sarfeh IJ, Soliman H, Waxman K *et al.* Impaired oxygenation of gastric mucosa in portal hypertension. Dig Dis Sci. 1989;34:225–8.
39. Larson MV, Ahlquist DA, Wiesner RH. Endoscopic assessment of gastric mucosal perfusion in patients with portal hypertension. Gastroenterology. 1989;96:287.
40. Larson MV, Ahlquist DA, Wiesner RH. Endoscopic assessment of gastric mucosal perfusion in patients before and after orthotopic liver transplantation. Hepatology. 1989;10:572.
41. C Piasecki, J Chin, Greenslade L *et al.* Endoscopic detection of ischaemia with a new probe indicates low oxygenation of gastric epithelium in portal hypertensive gastropathy. Gut. 1995;36:654–6.
42. Lamarque D, Levoir D, Duvoux C *et al.* Measurement of gastric intramucosal pH in patients with cirrhosis and portal hypertensive gastropathy. Gastroenterol Clin Biol. 1994;18:969–74.
43. Suit PF, Petras RE, Bauer TW *et al.* Gastric antral vascular ectasia. Am J Surg Pathol. 1987;11:750–7.
44. Gilliam JH, Geisinger KR, Wu WC. Endoscopic biopsy as diagnostic in gastric antral vascular ectasia: The watermelon stomach. Dig Dis Sci. 1989;34:885–8.
45. Hosking SW, Kennedy HJ, Seddon I *et al.*. The role of propranolol in congestive gastropathy of portal hypertension. Hepatology. 1987;7:437–41.
46. Benoit J, Barrowman JA, Harper SL *et al.* Role of humoral factors in the intestinal hyperemia associated with chronic portal hypertension. Am J Physiol. 1984;247:G486–93.
47. Kravetz D, Bosch J, Arderiu MT *et al.* Effects of somatostatin on splanchnic hemodynamics and plasma glucagon in portal hypertensive rats. Am J Physiol. 1988;254:G322–8.
48. Saperas E, Perez-Ayuso RM, Poca E *et al.* Increased gastric PGE_2 biosynthesis in cirrhotic patients with gastric vascular ectasias. Am J Gastroenterol. 1990;85:138–44.
49. Arakawa T, Satoh H, Kudukda T *et al.* Endogenous prostaglandin E_2 in gastric mucosa of patients with alcoholic cirrhosis and portal hypertension. Gastroenterology. 1987;93:135–40.
50. Weiler H, Weiler CH, Gerok W. Decreased prostaglandin E2 immunoactivity of gastric mucosa in portal hypertension. Neth J Med. 1991;38:4–12.
51. Ohta M, Hashizume M, Higashi H *et al.* Portal and gastric mucosal hemodynamics in cirrhotic patients with portal-hypertensive gastropathy. Hepatology. 1994;20:1432–6.
52. Pizcueta P, Pique JM, Fernandez M *et al.* Modulation of the hyperdynamic circulation of cirrhotic rats by nitric oxide inhibition. Gastroenterology. 1992;103:1909–15.
53. Sieber CC, Groszmann RJ. Nitric oxide mediates hyporeactivity to vasopressors in mesenteric vessels of portal hypertensive rats. Gastroenterology. 1992;103:235–9.
54. El-Newihi HM, Kanji VK, Mihas AA. Activity of gastric mucosal nitric oxide synthase in portal hypertensive gastropathy. Am J Gastroenterol. 1996;91:535–8.
55. Gostout CJ, Viggiano TR, Ahlquist DA *et al.* The clinical and endoscopic spectrum of the watermelon stomach. J Clin Gastroenterol. 1992;15:256–63.
56. Payen JL, Cales P, Voigt JJ *et al.* Severe portal hypertensive gastropathy and antral vascular ectasia are distinct entities in patients with cirrhosis. Gastroenterology. 1995;108:138–44.
57. Perez-Ayuso R, Pique J, Bosch J *et al.* Propranolol in prevention of recurrent bleeding from severe portal hypertensive gastropathy in cirrhosis. Lancet. 1991;337:1431–4.
58. Iwao T, Toyonaga A, Shigemori H *et al.* Vasopressin plus oxygen vs vasopressin alone in cirrhotic patients with portal hypertensive gastropathy: effects on gastric mucosal haemodynamics and oxygenation. J Gastroenterol Hepatol. 1996;11:216–22.
59. Panes J, Pique JM, Bordas JM *et al.* Drug therapy for acute bleeding from portal hypertensive gastropathy. Hepatology. 1994;19:55–60.
60. Pan-Ees J, Casadevall M, Fernandez M *et al.* Gastric microcirculatory changes of portal hypertensive rats can be attenuated by long-term estrogen–progestagen treatment. Hepatology. 1994;20:1261–70.
61. Tarnoue K, Tarnawski AS, Kishihara F *et al.* Effect of teprenone on portal hypertensive gastric mucosa. Digestion. 1996;57:35–40.
62. Thiruvengadam R, Gostout CJ. Congestive gastroenteropathy: an extension of nonvariceal upper gastrointestinal bleeding in portal hypertension. Gastrointest Endosc. 1989;35:504–7.
63. Nagral AS, Joshi AS, Bhatia SJ *et al.* Congestive jejunopathy in portal hypertension. Gut. 1993;34:694–7.
64. Hosking SW, Johnson AG, Smart HL *et al.* Anorectal varices, hemorrhoids, and portal hypertension. Lancet. 1989;1:349–52.

65. Foutch PG, Sivak MV. Colonic variceal hemorrhage after endoscopic injection sclerosis of esophageal varices: A report of three cases. Am J Gastroenterol 1984;79:756–60.
66. Kozarek R, Botoman V, Bredfeldt J *et al.* Portal colopathy: prospective study of colonoscopy in patients with portal hypertension. Gastroenterology. 1991;101:1192–7.
67. Ganguly S, Sarin SK, Bhatia V, Lahoti D. The prevalence and spectrum of colonic lesions in patients with cirrhotic and noncirrhotic portal hypertension. Hepatology. 1995;21:1225–31.
68. Misra SP, Dwivedi M, Misra V. Prevalence and factors influencing hemorrhoids, anorectal varices, and colopathy in patients with portal hypertension. Endoscopy. 1996;28:340–5.
69. Tseng-Nip T, Wai-Wah N, Shou-Dong L. Colonic mucosal changes in patients with liver cirrhosis. Gastrointest Endosc. 1997;42:408–12.
70. Munakata A, Nakajima H, Sasaki Y *et al.* Does portal hypertension modify colonic mucosal vasculature? Quantification of alteration by image processing and topology. Am J Gastroenterol. 1995;90:1997–2001.
70. Lam SK. Hypergastrinemia in cirrhosis of the liver. Gut. 1976;17:700–8.
71. Perez-Ayuso RM, Pique JM, Saperas E *et al.* Gastric vascular ectasias in cirrhosis: Association with hypoacidity not related to gastric atrophy. Scand J Gastroenterol. 1989;24:1073–8.
72. Pique JM, Leung FW, Kitahora T *et al.* Gastric mucosal blood flow and acid secretion in portal hypertensive rats. Gastroenterology. 1988;95:727–33.
73. Viggiano T, Gostout CJ, Carpenter HG *et al.* Congestive colopathy: endoscopic and histologic evidence. Am J Gastroenterol. 1990;85:1287.

25
Role of lipopolysaccharide and inducible nitric oxide synthase in gastrointestinal and hepatic disease: actions of selective inhibition of iNOS on microvascular integrity in the gut and liver

B. J. R. WHITTLE, S. M. EVANS and F. LÁSZLÓ

INTRODUCTION

Bacterial lipopolysaccharides (LPS) have been implicated in a large number of diseases of the gut and liver. These encompass not only the events during endotoxaemia that lead to multiple organ failure, but the disturbances of the circulation in disorders such as portal hypertension and cirrhosis, and in inflammatory diseases of the gut. Consideration of the microvascular changes that follow challenge with LPS, however, can give some insight into the processes that provoke tissue injury in a number of such conditions.

The most common origin of sepsis is the invasion of Gram-negative bacteria, frequently *Escherichia coli*, into the circulation[1]. The release of LPS from the cell wall of Gram-negative bacteria is responsible for many of the septic processes[2,3]. These acute effects may result from direct injurious actions of LPS on the vascular endothelium[4,5] or as a result of the release of tissue-damaging vasoactive mediators[2,3,6]. Subsequently, a widespread elevation of microvascular permeability occurs in many organs, including intestine and liver, several hours following LPS challenge[1-3]. The involvement of bacterial invasion has been implicated in the development of various diseases of the liver and the gut, including duodenal ulcer disease, inflammatory bowel disease and fulminant hepatic failure in cirrhosis[7-11].

CONSTITUTIVE NITRIC OXIDE

Nitric oxide (NO), formed from L-arginine, plays a dual role in the early and late phases of septic shock[12]. Under physiological circumstances the continuous production of NO by the Ca^{2+}-dependent constitutive NO synthase (NOS) isoenzyme in the vascular endothelium (eNOS) protects against endotoxin-provoked acute microcirculatory damage[13-15]. Inhibition of constitutive NOS at the time of administration of LPS provokes a rapid and substantial increase in vascular permeability in gastrointestinal tissue[15], an effect attenuated by the depletion of circulating neutrophils[16]. Moreover, administration of platelet-activating factor (PAF) receptor antagonists, thromboxane and leukotriene synthase inhibitors, protects against intestinal microvascular injury resulting from inhibition of eNOS[17,18]. Such results demonstrate that NO, synthesized by constitutive NOS, effectively counteracts the actions of injurious mediators in the early phase of LPS-induced tissue damage.

INDUCIBLE NITRIC OXIDE

Following *in-vitro* and *in-vivo* administration of endotoxin[19,20], however, subsequent vascular endothelial injury occurs in association with the expression of a Ca^{2+}-independent inducible isoenzyme of NOS (iNOS). In intestinal and hepatic tissues the activity of iNOS can be observed some 3 h after LPS administration[20-22]. In this later phase widespread cellular expression of iNOS occurs, involving the vascular endothelium[19,23], vascular smooth muscle cells[24], cardiac myocytes[25], pulmonary alveolar cells[26], renal juxtaglomerular cells[26,27], macrophages[28], neutrophils[29], hepatocytes[26] and intestinal epithelial cells[30]. This generalized overproduction of NO by iNOS is considered to be cytotoxic, not only as a consequence of its direct actions, but also through the interaction of NO with the superoxide anion to generate further reactive free radicals, such as peroxinitrite or the hydroxyl radical[31,32].

NITRIC OXIDE SYNTHASE INHIBITORS

A number of compounds that inhibit NO synthase have been used to investigate the role of NO in physiological and pathological processes. However, these agents, such as N^G-nitro-L-arginine methyl ester (L-NAME), N^G-monomethyl - L-arginine (L-NMMA), aminoguanidine or N^G-iminoethyl-L-ornithine (L-NIO) show little or no selectivity between the eNOS or iNOS isoenzymes *in vivo*[33-35]. Studies with such agents therefore require careful interpretation. In recent studies the bisisothiourea, N-(3-(aminomethyl)benzyl)acetamidine (1400W) has been shown to be a highly potent, tightly binding and selective inhibitor of iNOS[36]. The effect of this agent on the microvascular injury in the intestine and liver, that occurs following challenge with LPS, has therefore been examined.

ACTIONS OF ISOFORM SELECTIVE AND NON-SELECTIVE NOS INHIBITORS ON MICROVASCULAR INTEGRITY

1400W (a kind gift from Dr Richard Knowles, GlaxoWellcome Research, 0.1–10 mg/kg s.c.), aminoguanidine hemisulphate (Sigma, 25–50 mg/kg s.c.)

and L-NMMA (GlaxoWellcome Research; 25–50 mg/kg, s.c.) were injected concurrently with LPS (*E. coli* lipopolysaccharide 0111:B4, 3 mg/kg, i.v.) in rats. As a measure of vascular damage, leakage of [^{125}I]-human serum albumin was determined in the ileum 1 h after LPS challenge.

A single bolus injection of LPS (3 mg/kg i.v.) did not affect ileal albumin leakage over a 1 h period. Furthermore, concurrent administration of 1400W (1–10 mg/kg, s.c.) with endotoxin had no action on albumin leakage in the ileum after 1 h (Fig. 1). In contrast, concurrent administration of aminoguanidine (25–50 mg/kg s.c.) or L-NMMA (25–50 mg/kg s.c.) caused a significant dose-dependent increase in ileal albumin leakage in this early phase following LPS challenge (Fig. 1).

In further studies, 1400W (0.1–1 mg/kg s.c.), aminoguanidine (25–50 mg/kg s.c.) or L-NMMA (25–50 mg/kg s.c.) were administered 3 h after LPS challenge, and albumin leakage in the ileum was investigated 1 h later. All of these agents significantly inhibited LPS-provoked late-phase ileal albumin leakage ($p < 0.001$), as shown in Fig. 1.

In additional studies, 1400W (0.1–5 mg/kg s.c.) was administered concurrently with endotoxin, and albumin leakage in the ileum and liver was determined 5 h after LPS challenge. Under these conditions 1400W also significantly attenuated this late phase of ileal and hepatic microvascular damage provoked by LPS, by a maximum of 98 ± 2% and 87 ± 4%, respectively (n = 4–6, $p < 0.001$), as shown in Fig. 2.

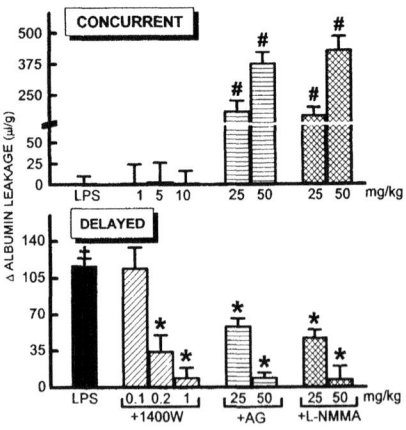

Figure 1 Actions of concurrent or delayed administration of 1400W (0.1–10 mg/kg s.c.), aminoguanidine (AG, 25–50 mg/kg s.c.) and L-NMMA (25–50 mg/kg s.c.) on the early phase (after 1 h) and late phase (after 4 h) of ileal albumin leakage (expressed as Δ μl/g tissue) following lipopolysaccharide (LPS; 3 mg/kg i.v.) administration in the rat. Nitric oxide synthase inhibitors were administered concurrently with (concurrent; upper panel), or 3 h after (delayed; lower panel), LPS challenge. Data are expressed as SEM, where (n) is at least 3; statistical significances are shown as increased albumin leakage induced by LPS (+ $p < 0.05$), potentiation (# $p < 0.05$) or inhibition (* $p < 0.05$) of LPS-induced vascular permeability

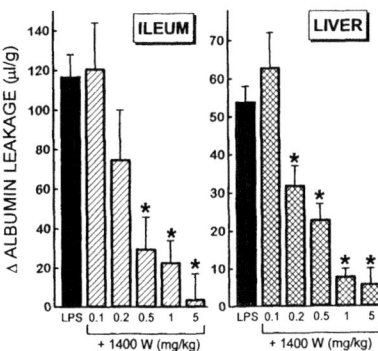

Figure 2   Effects of concurrent administration of 1400W (0.1–5 mg/kg s.c.) with lipopolysaccharide (LPS; 3 mg/kg i.v.) on albumin leakage (expressed as Δ μl/g tissue) 5 h after LPS in the rat ileum and liver. Data are expressed as SEM, where (*n*) is at least 5; statistical significances are shown as inhibition (* *p* < 0.05) of LPS-induced vascular permeability

DIVERGENT ACTIONS OF SELECTIVE AND NON-SELECTIVE NOS INHIBITORS

In this study, administration of NO synthase inhibitors, aminoguanidine or L-NMMA provoked microvascular damage in the small intestine in the early phase following LPS challenge. This augmentation of intestinal microvascular leakage presumably reflects the inhibition of eNOS by these agents, since in previous studies 1 h after LPS challenge, only constitutive NO synthase could be detected in various tissues, including the small intestine and the liver[20,21,26,30]. In contrast to the effects of these non-selective NO synthase inhibitors, the selective iNOS inhibitor, 1400W, had no effect in provoking vascular leakage when administered concurrently with LPS.

NO produced by eNOS might protect the microvasculature by inhibiting neutrophil adherence to the vascular endothelium[35,36], and possibly counteract the damaging actions of such mediators as PAF, thromboxanes and leukotrienes[17,18].

When the NO synthase inhibitors were administered 3 h after LPS challenge at a time of expression of iNOS, both the isoform non-selective (aminoguanidine, L-NMMA), and isoform selective (1400W) NO synthase inhibitors attenuated the intestinal albumin leakage. Furthermore, 1400W could protect the intestinal and hepatic microvasculature against late-phase injury, even when administered concurrently with LPS. These findings provide further evidence that the injurious actions of NO are a consequence of iNOS activity, confirming that iNOS is involved in the microcirculatory dysfunction in sepsis.

ROLE OF iNOS IN GASTROINTESTINAL INFLAMMATORY DISEASE

It is considered that iNOS plays a role in inflammatory bowel disease (IBD), the expression of iNOS being detected in the inflamed bowel of patients with ulcerative colitis[38,39]. In animal models of IBD, such as that provoked by trini-trobenzenesulphonic acid (TNBS) or in HLA-B27 transgenic rats, increased NO production or colonic iNOS activity also can be detected[40,41]. Pretreatment with L-NAME exacerbated the colonic damage produce by TNBS, suggesting a protective role for constitutive NOS, whereas administration of L-NAME, commencing at the time of iNOS expression, attenuated the colonic injury provoked by TNBS[42].

A single dose of the non-steroidal anti-inflammatory drug, indomethacin, leads to the induction of iNOS in the jejunum, detectable after 18 h, in association with the development of jejunal microvascular injury. Administration of L-NAME, at the time of iNOS expression, abolished the occurrence of jejunal injury, as did pretreatment with dexamethasone[9], which inhibits the expression of iNOS[23]. In addition, the broad-spectrum antibiotic, ampicillin, inhibited the development of iNOS activity and reduced intestinal inflammation following challenge[9]. These findings suggest that induction of iNOS following indomethacin administration involves local transmigration of gut bacteria, leading to microvascular injury in the gut. Further studies indicate that other non-steroidal anti-inflammatory agents, such as diclofenac or flurbiprofen, have similar actions in inducing iNOS and jejunal injury, an action that was inhibited by polymixin-B, which binds and inactivates LPS[43]. Thus the liberation of LPS in the jejunal tissue following bacterial invasion is likely to be involved in the induction of iNOS and the genesis of the microvascular injury and lesions. The evaluation of isoform-selective inhibitors such as 1400W in these models will give a better understanding of the role of iNOS in intestinal inflammation produced by non-steroidal anti-inflammatory agents.

Gastric mucosal infection with *Helicobacter pylori* is implicated as an important pathogenic factor in gastritis and duodenal ulcer disease. Extracts of *H. pylori* have been shown to cause expression of iNOS in macrophages and neutrophils *in vitro*[44,45]. Furthermore, it has been shown that *in-vivo* administration of *H. pylori* extracts, and more recently the purified LPS from *H. pylori*, leads to the expression of iNOS, associated with the reduction of cell viability in the rat duodenum[7,8]. These findings indicate that excess generation of NO by iNOS may play a role in development of gastritis and duodenal ulcer disease. Future studies with isoform selective NO synthase inhibitors in the *H. pylori*-infected mucosa will clarify the pathological actions of expression of iNOS in gastroduodenal ulceration.

PORTAL HYPERTENSION AND HEPATIC INJURY

The overproduction of NO has been suggested to contribute to the hyperdynamic circulation of portal hypertension and cirrhosis, a proposal based on the pharmacological findings with NO synthase inhibitors[10,11]. This excessive synthesis of NO may result from the expression of iNOS[46], which may be triggered by the elevated circulating levels of LPS found in cirrhotic patients[47,48]. However, in studies in rat models of portal hypertension, iNOS expression in splanchnic tissue could not be detected by radiochemical techniques[49]. The use of immunohistochemical and molecular techniques will clarify the involvement of iNOS expression under these conditions.

LPS is cytotoxic to hepatocytes *in vitro*[50] and is implicated in fulminant hepatic failure in cirrhotic patients[51]. Furthermore, *in vivo*, expression of iNOS can be detected in the whole liver tissue[21,22] and in hepatocytes[26] following LPS challenge. Induction of NO synthase has been shown to be associated with microcirculatory damage in the liver[22], and with direct cellular toxicity in hepatocytes[52].

In our present study the administration of the selective iNOS inhibitor, 1400W, reduced hepatic microvascular leakage provoked by LPS. This observation gives further support to the concept that expression of iNOS in the liver has harmful actions in LPS-related hepatic diseases, as elsewhere in the gut.

THERAPEUTIC IMPLICATIONS

Thus, selective iNOS inhibitors may provide a novel therapeutic approach in the treatment and prevention of inflammatory and cytotoxic processes that involve LPS. Such diseases may include gastroduodenal ulceration in *H. pylori* infection, intestinal lesions caused by non-steroidal anti-inflammatory agents, fulminant hepatic failure in liver cirrhosis, inflammation of the bowel and septic microcirculatory disturbances.

References

1. Root RK, Jacobs R. Septicemia and septic shock. In: Wilson JD, Braunwald E, Isselbacher KJ, editors. Harrison's principles of internal medicine. New York: Mc-Graw Hill; 1991:507–16.
2. Parillo JE. Septic shock in humans: advances in the understanding of pathogenesis, cardiovascular dysfunction and therapy. Ann Intern Med. 1990;113:227–42.
3. Bone RC. The pathogenesis of sepsis. Ann Intern Med. 1991;115:457–69.
4. Harlan JM, Harker LA, Reidy MA, Gajdusek CM, Schwartz SM, Striker GE. Lipopolysaccharide-mediated bovine endothelial cell injury *in vitro*. Lab Invest. 1983;48:269–74.
5. Meyrick BO, Ryan US, Brigham KL. Direct effects of *E. coli* endotoxin on structure and permeability of pulmonary endothelial monolayers and the endothelial layer of intimal explants. Am J Pathol. 1986;122:140–51.
6. Lefer AM, Lefer DJ. Pharmacology of the endothelium in ischaemia-reperfusion and circulatory shock. Annu Rev Pharmacol Toxicol. 1993;33:71–90.
7. Lamarque D, Tankovic J, Dutreuil C, Delchier JC, Whittle BJR. Induction of nitric oxide synthase by an extract of *Helicobacter pylori* (HP) in rat duodenum. Gastroenterology. 1995;108:A143.
8. Lamarque D, Kiss J, Tankovic J, Delchier JC, Whittle BJR. Relationship between induction of nitric oxide synthase and epithelial cell injury in rat duodenum by a *Helicobacter pylori* extract. Gastroenterology. 1996;110:A169.
9. Whittle BJR, László F, Evans SM, Moncada S. Induction of nitric oxide synthase and microvascular injury in the rat jejunum provoked by indomethacin. Br J Pharmacol. 1995;116:2286–90.
10. Whittle BJR. Nitric oxide in gastrointestinal physiology and pathology. In: Johnson LR, editor. Physiology of the gastrointestinal tract, 3rd edn. New York Raven Press; 1994:267–94.
11. Pizcueta P, Piqué JM, Fernández M *et al.* Modulation of hyperdynamic circulation of cirrhotic rats by nitric oxide inhibition. Gastroenterology. 1992;103:1909–15.
12. Moncada S, Higgs EA. Molecular mechanisms and therapeutic strategies related to nitric oxide, FASEB J. 1995;9:1319–30.

13. Hutcheson IR, Whittle BJR, Boughton-Smith NK. Role of nitric oxide in maintaining vascular integrity in endotoxin-induced acute intestinal damage in the rat. Br J Pharmacol. 1990;101:815–20.

14. Billiar TR, Curran RD, Harbrecht BG, Stuehr DJ, Demetris AJ, Simmons RL, Modulation of nitrogen oxide synthesis *in vivo*: NG-monomethyl-L-arginine inhibits endotoxin-induced nitrate/nitrite biosynthesis while promoting hepatic damage. J Leukocyte Biol. 1990;48:565–9.

15. László F, Whittle BJR, Moncada S. Time-dependent enhancement or inhibition of endotoxin-induced vascular injury in rat intestine by nitric oxide synthase inhibitors. Br J Pharmacol. 1994;111:1309–15.

16. László F, Whittle BJR, Moncada S. Attenuation by nitrosothiol NO donors of acute intestinal microvascular dysfunction in the rat. Br J Pharmacol. 1995;115:498–502.

17. László F, Whittle BJR, Moncada S. Interactions of constitutive nitric oxide with PAF and thromboxane on rat intestinal vascular integrity in acute endotoxaemia. Br J Pharmacol. 1994;113:1131–6.

18. László F, Whittle BJR. Colonic microvascular integrity in acute endotoxaemia: interactions between constitutive nitric oxide and 5-lipoxygenase products. Eur J Pharmacol. 1995;277:R1–3.

19. Palmer RMJ, Bridge L, Foxwell NA, Moncada S. The role of nitric oxide in endothelial cell damage and its inhibition by glucocorticoids. Br J Pharmacol. 1992;105:11–12.

20. Boughton-Smith NK, Evans SM, László F, Whittle BJR, Moncada S. The induction of nitric oxide synthase and intestinal vascular permeability by endotoxin in the rat. Br J Pharmacol. 1993;110:1189–95.

21. Salter M, Knowles RG, Moncada S. Widespread tissue distribution, species distribution and changes in activity of Ca^{2+}-dependent and Ca^{2+}-independent nitric oxide synthases. FEBS Lett. 1991;291:145–9.

22. László F, Whittle BJR, Evans SM, Moncada S. Association of microvascular leakage with induction of nitric oxide synthase: effects of nitric oxide synthase inhibitors in various organs. Eur J Pharmacol. 1995;283:47–53.

23. Radomski MW, Palmer RMJ, Moncada S. Glucocorticoids inhibit the expression of an inducible, but not the constitutive nitric oxide synthase in vascular endothelial cells. Proc Natl Acad Sci USA. 1990;87:10043–7.

24. Mitchell JA, Kohlhaas KL, Sorrentino R, Warner TD, Murad F, Vane JR. Induction by endotoxin of nitric oxide synthase in the rat mesentery: lack of effect of action of vasoconstrictors. Br J Pharmacol. 1993;109:265–70.

25. Brady AJB, Poole-Wilson PA, Harding SE, Warren JB. Nitric oxide production within cardiac myocytes reduces their contractility in endotoxemia, Am J Physiol. 1992;263:H1963–6.

26. Bandaletova T, Brouet I, Bartsch H, Sugimura T, Esumi H, Ohshima H. Immunohistochemical localization of an inducible form of nitric oxide synthase in various organs of rats treated with *Propionibacterium acnes* and lipopolysaccharide. APMIS. 1993;101:330–6.

27. Tojo A, Gross SS, Zhang L *et al.* Immunocytochemical localization of nitric oxide synthase in the juxtaglomerular apparatus of normal rat kidney. J Am Soc Nephrol. 1994;4:1438–47.

28. Marletta MA, Yoon PS, Iyengar R, Leaf CD, Wishnok JS. Macrophage oxidation of L-arginine to nitrite and nitrate: nitric oxide is an intermediate. Biochemistry. 1988;27:8706–11.

29. McCall TB, Boughton-Smith NK, Palmer RMJ, Whittle BJR, Moncada S. Synthesis of nitric oxide from L-arginine by neutrophils. Release and interaction with superoxide anion. Biochem J. 1989;261:293–6.

30. Tepperman BL, Brown JE, Korolkiewitz R, Whittle BJR. Nitric oxide synthase activity, viability and cyclic GMP levels in rat colonic epithelial cells. J Pharmacol Exp Ther. 1994;271:1477–82.

31. Beckman JS, Beckman TW, Chen J, Marshall PA, Freeman BA. Apparent hydroxyl radical production by peroxynitrate: implications for endothelial injury from nitric oxide and superoxide. Proc Natl Acad Sci USA. 1990;87:1620–4.

32. Hogg N, Darley-Usmar VM, Wilson MT, Moncada S. Production of hydroxyl radicals from the simultaneous generation of superoxide and nitric oxide. Biochem J. 1992;281:419–24.

33. Rees DD, Palmer RMJ, Shulz R, Moncada S. Characterisation of three inhibitors of endothelial nitric oxide *in vitro* and *in vivo*. Br J Pharmacol. 1990;101:746–52.

34. László F, Evans SM, Whittle BJR. Aminoguanidine inhibits both constitutive and inducible nitric oxide synthase isoforms in rat intestinal microvasculature *in vivo*. Eur J Pharmacol. 1995;272:169–75.

35. Lopez-Belmonte J, Whittle BJR. Aminoguanidine-provoked leukocyte adherence to rat mesenteric venules: role of constitutive nitric oxide synthase inhibition. Br J Pharmacol. 1995;116:2710–14.
36. Garvey EP, Oplinger JA, Furfine ES et al. 1400W is a slow, tight binding, and highly selective inhibitor of inducible nitric-oxide synthase in vitro and in vivo. J Biol Chem. 1997;21:4959–63.
37. Kubes P, Suzuki M, Granger DN. Nitric oxide: an endogenous modulator of leukocyte adhesion. Proc Natl Acad Sci USA. 1991;88:4651–5.
38. Boughton-Smith NK, Evans SM, Hawkey CJ et al. Nitric oxide synthase activity in ulcerative colitis and Crohn's disease. Lancet. 1993;342:338–40.
39. Middleton SJ, Shorthouse M, Hunter JD. Increased nitric oxide synthesis in ulcerative colitis. Lancet. 1993;341:465–6.
40. Aiko S, Grisham MB. Spontaneous intestinal inflammation and nitric oxide metabolism in HLA-B27 transgenic rats. Gastroenterology. 1995;109:142–50.
41. Boughton-Smith NK, Evans SM, Whittle BJR, Moncada S. Induction of colonic nitric oxide synthase in a rat model of colitis. Gastroenterology. 1992;102:A598.
42. Kiss J, Lamarque D, Delchier JC, Whittle BJR. Differential time-dependent effects of nitric oxide synthase inhibition on colonic inflammation induced by trinitrobenzene sulphonic acid in rats. Gastroenterology. 1996;110:A938.
43. Whittle BJR, Evans, SM, Laszlo F. Non steroidal antiinflammatory drugs induce nitric oxide synthase and microvascular injury in rat jejunum. Gastroenterology. 1996;110:A104.
44. Tsuji S, Kawano S, Tsuji M et al. Helicobacter pylori extract stimulates inflammatory nitric oxide production. Cancer Lett. 1996;108:195–200.
45. Wilson KT, Ramanujam KS, Mobley HL, Musselman RF, James SP, Meltzer SJ. Helicobacter pylori stimulates inducible nitric oxide synthase expression and activity in a murine macrophage cell line. Gastroenterology. 1996;111:1524–33.
46. Vallance P, Moncada S. Hyperdynamic circulation in cirrhosis: a role for nitric oxide? Lancet. 1991;337:776–8.
47. Lumsden AB, Henderson JM, Kutner MH. Endotoxin levels measured by a chromogenic assay in portal, hepatic and peripheral blood in patients with cirrhosis. Hepatology. 1988;8:232–6.
48. Guarner C, Soriano G, Tomas A et al. Increased serum nitrite and nitrate levels in patients with cirrhosis: relationship to endotoxemia. Hepatology. 1993;18:1139–43
49. Fernandez M, Garcia-Pagan J-C, Casadevall M et al. Evidence against a role for inducible nitric oxide synthase in the hyperdynamic circulation of portal hypertension. Gastroenterology. 1995;108:1487–95.
50. Hartung T, Wendel A. Endotoxin-inducible cytotoxicity in liver cell culture. Biochem Pharmacol. 1991;42:1129–35.
51. Wilkinson SP, Canalese J, Williams R. Consequences of Kupffer cell failure in fulminant hepatic failure and cirrhosis: with particular reference to endotoxemia. In: Liehr H, Grun M, editors, The reticuloendothelial system and the pathogenesis of liver disease. Amsterdam: Elsevier; 1980:337–40.
52. Curran RD, Ferrari FK, Kispert PH et al. Nitric oxide and nitric oxide-generating compounds inhibit hepatocyte protein synthesis. FASEB J. 1991;5:2085–92.

26
Bacterial overgrowth in the small intestine in chronic liver disease

F. CASAFONT, L. MARTIN and F. PONS-ROMERO

INTRODUCTION

Small intestinal bacterial overgrowth (SIBO) in the setting of chronic liver disease (CLD) was first reported by Martini, over 40 years ago[1]. Since then several other studies have confirmed a high prevalence among patients with liver disease, although the prevalence is different from study to study, ranging between 20% and 75%. In this chapter we summarize the current knowledge on the prevalence, the causes which may be involved and the consequences of SIBO in patients with CLD.

PREVALENCE OF SIBO IN PATIENTS WITH CLD

Several studies have been carried out, by different groups around the world, in which the relationship between SIBO and CLD has been assessed. The upper small bowel has been shown by Martini *et al.* to be contaminated in approximately 75% of patients with cirrhosis[1]. The organisms found in the duodenum and jejunum were coliforms and enterococci. In 1972 Lai *et al.* studied the microflora of the small intestine in 24 patients with biopsy-proven alcoholic cirrhosis by means of intestinal aspirate cultures[2]. Abnormal colonization of the upper small bowel was seen in 12 of these patients, including six with urea-splitting bacteria. Shindo *et al.* observed a 27% prevalence of SIBO in a group of cirrhotic patients[3]. The bacteria were composed mainly of species with the ability to deconjugate bile salts.

The types and number of bacteria were examined by Bode *et al.* in aspirates from the jejunum of 27 chronic alcoholics[4]. They found that the number of aerobic and anaerobic bacteria was higher in alcoholics than in a control group. In addition, coliform microorganisms, Gram-negative anaerobic bacteria and endospore-forming rods were cultured much more frequently from the jejunal fluid of alcoholics. No correlation was found between the number or types of microorganisms in the jejunum and the type or degree of liver disease in the alcoholics. In another study, performed by the same authors, a hydrogen breath test was used to investigate the incidence of SIBO in 45 chronic alcoholics[5]. In the group of patients with alcoholic liver disease, SIBO was more frequent (37.8%) than in a control group (13.3%). Although SIBO was more frequent in patients with cirrhosis (42.9%) than in those without cirrhosis (33.3%), this difference did not reach statistical significance.

In 1991 Chesta *et al.* published the results of their study carried out on 36 cirrhotic patients[6]. SIBO was demonstrated in 45% of the cirrhotics by means of a lactulose breath test, and in 64% by jejunal cultures. In this study SIBO was related to the severity of the liver disease, but not to the cause of the cirrhosis, the prevalence being similar in patients with alcoholic and those with non-alcoholic liver disease. We studied a group of 89 patients with alcoholic cirrhosis, 63 of them admitting regular alcohol consumption and 26 declaring abstinence[7]. SIBO was assessed by means of a glucose hydrogen breath test. We found that 30.3% of these patients had evidence of SIBO, and that this was not related either to the activity of liver disease or to the existence of regular alcohol consumption at the moment of the study (Fig. 1). There was a relationship between SIBO and the severity of cirrhosis, the prevalence being higher in patients in Child–Pugh class C (48.3%), than in those in class B (27%) or A (13.1%). In addition, SIBO was much more frequent in patients with ascites (37.1%) compared with patients without ascites (5.3%) (Fig. 2).

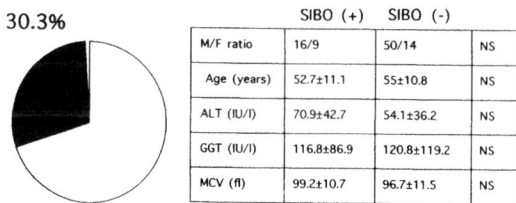

	SIBO (+)	SIBO (-)	
M/F ratio	16/9	50/14	NS
Age (years)	52.7±11.1	55±10.8	NS
ALT (IU/l)	70.9±42.7	54.1±36.2	NS
GGT (IU/l)	116.8±86.9	120.8±119.2	NS
MCV (fl)	99.2±10.7	96.7±11.5	NS

30.3%

Figure 1 Prevalence of small intestinal bacterial overgrowth (SIBO) in a group of patients with alcoholic cirrhosis

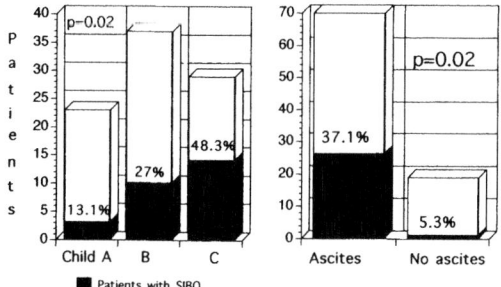

Figure 2 Relationship between small intestinal bacterial overgrowth (SIBO) and the severity of cirrhosis. Prevalence of SIBO among patients with and without ascites

All these studies confirm the high prevalence of SIBO in patients with CLD, although it is not clear whether it is related to the liver disease itself, and to the severity of liver injury, or to the cause of the CLD.

POSSIBLE CAUSES INVOLVED IN SIBO IN PATIENTS WITH CLD

There are several possible causes which may favour the development of SIBO in patients with CLD. For some authors SIBO would not be specific to CLD, because a similar prevalence has been observed among hospitalized patients without liver disease, which suggests that SIBO may be related to chronic illness and hospitalization[2]. Other authors think that SIBO is not related to the liver disease itself but to the cause of it, namely chronic alcoholism. However, SIBO has also been observed in alcoholics without liver disease, but with other associated diseases, such as chronic relapsing pancreatitis[8].

Several conditions can coincide in cirrhotic patients which would justify the high prevalence of SIBO. In a list of conditions which can induce SIBO it can be seen that several of them have been reported in cirrhotic patients (Table 1).

INTESTINAL MOTILITY DISTURBANCES

Several studies have demonstrated an altered proximal small bowel motility in patients with cirrhosis, which provokes a delay in mouth-to-caecum transit time[9,10]. Nevertheless, no clear relationship has been demonstrated between these motility disturbances and SIBO, in the setting of liver cirrhosis. Chesta et al. observed no significant differences in the small intestine motility pattern between cirrhotic patients with and without SIBO[10]. In contrast, there are indirect data which could support this association. Recently, Pardo et al. treated a group of cirrhotic patients who had evidence of SIBO, with a prokinetic drug[11]. They observed how the treatment accelerated the small intestine transit time and negativized the cultures from the jejunum, in all but one patient.

Further studies are necessary to clarify the role of intestinal motility disturbances in the development of SIBO, in patients with liver cirrhosis.

Table 1 Conditions favouring small intestinal bacterial overgrowth

Anatomical
    Blind loop, diverticula, fistulas, obstructions, resection of ileocaecal valve, etc.

Intestinal motility disorders
    Autonomic neuropathy, scleroderma, idiopathic intestinal pseudo-obstruction, etc.

Achlorhydria

Others
    Aged
    Malnutrition
    Local immunodeficiences
    Cirrhosis

ACHLORHYDRIA

It is known that acid secretion is one of the most important defence mechanisms against bacterial overgrowth. Although there are conflicting results, several studies have demonstrated a low acid gastric secretion in cirrhotics[12,13]. Thus, it is not surprising that several studies have found a relationship between SIBO and gastric hypoacidity in these patients[3,4]. Bode *et al.* found that the number of microorganisms in jejunal fluid correlated closely with the pH in gastric juice[4], and in the study carried out by Shindo *et al.* a good correlation between[14]CO_2 activity and gastric pH was also observed[3].

LOCAL IMMUNODEFICIENCIES

It is postulated that luminal IgA deficiency may exacerbate SIBO. On the other hand, it is known that there is a deficient intestinal production of secretory IgA in alcoholic cirrhosis[14]. This may be another possible contributory mechanism in the development of SIBO in these patients. However, this possibility has still not been confirmed.

MALNUTRITION

Malnutrition is a well-known cause of SIBO, and is a common finding in patients with cirrhosis – above all in those with advanced liver disease[15]. In the study we carried out in humans[7] we observed a tendency to poorer nutritional state in cirrhotic patients with SIBO, compared with those without SIBO, but this difference did not reach statistical significance. We are now studying, in our laboratory, this possible association between SIBO and malnutrition, in an experimental model of cirrhosis. Initially we have found a higher prevalence of SIBO in cirrhotic malnourished animals compared with that observed in well-nourished animals. However, the number of animals studied is still low, and we have to confirm these preliminary findings in a larger group.

CONSEQUENCES OF SIBO IN THE SETTING OF CLD

The possible consequences of SIBO in patients with CLD are not well established. Is it an incidental finding? Or could it have deleterious effects on the patient? The answer remains to be elucidated. Nevertheless, there are some data in the literature that suggest that it may have negative effects.

An elevated faecal fat excretion in some cirrhotic patients with SIBO, has been reported[3]. One of the manifestations of SIBO is malabsorption of different nutrients that can provoke a worsening of nutritional status. The above-mentioned findings, which we observed in humans and in the experimental study, could be interpreted as a consequence of the malnutrition, and not as a cause of it. Probably malnutrition is both a predisposing factor for malnutrition and a consequence of it, so forming a vicious circle.

SIBO could also have some influence on liver disease. It has been shown in experimental studies, and in humans, that SIBO can induce hepatobiliary injury resembling alcoholic liver disease[16,17]. Several mechanisms could explain the deleterious effect of SIBO on the liver: the accumulation of bacterial cell wall polymers derived from the intestinal bacterial overgrowth, inside the liver[15]; the overproduction of toxic bile acids such as lithocholic acid, due to bacterial overgrowth[3]; and the increased toxic effect of alcohol due to an elevated metabolization capacity of ethanol, it forming large amounts of acetaldehyde that is toxic to the liver[18]. Thus, SIBO may aggravate or perpetuate liver injury in patients who already have CLD. This may be the explanation for the relationship between SIBO and the severity of liver disease, observed by several authors.

An interesting result that we obtained in our study was the association between SIBO and the development of spontaneous bacterial peritonitis (SBP)[7]. Twelve of the 70 cirrhotic patients with ascites, whom we studied, developed an episode of SBP in the follow-up. The prevalence of SBP in patients with SIBO was higher (30.7%) than in those without bacterial overgrowth (9%) (Fig. 3). These results suggest that SIBO may be a predisposing factor for the development of SBP in patients with cirrhosis; but by which mechanism could SIBO induce the development of SBP? We think that one of the possible mechanisms is bacterial translocation (BT).

One of the conditions that favours BT is SIBO. In addition, several studies have demonstrated that BT is an important initial step in the pathogenesis of SBP in cirrhosis[19-22]. In an experimental model of cirrhosis we have observed a high prevalence of BT in animals with SIBO that is associated with the presence of SBP (Fig. 4). These results suggest that SIBO could predispose to BT, and BT would act as a permissive factor for SBP.

In summary, SIBO is common in patients with CLD, the cause probably being multifactorial and the consequences still awaiting elucidation, although an elevated risk of SBP may be expected.

References

1. Martini GA, Phear EA, Reubner B, Sherlock S. The bacterial content of small intestine in normal and cirrhotic subjects: relation to methionine toxicity. Clin Sci. 1956;16:35–51.
2. Lai D, Gorbach SL, Levitan R. Intestinal microflora in patients with alcoholic cirrhosis: urea-splitting bacteria and neomycin resistance. Gastroenterology. 1972;62:275–9.
3. Shindo K, Machida M, Miyakawa K, Fukumura M. A syndrome of cirrhosis, achlorhydria, small intestinal bacterial overgrowth, and fat malabsorption. Am J Gastroenterol. 1993;88:2084–91.
4. Bode JC, Bode C, Heidelbach R, Dürr HK, Martini GA. Jejunal microflora in patients with chronic alcohol abuse. Hepatogastroenterology. 1984;31:30–4.

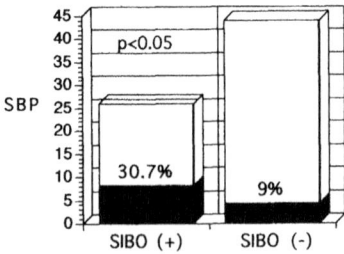

Figure 3 Prevalence of spontaneous bacterial peritonitis (SBP) in cirrhotic patients with and without small intestinal bacterial overgrowth (SIBO)

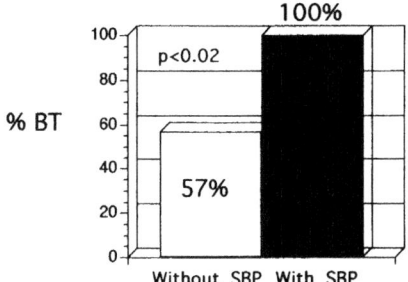

Figure 4   Prevalence of bacterial translocation (BT) in cirrhotic animals with and without spontaneous bacterial peritonitis (SBP)

5. Bode C, Kolepke R, Schafer K, Bode JC. Breath hydrogen excretion in patients with alcoholic liver disease. Evidence of small intestinal bacterial overgrowth. Z Gastroenterol. 1993;31:3–7.
6. Chesta J, Silva M, Thompson L, Del Canto E, Defilippi C. Small intestine bacterial overgrowth in patients with hepatic cirrhosis. Rev Med Chil. 1991;119:626–32.
7. Casafont F, de las Heras G, Martín L, López MJ, Ledesma F, Pons-Romero F. Small bowel bacterial overgrowth in patients with alcoholic cirrhosis. Dig Dis Sci. 1995;40:1252–6.
8. Lembcke B, Kraus B, Lankisch PG. Small intestinal function in chronic relapsing pancreatitis. Hepatogastroenterology. 1985;32:149–51.
9. Van Thiel DH, Fagiuoli S, Wright HI, Chien M, Gavaler JS. Gastrointestinal transit in cirrhotic patients: effect of hepatic encephalopathy and its treatment. Hepatology. 1994;19:67–71.
10. Chesta J, Defilippi C, Defilippi C. Abnormalities in proximal small bowel motility in patients with cirrhosis. Hepatology. 1993;17:828–32.
11. Pardo A, Viñado B, Santos J et al. Effect of cisapride on intestinal bacterial overgrowth due to gramnegative organisms in cirrhosis. A pilot, randomized, controlled trial. J Hepatol. 1997;26:103 (abstract).
12. Fraser AG, Pounder RE, Burroughs AK. Gastric secretion and peptic ulceration in cirrhosis. J Hepatol. 1993;19:171–82.
13. Gaur SK, Vij JC, Sarin SK, Anand BS. Gastric secretion in cirrhosis and non-cirrhotic portal fibrosis. Digestion. 1988;39:151–5.
14. Pelletier G, Briantais MJ, Buffet C, Pillot J, Etienne JP. Serum and intestinal secretory IgA in alcoholic cirrhosis of the liver. Gut. 1982;23:475–80.
15. Ledesma F, Casafont F, Martín L, Sánchez E, Ordóñez J, Pons-Romero F. Influencia del estado nutricional sobre las características del líquido ascítico en cirrosis hepática alcohólica. Nutr Hosp. 1996;11:238–44.
16. Lichtman SN, Keku J, Schwab JH, Sartor RB. Hepatic injury associated with small bowel bacterial overgrowth in rats is prevented by metronidazole nd tetracycline. Gastroenterology. 1991;100:513–19.
17. Hocking MP, Duerson MC, O'Leary JP, Woodward ER. Jejuno-ileal bypass for morbid obesity. N Engl J Med. 1983;308:995–9.
18. Baraona E, Julkunen R, Tannenbaum L, Lieber CS. Role of intestinal bacterial overgrowth in ethanol production and metabolism in rats. Gastroenterology. 1986;90:103–10.
19. Runyon BA, Squier S, Borzio M. Translocation of gut bacteria in the rat with cirrhosis to mesenteric lymph nodes partially explains the pathogenesis of spontaneous bacterial peritonitis. J Hepatol. 1994;21:792–6.
20. García-Tsao G, Lee F, Barden GE, Cartun R, West AB. Bacterial translocation to mesenteric lymph nodes is increased in cirrhotic rats with ascites. Gastroenterology. 1995;108:1835–41.
21. Lovet JM, Bartolí R, Planas R et al. Bacterial translocation in cirrhotic rats. Its role in the development of spontaneous bacterial peritonitis. Gut. 1994;35:1648–52.
22. Casafont F, Sánchez E, Martín L, Agüero J, Pons-Romero F. Influence of malnutrition on the prevalence of bacterial translocation and spontaneous bacterial peritonitis in experimental cirrhosis. Hepatology. 1997 (In press).

Section VI
Spontaneous bacterial peritonitis in cirrhotics

27
Spontaneous bacterial peritonitis: incidence, diagnosis and clinical course

A. OCHS

INTRODUCTION AND DEFINITION OF SPONTANEOUS BACTERIAL PERITONITIS

Spontaneous bacterial peritonitis (SBP) is a common and life-threatening complication of decompensated cirrhosis[1]. SBP is defined as an intra-abdominal infection in the absence of a surgically treatable source such as perforation or abscesses. Although SBP was recognized early in this century, Conn coined the term in 1964[2]. Since then an explosion of information has been accumulated on the pathophysiology, diagnosis, treatment and survival of this complication[3–11].

This chapter summarizes recent articles, focusing on the incidence, diagnosis, differential diagnosis and clinical course of this entity.

Several subtypes of SBP have been defined (Table 1). SBP has to be distinguished from secondary bacterial peritonitis, since the treatment differs, and operations on patients with SBP have a mortality of 90%[12]. In cirrhotic patients with infected ascites 90% will present with SBP and 10% with secondary bacterial peritonitis.

EPIDEMIOLOGY

According to early reports from Conn and co-workers[2] SBP was a rare event, predominantly diagnosed at autopsy with an estimated prevalence of 7.2% between 1971 and 1979[3]. Nine studies published between 1980 and 1990, with 1330 patients, showed a mean prevalence of 14.9% (range 10–21%)[3]. If cases of culture-negative neutrocytic ascites (CNNA) were considered as SBP, this number increased to 19% (range 12–26%)[3,15,16]. In up to 20% of patients admitted with ascites SBP can be diagnosed. The 1-year probability to develop the first episode of SBP in patients with hepatic ascites amounts to 11%[14,17,18]. Poor liver function (e.g. a serum bilirubin of >2.5 mg/100 ml) or a low ascitic fluid protein concentration (<1 g/100 ml) increase the probability to 29–33% at 1 year[18,19].

Table 1 Definition and features of SBP and several subtypes of ascitic infection

Description	Culture of ascitic fluid	PMN*/μl (ascitic fluid)	Characteristics
Spontaneous bacterial peritonitis	Positive	>250	Needs immediate antibiotic treatment, spontaneous resolution rare, very low germ concentration
Culture-negative neutrocytic ascites (CNNA)	Negative	>250	Requires antibiotic treatment, may be caused by suboptimal culture technique, spontaneous resolution rare, less serious variant of SBP?[9]
Monomicrobial non-neutrocytic bacterascites (MNBA) (asymptomatic bacterascites)	Positive	<250	Needs careful observation with clinical symptoms present[4,13]; may progress to SBP[14]; may resolve spontaneously
Secondary bacterial peritonitis	Positive (single or multiple organisms)	>250	Clinical symptoms of limited value[4]
Polymicrobial bacterascites	Positive (multiple organisms)	<250	Consequence of incidental gut puncture during paracentesis[7]

* PMN = polymorphonuclear count.

342

Approximately 60% of cases of SBP are community-acquired; the remaining cases develop during hospitalization[19].

The underlying disease is predominantly cirrhosis of any aetiology[1,3-6]. Some cases have been reported in children with nephrotic syndrome[20]. The incidence is lower in patients with cardiac failure, the Budd–Chiari syndrome, or with liver metastases. These instances share a much higher ascitic protein concentration as compared to ascites due to portal hypertension[1].

PATHOPHYSIOLOGY

Figure 1 summarizes the current view of the pathophysiology of SBP. Portal hypertension due to cirrhosis, and to a lesser extent due to acute hepatitis, causes ascites and mediates translocation of gut bacteria to mesenteric lymph nodes. This process is facilitated by intestinal congestion, bacterial overgrowth of small intestine and impaired function of the intestinal immune defence[7,21-23]. Direct migration of microbia from the gut into the abdominal cavity is unlikely, since usually SBP is a monomicrobial infection[4]. From infected lymph nodes blood is contaminated and prolonged bacteraemia is induced by an impaired reticulo-endothelial system, portosystemic shunts and reduced opsonic and phagocytic activity of the serum. Low protein ascites with reduced concentrations of opsonins and complement, and impaired function of polymorphonuclear neu-trophil leucocytes (PMN)[24], is prone to bacterial colonization (bacterascites) which may progress to SBP. Other sources of prolonged bacteraemia are urinary and respiratory tract infections and invasive medical interventions[3-6].

MICROBIA

In 92% of cases with SBP a single organism is isolated. Table 2 lists the distrib-ution of isolated species compiled from the literature[3,5,6,19,25-30]. In 50–72% of

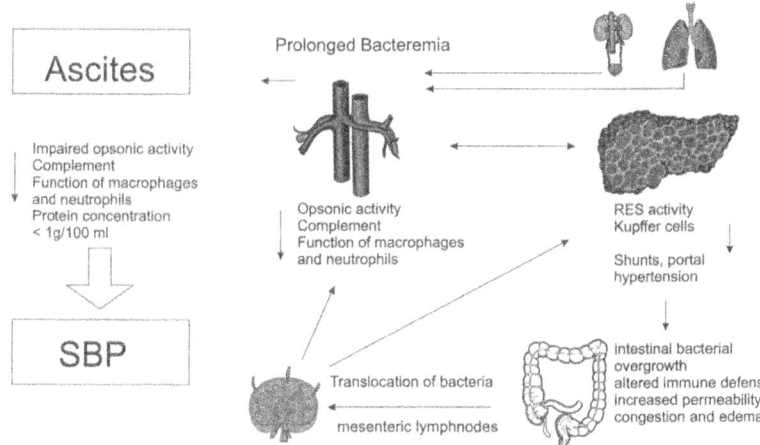

Figure 1 Current view of the pathophysiology of SBP

Table 2 Spectrum of microbia isolated from ascitic fluid of patients with SBP[3,5,6,19,25-30]

	Type of bacteria			
	Gram-positive (%)	Gram-negative (%)	Anaerobes (%)	Miscellaneous (%)
Frequency	50–72	25–30	3–5	2
	E. coli (50)	Streptococcus spp. (15–20)	Bacteroides spp.	Diphtheroids
	Klebsiella spp. (10–15)	Str. pneumoniae (5–7)	Clostridium spp.	Listeria monocytogenes,
	Enterobacter (13)	Enterococcus spp. (7–12)		Neisseria spp.,
				Bacillus spp.
	Others such as Serratia spp., Citrobacter spp., Acinetobacter spp., Salmonella spp., Pseudomonas aeruginosa, Proteus spp.	Staphylococcus spp. (2–4)		

the cases Gram-negative bacteria can be found. *Escherichia coli* with 50%, *Klebsiella* spp. (13%) and *Enterobacter* spp. (13%) are the most frequently isolated microorgansims in this group. Gram-positive cocci account for 25–30% of the cases. In only 3–5% anaerobes can be found, which may be due to the high oxygen tension within the ascitic fluid. By contrast, in cases of secondary bacterial peritonitis, anaerobes can be detected in up to 90% of cases.

Prophylactic antibiotic treatment changes the spectrum of microorganisms, and Gram-positive cocci occur in 70% of cases, as opposed by 14.3% of Gram-negative bacteria[31].

PREDISPOSING FACTORS

A major risk factor to develop an episode of SBP is impaired liver function (Table 3). Seventy per cent of patients with SBP are in Child–Pugh (CP) class C. Patients with CP class C are likely to develop an episode within 1 year in up to 71% of cases[19]. Poor nutritional status, a serum bilirubin concentration of >2.5 mg/100 ml, a prothrombin time ratio of <40% and the presence of hepatic encephalopathy (HE) will increase the likelihood of an episode to 20–36%[4,15,17,19].

Gastrointestinal (GI) bleeding is associated with bacteraemia, especially when sclerotherapy is performed. Whether bacteraemia justifies antibiotic treatment is debated[32]. More than 20% of ascitic patients with GI bleeding present with infections at admission, and an additional 30% will develop bacterial infections during hospitalization. Elective or prophylactic sclerotherapy, or rubber-band ligation, are not associated with an increased risk to develop an episode of SBP[33,34]. Three per cent of patients with emergency sclerotherapy will develop SBP; of those 90% are in CP class C[33,34]. Overall 25% of CP class C patients undergoing emergency sclerotherapy will develop a bacterial infection.

An ascitic protein concentration of <1 g/L increases the incidence of an episode of SBP within 1 year to 20%, as opposed to 4% in patients with higher protein concentrations[4,17,35–37].

Table 3 Possible risk factors to develop an episode of SBP and instances not commonly associated with SBP[3–6,8]

Increased frequency of SBP
Child–Pugh (CP) class C
Gastrointestinal bleeding in CP class C with or without sclerotherapy
Ascitic fluid protein concentration <1 g/L
Urinary or respiratory tract infections
Intravascular catheters
Previous episode of SBP
Large-volume paracentesis?

Risk of SBP not increased
Diagnostic paracentesis
Elective or prophylactic sclerotherapy/ligation
Hepatocellular carcinoma

Diagnostic paracentesis is not a risk factor for SBP. Diuretic treatment of ascites increases ascitic fluid protein concentrations and opsonin activity[38,39], whereas therapeutic paracentesis may lower protein and opsonin concentrations[24,38,40]. In a clinical randomized trial, however, the 1-year probability to develop SBP was 18.6% in the paracentesis group and 24% in patients treated with diuretics[41]. It has been argued that, in this study, infrequent paracentesis was sufficient to control ascites[39].

CLINICAL SYMPTOMS

Classical signs of peritonitis such as a rigid abdomen are often lacking or difficult to detect. Rebound tenderness may be prevented by the presence of ascites, and can be found in 30–47% of cases, usually in a mild form. Table 4 shows differences in clinical symptoms and signs of ascitic patients with and without SBP[29]. Interestingly, the frequency of GI bleeding or diarrhoea was not different between the groups.

Up to 10% of patients with SBP are completely asymptomatic. In 25–40% of cases hepatic encephalopathy (HE) is present, or worsens during the course of the disease. HE or fever may represent the only symptom in 10% and 50%, respectively. In 20% of cases with SBP GI bleeding occurs, and kidney function may deteriorate in 33–46% of cases[9,30,31,42]

DIAGNOSIS

Diagnostic paracentesis

This safe procedure should be performed with a very low threshold of suspicion. In our institution every patient admitted with clinically detectable ascites undergoes diagnostic paracentesis routinely. The risk of intra-abdominal bleeding is lower than 1%. Perforation of the gut was reported to occur in 0.6% of 1578 diagnostic taps leading to polymicrobial bacterascites. In only one patient did a non-fatal peritonitis develop[1].

Determination of ascitic protein, cholesterol concentrations and cytology are helpful to distinguish transudate from exudate and benign from malign ascites[43-47]. Table 5 shows the sensitivity, specificity, and accuracy of various parameters determined in ascitic fluid analysis. It is now widely accepted that a

Table 4 Comparison of symptoms and clinical signs of ascitic patients with and without SBP

	SBP (68 patients) (%)	Sterile ascites (108 patients)
Abdominal pain	82	61*
Malaise	86	64*
Nausea/vomiting	51	24*
Altered mental status	50	34
Fever	53	10*
Chills	43	8*

* Significant differences, (modified after ref. 29).

Table 5 Sensitivity, specificity and accuracy of various parameters obtained from ascitic fluid[3,43,48]

	Sensitivity (%)	Specificity (%)	Accuracy (%)
PMN > 500/μl	80–93	91–97	92
PMN > 250/μl	84–93	86–93	88–90
pH	54	96	85
Lactate	58	93	86

threshold of $\geq$250/μl PMN count establishes the diagnosis of SBP without compromising specificity, in comparison to a threshold of >500 PMN/μl. PMN count is superior to white blood cell count. Diuretic treatment increases the leucocyte count in ascitic fluid. PMN count increases only in the presence of infection. Ascitic fluid pH and lactate concentrations have a low sensitivity.

The yield of conventional culture techniques is low, and rarely exceeds 40%. Inoculation of ascites into blood culture bottles at the patient's bedside improves the sensitivity to a range of 50–93%[27,29,42,49–51]. Reasons for negative ascitic cultures in SBP are the low microbial concentrations of one or two organisms/ml, inadequate culture techniques or spontaneous resolution of an episode. Usually 12–72 h may elapse before cultures become positive. BacT/ALERT, a colorimetric method to demonstrate bacteria, has been reported to become positive within 13 h, with a comparable sensitivity to blood culture techniques[35].

Blood cultures obtained simultaneously demonstrate the same microorganism as in ascites in 19–53% of cases with positive ascitic cultures[3,9,27,29,30,52].

In the remaining cases CNNA is diagnosed. Simultaneously collected blood cultures are positive in 7.5–33% of the cases with CNNA[27,28,31,42]. Additional positive cultures can be obtained from the urinary or respiratory tract[3,29]. Patients with SBP have positive urine cultures in 51% of cases as compared to 10% in patients with sterile ascites[29].

Ascites rich in lymphocytes is suspicious for tuberculosis, fungal infection or *Chlamydia trachomatis*[4,53]. The diagnosis of tuberculous peritonitis is still difficult, and may require laparoscopy. Polymerase chain reaction is not recommended routinely; the value of ascitic pH or lactate determination has been questioned[54]. The determination of adenosine deaminase, an enzyme secreted by proliferating lymphocytes, has been advocated for the diagnosis of tuberculous ascites; however, this test is less reliable in patients with cirrhosis[53,54]. Patients with cirrhosis and infection with the human immunodeficiency virus should be carefully evaluated for fungal and tuberculous peritonitis. Diagnostic paracentesis in HIV patients is safe[55].

Secondary bacterial peritonitis occurs in 5–15% of cases with infected ascites[5,56,57]. Secondary bacterial peritonitis should be distinguished from SBP, since surgery in the latter has a mortality of 90%[56,58]. Clinical symptoms are of minor use, since a rigid abdomen or rebound tenderness are often lacking in both instances. Table 6 shows typical features of patients with secondary peritonitis[56–58]. Secondary bacterial peritonitis is likely if two or more parameters are present. Typically, ascites in secondary peritonitis reveals polymicrobial cultures. Anaerobic bacteria are present in 90% of cases as opposed to only 4% in

Table 6 Typical features of SBP and secondary bacterial peritonitis

	SBP	*Secondary peritonitis*
Ascitic total protein concentration	<1 g/100 ml	>1 g/100 ml
Glucose	As in serum	<50 mg/100 ml
Serum lactate dehydrogenase	<100 U/ml	>225 U/L
Ascitic culture	Monomicrobial	More than two species of microorganisms
Anaerobic bacteria in ascites	4%	>80%
Response to antibiotic treatment	Within 48 h	Absent

cases of SBP. The criteria of Table 6 work better in cases of free perforation as opposed to non-perforating secondary bacterial peritonitis[7].

Radiographic testing in the search for gut perforation or loculated pus is mandatory after secondary bacterial peritonitis is suspected[57]. An ascitic fluid bilirubin concentration of >6 mg/100 ml, and an ascitic fluid/serum bilirubin gradient of >1, is suggestive of biliary perforation[57]. Other sources of secondary peritonitis are ruptured umbilical hernias or diverticulitis.

CLINICAL COURSE AND PROGNOSTIC FACTORS

The hospital mortality of patients with SBP is 10 times higher than that of patients with uninfected ascites[1]. Even in the 1990s, SBP is still a severe and life-threatening complication of cirrhosis. Recent studies reported a better outcome in terms of both resolution of SBP and the hospital mortality. Table 7 summarizes data on resolution and survival before 1980, 1980–1990 and 1990 to the present. In the studies of Conn, resolution was absent and survival was poor[2]. This figure has improved in recent studies. Infection is controlled in up to 92% and the overall hospital mortality of an episode amounts to 17–27%. Better outcome is thought to be caused by a diagnostic threshold of >250 ascitic PMN/μl to diagnose SBP, frequent diagnostic paracentesis on suspicion and non-nephrotoxic antibiotics. The natural course of the disease cannot be determined, since every patient is treated with antibiotics after the diagnosis of SBP is established. However, spontaneous resolution of SBP is very unlikely. A retap performed 4 h after the initial diagnostic paracentesis, and prior to commencement of antibiotic treatment, confirms an elevated PMN count in all cases, and cultures demonstrate the same microorganisms in 85% of cases[1].

Hospital mortality is influenced by the presence of additional risk factors and complications (Table 8). In the absence of risk factors survival is favourable. Community-acquired episodes have a better prognosis than nosocomial SBP,

Table 7 Resolution and hospital mortality rates (percentages), compiled from the literature[4,5,9,25,26,31,42,59-63]

	1970 and earlier	*1980–1990*	*1990 to present*
Resolution of SBP	Absent	50–87	74–92
Hospital mortality	>90	26–60	17–27

Table 8 Prognostic factors influencing the hospital mortality of patients admitted for an episode of SBP (percentages)

	Uncomplicated SBP (no bleeding, hepatic encephalopathy, or renal failure)	Community-acquired / nosocomial SBP	Gastrointestinal bleeding	Renal failure progressive/steady/ transient	Septic shock at admission or shortly after commencement of antibiotic therapy
Hospital mortality	0	27/50	38	100/31/5	100

since the latter frequently develops as a consequence of emergency treatments such as sclerotherapy or invasive medical interventions[64]. Follo and co-workers have shown that 33% of patients with SBP will develop renal impairment. Progressive renal failure[65] or septic shock at admission, or shortly after start of antibiotic treatment[5,25,42] is associated with 100% mortality.

Additional positive predictive factors of survival and resolution are transaminases less than 4 times elevated, younger age, preserved liver function, and the absence of ileus[5,42,60].

CNNA has a slightly better prognosis than culture-positive SBP; the reasons are unknown[3]. Causes of death are listed in Table 9. Only one-third of the patients will die from infection.

The long-term survival is poor after the first episode of SBP. Tito and co-workers found that patients with sterile ascites had a 1-year survival of 57% as opposed to 38% in patients with SBP[19,61,62]. After survival of an episode the 1-year probability of recurrence ranges between 32% and 69% of cases[61,62]. Predictors of recurrence are poor liver function and a low ascitic protein concentration[62].

SUMMARY

SBP is a serious complication of patients with cirrhosis, and is defined as infection of ascites in the absence of a surgically treatable source. The diagnosis is established if the PMN count of ascitic fluid exceeds $250/\mu l$. Monomicrobial bacterial cultures become positive in 60% of cases. Gram-negative bacteria of enteric origin can be demonstrated in 70% of cases with positive cultures; anaerobes are an exception. In secondary bacterial peritonitis, multiple organisms can be found and the ascitic protein concentration exceeds 1 g/100 ml. The incidence of SBP amounts to 10–21% and is particularly high in patients with poor liver function and low ascitic protein concentrations. In patients admitted with ascites nosocomial SBP will develop in 10–32% of cases. Approximately 20% of patients die during hospitalization. Survival is poor if progressive renal failure, septic shock, or GI bleeding occur. Community-acquired SBP has a better prognosis than nosocomial cases. Main causes of death are liver failure and septicaemia. The 1-year survival amounts to 38% after the first episode of SBP, and in 69% of cases SBP recurs within 1 year. Recurrence of SBP can be prevented by prophylactic antibiotic treatment, but survival is not significantly

Table 9 Causes of death of patients with SBP

Causes of death	Percentage of cases
Liver failure	30–44
Septicaemia	25–30
Multiorgan failure	20–30
Gastrointestinal bleeding	10–18
Other infections	10–20

influenced. Poor survival and high recurrence of SBP necessitate early consideration of liver transplantation in patients who have survived an episode.

References

1. Runyon BA. Spontaneous bacterial peritonitis: an explosion of information. Hepatology. 1988;8:171–5.
2. Conn HO. Spontaneous peritonitis and bacteremia in Laennec's cirrhosis caused by enteric organisms. Ann Intern Med. 1964;60:568–80.
3. Garcia-Tsao G. Spontaneous bacterial peritonitis. Gastroenterol Clin N Am. 1992;21:257–75.
4. Guarner C, Runyon BA. Spontaneous bacterial peritonitis: pathogenesis, diagnosis, and management. Gastroenterologist. 1995;3:311–28.
5. Planas R, Arroyo V. Spontaneous bacterial peritonitis. Acta Gastroenterol Belg. 1995;58:297–310.
6. Propst T, Propst A, Schauer G, Judmaier G, Braunsteiner H, Vogel W. Spontaneous bacterial peritonitis in chronic liver disease with ascites. Dtsch Med Wochenschr. 1993;118:943–6.
7. Runyon BA, Squier S, Borzio M. Translocation of gut bacteria in rats with cirrhosis to mesenteric lymph nodes partially explains the pathogenesis of spontaneous bacterial peritonitis. J Hepatol. 1994;21:792–6.
8. Arroyo V, Navasa M, Rimola A. Spontaneous bacterial peritonitis in liver cirrhosis: treatment and prophylaxis. Infection. 1994;22(Suppl. 3):S167–75.
9. al Amri SM, Allam AR, al Mofleh IA. Spontaneous bacterial peritonitis and culture negative neutrocytic ascites in patients with non-alcoholic liver cirrhosis. J Gastroenterol Hepatol. 1994;9:433–6.
10. Ginès P, Navasa M. Management of ascites, hepatorenal syndrome, and spontaneous bacterial peritonitis in cirrhosis. Curr Opin Gastroenterol. 1995;11:233–7.
11. Bhuva M, Ganger D, Jensen D. Spontaneous bacterial peritonitis: an update on evaluation, management, and prevention. Am J Med. 1994;97:169–75.
12. Garrison RN, Cryer HM, Howard DA, Polk HC Jr. Clarification of risk factors for abdominal operations in patients with hepatic cirrhosis. Ann Surg. 1984;199:648–55.
13. Runyon BA. Monomicrobial nonneutrocytic bacterascites: a variant of spontaneous bacterial peritonitis. Hepatology. 1990;12:710–15.
14. Chu CM, Chang KY, Liaw YF. Prevalence and prognostic significance of bacterascites in cirrhosis with ascites. Dig Dis Sci. 1995;40:561–5.
15. Almdal TP, Skinhoj P. Spontaneous bacterial peritonitis in cirrhosis. Incidence, diagnosis, and prognosis. Scand J Gastroenterol. 1987;22:295–300.
16. Storgaard JS, Svendsen JH, Hegnhoj J, Krintel JJ, Nielsen PB. Incidence of spontaneous bacterial peritonitis in patients with ascites. Diagnostic value of white blood cell count and pH measurement in ascitic fluid. Liver. 1991;11:248–52.
17. Llach J, Rimola A, Navasa M et al. Incidence and predictive factors of first episode of spontaneous bacterial peritonitis in cirrhosis with ascites: relevance of ascitic fluid protein concentration. Hepatology. 1992;16:724–7.
18. Novella M, Sola R, Soriano G et al. Continuous versus inpatient prophylaxis of the first episode of spontaneous bacterial peritonitis with norfloxacin. Hepatology. 1997;25:532–6.
19. Andreu M, Sola R, Sitges-Serra A et al. Risk factors for spontaneous bacterial peritonitis in cirrhotic patients with ascites. Gastroenterology. 1993;104:1133–8.
20. Ackerman Z. Ascites in nephrotic syndrome. Incidence, patients' characteristics, and complications. J Clin Gastroenterol. 1996;22:31–4.
21. Llovet JM, Bartoli R, Planas R et al. Bacterial translocation in cirrhotic rats. Its role in the development of spontaneous bacterial peritonitis. Gut. 1994;35:1648–52.
22. Schimpl G, Pesendorfer P, Steinwender G, Feierl G, Ratschek M, Hollwarth ME. Allopurinol and glutamine attenuate bacterial translocation in chronic portal hypertensive and common bile duct ligated growing rats. Gut. 1996;39:48–53.
23. Casafont Morencos F, de las Heras Castano G, Martin Ramos L et al. Small bowel bacterial overgrowth in patients with alcoholic cirrhosis. Dig Dis Sci. 1996;41:552–6.
24. Lebrun L, Pelletier G, Briantais MJ, Galanaud P, Etienne JP. Impaired functions of normal peripheral polymorphonuclear leukocytes in cirrhotic ascitic fluid. J Hepatol. 1992;16:98–101.

25. Henz S, Bühler H, Pirovino M. Die spontane bakterielle Peritonitis: diagnostische und prognostische Aspekte. Schweiz Med Wochenschr. 1995;125:2379–86.
26. Kaymakoglu S, Eraksoy H, Ökten A et al. Spontaneous ascitic infection in different cirrhotic groups: prevalence, risk factors and the efficacy of cefotaxime therapy. Eur J Gastroenterol Hepatol. 1997;9:71–6.
27. Navasa M, Follo A, Llovet JM et al. Randomized, comparative study of oral ofloxacin versus intravenous cefotaxime in spontaneous bacterial peritonitis. Gastroenterology. 1996;111:1011–17.
28. Pawar GP, Gupta M, Satija VK. Evaluation of culture techniques for detection of spontaneous bacterial peritonitis in cirrhotic ascites. Indian J Gastroenterol. 1994;13:139–40.
29. Ho H, Zuckerman MJ, Ho TK, Guerra LG, Verghese A, Casner PR. Prevalence of associated infections in community-acquired spontaneous bacterial peritonitis. Am J Gastroenterol. 1996;91:735–42.
30. Boixeda D, De Luis DA, Aller R, De Argila CM. Spontaneous bacterial peritonitis. Clinical and microbiological study of 233 episodes. J Clin Gastroenterol. 1996;23:275–9.
31. Llovet JM, Rodriguez-Iglesias P, Moitinho E et al. Spontaneous bacterial peritonitis in patients with cirrhosis undergoing selective intestinal decontamination – a retrospective study of 229 spontaneous bacterial peritonitis episodes. J Hepatol. 1997;26:88–95.
32. Schlaeffer F, Riesenberg K, Mikolich D, Sikuler E, Niv Y. Serious bacterial infections after endoscopic procedures. Arch Intern Med. 1996;156:572–4.
33. Bac DJ, de Marie S, Siersema PD, Snobl J, van Buuren HR. Post-sclerotherapy bacterial peritonitis: a complication of sclerotherapy or of variceal bleeding? Am J Gastroenterol. 1994;89:859–62.
34. Lo GH, Lai KH, Shen MT, Chang CF. A comparison of the incidence of transient bacteremia and infectious sequelae after sclerotherapy and rubber band ligation of bleeding esophageal varices. Gastrointest Endosc. 1994;40:675–9.
35. Ortiz J, Soriano G, Coll P et al. Early microbiologic diagnosis of spontaneous bacterial peritonitis with BacT/ALERT. J. Hepatol. 1997; 26:839–44.
36. Runyon BA. Low-protein-concentration ascitic fluid is predisposed to spontaneous bacterial peritonitis. Gastroenterology. 1986;91:1343–6.
37. Hurwich DB, Lindor KD, Hay JE, Gross JB, Jr Kaese D, Rakela J. Prevalence of peritonitis and the ascitic fluid protein concentration among chronic liver disease patients. Am J Gastroenterol. 1993;88:1254–7.
38. Ljubicic N, Bilic A, Kopjar B. Diuretics vs. paracentesis followed by diuretics in cirrhosis: effect on ascites opsonic activity and immunoglobulin and complement concentrations. Hepatology. 1994;19:346–53.
39. Runyon BA, Van Epps DE. Diuresis of cirrhotic ascites increases its opsonic activity and may help prevent spontaneous bacterial peritonitis. Hepatology. 1986;6:396–9.
40. Runyon BA, Antillon MR, Montano AA. Effect of diuresis versus therapeutic paracentesis on ascitic fluid opsonic activity and serum complement. Gastroenterology. 1989;97:158–62.
41. Sola R, Andreu M, Coll S, Vila MC, Oliver MI, Arroyo V. Spontaneous bacterial peritonitis in cirrhotic patients treated using paracentesis or diuretics: results of a randomized study. Hepatology. 1995;21:340–4.
42. Llovet JM, Planas R, Morillas R et al. Short-term prognosis of cirrhotics with spontaneous bacterial peritonitis: multivariate study. Am J Gastroenterol. 1993;88:388–92.
43. Wang SS, Lu CW, Chao Y et al. Malignancy-related ascites: a diagnostic pitfall of spontaneous bacterial peritonitis by ascitic fluid polymorphonuclear cell count. J Hepatol. 1994;20:79–84.
44. Runyon BA, Hoefs JC, Morgan TR. Ascitic fluid analysis in malignancy-related ascites. Hepatology. 1988;8:1104–9.
45. Jüngst D, Xie Y, Gerbes AL. Pathophysiology of elevated ascites fluid cholesterol in malignant ascites. Increased ascites to serum relation of proteins and lipoproteins in patients with peritoneal carcinomatosis as compared to patients with cirrhosis of the liver. J Hepatol. 1992;14:244–8.
46. Lee HH, Carlson RW, Bull DM. Early diagnosis of spontaneous bacterial peritonitis: values of ascitic fluid variables. Infection. 1987;15:232–6.
47. Runyon BA. Malignancy-related ascites and ascitic fluid 'humoral tests of malignancy'. J Clin Gastroenterol. 1994;18:94–8.

48. Albillos A, Cuervas-Mons V, Millan I *et al.* Ascitic fluid polymorphonuclear cell count and serum to ascites albumin gradient in the diagnosis of bacterial peritonitis. Gastroenterology. 1990;98:134–40.
49. Runyon BA, Canawati HN, Akriviadis EA. Optimization of ascitic fluid culture technique. Gastroenterology. 1988;95:1351–5.
50. Puri AS, Puri J, Ghoshal UC *et al.* Frequency, microbial spectrum and outcome of spontaneous bacterial peritonitis in North India. Indian J Gastroenterol. 1996;15:86–9.
51. Castellote J, Xiol X, Verdaguer R *et al.* Comparison of two ascitic fluid culture methods in cirrhotic patients with spontaneous bacterial peritonitis. Am J Gastroenterol. 1990;85:1605–8.
52. Schölmerich J, Gerbes AL, Andus T, Leser HG. Spontaneous bacterial peritonitis in liver cirrhosis with ascites. Dtsch Med Wochenschr. 1995;120:454–61.
53. Hillebrand DJ, Runyon BA, Yasmineh WG, Rynders GP. Ascitic fluid adenosine deaminase insensitivity in detecting tuberculous peritonitis in the United States. Hepatology. 1996;24:1408–412.
54. Sanchez-Lombrana JL, de la Vega J, Fernandez E *et al.* Tuberculous peritonitis: diagnostic value of ascitic fluid pH and lactate. Scand J Gastroenterol. 1995;30:87–91.
55. Cappell MS, Shetty V. A multicenter, case-controlled study of the clinical presentation and etiology of ascites and of the safety and clinical efficacy of diagnostic abdominal paracentesis in HIV seropositive patients. Am J Gastroenterol. 1994;89:2172–7.
56. Runyon BA, Hoefs JC. Spontaneous vs secondary bacterial peritonitis. Differentiation by response of ascitic fluid neutrophil count to antimicrobial therapy. Arch Intern Med. 1986;146:1563–5.
57. Akriviadis EA, Runyon BA. Utility of an algorithm in differentiating spontaneous from secondary bacterial peritonitis. Gastroenterology. 1990;98:127–33.
58. Pacelli F, Doglietto GB, Alfieri S *et al.* Prognosis in intra-abdominal infections. Multivariate analysis on 604 patients. Arch Surg. 1996;131:641–5.
59. Caly WR, Strauss E. A prospective study of bacterial infections in patients with cirrhosis. J Hepatol. 1993;18:353–8.
60. Toledo C, Salmeron JM, Rimola A *et al.* Spontaneous bacterial peritonitis in cirrhosis: predictive factors of infection resolution and survival in patients treated with cefotaxime. Hepatology. 1993;17:251–7.
61. Silvain C, Besson I, Ingrand P, Mannant PR, Fort E, Beauchant M. Prognosis and long-term recurrence of spontaneous bacterial peritonitis in cirrhosis (letter). J Hepatol. 1993;19:188–9.
62. Tito L, Rimola A, Gines P, Llach J, Arroyo V, Rodes J. Recurrence of spontaneous bacterial peritonitis in cirrhosis: frequency and predictive factors. Hepatology. 1988;8:27–31.
63. Rolachon A, Cordier L, Bacq Y *et al.* Ciprofloxacin and long-term prevention of spontaneous bacterial peritonitis: results of a prospective controlled trial. Hepatology. 1995;22:1171–4.
64. Carey WD, Boayke A, Leatherman J. Spontaneous bacterial peritonitis: clinical and laboratory features with reference to hospital-acquired cases. Am J Gastroenterol. 1986;81:1156–61.
65. Follo A, Llovet JM, Navasa M *et al.* Renal impairment after spontaneous bacterial peritonitis in cirrhosis: incidence, clinical course, predictive factors and prognosis. Hepatology. 1994;20:1495–501.

28
Treatment and prophylaxis of spontaneous bacterial peritonitis

A. RIMOLA, M. NAVASA and J. RODÉS

INTRODUCTION

Spontaneous bacterial peritonitis (SBP) is the infection of a previously sterile ascitic fluid, with no apparent intra-abdominal source of infection. Although spontaneous bacterial peritonitis can theoretically appear in any patient with ascites, this type of infection is presented almost exclusively by cirrhotics with ascites. SBP usually occurs in cirrhotic patients with advanced liver disease.

PATHOGENESIS

It is possible that secondary bacteraemia in cirrhosis could be favoured by disturbances in the defensive mechanisms normally acting against localized infections, such as neutrophil dysfunction and the reduction of humoral defensive factors present in most of these patients. The other 50% of bacteraemic episodes are spontaneous. Since spontaneous bacteraemia is caused predominantly by enteric organisms, the most accepted pathogenic mechanisms for this type of infection are the following: (a) the depression of the hepatic reticuloendothelial system, which represents a failure of the liver in 'filtering' these bacteria, thereby allowing the passage of microorganisms from the bowel lumen to the systemic circulation via the portal vein; (b) the relative increase of aerobic Gram-negative bacilli in the jejunal flora in cirrhosis, and the possible alteration in the intestinal barrier caused by circumstances decreasing mucosal blood flow (e.g. acute hypovolaemia or splanchnic vasoconstrictor drugs); and (c) bacterial translocation, or the process by which enteric bacteria can cross the mucosa and infect the mesenteric lymph nodes, and reach the blood stream through the intestinal lymphatic circulation. To explain the mechanism of spontaneous bacteraemia caused by non-enteric bacteria, it can reasonably be assumed that these microorganisms enter the circulation from the skin or the upper respiratory tract, this pathogenesis being favoured in many cases by therapeutic or diagnostic procedures which rupture the natural mucocutaneous barriers. Whatever the source of the bacteria reaching the blood stream, a bacteraemic event could be more prolonged, and therefore could more readily become clinically significant in cirrhotic patients than in non-cirrhotic subjects, because of the marked depression of the reticuloendothelial system in the former. This assumption is supported by experimental data demonstrating that cirrhotic rats had more prolonged bacteraemia than normal animals after intravenous injection of *Escherichia coli*[1-5].

According to the most accepted hypothesis on the pathogenesis of SBP, the mechanisms by which cirrhotic patients with ascites develop this type of infection is the colonization of the ascitic fluid from an episode of bacteraemia[1]. Although the passage of microorganisms from the blood stream to the ascites has never been documented, it can be assumed that bacteria present in the circulation may easily reach the ascites because of the constant fluid exchange between these two compartments. Once microorganisms have colonized the ascites the development of peritonitis would depend on the defensive capacity of ascitic fluid. Patients with a decreased antimicrobial activity of ascitic fluid would develop SBP. The passage of enteric organisms from the bowel lumen to the peritoneal cavity through the intestinal wall, another theoretical mechanism for development of spontaneous bacterial peritonitis, has never been clinically or experimentally demonstrated.

CLINICAL AND LABORATORY DATA

The clinical picture of SBP has been described in detail in several excellent articles including a large number of patients with this infection[1-6]. Abdominal pain and fever are the most frequent signs presented by cirrhotics with SBP. The majority of patients complain of diffuse abdominal pain, often with rebound tenderness. However, it is important to point out that in some cases abdominal pain is localized or absent, particularly in patients seen in early stages of the infection or in patients with hepatic encephalopathy, leading to the possibility of misdiagnosis. Fever, although present in most cases, is not usually a prominent sign. Other clinical data frequently observed in patients with SBP are hepatic encephalopathy, gastrointestinal motility disturbances (vomiting, diarrhoea, or ileus), oliguria and septic shock. The development of septic shock in subjects with SBP has very poor prognostic significance. The frequency of presentation of these signs mainly depends on when SBP is diagnosed; the clinical picture in patients with early diagnosis is usually less expressive. In this setting it is important to note that approximately 10% of cirrhotic patients with SBP are completely asymptomatic at the time of the diagnosis of infection[3].

The most outstanding laboratory finding in patients with SBP is an increase in the ascitic fluid leucocyte count exclusively due to a marked rise in the number of polymorphonuclear leucocytes. The average polymorphonuclear cell count in ascitic fluid in cirrhotics with SBP reported in recent studies[6,7] is approximately 7000/ml. Nevertheless, although most patients with SBP show an undoubtedly increased ascitic fluid polymorphonuclear count, the minimum polymorphonuclear count capable of discriminating between infected ascites and non-infected ascites in cirrhosis has been debated for years. At present there is general agreement on the fact that 250 polymorphonuclear leucocytes/ml of ascitic fluid can be reasonably used as this cut-point and, therefore, can be useful for establishing the diagnosis of SBP and, more importantly, for making the decision to start antibiotic therapy, since this figure has a good sensitivity, specificity and diagnostic accuracy in cirrhotics with ascites[2,8]. Several authors have also reported a decrease in pH and an increase in lactate concentration in ascitic fluid from patients with SBP. The pH of ascitic fluids has been found to be lower than 7.35, and the arterial blood ascitic fluid pH gradient higher than 0.10 in most cases of SBP. Similarly, a considerable proportion of patients with SBP show a lactate concentration in ascitic fluid >25 mg/dl, and an ascitic fluid-arterial lactate gradient >20 mg/dl[8,9]. However, since the incidence and magnitude of the changes in ascitic fluid pH and lactate concentration vary greatly in patients with SBP studied by different authors, these alterations are difficult to interpret, thus limiting their diagnostic value.

MICROBIOLOGICAL DATA

Most cases of SBP in cirrhosis are caused by bacteria normally present in the intestinal flora. Individually, *E. coli* is the most common organism isolated from patients with these types of infection. However, ascitic fluid cultures are negative in a high proportion of patients with a clinical and laboratory picture of SBP, a condition called 'culture-negative neutrocytic ascites', which is currently considered as a variant of SBP[10,11]. This is mainly due to the fact that the number of bacteria in ascitic fluid in patients with SBP is usually very small (the concentration of organisms is lower than one per millilitre in most patients[12]). For increasing the probability of isolating causative organisms in this infection it is recommendable that media normally used for blood culture (aerobic and anaerobic bottles) are bedside inoculated with a large volume of ascitic fluid (10 ml or more)[12]. Nevertheless, approximately 30–50% of patients with SBP reported in recent large series have negative cultures regardless of the use of the most accurate microbiological methods[6,7,13,14].

Positive ascitic fluid cultures are obtained in approximately 5% of cirrhotic patients with ascites without clinical or biological signs of SBP when ascitic fluid is routinely cultured. The significance of this condition, usually called 'asymptomatic bacteriascites', is unclear, although it represents the stage of bacterial colonization of ascitic fluid. Some cases of asymptomatic bacteriascites progress to authentic SBP, while others may resolve spontaneously.

The same bacteria are isolated from ascitic fluid and blood cultures in 30–40% of patients with SBP[5,13]. In other patients blood cultures are positive but ascitic fluid culture is negative. In these cases, as in non-cirrhotic patients with haematogenous infections, it is reasonable to accept that the bacteria isolated from blood cultures are the causative organisms of SBP.

DIAGNOSIS

The existence of SBP should always be suspected when a cirrhotic patient develops fever, hepatic encephalopathy with unclear precipitating factor, acute renal function impairment without any apparent cause, or shock unrelated to a hypo-volaemic event. The appearance of abdominal pain in a cirrhotic patient with ascites must always be considered as a high index of suspicion of SBP. Therefore, whenever these signs appear, blood samples for cultures and total and differential white blood cell count, and ascitic fluid samples for cultures and cell count, should immediately be taken and processed. Since most SBP are present at the time of admission in patients referred to hospital for ascites, the aforementioned tests in ascitic fluid should also be performed on admission in ascitic cirrhotics. Urine culture and sediment and (in patients with hepatic encephalopathy) chest radiography should also be performed, since most urinary tract infections occur without signs suggesting urinary tract involvement, and pneumonia can be clinically inapparent in patients with profound encephalopathy.

Almost all episodes of peritonitis in cirrhotic patients with ascites are sponta-neous. Therefore, infection of the ascitic fluid in these patients should always be considered as SBP unless there are clinical or laboratory features indicating the possibility of a secondary peritonitis. This should be suspected when a patient shows one of the following features: (a) selective and persistent localized abdominal pain; (b) total protein concentration >1 g/dl, glucose <50 mg/dl, or lactic dehydrogenase greater than the upper limit of normal for serum, or (c) the isolation of more than one type of microorganism in the ascitic fluid culture, particularly when cultures grow anaerobic bacteria[5,15].

TREATMENT

Until the last decade the development of a serious bacterial infection in patients with advanced liver disease usually had ominous prognostic significance. This is no longer so. In our unit we have shown a progressive increase in the rate of res-olution of infection, and in survival, in different series of cirrhotics with SBP treated with therapeutic regimes over the past two decades. Although improved general management of patients with advanced liver failure may have played a role in the improvement of the prognosis of cirrhotics with severe bacterial infections, other important reasons could be earlier diagnosis of infective com-plications (and, therefore, earlier commencement of antimicrobial therapy) and better selection of antibiotics to be used in these patients. The importance of the early diagnosis, and the symptoms and signs on which the suspicion of severe infection must be established, has been stressed beforehand.

Since SBP is a severe infection, antimicrobial therapy must be started imme-diately it is suspected and, thus, before identification of the causative organism and knowledge of its *in-vitro* sensitivity. Until the decade of the 1980s, combin-ations of aminoglycosides and ampicillin, or first or second-generation cephalosporins, were the antibiotic regimes habitually used in these patients. However, these regimes were associated with a relatively low efficacy and a high risk of nephrotoxicity[16,17]. In 1984 a prospective, randomized trial compar-ing the efficacy and safety of tobramycin combined with ampicillin versus cefo-taxime in cirrhotic patients with severe infections (mostly SBP) demonstrated the superiority of cefotaxime administration in terms of higher infection resolution rate, lower incidence of side-effects and greater survival[18]. Since then, cefotaxime has been considered as one of the first-choice antibiotics for initial empirical therapy in severely infected cirrhotics. It is important to note that, according to the results of several studies reassessing the usefulness of cefotaxime in patients with SBP, the high efficacy and safety of this antimicrobial agent has remained almost unmodified up to the present in these patients, regardless of its wide use and the progressive reduction in its dosage[6,7,13,18-20]. The usefulness of other antibiotics has also been investigated in patients with SBP: several second- and third-generation cephalosporins (ceftriaxone, ceftizoxime and cefonicid), aztreonam, amoxicillin-clavulanic acid and different quinolones. All of them, with the exception of aztreonam, have shown adequate therapeutic efficacy and safety, although regimes including penicillin derivatives are associated with a relatively high incidence of superinfections[21-26]. Interestingly, in a recent study it has been reported that oral administration of ofloxaxin (a quinolone very effective against organisms commonly causing peritonitis in cirrhosis, with high bioavailability and adequate distribution to ascitic fluid after oral administration) is as effective as intravenous cefotaxime in uncomplicated SBP[27].

It is important to note that, in spite of the high rate of infection resolution obtained with the current antibiotic regimes, the mortality rate in patients with severe bacterial infection still remains relatively high. Approximately 20–40% of patients with SBP died while hospitalized. Prognostic factors in patients with this type of infection have recently been investigated in several studies[6,14,20], the most important clinical features adversely influencing the prognosis being nosocomial acquisition of the infection, advanced degree of severity of the underlying liver disease, and the existence of complications related to the peritonitis, such as shock, ileus or renal dysfunction. Furthermore, patients with SBP with markedly increased inflammatory response secondary to the ascitic fluid infection (estimated by high circulating and ascitic fluid levels of tumour necrosis factor-α (TNF-α) and interleukin 6 (IL-6), two cytokines involved in the initial steps of inflammation) showed a greater hospital mortality rate and a higher incidence of renal failure during the infectious episode than those with lower levels of these cytokines. These results raise the future possibility of modulating the inflammatory response as a co-adjuvant therapy in severely infected cirrhotics.

Another important feature concerning the outcome of patients with SBP is their poor mid- and long-term prognosis. The cumulative survival of patients recovering from the first episode of SBP has been estimated as low as 38% at 1 year and 16% at 3 years of follow-up[28]. Therefore, since the current survival probability in cirrhotic patients undergoing liver transplantation is much better than these figures, this therapeutic procedure should be considered in cirrhotics after resolving the first episode of this infection.

PROPHYLAXIS

Several groups of cirrhotics have been identified as being at particular risk of acquiring SBP. The most important of these groups are patients with marked derangements in the defensive mechanism, patients with circumstances (particularly gastrointestinal bleeding) contributing to the impairment of these mechanisms, patients with previous episodes of severe infections, and patients who undergo invasive procedures[28-32]. It is therefore logical that most studies investigating the possibility of prevention of infection in cirrhosis have involved the cirrhotic populations mentioned above.

Since bacterial infections in cirrhosis are predominantly caused by bacteria of enteric origin, most of these studies have been addressed to assess the efficacy of intestinal decontamination in these patients. The pioneer study consisted of a prospective, randomized, controlled trial on the prophylactic effect of 6-hourly administration of oral non-absorbable antibiotics (gentamicin; neomycin, colistin, vancomycin and nystatin, in different combinations) in a large series of cirrhotic patients with gastrointestinal haemorrhage[33]. Patients prophylactically treated with oral non-absorbable antibiotics showed a lower incidence of infection than those who did not receive these drugs (16% vs 35% respectively), this difference being particularly apparent when only infections caused by enteric organisms were considered (4% vs 21%, respectively). Infections caused by non-enteric bacteria were observed with a similar frequency in both groups of patients. These results indicate that intestinal decontamination is useful in preventing infection in cirrhotics with gastrointestinal bleeding.

However, the high frequency of administration and cost of the antibiotic regimes described above led to the investigation of other antimicrobial agents for the prevention of infection in cirrhotic patients. In this setting norfloxacin, a quinolone antibiotic poorly absorbed when orally administered, very effective *in vitro* against enterobacteria and capable of producing selective intestinal decontamination (that is, the elimination of aerobic Gram-negative bacilli from the faecal flora without changes in other microorganisms) in cirrhotic patients after a few doses of antibiotic has been investigated in several controlled studies. In one of these studies the oral administration of 400 mg/12 h of norfloxacin was very useful in reducing the incidence of infection in cirrhotic patients with gastrointestinal haemorrhage[34]. In this investigation bacterial infectious complications occurred in 10% of the patients receiving norfloxacin, and in 37% of the patients from the control group. This difference was due to a reduced incidence of infections caused by enteric bacteria in the treated group. In another study a markedly low incidence of in-hospital SBP was reported in ascitic cirrhotics with low ascitic fluid protein content when prophylactically treated with 400 mg/day of norfloxacin during the whole period of hospitalization (0% in the treated group versus 22% in the control group)[35]. Finally, in a multicentre, double-blind, placebo-controlled trial, long-term administration of 400 mg/day of norfloxacin was very effective in reducing the probability of SBP recurrence in patients who had recovered from an episode of this type of infection (20% in the treated group versus 68% in the placebo group at 1 year[36]. The 1-year probability of recurrence of SBP caused by Gram-negative bacilli was only 3% in the treated group, whereas it was 60% in the placebo group. Interestingly, in this study norfloxacin administration caused selective intestinal decontamination throughout the study period (mean follow-up period of 6 months, with a range of 1–19 months) without any association with overgrowth of resistant, potentially pathogenic bacteria or with increased faecal concentration of *Candida* spp.

More recently the effectiveness of antibiotics other than norfloxacin has also been investigated. In two studies, cirrhotics with ascites receiving long-term oral administration of ciprofloxacin (750 mg once a week)[37] or trimethoprim-sulphamethoxazole (one double strength tablet five times a week)[38], respectively, showed a reduced incidence of SBP as compared to patients not receiving this prophylaxis. In these investigations the incidence of the infection was approximately 3% in treated patients and 25% in control patients. In another controlled study systemic antibiotic therapy consisting of 10-day administration of ofloxacin (400 mg/day, first intravenously, then orally), plus intravenous amoxicillin–clavulanic acid before each endoscopic examination was also effective in preventing bacterial infection in cirrhotic patients with gastrointestinal haemorrhage (20% in the treated group versus 66% in the control group)[39].

References

1. Hoefs JC, Runyon BA. Spontaneous bacterial peritonitis. Disease-a-month. 1985;31:1–48.
2. Pinzello G, Simonetti RG, Craxi A, DiPiazza S, Spano C, Pagliaro L. Spontaneous bacterial peritonitis: a prospective investigation in predominantly nonalcoholic cirrhotic patients. Hepatology. 1983;3:545–9.
3. García-Tsao G. Spontaneous bacterial peritonitis. Gastroenterol Clin N Am. 1992;21:257–75.
4. Correia JP, Conn HO Am. Spontaneous bacterial peritonitis. Endemic or epidemic? Med Clin N Am. 1975;59:963–81.
5. Hoefs JC, Canawati HN, Sapico FL, Hopkins RR, Weiner J, Montgomery JZ. Spontaneous bacterial peritonitis. Hepatology. 1982;2:399–407.
6. Toledo C et al. Spontaneous bacterial peritonitis in cirrhosis: predictive factors of infection resolution and survival in patients treated with cefotaxime. Hepatology. 1993;17:251–7.
7. Rimola A et al. Two different dosages of cefotaxime in the treatment of spontaneous bacterial peritonitis in cirrhosis: results of a prospective, randomized, multicenter study. Hepatology. 1995;21:674–9.
8. Albillos A et al. Ascitic fluid polymorphonuclear cell count and serum to ascitis albumin gradient in the diagnosis of bacterial peritonitis. Gastroenterology. 1990;98:134–40.
9. Attali P, Turner K, Pelletier G, Ink O, Etienne JP. pH of ascitic fluid: diagnostic and prognostic value in cirrhotic and noncirrhotic patients. Gastroenterology. 1986;90:1255–60.
10. Runyon BA, Hoefs JC. Culture-negative neutrocytic ascites: a variant of spontaneous bacterial peritonitis. Hepatology. 1984;4:1209–11.
11. Terg R et al. Analysis of clinical course and prognosis of culture-positive spontaneous bacterial peritonitis and neutrocytic ascites. Evidence of the same disease. Dig Dis Sci. 1992;37:1499–504.
12. Runyon BA, Canawati HN, Akriviadis EA. Optimization of ascitic fluid culture technique. Gastroenterology. 1988;95:1351–5.
13. Runyon BA, McHutchison JG, Akriviadis EA, Montano AA. Short-course versus long-course antibiotic treatment of spontaneous bacterial peritonitis. A randomized controlled study of 100 patients. Gastroenterology. 1991;100:1737–42.
14. Llovet JM et al. Short-term prognosis of cirrhotics with spontaneous bacterial peritonitis: multivariate study. Am J Gastroenterol. 1993;88:388–92.
15. Runyon BA, Hoefs JC. Ascitic fluid analysis in the differentiation of spontaneous bacterial peritonitis from gastrointestinal tract perforation into ascitic fluid. Hepatology. 1984;4:447–50.
16. Cabrera J et al. Aminoglycoside nephrotoxicity in cirrhosis: value of urinary beta$_2$-microglobulin to discriminate functional renal failure from acute tubular damage. Gastroenterology. 1982;82:97–105.
17. Moore RD, Smith CR, Lietman PS. Increased risk of renal dysfunction due to interaction of liver disease and aminoglycosides. Am J Med. 1986;80:1093–7.
18. Felisart J et al. Cefotaxime is more effective than is ampicillin–tobramycin in cirrhotics with severe infections. Hepatology. 1985;5:457–62.
19. Ariza J et al. Aztreonam vs cefotaxime in the treatment of Gram-negative spontaneous bacterial peritonitis in cirrhotic patients. Hepatology. 1991;14:91–8.

20. Follo A et al. Renal impairment after spontaneous bacterial peritonitis in cirrhosis: incidence, clinical course, predictive factors and prognosis. Hepatology. 1994;20:1495–501.
21. Ariza J et al. Evaluation of aztreonam in the treatment of spontaneous bacterial peritonitis in patients with cirrhosis. Hepatology. 1986;6:906–10.
22. Mercader J. Gómez J, Ruiz J, Garre MC, Valdés M. Use of ceftriaxone in the treatment of bacterial infections in cirrhotic patients. Chemotherapy. 1989;35(Suppl. 2):23–6.
23. Gómez-Jiménez J et al. Randomized trial comparing ceftriaxone with cefonicid for treatment of spontaneous bacterial peritonitis in cirrhotic patients. Antimicr Ag Chem. 1993;37:1587–92.
24. Rimola A et al. Efficacy of ceftizoxime in the treatment of severe bacterial infections in patients with cirrhosis. Drug Invest. 1992;4:(Suppl. 1):35–7.
25. Granje JD et al. Amoxycillin–clavulanic acid therapy of spontaneous bacterial peritonitis: a prospective study of twenty-seven cases in cirrhotic patients. Hepatology. 1990;11:360–4.
26. Silvain C, Breux JP, Grollier G, Rouffineau J, Bezq-Giraudon B, Beauchant M. Les septicémies et les infections du liquide d'ascite du cirrhotique peuvent-elles être traitées exclusivement par voie orale? Gastroent Clin Biol. 1989;13:335–9.
27. Navasa M et al. Randomized, comparative study of oral norfloxacin versus intravenous cefotaxime in spontaneous bacterial peritonitis. Gastroenterology. 1996;111:1011–17.
28. Titó L, Rimola A, Ginés P, Llach J, Arroyo V, Rodés J. Recurrence of spontaneous bacterial peritonitis in cirrhosis: frequency and predictive factors. Hepatology. 1988;8:27–31.
29. Rimola A, Soto R, Bory F, Arroyo V, Piera G, Rodés J. Reticuloendothelial system phagocytic activity in cirrhosis and its relation to bacterial infections and prognosis. Hepatology. 1984;4:53–8.
30. Runyon BA. Low-protein concentration ascitic fluid is predisposed to spontaneous bacterial peritonitis. Gastroenterology. 1986;91:1343–6.
31. Llach J et al. Incidence and predictive factors of the first episode of spontaneous bacterial peritonitis in cirrhosis with ascites: relevance of ascitic fluid protein concentration. Hepatology. 1992;16:724–7.
32. Andreu M et al. Risk factors for spontaneous bacterial peritonitis in cirrhotic patients with ascites. Gastroenterology. 1993;104:1133–8.
33. Rimola A et al. Oral, nonabsorbable antibiotics prevent infection in cirrhosis with gastrointestinal hemorrhage. Hepatology. 1985;5:463–7.
34. Soriano G et al. Norfloxacin prevents bacterial infection in cirrhotics with gastrointestinal hemorrhage. Gastroenterology. 1992;103:1267–72.
35. Soriano G et al. Selective intestinal decontamination prevents spontaneous bacterial peritonitis. Gastroenterology. 1991;100:477–81.
36. Ginés P et al. Norfloxacin prevents spontaneous bacterial peritonitis recurrence in cirrhosis: results of a double-blind, placebo-controlled trial. Hepatology. 1990;12:716–24.
37. Rolanchon A et al. Ciprofloxacin and long-term prevention of spontaneous bacterial peritonitis: results of a prospective controlled trial. Hepatology. 1995;22:1171–4.
38. Singh N, Gayoswski T, Yu VL, Wagener MM. Trimethroprim-sulfamethoxazole for the prevention of spontaneous bacterial peritonitis in cirrhosis: a randomized trial. Ann Intern Med. 1995;122:595–8.
39. Blaise M, Pateron D, Trinchet JC, Levacher S, Beaugrand M, Pourriat JL. Systemic antibiotic therapy prevents bacterial infection in cirrhotic patients with gastrointestinal hemorrhage. Hepatology. 1994;20:34–8.

Section VII
Liver injury in patients with diseases of the gastrointestinal tract

29
Haemochromatosis: a defect in gut transport leads to liver injury

W. STREMMEL, C. SMOLAREK and S. GEHRKE

INCIDENCE AND GENETIC DEFECT

Genetic haemochromatosis is a common inherited disorder of iron metabolism. The mode of inheritance of the haemochromatosis trait is autosomal recessive. The gene defect has been localized to chromosome 6 in proximity to the HLA-A histocompatibility locus[1]. Based on pedigree analysis and HLA typing carried out in Europe, the USA, and Australia it was shown that HLA-A3 occurred in about 75% of patients with haemochromatosis compared to 28–30% in controls[1]. In various studies it was estimated that the gene frequency is 5–7%, and that about 0.3–0.45% of the population is homozygous for the haemochromatosis allele[1,2]. Recently the gene most likely responsible for genetic haemochromatosis, termed HFE (haemochromatosis Fe), has been identified[3]. It resembles a protein related to the MHC class I family localized on the short arm of chromosome 6 (Fig. 1). In about 80% of haemochromatotic patients a common mutation of the gene was identified at nucleotide 845 by a G to A transition. The resulting cysteine-to-tyrosine substitution at the amino acid position 282 (C282Y mutation) could result in disruption of the characteristic HFE structure (Fig. 1). This opens an intramolecular disulphide bridging which is essential for interaction with β2-microglobulin. Since β2-microglobulin is essential for export of MHC proteins and their insertion into the cell membrane, the C282Y mutation would prevent surface presentation of HFE. How this may induce iron overload in specific organs is still unknown. A hint may be given by the observation that β2-microglobulin knockout mice reveal severe iron overload[4]. However, the resulting biochemical defect is still not defined.

Another predominant point mutation in HFE can be found at amino acid position 63 (H63D mutation). This second mutation is not obviously involved in cellular iron accumulation[3]. It is still unclear how both mutations are involved in the pathogenesis of haemochromatosis. It is interesting to speculate whether the immune system may also play a role in the development of the disease.

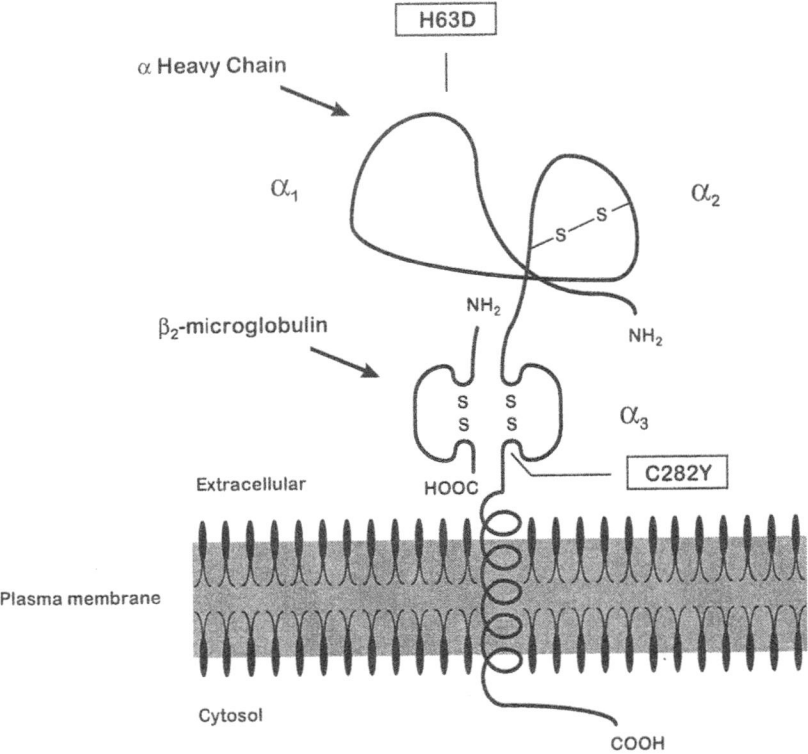

Figure 1 Hypothetical model of the HFE protein (from ref. 3)

PHYSIOLOGY OF IRON METABOLISM

The net pathophysiological effect of homozygosity of the haemochromatosis allele is iron overload of the organism. In advanced symptomatic disease total body storage iron may be increased to 20–40 g, compared to approximately 3–4 g of storage iron in normal subjects[5].

Under physiological conditions iron balance is regulated through control of iron absorption. Absorbed iron is highly conserved by the organism since no specific mechanisms for iron excretion are available except the obligatory losses through exfoliation of gastrointestinal mucosal cells, with smaller amounts being lost through bile, urine and skin[6]. These losses of 0.5–2 mg per day are balanced by controlled absorption of 0.5–2 mg of iron per day by the upper intestinal mucosa from a diet containing 10–20 mg of iron[7,8]. Iron stores and iron absorption appear to be reciprocally related: as iron stores decline absorption increases, and vice versa[8–14]. Similarly, increased plasma iron turnover is associated with increased iron absorption. Despite these phenomena the mechanisms of regulation of iron absorption, including signal transduction and involved mediators, are not known.

Absorption of dietary iron

In Western diets iron is present in equal amounts as haem iron (haemoglobin and myoglobin in meat) and non-haem iron (vegetables, fruits, cereals). Haem iron is taken up by the mucosal cells via endocytosis. The haem complex is then degraded by haem oxygenase, and Fe^{2+} is released for absorption in the body[15,16]. Non-haem iron is solubilized in the acid milieu of the stomach. This ionized iron (predominantly ferric iron) is complexed to small molecules such as ascorbic acid, citric acid, peptides, amino acids, sugars, fatty acids, and bile acids serving to prevent iron from precipitation[6,7,17]. This is of particular importance in the pH-neutral environment of the duodenum where the actual absorption process takes place[18].

Uptake of iron by mucosal cells involves several steps: (a) presentation of chelated iron to the cell surface; (b) binding and translocation across the microvillous membrane of the mucosal cell; (c) intracellular transport bound to an intracytoplasmic iron binding factor; (d) release at the basolateral site of the plasma membrane. In studies with human microvillous plasma membrane vesicles from duodenum it was shown that initially a reduction to Fe^{2+} by a membrane ferrireductase has to occur. This is followed by the essential step of translocation across the apical plasma membrane representing a facilitated, high-affinity transport system[19]. Several putative membrane proteins involved in this process have been identified[19-21]; however, definite proof of those as responsible membrane iron transporters is still missing. Recently, a new divalent cation transport protein (DCT1) of the Nramp family has been suggested as the iron membrane carrier protein[21]. After translocation across the plasma membrane, iron has to be complexed to an intracytoplasmic iron-binding factor, or ferritin itself, to prevent cell damage by the formation of hydroxyl radicals. Whether this factor represents a protein or a suitable organic chelator is still unclear. The cytoplasmic transit-iron pool is of significance for intracellular iron metabolism, because it co-ordinates the distribution of intracellular iron according to the cellular needs[22].

Iron storage proteins

Intracellular iron storage proteins are ferritin and haemosiderin, which are of particular importance in the liver[23,24]. Ferritin is a soluble cytoplasmic protein serving as pure iron storage protein with the ability of rapid accumulation and release of iron by a yet-unknown molecular mechanism[25]. Structurally, ferritin is a spheric complex composed of 24 apoferritin monomers of the isotypes H (heavy, 21 kDa) and/or L (light, 19 kDa) with a total apparent molecular weight of 450 000. To a small extent the complex ferritin molecule is released in plasma from which it is taken up by a specific ferritin receptor into certain cell types, e.g. hepatocytes[26,27]. Haemosiderin is present as an insoluble complex in secondary lysosomes, particularly in liver, serving as long-term or even final storage form of iron. It is assumed that haemosiderin is a proteolytic degradation product of ferritin[28]. Although this amorphous haemosiderin may remain relatively inert, it may be one major source of the labile iron thought to be of significance for cellular toxicity[29]. At the light microscopy level, excess soluble ferritin appears as a blue homogeneous coloration of the cytosol on Perl's

Prussian blue staining, while haemosiderin is identified by the same stain as blue granular deposits localized most densely around the biliary canaliculi of hepatocytes.

Transport of iron from gut to liver

The excretion mechanism of iron at the basolateral site of the mucosal cells is not completely understood. It is thought to involve the enzymatic formation of Fe^{2+} which passes plasma membranes easier than Fe^{3+} does[30]. After release from the basolateral site of the plasma membrane the toxic effects of Fe^{2+} (initiation of lipid peroxidation, oxidation of catecholamines) have to be prevented. It is postulated that Fe^{2+} has to be oxidized to Fe^{3+}. The responsible mechanism could involve ceruloplasmin. Iron can be transported via the portal blood to the liver by binding to low molecular weight natural chelating agents (amino acids, ascorbic acid, etc.). This non-transferrin-bound iron may be taken up by the hepatocytes by a membrane iron transport system similar to the one in apical membranes at mucosal cells (possibly DCT1).

The transferrin-bound iron is taken up by hepatocytes and other cells by the transferrin receptor endosomal pathway[24,31]. In addition a non-endosomal pathway for uptake of transferrin-bound iron was suggested[32,33]. It was thought to involve reduction of Fe^{3+}-transferrin at the transferrin receptor site with labilization of Fe^{2+} binding, translocation across the membrane and rapid incorporation into cytosolic ferritin. However, there were methodological problems with this study, and the concept of hepatic iron uptake by an iron reduction process is questionable[34].

Transferrin is a glycoprotein which, like other plasma glycoproteins, can be desialylated by liver endothelial cells[35]. This asialotransferrin may then be taken up into hepatocytes by asialoglycoprotein receptors and enter an endosomal compartment[36]. In contrast to the pathway of normal (sialylated) transferrin, asialotransferrin does not recycle to the plasma membrane, but is degraded in the lysosomal compartment[36]. While, under physiological conditions, this pathway is of not of major relevance, in alcoholism asialotransferrin is markedly increased, and correlates with the hepatic iron content and fibrosis, as well as with the amount of alcohol consumed (means for detection of alcohol abuse)[37,38].

In addition there are endocytotic pathways for hepatocellular incorporation of haem. Haem is taken up in the form of haemoglobin–haptoglobin complexes[39], as haem–haemopexin complexes[40] and possibly directly from haem–albumin complexes[41].

IRON METABOLISM IN HAEMOCHROMATOSIS

Definition and classification of haemochromatosis

The term 'haemochromatosis' defines the pathological deposition of excessive iron in the parenchymal cells of many organs, leading to cellular toxicity and damage followed by functional insufficiency. In genetic haemochromatosis the increase in total body iron stores is due to an inappropriately high level of intestinal iron absorption resulting from an inherited autosomal recessive abnormality in iron metabolism. When the accumulation of excess iron is due to other conditions, the term 'secondary iron overload syndrome' is used. Of particular importance are diseases associated with disordered erythropoiesis, usually thalassaemia or sideroblastic anaemia. In addition to the defect in iron utilization and increased intestinal iron absorption, those conditions are also complicated by a parenteral iron overload component due to the requirement of multiple blood transfusions. This latter component leads to excessive iron deposition initially confined to the reticuloendothelial system. In later stages iron is also transferred to the parenchymal cells resembling the organ distribution pattern in genetic haemochromatosis. The clinical features of advanced symptomatic haemochromatosis are characteristic. Patients usually present with lethargy, loss of libido, joint pain, symptoms related to the onset of diabetes mellitus or upper abdominal pain. Hepatomegaly, skin pigmentation, testicular atrophy/amenorrhoea, and arthropathy are the most prominent physical signs[42]. The clinical and biochemical expression of the disease varies, depending on such factors as age, sex, and chronic blood loss. The lower prevalence of symptomatic disease among females (1:10) is attributed to physiological iron losses and lower intake of dietary iron. Young patients, identified by family screening, are often asymptomatic[42]. They rarely present with advanced haemochromatosis. In these cases cardiomyopathy is a relatively frequent clinical feature.

Heterozygous carriers of the haemochromatosis gene may reveal minor biochemical expression of the disease with a slightly increased level of iron absorption in 20–30% of cases[43–45]. However, progressive iron overload with full clinical and biochemical expression is not a feature of heterozygous subjects; not even in subjects who have an excessive intake of alcohol[46–48].

Speculation concerning the underlying metabolic defect in genetic haemochromatosis

The genetic defect in genetic haemochromatosis leads to an inappropriate 2–4-fold increase in iron absorption. This indicates a disorder in the regulation of the iron absorption process.

Regulation of proteins involved in iron metabolism

The first question is whether a defect in the regulation of transferrin, transferrin receptor and ferritin, as key proteins of iron metabolism, is responsible for increased iron absorption from the gut. The transferrin receptor, although not involved in the uptake of iron at the luminal brushborder plasma membrane[49], was shown to be present at the basolateral site of duodenal mucosal cells[50–53]. At this site the transferrin receptor facilitates entry of iron into the mucosal cell from plasma by internalizing plasma-derived diferric transferrin. Transferrin receptors are increased in anaemia, particularly in iron-deficient states[54]. It is assumed that, under these conditions, iron is absorbed in greater amounts by the enterocyte and rapidly diverted to the blood stream. The reduction of the intracellular iron pool may activate mechanisms in an attempt to restore the iron balance of the organism. Concomitant with this activation of transferrin receptor gene expression, a decrease in ferritin mRNA was observed[54]. On the other hand, secondary iron overload conditions reveal a down-regulation of duodenal transferrin receptor and a significantly higher ferritin H- and L-subunit gene expression[54]. Both situations represent the physiological response of epithelial cells to iron deficiency and iron overload, accomplished by the concerted post-transcriptional regulation of the mRNAs for ferritin and transferrin receptor[55]. The expression of ferritin and transferrin receptor is regulated in response to changing levels of iron by alteration in mRNA translation efficiency and stability, respectively (Fig. 2). Excess of iron results in an increase in the translation of ferritin mRNA, whereas iron limitation decreases ferritin mRNA translation. The synthesis of transferrin receptor is regulated in the opposite direction: due to changes in mRNA stability an increase in iron deficiency and a decrease in excess of iron can be observed. Transferrin receptor regulation allows for modulation of iron uptake, and ferritin regulation allows for the adequate sequestration of excess iron and minimizes sequestration when iron is limited. The opposite but co-ordinate regulation of these two genes is mediated by similar cis-acting RNA sequence/structure motifs forming moderately stable stem-loop configurations in the untranslated regions of both mRNAs (iron responsive elements, IRE)[56]. While for ferritin the IRE is localized in the 5′-untranslated region of the mRNA, and controls translation initiation, the IRE of the transferrin receptor is localized at the 3′-untranslated region of the mRNA[56]. A common trans-acting RNA-binding protein (IRE-BP, also called iron regulatory protein IRP) serves as key participant in the regulation of both genes[57,58]. This IRP binds under iron-deficient conditions to the IRE of both mRNA. This binding is mediated by a complex mechanism ('iron–sulphur switch') controlled by the cellular iron status[59,60]. Binding to the IRE at the 5′-untranslated region of the ferritin mRNA inhibits translation, while binding to the 3′ IRE of the transferrin receptor mRNA stabilizes the message. The net result is that, in iron deficiency, ferritin biosynthesis is decreased while transferrin receptor expression is increased. The reverse mechanism acts in secondary iron overload, in which ferritin expression is high and transferrin receptor expression is low.

Pattern of protein expression in genetic haemochromatosis

High ferritin and low transferrin receptor expression is also observed in the liver of patients with untreated genetic haemochromatosis[61,62]. However, in the duodenal mucosa of these patients no decrease in transferrin receptor mRNA was seen, although it was expected on the basis of the increased body iron stores[54]. In addition a low level of ferritin transcripts was detected[54]. Thus, in subjects with genetic haemochromatosis, duodenal ferritin and transferrin receptor mRNA are still modulated in concert. Low ferritin and high transferrin receptor concentrations (high IRP activity) in genetic haemochromatosis trigger the intestinal mucosa as iron-deficient (low mucosal iron content), as observed in anaemic and sideropenic patients, although body iron stores are increased ('paradoxical' mucosal iron deficiency). This low mucosal iron situation may induce an accelerated transfer of iron to the blood, and may represent the key pathogenetic feature in haemochromatosis. The mechanism by which the duodenal mucosa is sensed as iron-deficient in genetic haemochromatosis is still unclear.

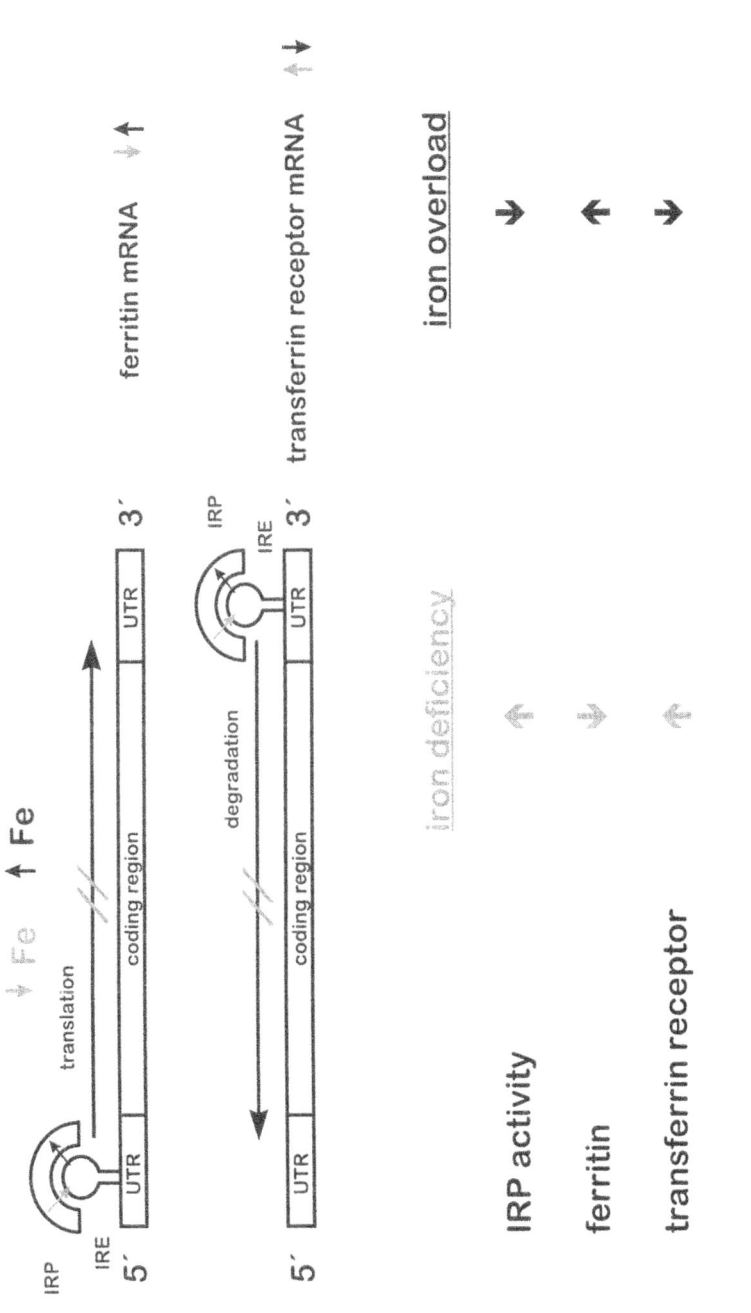

Figure 2 Iron-dependent post-transcriptional regulation of messenger RNA of ferritin and transferrin receptor by iron-responsive element (IRE) and iron regulatory protein (IRP)

Here the candidate gene for haemochromatosis comes into play. Very recent observations indicate that HFE is expressed in mucosal cells of the intestine[63]. The presence at the basolateral site of the mucosal cells could sense interaction with HFE-detecting cells of the lymphatic system or macrophages. They could signal the iron status of the body to enterocytes: high iron content of these cells may, by an unknown mechanism, trigger low IRP activity (high ferritin, low transferrin receptor, Fig. 2) thus prohibiting iron absorption. Low iron concentrations in HFE-detecting cells would induce high iron absorption (IRP activity increased). In genetic haemochromatosis there may be no signalling of iron to mucosal cells because of lack of HFE membrane expression. As a result IRP activity is up-regulated. Whether it is indeed the lack of iron signalling to the mucosal cells remains to be established.

The following hypothesis concerning the pathogenesis in genetic haemochromatosis can be proposed. The missing interaction of HFE-presenting mucosal cells with lymphocytes/macrophages sensing the body iron status results in high IRP activity (Fig. 3). This induces an iron-deficiency situation in mucosal cells, triggering increased absorption of iron. This is rapidly translocated across the enterocyte and, as non-transferrin-bound iron, transported via portal venous blood to the liver. Here, with time, an iron overload situation is created by trapping of excess iron. Consequently IRP activity is reduced with high ferritin and low transferrin receptor levels (Fig. 2).

Pathophysiological consequences of iron overload

Increased iron absorption leads to a positive iron balance and accumulation of excess body iron in genetic haemochromatosis. It is interesting that only specific organs are affected by iron loading. Those include liver, pancreas and, to a lesser extent, endocrine glands, particularly the pituitary, as well as heart and joints.

The dark pigmentation of the skin, although a typical clinical feature, is not alone due to iron deposits. The epidermis of the skin is thin, and increased melanin is found in the cells of the basal layer.

Deposits of iron are observed around the synovial lining cells of joints, and calcium pyrophosphate crystals may be seen within deposits of calcium embedded in the synovial tissue. This arthropathy develops in 25–30% of patients at any stage of the disease[64]. The small joints of the hands (second and third

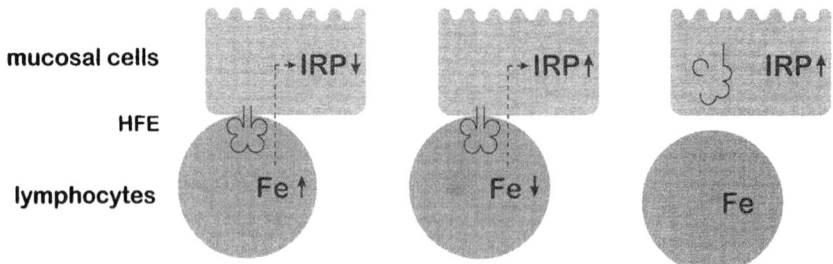

Figure 3 Hypothetical interaction of lymphocytes with mucosal cells presenting wild-type forms of HFE and lack of interaction in mutant forms (C282Y) of HFE

metacarpophalangeal joints) are the first joints to be involved. A progressive polyarthritis involving wrists, hips, and knees may ensue. Roentgenological manifestations consist of subchondral sclerosis and cystic changes, loss of articular cartilage, diffuse demineralization, hypertrophic bone proliferation and calcification of the synovium.

The parenchymal deposits of iron in the liver of patients with genetic haemochromatosis consist of ferritin and haemosiderin. In early stages these deposits are found in the periportal parenchymal cells, especially within lysosomes in the pericanalicular cytoplasm of the hepatocytes. This stage progresses to perilobular fibrosis and deposition of iron in the bile duct epithelium, Kupffer cells, and fibrous septa. In advanced disease the pattern of cirrhosis is characterized by broad fibrous septa surrounding large areas of comparatively normal parenchyma. Hepatocellular carcinoma without iron deposition in tumour cells is observed in about 30% of cirrhotic patients, even after removal of excess body iron stores by phlebotomy therapy[42]. The pathogenesis of hepatocellular carcinoma is uncertain. One hypothesis suggests a relation to increased oxidative stress produced by iron with oxidant damage to the DNA, acting as initiator or promotor of carcinogenesis[65,66]. The suggestion that there may be a link to concomitant HBV infection with integration of HBV DNA into the host's genome is intriguing, but not yet conclusively proven[67].

Although iron deposits in the pancreas are predominantly localized in the exocrine parenchyma, with development of tissue fibrosis, functional impairment of digestive enzyme secretion is a rare clinical feature. However, the selective accumulation of iron in B cells of the endocrine pancreas in advanced disease contributes to the diabetes often observed in these patients[42]. Along with the component of impaired insulin secretion by damaged B cells, there is an almost obligatory insulin resistance observed in iron overload disease[68]. This is due to an insulin receptor/post-receptor defect in the iron loaded liver, which is – in contrast to the destruction of the B cells – reversible after completion of the phlebotomy therapy[68].

Iron deposition in the heart is observed in 15% of patients. Those deposits are more extensive in ventricular than in atrial myocardium, resulting in intracellular disruption[69]. The ensuing haemodynamic derangement is generally designated as dilated cardiomyopathy, but some patients may have a pattern of myocardial restriction[70].

Another cell type which selectively accumulates iron in genetic haemochromatosis is the hypogonadotropic cell of the pituitary gland. Iron-induced cell damage leads to impaired secretion of follicle-stimulating hormone and luteinizing hormone, which results in the clinical manifestation of hypogonadotropic hypogonadism with impotence in males and amenorrhoea in females[68]. Despite secondary low testosterone levels in male patients, peripheral sexual hormone metabolism remains unaltered[68].

Why certain organs and cells are particularly affected by excessive iron accumulation remains unclear. It is not the expression of transferrin receptors or ferritin receptors which is responsible for the specific distribution of excessive iron deposition in certain cell types.

Interestingly, in patients with haemochromatosis there is a significant fraction of non-transferrin-bound iron in plasma, which gradually decreases during the course of phlebotomy treatment[71,72]. This represents iron ions ligated to low-molecular mass organic molecules such as citrate, which do not exchange to a significant extent with the free binding sites on the transferrin molecule[71]. This source of iron is not obviously correlated with the concentration of total plasma non-haem iron, with the exception that it is usually present when plasma iron is greater than 40 μmol/L[71]. Although this non-transferrin-bound iron does not strongly correlate with the transferrin saturation in plasma, there may be a correlation to the serum ferritin concentration. It has been implied that, in haemochromatosis, this low-molecular mass iron complex enters the circulation from the gut[73]. Studies in rats and mice have shown that the liver has an effective uptake system for these non-transferrin-bound iron ions[74-76].

Mechanisms of iron-induced cellular toxicity

Why does iron overload of cells induce cell damage and cell death, with the consequence of functional impairment and structural organ damage? This will be discussed using the example of liver cell injury. Several mechanisms whereby excess hepatic iron causes cellular injury with resultant fibrosis and cirrhosis have been proposed. Iron-induced peroxidative injury to phospholipids of organelle membranes, in particular of lysosomes and mitochondria, is the key pathogenetic factor[77,78]. Additional mechanisms may represent iron-stimulated depletion of vitamin E and C stores[79,80], and possibly low glutathione levels[81], as well as a direct stimulation of collagen synthesis by iron[82]. It is well established that ionic iron forms highly reactive free radicals, especially from oxygen. In order to exert potent oxidizing effects, iron must be present in a reactive and presumably low molecular weight form because ferritin- or transferrin-bound iron is relatively unreactive[83,84]. One candidate for this source of iron may be the non-transferrin-bound iron which is complexed, e.g. to citrate. This is present in significant concentration in the circulation of haemochromatotic patients[71], and readily taken up by hepatocytes (see above). Alternatively it is possible that cellular reductants are capable of enhancing the mobilization of iron from cellular ferritin stores[29]. Moreover, at pH 4.5 (found within lysosomes) iron from haemosiderin is available for initiation of lipid peroxidation without addition of reductants[29]. Such low molecular chelate or free ionic iron may play a catalytic role in the initiation of peroxidative injury, either by the Fenton reaction:

$$Fe^{2+} + O_2 \longrightarrow Fe^{3+} + \cdot O_2$$
$$\cdot O_2 + O_2 \xrightarrow{+2H+} H_2O_2$$
$$Fe^{2+} + H_2O_2 \longrightarrow Fe^{3+} + OH^- + \cdot OH$$

or by the iron-catalysed Haber–Weiss reaction:

$$Fe^{3+} \text{ complex} + O_2^- \longrightarrow Fe^{2+} \text{ complex} + O_2$$
$$Fe^{2+} \text{ complex} + H_2O_2 \longrightarrow Fe^{3+} \text{ complex} + OH^- + \cdot OH$$

Net reaction: $O_2 + H_2O_2 \xrightarrow{\text{Fe-complex}} O_2 + OH^- + \cdot OH$

The derived hydroxyl radical ($\cdot$ OH) is highly reactive and capable of initiating numerous free radical cascades and oxidations. Others[85] have questioned the involvement of hydroxyl radicals, and proposed the initiation of lipid peroxidation by Fe^{2+} and H_2O_2 in a reaction mediated by an oxidant requiring both Fe^{3+} and Fe^{2+}.

Regardless of the initiating species the consequence is a peroxidative decomposition of polyunsaturated fatty acids of organelle membrane phospholipids. This damage to cellular organelle membranes causes loss of fluidity, changes in membrane potential, increased permeability to ions, and eventual rupture leading to release of cell and organelle content[77,78].

Increased lability of iron-loaded lysosomes leads to increased autophagy of hepatocytes, accounting for the characteristic changes in liver biopsy specimens from haemochromatotic patients[86]. In mitochondria iron-induced lipid peroxidation impairs, among other enzymes, the activity of cytochrome oxidase, the terminal enzyme of the mitochondrial electron transport chain[77]. Microsomal lipid peroxidation is associated with a decrease in the concentration and activity of cytochrome P450[81].

In addition, tissue concentrations of vitamin C and E, to physiological antioxidants, are often decreased in haemochromatosis, perhaps due to increased vitamin oxidation catalysed by iron[78,80]. Therefore it is conceivable that the deficiency of these two antioxidants may be of relevance in perpetuating the lipid peroxidation process. Moreover, glutathione, the key compound in protecting cells against numerous toxins and oxidative stress, was found to be significantly decreased in experimentally iron-overloaded rats[81]. However, this could not yet be detected in liver biopsy specimens of patients with genetic haemochromatosis[87].

Lipid peroxidation induces cell degeneration and cell death. This continuous process is followed by permanent regeneration of hepatocytes and proliferation of fibroblasts with increased synthesis of collagen leading to cirrhosis. In addition, it was proposed that excess tissue iron may provide a direct stimulus to collagen biosynthesis, leading to the development of fibrosis without preceeding iron-mediated cellular injury[82].

LIVER TRANSPLANTATION IN GENETIC HAEMOCHROMATOSIS

The above-described mechanisms favour the hypothesis that genetic haemochromatosis is due to increased intestinal iron absorption. This may be the result of a mutation in the HFE gene, preventing interaction with iron-sensing lymphocytes or macrophages and intestinal mucosal cells. If the genetic defect were located to the intestine, liver transplantation could not cure the disease. Indeed, in a series of liver-transplanted patients with haemochromatosis there was evidence for recurrent iron accumulation in the liver[88]. Due to incomplete documentation and a short period of follow-up conclusive evidence may not be drawn at this time. The observed poor outcome of liver transplantation in these patients is also of interest (Fig. 4). This may be explained by free radical injury due to increased presentation of non-transferrin-bound iron (increased iron absorption) to the transplanted liver. The data are compatible with the hypothesis that the metabolic defect is localized in the gut.

Interesting observations result from accidental transplantation of haemochromatotic livers in patients with acute hepatic failure. In these situations increased

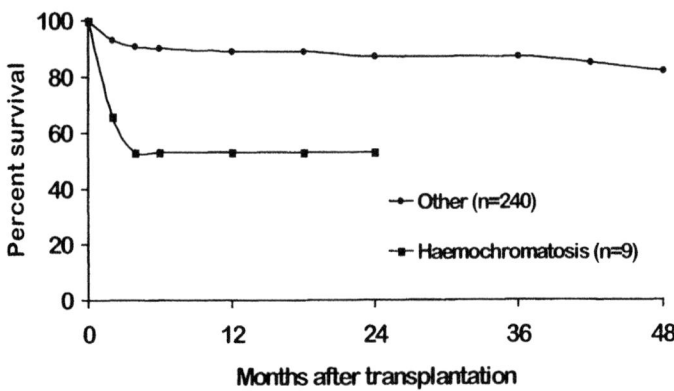

Figure 4 Survival of patients with haemochromatosis after liver transplantation (modified from ref. 88)

serum ferritin levels dropped to normal, and the high liver iron levels normalized with time (Figs 5 and 6)[89,90]. These observations do not favour the hypothesis that the defect is localized in the liver. Although these results of case reports in liver-transplanted patients have circumstantial character, they may be taken as indirect evidence for the proposed hypothesis that genetic haemochromatosis is due to a metabolic defect of iron metabolism in the gut, rendering the mucosal cells iron-deficient, and leading to increased iron absorption in these patients.

Acknowledgement

This work was supported by grants STR 92/4, 216/4–1 and SFB 1628 from the Deutsche Forschungsge-meinschaft.

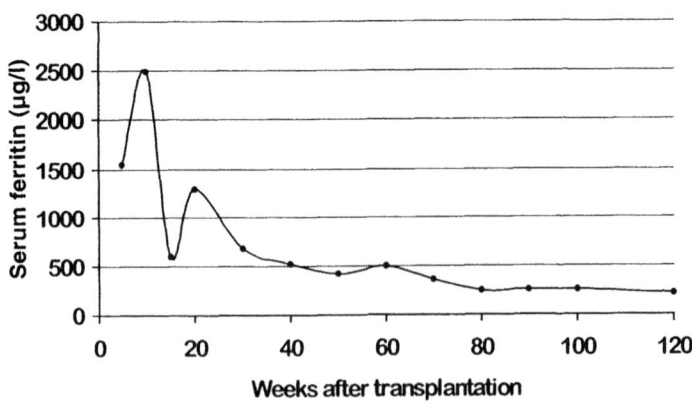

Figure 5 Serum ferritin after transplantation of a donor liver with haemochromatosis (modified from ref. 90)

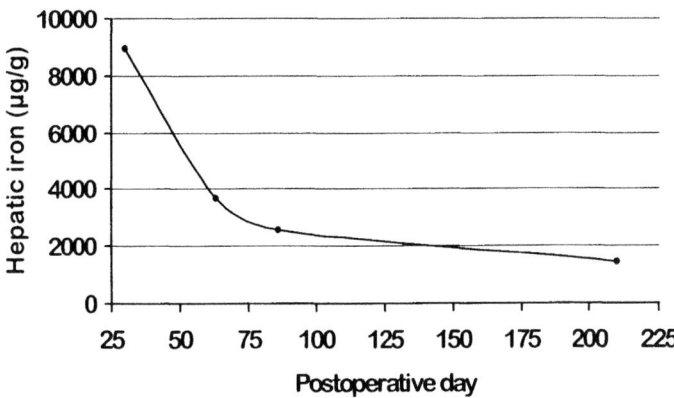

Figure 6 Hepatic iron content after transplantation of a donor liver with haemochromatosis (modified from ref. 89)

References

1. Simon M, LeMignon L, Fauchet R *et al.* A study of 609 HLA haplotypes marking the hemochromatosis gene (1) mapping of the gene near the HLA-A locus and characters required to define a heterozygous population and (2) hypothesis concerning the underlying cause of hemochromatosis HLA association. Am J Hum Genet. 1987;41:89–105.
2. Edwards CQ, Griffen LM, Goldgar D, Drummond C, Skolnick MH, Kushner JP. Prevalence of hemochromatosis among 11,065 presumably healthy blood donors. N Engl J Med. 1988;318:1355–62.
3. Feder J, Gnirke W, Thomas W *et al.* A novel MHC class I-like gene is mutated in patients with hereditary haemochromatosis. Nature Genet. 1996;13:399–408.
4. Rothenberg BE, Volands JR. β_2 Knockout mice develop parenchymal iron overload: a putative role for class I genes of the major histocompatibility complex in iron metabolism. Proc Natl Acad Sci USA. 1996;93:1529–34.
5. Bomford A, Williams R. Long term results of venesection therapy in idiopathic haemochromatosis. Q J Med. 1976;45:611–23.
6. Powell LW, Halliday JW. Iron absorption and iron overload. Clin Gastroenterol. 1982;10:707–35.
7. Charlton RW, Bothwell TH. Iron absorption. Annu Rev Med. 1983;34:55–68.
8. Strohmeyer GW, Miller SA, Scarlata RW, Moore EW, Greenberg MS, Chalmers TC. Effect of hypoxia on iron absorption and mobilization in the rat. Am J Physiol. 1964;207:55–60.
9. Conrad ME, Parmley RT, Osterloh K. Small intestinal regulation of iron absorption in the rat. J Lab Clin Med. 1987;110:416–26.
10. Raja KB, Bjarnason I, Simpson RJ, Peters TJ. *In vitro* measurement and adaptive response of Fe^{3+} uptake by mouse intestine. Cell Biochem Funct. 1987;5:69–76.
11. Hahn PF, Bale WF, Ross JR, Balfour WM, Whipple GH. Radioactive iron absorption by gastro-intestinal tract. J Exp Med. 1943;78:169–88.
12. Reynafarje C, Ramos J. Influence of altitude changes on intestinal iron absorption. J Lab Clin Med. 1961;57:848–55.
13. Brissot P, Campion JP, Guillouzo A *et al.* Experimental hepatic iron overload in the baboon: results of a two year study. Dig Dis Sci. 1983;28:616–24.
14. Huebers HA, Brittenham GM, Sciba E, Finch CA. Absorption of carbonyl iron. J Lab Clin Med. 1986;108:473–8.
15. Grasbeck R, Kouvonen I, Lundberg M, Tenhunen R. An intestinal receptor for heme. Haematologia. 1979;23:5–9.
16. Raffin SB, Woo CH, Rooste KT, Prince DM, Schmid R. Intestinal absorption of hemoglobin iron–heme cleavage by mucosal heme oxygenase. J Clin Invest. 1974;54:1344–52.

17. Bezkorovainy A. Biochemistry of nonheme iron in man. II. Absorption of iron. Clin Physiol Biochem. 1989;7:53–69.
18. Hungerford DM, Linder M. Interactions of pH and ascorbate in intestinal iron absorption. J Nutr. 1983;113:2615–22.
19. Teichmann R, Stremmel W. Iron uptake by human upper small intestine microvillus membrane vesicles: indication for a facilitated transport mechanism mediated by a membrane iron-binding protein. J Clin Invest. 1990;86:2145–53.
20. Conrad ME, Umbrelt JN. A concise review: iron absorption – the mucin–mobilferrin-integrin pathway. Am J Hematol. 1993;42:67–73.
21. Gunshin H, Mackenzie B, Berger UV, et al. Cloning and characterization of a mammalian proton-coupled metal-ion transporter. Nature. 1997;388:482–7.
22. Jacob A. Low molecular weight intracellular iron transport compounds. Blood. 1977;50:433–9.
23. Theil EM. Ferritin: structure, gene regulation, and cellular function in animals, plants and microorganisms. Annu Rev Biochem. 1987;56:289–315.
24. Bezkorovainy A. Biochemistry of nonheme iron in man. I. Iron proteins and cellular iron metabolism. Clin Physiol Biochem. 1989;7:1–17.
25. Halliday JW, Powell LW. Ferrin metabolism and the liver. Semin Liver Dis. 1984;4:207–16.
26. Mack U, Powell LW, Halliday JW. Detection and isolation of a hepatic membrane receptor for ferritin. J Biol Chem. 1983;258:4672–5.
27. Mack U, Storey EL, Powell LW, Halliday JW. Characterization of the binding of ferritin to the rat liver ferritin receptor. Biochim Biophys Acta. 1985;843:164–70.
28. Peters TJ, Ward RJ, Dickson DPE, Mann S. The haemosiderins. International conference on proteins of iron transport and storage. Brisbane, Australia, 1989 (abstract).
29. O'Connell MJ, Ward JR, Baum H. The role of iron in ferritin and hemosiderin-mediated lipid peroxidation in lysosomes. Biochem J. 1985;229:135–9.
30. Eastham EJ, Bell JI, Douglas AP. Iron-transport characteristics of vesicles of brush-border and basolateral plasma membrane from the rat enterocyte. Biochem J. 1977;164:289–94.
31. Dautry-Varsat A, Ciechanover A, Lodish HF. pH and the recycling of transferrin during receptor-mediated endocytosis. Proc Natl Acad Sci USA. 1983;80:2258–62.
32. Thorstensen K, Romslo I. Uptake of iron from transferrin by isolated rat hepatocytes. A redox-mediated plasma membrane process. J Biol Chem. 1988;263:8844–50.
33. Thorstensen K, Romslo I. The role of transferrin in the mechanism of cellular iron uptake. Biochem J. 1990;271:1–10.
34. Thorstensen K, Aisen P. Release of iron from diferric transferrin in the presence of rat liver plasma membranes: no evidence of a plasma membrane diferric transferrin reductase. Biochem Biophys Acta. 1990;1052:29–35.
35. Irie S, Kishimoto R, Tavassoli M. Desialylation of transferrin by rat liver endothelium. J Clin Invest. 1988;82:508–13.
36. Ashwell G, Morell AG. The role of surface carbohydrates in the hepatic recognition and transport of circulating glycoproteins. Adv Enzymol Relat Areas Mol Biol. 1987;41:99–128.
37. Regoeczi E, Chindemi PA, Debanne MT. Transferrin glycans: a possible link between alcoholism and hepatic siderosis. Alcohol Clin Exp Res. 1984;8:287–92.
38. Stibler H, Borg S. Evidence of reduced sialic acid content in serum transferrin in male alcoholics. Alcohol Clin Exp Res. 1981;5:545–9.
39. Kino K, Tsunoo H, Higa Y, Takami M, Hamaguchi H, Nakajima H. Hemoglobin-haptoglobin receptor in rat liver plasma membrane. J Biol Chem. 1980;255:9616–20.
40. Smith A, Morgan WT. Haem transport to the liver by haemopexin. Receptor-mediated uptake with recycling of the protein. Biochem J. 1979;82:47–54.
41. Sinclair PR, Bement WJ, Gorman N, Liem HH, Wolkoff AW, Müller-Eberhard U. Effect of serum proteins of haem uptake and metabolism in primary cultures of liver cells. Biochem J. 1988;256:159–65.
42. Niederau C, Fischer R, Sonnenberg A, Stremmel W, Trampisch HJ, Strohmeyer G. Survival and causes of death in cirrhotic and noncirrhotic patients with primary hemochromatosis. N Engl J Med. 1985;313:1256–62.
43. Beaumont C, Simon M, Fauchet R. Serum ferritin as a possible marker of the hemochromatosis allele. N Engl J Med. 1979;301:169–74.
44. Cartwright G, Edwards C, Kravitz K. Hereditary hemochromatosis: phenotypic expression of the disease. N Engl J Med. 1979;301:175–9.

45. Valberg LS, Lloyd DA, Ghent CN. Clinical and biochemical expression of the genetic abnormality in idiopathic hemochromatosis. Gastroenterology. 1980;79:884–92.
46. Bassett ML, Halliday JW, Powell LW. Value of hepatic iron measurements in early hemochromatosis and determination of the critial iron level associated with fibrosis. Hepatology. 1986;6:24–9.
47. Simon M, Bourtel M, Genetet B. Idiopathic hemochromatosis and iron overload in alcoholic liver disease: differentiation by HLA phenotype. Gastroenterology. 1977;73:655–8.
48. Tavill AS, Bacon BR. Hemochromatosis: iron metabolism and the iron overload syndromes. In: Zakim D, Boyer TD, editors. Hepatology: a textbook of liver disease. Philadelphia, PA: WB Saunders; 1989;1273–99.
49. Peters TJ, Raja BK, Simpson RJ, Snape S. Mechanisms and regulation of intestinal iron absorption. Ann NY Acad Sci. 1989;189:141–7.
50. Levine JS, Seligman PA. The ultrastructural immunocytochemical localization of transferrin receptor (TFR) and transferrin (TF) in the gastrointestinal tract of man. Gastroenterology. 1984;86:1161.
51. Parmeley RT, Barton CJ, Conrad ME. Ultrastructural localization of transferrin, transferrin receptor and iron binding sites in human placental and duodenal microvilli. Br J Haematol. 1985;60:81–9.
52. Banerjee D, Flanagan PR, Cluett J, Valbert LS. Transferrin receptors in the human gastrointestinal tract. Relationship to body iron stores. Gastroenterology. 1986;91:861–9.
53. Mattia E, den Blaauwen J, van Renswoude J. Role of protein synthesis in the accumulation of ferritin mRNA during exposure of cells to iron. Biochem J. 1990;267:553–5.
54. Pietrangelo A, Rocchi E, Casalgrandi G et al. Regulation of transferrin, transferrin receptor, and ferritin genes in human duodenum. Gastroenterology. 1990;102:802–9.
55. Theil CE. Regulation of ferritin and transferrin receptor mRNAs. J Biol Chem. 1990;265:4771–4.
56. Hentze MW, Caughman SW, Casey JL et al. A model for the structure and functions of iron-responsive elements. Gene. 1988;72:201–8.
57. Leibold EA, Munro HB. Cytoplasmic protein binds in vitro to a highly conserved sequence in the 5′ untranslated region of ferritin heavy- and light-subunit mRNAs. Proc Natl Acad Sci USA. 1988;85:2171–5.
58. Rouault TA, Hentze MW, Caughman SW, Harford JB, Klausner RD. Binding of a cytosolic protein to the iron-responsive element of human ferritin messenger RNA. Science. 1988;241:1207–10.
59. Haile DJ, Hentze MW, Rouault RA, Harford JB, Klausner RD. Regulation of interaction of the iron-responsive element binding protein with iron-responsive RNA elements. Mol Cell Biol. 1989;9:5055–61.
60. Hentze MW, Rouault RA, Harford JB, Klausner RD. Oxidation–reduction and the molecular mechanism of a regulatory RNA–protein interaction. Science. 1989;244:357–9.
61. Pietrangelo A, Casalgrandi G, Gualdi R, Cairo G, Ventura E. Studies on the regulation of liver gene expression in experimental and human siderosis. J Hepatol. 1991;31:60.
62. Sciot R, Paterson A, Van den Oord JJ, Desmet V. Lack of hepatic transferrin receptor expression in hemochromatosis. Hepatology. 1987;7:831–7.
63. Parkkila S, Waheed A, Britton RS et al. Immunohistochemistry of HLA-H, the protein defective in patients with hereditary hemochromatosis. Proc Natl Acad Sci USA. 1997;94:2534–9.
64. Hamilton EBD, Bomford AB, Laws JW, Williams R. The natural history of arthritis in idiopathic hemochromatosis: progression of the clinical and radiologic features over ten years. QJ Med. N.S., 1982;199:321–9.
65. Gutteridge JMC, Rowley DA, Griffiths E, Halliwell B. Low-molecular-weight iron complexes and oxygen radical reactions in idiopathic haemochromatosis. Clin Sci. 1985;68:463–71.
66. Halliwell B, Gutteridge JMC. Oxygen free radicals and iron in relation to biology and medicine. Some problems and concepts. Arch Biochem Biophys. 1986;246:501–11.
67. Blumberg BS. Hepatitis B virus, iron and iron-binding proteins. In: Szentivanyi A, Friedman H, editors. Viruses, immunity and immunodeficiency. London: Plenum Press; 1986;110–20.
68. Stremmel W, Niederau C, Berger M, Kley HK, Krüskemper HL, Strohmeyer G. Abnormalities in estrogen, androgen, insulin metabolism in idiopathic hemochromatosis. Ann NY Acad Sci. 1988;526:209–23.
69. Buja LM, Robert WC. Iron in the heart, etiology and clinical significance. Am J Med. 1971;51:209–21.

70. Dabestani A, Child JS, Henze E *et al.* Primary hemochromatosis: anatomic and physiologic characteristics of the cardiac ventricles and their response to phlebotomy. Am J Cardiol. 1984;54:153–9.
71. Arouma OI, Bomford A, Polson RJ, Halliwell B. Nontransferrin-bound iron in plasma from hemochromatosis patients: effect of phlebotomy therapy. Blood. 1988;72:1416–19.
72. Grootveld M, Bell JD, Halliwell B, Okezie IA, Bomford A, Sadler PJ. Non-transferrin-bound iron in plasma or serum from patients with idiopathic hemochromatosis. J Biol Chem. 1989;264:4417–22.
73. Batey RG, Fong LC, Shamir S, Sherlock S. A non-transferrin-bound serum iron in idiopathic hemochromatosis. Dig Dis Sci. 1980;25:340–9.
74. Wright TL, Brissot P, Ma WL, Weisiger RA: Characterization of non-transferrin-bound iron clearance by rat liver. J Biol Chem. 1986;261:10909–10.
75. Craven CM, Alexander J, Eldrige M, Kushner JP, Bernstein S, Kaplan J. Tissue distribution and clearance kinetics of non-transferrin-bound iron in the hypotransferrinemic mouse: a rodent model for hemochromatosis. Proc Natl Acad Sci USA. 1987;84:3457–64.
76. Brissot P, Wright TL, Ma WL, Weisiger RA. Efficient clearance of non-transferrin-bound iron by rat liver: implications for hepatic iron loading in iron overload states. J Clin Invest. 1985;76:1463–70.
77. Bacon BR, Britton RS. The pathology of hepatic iron overload: a free radical-mediated process? Hepatology. 1990;11:127–370.
78. Britton RS, Bacon BR, Recknagel RO. Lipid peroxidation and associated hepatic organelle dysfunction in iron overload. Chem Phys Lipids. 1987;45:207–39.
79. Bacon BR, Britton RS, O'Neill R. Effects of vitamin E deficiency on hepatic mitochondrial lipid peroxidation and oxidative metabolism in rats with chronic dietary iron overload Hepatology. 1989;9:398–404.
80. Mak IT, Weglicki, WB. Characterization of iron-mediated peroxidative injury in isolated hepatic lysosomes. J Clin Invest. 1985;75:58–63.
81. Bacon BR, Healey FJ, Brittenham GM *et al.* Hepatic microsomal function in rats with chronic dietary iron overload. Gastroenterology. 1986;90:1844–53.
82. Weintraub LR, Goral A, Grasso J. Pathogenesis of hepatic fibrosis in experimental iron overload. Br J Haematol. 1985;59:321–31.
83. Halliwell B, Gutteridge JMC. The importance of free radicals and catalytic metal ions in human diseases. Molec Aspects Med. 1985;8:89–95.
84. Aruoma OI, Halliwell B. Superoxide-dependent and ascorbate-dependent formation of hydroxyl radicals from hydrogen peroxide in the presence of iron. Are lactoferrin and transferrin promoters of hydroxyl radical generation? Biochem J. 1987;241:273–85.
85. Minott G, Aust SD. The requirement of iron III in the initiation of lipid peroxidation by iron III and hydrogen peroxide. J Biol Chem. 1987;262:1098–104.
86. Seymour CA, Peters TJ. Organelle pathology in primary and secondary haemochromatosis with special reference to lysosomal changes. Br J Haematol. 1978;40:239–53.
87. Selden C, Seymour CA, Peters TJ. Activities of some free-radical scavenging enzymes and glutathione concentrations in human and rat liver and their relationship to the pathogenesis of tissue damage in iron overload. Clin Sci. 1980;58:211–19.
88. Farrell FJ, Nguyen M, Woodley S *et al.* Outcome of liver transplantation patients with hemochromatosis. Hepatology. 1994;20:404–10.
89. Adams PC, Ghent CN, Grant DR, Frei JV, Wall WJ. Transplantation of a donor liver with haemochromatosis: evidence against an inherited intrahepatic defect. Gut. 1991;32:1082–3.
90. Dabkowski PL, Angus PW, Smallwood RA, Ireton J, Jones RM. Site of metabolic defect in idiopathic haemochromatosis: insights from transplantation of an affected organ. Br Med J. 1993;306:1726.

30
Liver and biliary abnormalities in ulcerative colitis and Crohn's disease

R. H. WIESNER

INTRODUCTION

Diseases of the liver and bile ducts are the most common extraintestinal conditions associated with inflammatory bowel disease (IBD). Indeed, hepatobiliary disease affects as many as 10–15% of patients having IBD[1–3]. Furthermore, a broad spectrum of hepatobiliary disorders have been found in patients with IBD, some of which occur specifically with chronic ulcerative colitis (CUC), some with Crohn's disease, and some with both (Table 1). The incidence and significance of the various hepatobiliary disorders vary considerably. In addition, the pathogenesis of most of these disorders has been poorly defined. In this chapter the incidence, epidemiology, diagnosis, pathogenesis, pathology, and treatment of the various hepatobiliary disorders that are seen in association with IBD are reviewed.

Table 1 Hepatobiliary disorders that occur in association with ulcerative colitis and Crohn's disease

Ulcerative colitis and Crohn's disease	Crohn's disease alone
Primary sclerosing cholangitis	Gallstones
Cholangiocarcinoma	Granulomas
Autoimmune chronic hepatitis	Amyloidosis
Fatty infiltration	
Cryptogenic cirrhosis	
Primary biliary cirrhosis	
Hepatitis C	
Hepatic abscess	
Sarcoidosis	
Portal vein thrombosis	

BILIARY DISORDERS

Primary sclerosing cholangitis

Primary sclerosing cholangitis (PSC) is a syndrome of unknown aetiology characterized by fibrosis and inflammation of the intrahepatic and extrahepatic bile ducts[4–6]. It is the most common hepatobiliary disorder associated with IBD, and is seen most commonly in patients with CUC. The diagnosis is made on the basis of a cholangiogram that shows 'beading' and irregularity of the extrahepatic and intrahepatic biliary tree, or both (Fig. 1). The term 'primary' is used to distinguish this entity from bacterial cholangitis or biliary cirrhosis secondary to choledocholithiasis, congenital abnormalities of the biliary tree, previous biliary surgery, or other insults causing stricturing of the biliary tree. Criteria commonly used for the diagnosis are shown in Table 2.

PSC is associated with other autoimmune disorders; particularly IBD, idiopathic fibrosing processes such as Riddle's thyroiditis, retroperitoneal fibrosis, and mediastinal fibrosis (Table 3); approximately 75% of PSC patients have associated IBD, most commonly CUC.

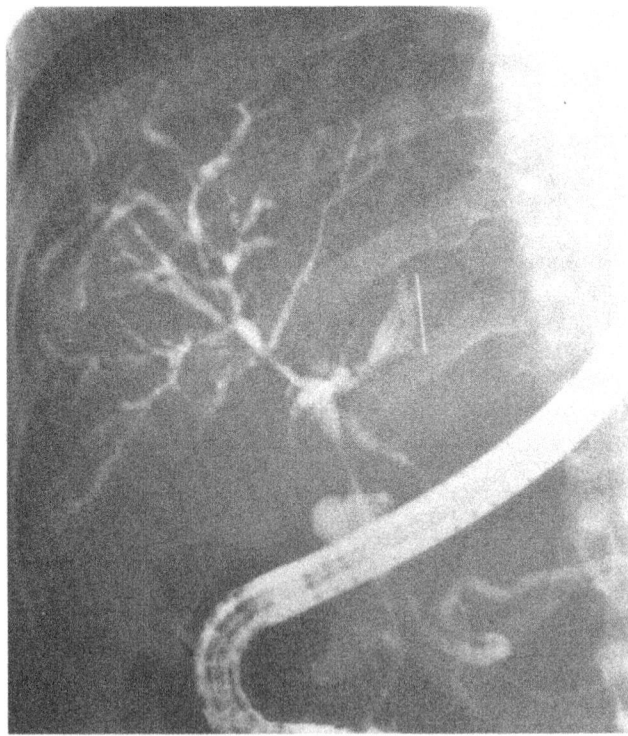

Figure 1 Classic beading and irregularity of both the intrahepatic and extrahepatic bile ducts which is diagnostic of primary sclerosing cholangitis, particularly in the setting of inflammatory bowel disease

Table 2 Criteria for the diagnosis of primary sclerosing cholangitis

Feature	Inclusion	Exclusion
Clinical	History of IBD, history of chronic cholestasis	Immune deficiency syndrome; trauma or ischaemia; toxic injury – drug
Laboratory	Increased alkaline phosphatase, increased bilirubin	
Cholangiogram	Beading and narrowing of intrahepatic and/or extrahepatic bile ducts	Choledocholithiasis, congenital bile duct disease, previous biliary surgery
Histological	Periductal inflammation and/or fibrosis, ductopenia, obliterative fibrosis of bile ducts, biliary cirrhosis	Florid duct lesion of PBC
Serology	pANCA	High-titre antimitochondrial antibody

Table 3 Diseases associated with primary sclerosing cholangitis

Inflammatory bowel disease	Chronic pancreatitis
Coeliac disease	Rheumatoid arthritis
Retroperitoneal fibrosis	Peyronie's disease
Thyroiditis	Bronchiectasis
Sjögren's syndrome	Systemic sclerosis
Autoimmune chronic hepatitis	Membranous nephropathy
Lupus erythematosus	Pseudotumour of orbit
Vasculitis	Autoimmune haemolytic anemia
Immune thrombocytopenic purpura	Angioblastic lymphadenopathy
Histiocytosis-X	Cystic fibrosis
Gallbladder disease	Eosinophilia
Intra-abdominal adenopathy	

The prevalence of PSC in patients with IBD has been estimated to be about 4%. Recently these estimates have been supported by epidemiological studies from Sweden in which the prevalence of CUC was found to be 171 cases per 100 000 patients, of which 3.7% had documented PSC[7]. The incidence of PSC was 5.5% in patients with pancolitis and only 0.5% in those with distal colitis. These results probably underestimate the true prevalence of PSC because it can occur in patients with normal serum alkaline phosphatase levels and can occur in the absence of IBD. Abnormal levels of serum alkaline phosphatase in a patient with IBD usually prompts suspicion for PSC, and usually leads to the diagnosis if a cholangiogram is performed.

Pathogenesis of PSC

The cause of PSC remains unknown; however, genetic factors, acquired factors, or both could be involved[1,6]. Potential causative factors for PSC are listed in Table 4. Although it is tempting to consider portal bacteraemia, absorbed colon

Table 4 Potential aetiopathological factors in primary sclerosing cholangitis

Portal bacteraemia	Viral infection
Absorption of colon toxins	Genetic predisposition
Toxic bile acids	Ischaemic arteriolar damage
Copper toxicity	Immunological mechanisms

toxins, and toxic bile acids as a cause for PSC, the evidence to support these aetiologies is meagre[8–10]. Furthermore, we and others have demonstrated that copper accumulation in the liver is a secondary phenomenon[11]. Therefore, copper hepatotoxicity is unlikely to play a major role in the pathogenesis of this disorder.

Several findings are compatible with an important role for genetic and immunological factors in the pathogenesis of PSC. One such finding is the high frequency of the occurrence of HLA-B8 and HLA-DR3 in PSC patients[12,13]. In addition, the increased incidence of PSC in family members has been demonstrated, suggesting that genetic factors may be important[14,15].

Currently, the pathogenesis of PSC is believed to be most closely linked to alterations in immune regulation. Like primary biliary cirrhosis, a disease thought to be a model autoimmune disease, PSC is characterized by lymphocytic bile duct destruction, the presence of hypergammaglobulinaemia, and association with other autoimmune disease, particularly CUC[1]. More recently, PSC patients have been found to have a high incidence of circulating anticolon antibodies, antinuclear antibodies, and antineutrophilic cytoplasmic antibodies[16–23]. While the presence of antineutrophilic cytoplasmic antibodies has been a curious finding, a direct pathogenic role has not been demonstrated to date.

Indeed, to date the most popular theory on the aetiopathogenesis of PSC supports an immunological basis; however, the specific details remain poorly defined at this point in time.

Clinical manifestations

Patients with PSC most commonly are young men, and often clinically present with pruritus, jaundice, right upper quadrant pain, fever, weight loss, and malaise[6]. Less frequently, PSC patients present with complications of portal hypertension, such as ascites and oesophageal variceal bleeding. Increasingly, the diagnosis of PSC is made in patients with IBD who are asymptomatic with regard to their liver disease, but who are found incidentally to have an increase in serum alkaline phosphatase level.

In general, laboratory findings reveal a chronic cholestatic biochemical profile with an elevated serum alkaline phosphatase level that is usually two to three times the upper limit of normal, and an elevated aminotransferase level that is generally up to two times the upper limit of normal[1]. These biochemical abnormalities are usually persistent, and present for 6 months or more before an evaluation for PSC is pursued. Serum bilirubin levels can be elevated but most often are in the normal range at the time PSC is diagnosed. Traditional autoantibodies are conspicuous by their absence, with less than 25% of patients having antinuclear antibodies, antismooth muscle antibodies, or antimitochondrial antibodies.

The diagnosis of PSC is made on the basis of a cholangiogram showing beading and irregularity of the extrahepatic and intrahepatic biliary tree[1]. Liver histological findings, although helpful in confirming the diagnosis and excluding other causes of liver disease, rarely reveal specific findings that allow the diagnosis of PSC to be made confidently on the basis of liver biopsy alone. However, histological staging has been shown to have a prognostic utility[2] (Table 5 and Fig. 2). When present, however, the obliterative bile duct lesion is almost pathognomonic of PSC (Fig. 3). PSC has been found in association with a number of diseases other than IBD, which are listed in Table 3.

Natural history

Information regarding the natural history of PSC continues to emerge. Given our lack of knowledge of the pathogenesis of PSC, the unavailability of

Table 5 Histological staging criteria for chronic hepatitis associated with primary sclerosing cholangitis

Stage	Criteria
Stage I (portal stage)	Portal hepatitis or bile duct abnormalities, with little or no periportal inflammation and fibrosis
Stage II (periportal stage)	Periportal fibrosis, with or without periportal hepatitis, or prominent enlargement of portal tracts with intact limiting plates
Stage III (septal disease)	Septal fibrosis, bridging necrosis, or both. Bile ducts are often absent or damaged. In the parenchyma there is biliary and fibrosing piecemeal necrosis with associated copper deposition
Stage IV (cirrhotic stage)	Biliary cirrhosis. Bile ducts have often disappeared; ductopenia

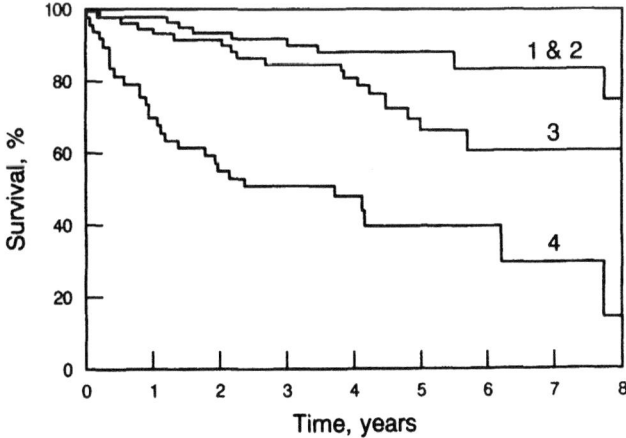

Figure 2 Kaplan–Meier estimated survival by histological stage on liver biopsy at time of PSC diagnosis

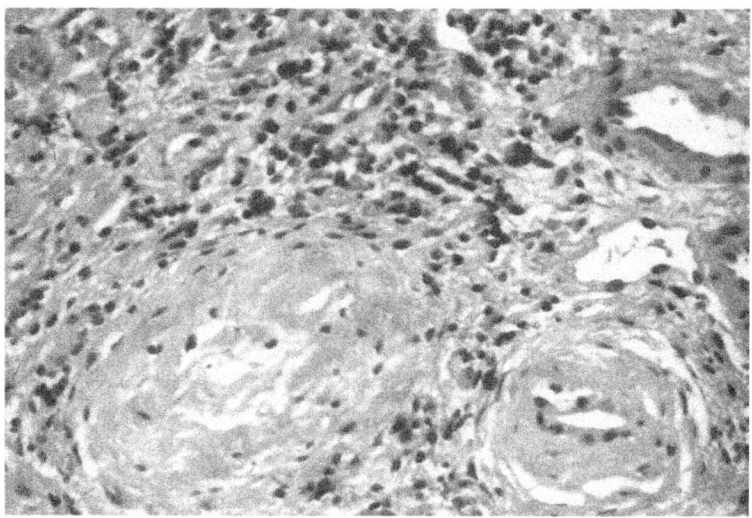

Figure 3 Fibrosing obliterative duct lesion which is nearly pathognomonic of primary sclerosing cholangitis

serological markers for diagnosis, and the unpredictable nature of the syndrome, defining the natural history and prognosis of PSC can be extremely difficult. Nevertheless, on the basis of a number of prospective studies, growing evidence indicates that PSC is frequently a progressive disease. In the largest series of PSC patients reported from the Mayo Clinic, with a mean follow-up of 6 years, median survival from the time of diagnosis was 11.9 years, and both symptomatic and asymptomatic patients had a reduced survival compared to a United States controlled population matched for age, gender, and race[24] (Fig. 4). These

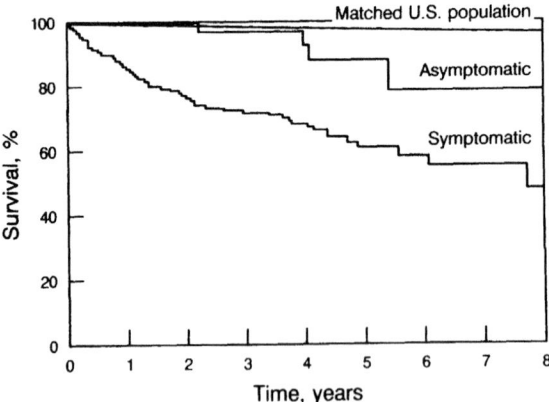

Figure 4 Kaplan–Meier estimated survival curves for asymptomatic and symptomatic primary sclerosing cholangitis patients. For comparison, the survival curve of the United States population matched for age, sex, and race to the asymptomatic population is also shown. For differences in survival: asymptomatic versus controlled ($p < 0.0001$), symptomatic versus asymptomatic ($p < 0.003$)

findings have been further confirmed by other centres, which have reported median survival times ranging between 9 and 17 years[25].

From these natural history studies we and others have created a survival model which can estimate patient survival at any point in the disease course. In these models patients age, serum bilirubin, histological stage, and the presence or absence of splenomegaly can be used to estimate long-term survival[26] (Fig. 5). These survival models have been helpful not only for prognosis, but also for selection and timing for liver transplantation.

Treatment

Although a number of experimental therapies, including controlled clinical trials using D-penicillamine, cyclosporin, methotrexate, and ursodeoxycholic acid, have been performed, none of these therapies has been associated with a beneficial clinical, biochemical, or histological response[27–29]. Furthermore, a recent study reported from the Mayo Clinic indicates that ursodeoxycholic acid therapy has a minimal impact on preventing disease progression and prolonging survival free of death or liver transplantation[30]. Similar studies evaluating methotrexate have also failed to show a major impact on preventing disease progression[31].

While several centres have advocated biliary tract surgery for bile duct stricturing, we believe that biliary surgery should be considered only as a palliative measure aimed at relieving symptoms of jaundice, pruritus, and bacterial cholangitis, and not meant as a treatment for underlying liver disease. Consensus is growing that biliary surgery is of little or no value in patients with PSC who have cirrhosis, particularly in those who have severe intrahepatic bile duct stricturing.

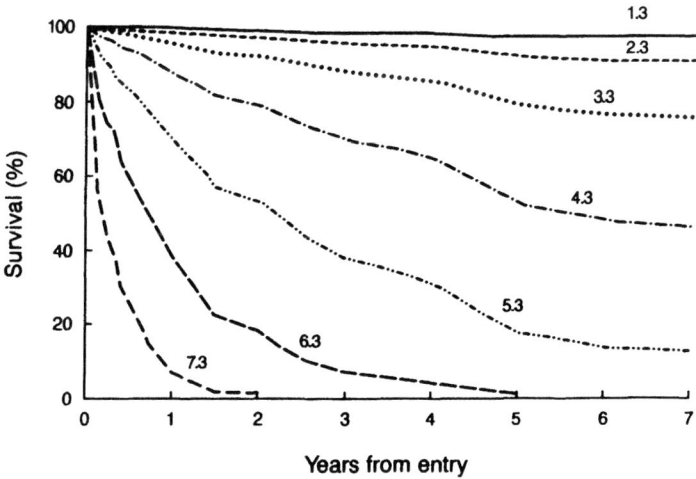

Figure 5 The estimated survival for primary sclerosing cholangitis patients transplanting the Mayo PSC risk score based on age, serum bilirubin level, histological stage, and the presence or absence of splenomegaly into a survival function. Using the risk score one can estimate survival for the individual patient at any point in the disease course

For patients who have a dominant stricture of the biliary tract associated with the acute onset of jaundice, pruritus, or bacterial cholangitis, percutaneous endoscopic balloon dilatation of the stricture, with removal of biliary sludge, is frequently effective in alleviating jaundice and pruritus, and decreasing the frequency and severity of bacterial cholangitic episodes. These procedures are the most effective in patients whose symptoms have been of recent onset, and less effective in those with long-standing jaundice or in those who have a long-standing history of recurrent episodes of bacterial cholangitis[32]. Furthermore, patients with PSC and severe intrahepatic bile duct stricturing appear to benefit less from balloon dilatation of dominant strictures of the common bile duct than those who have only minimal changes in the intrahepatic bile ducts.

Proctocolectomy appears to have no effect on the clinical course of PSC, and therefore should be considered only for patients who have severe IBD or who have developed premalignant or malignant lesions of the colon[33]. A proctocolectomy should not be considered a therapeutic option for the treatment of PSC alone. In addition, patients undergoing proctocolectomy with the construction of an ileal stoma are at risk for developing peristomal varices, which often bleed profusely[34]. This complication can be prevented by performing an ileal rectal pull-through procedure which eliminates the formation of an ileal stoma and therefore the formation of peristomal varices[35].

Finally, for patients with end-stage PSC, liver transplantation is the only viable lifesaving therapeutic alternative. The results of liver transplantation in PSC patients have been excellent, and seem to be improving, with the most recent reports indicating an 80–85% 3-year survival[6,36,37]. Unfortunately, it appears that PSC does recur in the hepatic allograft in approximately 20–25% of patients, and can lead to severe stricturing, biliary cirrhosis, and the need for retransplantation[38].

Cholelithiasis

Gallstones occur in up to 11% of the general population[1]. However, in patients with ileal Crohn's disease, up to 35% may experience cholesterol gallstones[39–42]. This is felt to be related to decreased absorption of bile acids because of distal ileal disease frequently found in Crohn's disease. The occurrence of cholesterol gallstones in Crohn's disease correlates directly with the extent of ileal disease.

In patients with CUC there does not appear to be an increased incidence of cholesterol gallstones. However, in patients with PSC and CUC, cholelithiasis and choledocholithiasis occur in 25–30%[43]. Because PSC occurs primarily in young males this probably represents an increased incidence of cholelithiasis. Chronic cholestasis is known to predispose to the formation of cholesterol gallstones, and bile stasis associated with bacterial cholangitis predisposes patients to the development of pigment stones, which are most often found in patients with PSC.

For patients who are symptomatic from gallstone disease, laparoscopic cholecystectomy appears to be the procedure of choice. However, because of the high frequency of pigment stones seen in patients with PSC, a cholangiogram is indicated at the time of cholecystectomy to exclude the presence of stones in the biliary tree.

Cholangiocarcinoma

Carcinoma of the biliary tract is more common in patients with CUC than in the general population[44]. Furthermore, it has been detected in patients with Crohn's disease. Bile duct carcinoma in patients with IBD usually develops in those who also have PSC. In fact, many investigators believe PSC may be a prerequisite for the development of bile duct cancer in this group of patients. It is now established that cholangiocarcinoma may develop during the course of disease in up to 30% of patients with PSC[45]. The PSC patients at highest risk for the development of cholangiocarcinoma are those with long-standing CUC and those with histological cirrhotic-stage disease on liver biopsy. Indeed, many consider PSC to be a premalignant condition of the biliary tree, just as CUC is a premalignant condition of the colon. We have recently documented multiple areas of bile duct dysplasia with carcinoma *in situ* in patients undergoing liver transplantation for long-standing PSC.

Unfortunately, the diagnosis of bile duct carcinoma has been difficult in PSC patients because no serological markers exist, and biliary cytological findings have not always been helpful in the early diagnosis of cholangiocarcinoma. The difficulty in making the diagnosis of cholangiocarcinoma in a patient with PSC is supported by a report from the University of Pittsburgh, in which 10% of patients with PSC undergoing liver transplantation were found to have an unsuspected cholangiocarcinoma.

Recent reports suggest that the measurement of serum CA 19–9 level may be helpful in diagnosing cholangiocarcinoma in the setting of PSC[46]. Indeed, CA 19–9 levels are elevated in those patients with established cholangiocarcinoma, but this has not been shown to be helpful as an early marker, or in those who are predisposed to developing cholangiocarcinoma[47,48].

Operative management, chemotherapy, and radiation therapy have all been associated with dismal results, and have made little impact on the natural history of cholangiocarcinoma in the setting of PSC. In addition, in patients with PSC and concomitant cholangiocarcinoma undergoing liver transplantation, bile duct carcinoma has recurred almost uniformly, leading to a 3-year survival of less than 15%[49]. Therefore, at this time many transplant centres consider the diagnosis of cholangiocarcinoma a contraindication to performing liver transplantation.

Primary biliary cirrhosis

The concomitant diagnosis of IBD and primary biliary cirrhosis (PBC) has rarely been described[50]. Although PSC and PBC may have some clinical, biochemical, and histological overlap, these two chronic cholestatic liver diseases can be readily differentiated by means of cholangiography. Whether a true association between PBC and IBD exists, or whether these reported cases occurred by chance, remains unanswered at this time.

HEPATIC DISORDERS

Autoimmune chronic hepatitis

It is important to emphasize that morphological features of chronic hepatitis may occur in patients with PSC, thus confusing the diagnosis[51]. Therefore, definition of the true frequency of chronic hepatitis in patients with IBD requires exclusion of stricturing of the intrahepatic and extrahepatic biliary tree by cholangiography. In previous studies a substantial proportion of patients with PSC was incorrectly diagnosed as having chronic hepatitis on the basis of liver biopsy alone. However, when strict histopathological and cholangiographic criteria are utilized for the diagnosis of autoimmune chronic hepatitis, a definite association with IBD appears to exist[52]. This has recently been described by Boberg et al., who defined clinical features for autoimmune chronic hepatitis patients who have PSC[53]. Indeed, many investigators believe an overlap syndrome does exist, in which patients have features of both autoimmune chronic hepatitis and PSC. Diagnostic features of autoimmune chronic hepatitis in PSC patients, and a scoring system, are shown in Table 6. In addition, because many patients with IBD have undergone previous operative procedures, or have required blood transfusions, hepatitis B and C must be excluded when features of chronic hepatitis are present.

The incidence of autoimmune chronic hepatitis in patients with IBD has been shown to be between 15% and 20%[54]. On the other hand, the incidence of CUC in large populations of patients with established autoimmune chronic hepatitis has been shown to be approximately 16%[52,55].

Pathogenesis

The pathogenesis of autoimmune chronic hepatitis associated with IBD remains poorly defined. The most popular hypothesis is that chronic hepatitis occurs as a consequence of abnormal autoimmune responsiveness. However, whether the immunopathological mechanisms of autoimmune chronic hepatitis with IBD are

Table 6 Features suggesting a diagnosis of autoimmune chronic hepatitis in patients with primary sclerosing cholangitis (scoring points)

Gender (female)	+2
Alkaline phosphatase/AST <3	+2
Gammaglobulin >2×	+3
Antinuclear antibody, antismooth muscle antibody, anti-LKM >1:80	+3
Other autoimmune disease	+1
HLA-B8 and HLA-DR3	+1
Piecemeal/artery necrosis	+3
Antimitochondrial antibody negative	0
Viral marker negative	+3
Alcohol <25 g/day	+2
No hepatotoxic medications	+1

Criteria for diagnosis of autoimmune chronic hepatitis: score ≥15 definite; 10–14 probable; <10 not. Details from ref. 53.

Table 7 Comparison of autoimmune chronic hepatitis and primary sclerosing cholangitis associated with inflammatory bowel disease

	ACH	PSC
Age (years)	30–40	30–40
Gender (male)	2/3	2/3
Alkaline phosphatase	<2 × normal	>2 × normal
Gamma globulin (g/dl)	>2.5	<2.5
Alanine aminotransferrin (U/L)	>300	<300
Antinuclear antibody	100%	20%
HLA-B8, HLA-DR3	Yes	Yes
Other autoimmune disease	70%	30%

the same mechanisms that are involved in patients without IBD has not been evaluated.

Clinical manifestations

A comparison of patients with autoimmune chronic hepatitis and PSC associated with IBD is shown in Table 7[52]. Similar to PSC, autoimmune chronic hepatitis associated with IBD usually occurs in men (70%) and presents in the third and fourth decade of life. The duration of IBD before recognition of chronic hepatitis is variable; in most reports the activity and prognosis of chronic hepatitis do not seem to correlate with the extent of involvement or the severity of IBD. Most patients have non-specific symptoms such as fatigue and malaise, and physical examination may show hepatosplenomegaly or other stigmata of chronic liver disease. Biochemical liver function tests meet the criteria set forth for moderate-to-severe autoimmune chronic hepatitis; namely, aminotransferase levels are five or more times the upper limit of normal, and gammaglobulin levels are over twice the upper limit of normal. Antinuclear antibodies, anti-smooth muscle antibodies, anti-LKM, or a variety of combinations are present in almost all cases. Frequently these patients have evidence of other autoimmune diseases such as polyarthritis, thyroiditis, and keratoconjunctivitis sicca, all of which are infrequently seen in patients with PSC.

Pathology

Histological findings in autoimmune chronic hepatitis with IBD are similar to those seen in autoimmune chronic hepatitis without IBD. The disease is characterized by periportal and portal inflammation, with piecemeal and bridging necrosis with or without the presence of cirrhosis[53]. This compares to PSC, in which one sees periductal fibrosis, obliterative fibrosis of the bile ducts, ductopenia, and biliary cirrhosis[51]. Indeed, a number of patients may have features of both entities, and this condition falls into what most investigators call the 'overlap syndrome'[53]. Patients with autoimmune chronic hepatitis associated with IBD should be treated with corticosteroid therapy in an attempt to relieve symptoms, improve biochemical parameters, and improve histology.

Table 8 Response to corticosteroid therapy in patients with autoimmune chronic hepatitis with or without inflammatory bowel disease and features of primary sclerosing cholangitis

Response to corticosteroids	ACH + PSC + IBD	ACH + IBD	ACH alone
Remission (%)	20	67	94
Duration of therapy (months)	57	22	21
Treatment failure (%)	80	14	6
Progression to cirrhosis (%)	75	60	25

A recent study of patients with severe autoimmune chronic hepatitis assessed the prevalence and impact of CUC, and the frequency of cholangiographic or histological features of PSC, in those patients with CUC[52]. Seventeen of 105 patients (16%) with autoimmune chronic hepatitis who had a screening colonoscopy had evidence of CUC. This study evaluated the response to corticosteroid therapy in patients with autoimmune chronic hepatitis who had IBD with and without features of PSC on cholangiography (Table 8). Results of this study revealed that patients with autoimmune chronic hepatitis and CUC without features of PSC responded well to immunosuppressive therapy, and similar to patients with autoimmune chronic hepatitis who did not have IBD. However, patients with autoimmune chronic hepatitis with IBD who had cholangiographic features of PSC went into remission less frequently, failed treatment more commonly, and progressed to cirrhosis more often than their counterparts who did not have evidence of PSC. Furthermore, in those with IBD who did respond, the duration of therapy to induce a remission was $2\frac{1}{2}$ times longer compared to those without IBD.

These findings suggest that patients who have the overlap syndrome (i.e. those patients with autoimmune chronic hepatitis with features of PSC) will respond poorly to corticosteroids, and may have a more aggressive course. As noted previously, ursodeoxycholic acid therapy appeared to have no effect on disease progression in PSC in general; however, ursodeoxycholic acid therapy has not been evaluated in this particular subset of patients to date[30].

Cryptogenic cirrhosis

The overall prevalence of cirrhosis appears to be 1–5% in patients with both CUC and Crohn's disease[1]. Most of these patients are classified as having biliary cirrhosis, most likely related to undiagnosed PSC. However, as noted above, many of these patients have had previous operations and transfusions and, indeed, hepatitis C may have been the cause of cirrhosis in a number of previous reports. In general, hepatitis B markers have been absent in these patients.

Clinical manifestations

Patients with cirrhosis in association with IBD present clinically with the usual symptoms of end-stage liver disease, including jaundice, ascites, encephalopathy, and variceal bleeding. On the other hand, many patients have compensated cirrhosis, which is an incidental finding at the time of autopsy.

Treatment

Once cirrhosis has developed, treatment is limited to managing the complications associated with portal hypertension. Patients with variceal bleeding should undergo sclerotherapy or banding, instead of undergoing a surgical portacaval shunt, since they often will become candidates for liver transplantation. The transjugular intrahepatic portosystemic shunt is often used as a bridge to control variceal bleeding until transplantation can be carried out. A special consideration is the need for proctocolectomy in a patient who has clinical evidence of portal hypertension. In such cases an abdominal stoma may lead to the formation of peristomal varices, which can be associated with a high risk of bleeding. In this situation, as in PSC, we recommend that an ileoanal procedure be performed, to avoid the high risk of developing peristomal varices. When life-threatening complications of portal hypertension occur, or the quality of life is significantly diminished, liver transplantation has become an excellent therapeutic alternative, with most transplant centres achieving an 80% 2-year survival.

Fatty infiltration

Fatty infiltration, usually microvesicular in nature, has been reported in up to 80% of patients with IBD[1]. Fatty liver is defined as an acquired disorder of metabolism resulting in accumulation of triglycerides within hepatocytes in quantities sufficient to be visible on microscopy. Frequently the accumulation of fat within the hepatocytes does not result in necrosis, inflammation, fibrosis, or cirrhosis, and is potentially reversible.

Fatty liver occurs in most patients with CUC and Crohn's disease[3,54]. The fat appears to be contained in large vesicles, and is typically diffusely distributed in the lobule, although some reported preferential distribution in the central lobular or periportal areas. Rarely, Mallory's highland has been found. Fat is often present concurrently with other histological lesions, which makes interpretation of the clinical and biochemical significance of fatty liver more difficult.

In general, most patients with fatty liver are asymptomatic with respect to their liver disease[56]. The physical examination usually shows no abnormalities, except for hepatomegaly. Results of laboratory investigations in patients with fatty liver are normal, or show minimal abnormalities in aspartate aminotransferase and alanine transaminase levels.

The fatty infiltration may subside in seriously ill patients who respond to therapy for IBD and malnutrition. Persistence of fat, however, has been documented in several instances when repeat biopsies have been obtained. The presence of fat alone does not appear to be associated with progressive hepatic damage in patients with IBD, but progression to fibrosis may occur when fatty liver coexists with severe inflammatory lesions[1].

Treatment should be directed towards IBD itself, and restoration of protein–calorie nutrition. Resection of the bowel is neither beneficial nor indicated, for hepatic lesions. One investigator showed that the frequency of fatty liver was the same 3–7 years after colectomy for CUC as it had been at the time of bowel resection[57].

Hepatic granulomas

Hepatic granulomas have been reported in several series of IBD patients[56,58,59]. The majority of hepatic granulomas have been found in Crohn's disease; although they are also seen in association with CUC. The frequency in reported series ranges from 0% to 15%[60]. A recent series reported from the Mayo Clinic showed granulomas to be present in 4% of patients with IBD, and these were most frequently attributed to concurrent sarcoidosis[61].

From a pathological standpoint the granulomas are usually non-caseating and are located in both the portal tracts and the parenchyma. Multinucleated giant cells have occasionally been present.

Overall, the prognosis for patients with hepatic granulomas in the presence of IBD is good. Such patients have not developed progressive liver disease or cirrhosis; thus, no specific therapy has been proposed for hepatic granulomas found in patients with IBD. Treatment, again, should be directed towards the IBD itself. The role of colectomy in the management of patients with hepatic granulomas remains unknown, but seems to be contraindicated, since it is generally a benign disease.

MISCELLANEOUS DISORDERS

Amyloidosis

Amyloid infiltration of the liver has been reported to occur in patients with both CUC and Crohn's disease[1]. Amyloidosis has been suspected generally on the basis of extrahepatic manifestations such as nephropathy; although in several reports amyloid was disclosed by liver biopsy in the absence of any previous clinical suspicion.

Amyloidosis of the liver or other organs is rare among patients with IBD, and occurs in 1–3% of patients, particularly in those having Crohn's disease with fistula and perianal disease[1].

Clinical features have not been reported in most reviews of amyloidosis in IBD patients, except for the fact that there is a frequent occurrence of proteinuria. It is also important to note that the majority of patients with IBD who have amyloidosis have foci of chronic suppuration as extraintestinal complications of their IBD. Furthermore, most patients have a connective tissue disorder, such as rheumatoid arthritis or ankylosing spondylitis. From a laboratory standpoint only slight elevations of serum alkaline phosphatase levels are noted, and rarely are serum bilirubin levels increased.

Regarding pathogenesis, amyloid deposition in the liver is presumed to be secondary to chronic inflammation most often related to a chronic suppurative process. The mechanisms remain unknown, however.

Amyloidosis, if progressive, is fatal. In reactive systemic amyloidosis the nature of the underlying liver disease, and the rate of amyloid deposition, determine the prognosis. Control of the underlying liver disease in certain circumstances has led to complete recovery, but the applicability of this observation to patients with IBD remains ill-defined. In experimental models of reactive systemic amyloidosis, deposition can be increased with corticosteroid therapy.

Despite these data it seems unreasonable to withhold the use of corticosteroids if they are needed for the management of IBD. There presently is no information concerning the usefulness of colchicine therapy in the treatment of hepatic amyloidosis associated with IBD.

Hepatic abscess

Prior to the availability of broad-spectrum antimicrobial therapy, pyelophlebitis and pyogenic liver abscesses were frequently associated with severe IBD. Today, hepatic abscesses in patients at the time of liver disease are rare.

Portal vein thrombosis

One investigator reported four patients with Crohn's disease who developed thrombosis of the portal vein. In addition, Stauffer *et al.* found this complication in a patient with CUC[62]. Overall, this is a rare complication most often related to previous untreated microbial sepsis.

Sarcoidosis

Sarcoidosis of the liver has been reported in four patients with CUC, and we have described six patients with sarcoidosis in conjunction with PSC. This is usually diagnosed on the basis of portal granulomas present in the liver[63].

References

1. Vierling JM. Hepatobiliary complications of ulcerative colitis and Crohn's disease. In: Zakim D, Boyer TD, editors. Hepatology: a textbook of liver disease, 3rd edn. Philadelphia, PA: Saunders; 1996:1366–404.
2. Harmatz A. Hepatobiliary manifestations of inflammatory bowel disease. Med Clin N Am. 1994;78:1387.
3. Wiesner RH. Hepatobiliary diseases associated with inflammatory bowel disease. In: Gitnick G, editor. Principles and practices of gastroenterology and hepatology, 2nd edn. Norwalk, CT: Appleton and Lange; 1994:909–15.
4. Wiesner RH, LaRusso NF. Clinicopathologic features of the syndrome of primary sclerosing cholangitis. Gastroenterology. 1980;79:200.
5. Chapman RWG, Marborgh BA, Rhodes JM *et al.* Primary sclerosing cholangitis: a review of its clinical features, cholangiography, and hepatic histology. Gut. 1980;21:870.
6. Wiesner RH. Current concepts in primary sclerosing cholangitis. Mayo Clin Proc. 1996;69:969–82.
7. Olsson R, Danielsson A, Jarnerot G *et al.* Prevalence of primary sclerosing cholangitis in patients with ulcerative colitis. Gastroenterology. 1991;100:1319–23.
8. Eade MM, Brooke BN. Portal bacteremia in cases of ulcerative colitis submitted to colectomy. Lancet. 1969;1:1008–9.
9. Vinnik IE, Kern F Jr, Struthers JE Jr *et al.* Experimental chronic portal vein bacteremia. Proc Soc Exp Biol Med. 1964;115:311–14.
10. Wiesner RH. Etiopathogenesis of primary sclerosing cholangitis. In: Gentilini P, Arias IM, McIntyre N, Rodes J, editors. Cholestasis. Amsterdam: Excerpta Medica; Elsevier; 1994:153–60.
11. Gross JB, Ludwig J, Wiesner RH *et al.* Abnormalities in tests of copper metabolism in primary sclerosing cholangitis. Gastroenterology. 1985;89:272.
12. Chapman RW, Varglese Z, Gaul R *et al.* Association of primary sclerosing cholangitis with HLA-B8. Gut. 1983;24:38–41.
13. Schrumpf E, Fausa O, Forre O. HLA antigens and immunoregularity T cells in ulcerative colitis associated with hepatobiliary disease. Scand J Gastroenterol. 1982;17:187–91.

14. Jorge AD, Esley C, Ahumada J. Family incidence of primary sclerosing cholangitis associated with immunologic diseases. Endoscopy. 1987;19:114–17.

15. Quigley EM, LaRusso NF, Ludwig J et al. Familial occurrence of primary sclerosing cholangitis and ulcerative colitis. Gastroenterology. 1983;85:1160–5.

16. Chapman RW, Cottone M, Selby WS et al. Serum autoantibodies, ulcerative colitis, and primary sclerosing cholangitis. Gut. 1986;27:86–91.

17. Snook JA, Chapman RW, Fleming K, Jewell DP. Antineutrophil nuclear antibody in ulcerative colitis. Crohn's disease and primary sclerosing cholangitis. Clin Exp Immunol. 1989;76:30–3.

18. Duerr RH, Targan SR, Landers CJ et al. Neutrophil cytoplasmic antibodies: a link between primary sclerosing cholangitis and ulcerative colitis. Gastroenterology. 1991;100:1385–91.

19. Das KM, Vecchi M, Sakamaki S. A shared and unique epitope(s) on human colon, skin, and biliary epithelium detected by a monoclonal antibody. Gastroenterology. 1990;98:464–9.

20. Lo SK, Fleming KA, Chapman RW. Prevalence of antineutrophil antibody in primary sclerosing cholangitis and ulcerative colitis using an alkaline phosphatase technique. Gut. 1992;33:1370–5.

21. Klein R, Eisenburg J, Weber P et al. Significance and specificity of antibodies to neutrophils detected by Western blotting for the serological diagnosis of primary sclerosing cholangitis. Hepatology. 1991;14:1147–52.

22. Seibold F, Weber P, Klein R et al. Clinical significance of antibodies against neutrophils in patients with inflammatory bowel disease and primary sclerosing cholangitis. Gut. 1992;33:657–62.

23. Halbwachs-Mecarelli L, Nusbaum P, Noel LH et al. Antineutrophil cytoplasmic antibodies (ANCA) directed against cathepsin G in ulcerative colitis, Crohn's disease, and primary sclerosing cholangitis. Clin Exp Immunol. 1992;90:79–84.

24. Wiesner RH, Grambsch PM, Dickson ER et al. PSC: natural history, prognostic factors, and survival analysis. Hepatology. 1989;10:430–6.

25. Farrant JM, Hayllar KM, Wilkinson ML et al. Natural history and prognostic variables in primary sclerosing cholangitis. Gastroenterology. 1991;100:1710–17.

26. Dickson ER, Mutaugh PA, Wiesner RH et al. Primary sclerosing cholangitis: refinement and validation of survival models. Gastroenterology. 1992;103:1893–901.

27. LaRusso NF, Wiesner RH, Ludwig J et al. Prospective trial of penicillamine in primary sclerosing cholangitis. Gastroenterology. 1988;95:1036–42.

28. Lindor KD, Wiesner RH, Colwell L et al. The combination of prednisone and colchicine in patients with primary sclerosing cholangitis. Am J Gastroenterol. 1991;86:57–61.

29. Wiesner RH, Steiner B, LaRusso NF et al. A controlled clinical trial evaluating cyclosporine in the treatment of primary sclerosing cholangitis. Hepatology. 1991;14(Suppl.):abstract 63A.

30. Lindor KD for Mayo PSC Study Group. Ursodiol for primary sclerosing cholangitis. N Engl J Med. 1997;336:691–5.

31. Knox TA, Kaplan MM. A double-blind controlled trial of oral-pulse methotrexate therapy in the treatment of primary sclerosing cholangitis. Gastroenterology. 1994;106:494–9.

32. Bender CE, Wiesner RH, LeRoy AJ et al. Long-term benefit of percutaneous dilatation of dominant bile duct strictures in primary sclerosing cholangitis. Hepatology. 1991;14:abstract 191A.

33. Cangemi JR, Wiesner RH, Beaver SJ et al. Effect of proctocolectomy for chronic ulcerative colitis on the natural history of primary sclerosing cholangitis. Gastroenterology. 1989;96:790–4.

34. Wiesner RH, LaRusso NF, Dozois RR, Beaver SJ. Peristomal varices after proctocolectomy in patients with primary sclerosing cholangitis. Gastroenterology. 1986;90:316–22.

35. Kartheuser AH, Dozois RR, Wiesner RH et al. Complications and risk factors after ileal pouch-anal anastomosis for ulcerative colitis associated with primary sclerosing cholangitis. Ann Surg. 1993;217:314–20.

36. Narumi S, Roberts JP, Emond JC et al. Liver transplantation for sclerosing cholangitis. Hepatology. 1995;22:451–7.

37. McEntee G, Wiesner RH, Rosen C et al. A comparative study of patients undergoing liver transplantation for primary sclerosing cholangitis and primary biliary cirrhosis. Transplant Proc. 1991;23:1563–4.

38. Sheng R, Campbell WL, Zajko AB, Baron RL. Cholangiographic features of biliary strictures after liver transplantation for primary sclerosing cholangitis: evidence of recurrent disease. Am J Roentgenol. 1996;166:1109–13.

39. Greenstein AJ, Janowitz HD, Sachar DB. The extraintestinal complications of Crohn's disease and ulcerative colitis: a study of 700 patients. Medicine. 1976;55:401.
40. Cohen S, Kaplan M, Gottlieb L *et al.* Liver disease and gallstones in regional enteritis. Gastroenterology. 1971;60:237.
41. Baker AL, Kaplan MM, Norton RA *et al.* Gallstones in inflammatory bowel disease. Dig Dis. 1974;19:109.
42. Heaton KW, Read AE. Gallstones in patients with disorders of the terminal ileum and disturbed bile salt metabolism. Br Med J. 1969;3:494.
43. Brandt DJ, MacCarty RL, Charboneau JW *et al.* Gallbladder disease in patients with primary sclerosing cholangitis. Am J Roentgenol. 1988;150:571–4.
44. Rosen CB, Nagorney DM, Wiesner RH *et al.* Cholangiocarcinoma complicating primary sclerosing cholangitis. Ann Surg. 1991;213:21–5.
45. Farges O, Malassagne B, Sebaugh M *et al.* Primary sclerosing cholangitis: liver transplantation or biliary surgery. Surgery. 1995;117:146–55.
46. Nichols JC, Gores GJ, LaRusso NF *et al.* Diagnostic role of serum CA 19-9 for cholangiocarcinoma in patients with primary sclerosing cholangitis. Mayo Clin Proc. 1993;68:874–9.
47. Fisher A, Theise ND, Min A *et al.* CA 19-9 does not predict cholangiocarcinoma in patients with primary sclerosing cholangitis undergoing liver transplantation. Liver Transplant Surg. 1995;1:94–8.
48. Ramage JK, Donaghy A, Farrant JM, Williams R. Serum tumor markers for the diagnosis of cholangiocarcinoma in primary sclerosing cholangitis. Gastroenterology. 1995;108:865–9.
49. Piclmayr R, Lamesch P, Weimann A *et al.* Surgical treatment of cholangiocellular carcinoma. World J Surg. 1995;19:83–8.
50. Ludwig J, LaRusso NF. Primary biliary cirrhosis in a patient with chronic ulcerative colitis. In: Ishak KG, editor. Hepatopathology 1985. NJ: American Association for the Study of Liver Diseases. 1985:197.
51. Ludwig J, Barham SS, LaRusso NF *et al.* Morphologic features of chronic hepatitis associated with primary sclerosing cholangitis and chronic ulcerative colitis. Hepatology. 1981;1:632.
52. Perdigoto R, Carpenter HA, Czaja AJ. Frequency and significance of chronic ulcerative colitis in severe corticosteroid-treated autoimmune hepatitis. J Hepatol. 1992;14:325.
53. Boberg KM, Fausa O, Haaland T *et al.* Features of autoimmune hepatitis in primary sclerosing cholangitis: an evaluation of 114 primary sclerosing cholangitis patients according to a scoring system for the diagnosis of autoimmune hepatitis. Hepatology. 1996;23:1369–76.
54. Vierling JM. Hepatobiliary diseases in patients with inflammatory bowel disease. In: Targan S, Shanahan F, editors. Inflammatory bowel diseases: from bench to bedside. Baltimore, MD: Williams & Wilkins; 1994:654.
55. Olsson R, Hulten L. Concurrence of ulcerative colitis and chronic active hepatitis: clinical courses and results of colectomy. Scand J Gastroenterol. 1975;10:331.
56. Dordal E, Glagov S, Kirsner JB. Hepatic lesions in chronic inflammatory bowel disease: clinical correlations with liver biopsy diagnoses in 103 patients. Gastroenterology. 1967;52:239.
57. Eade MN, Cooke WT, Brooke BN. Liver disease in ulcerative colitis: the long-term effect of colectomy. Ann Intern Med. 1970;72:489.
58. Wewer V, Gluud C, Schlicting P *et al.* Prevalence of hepatobiliary dysfunction in a regional group of patients with chronic inflammatory bowel disease. Scand J Gastroenterol. 1991;26:97.
59. Dew MJ, Thompson H, Allain RN. The spectrum of hepatic dysfunction in inflammatory bowel disease. Q J Med. 1979;48:113.
60. Eade MN. Liver disease in ulcerative colitis: analysis of operative liver biopsy in 138 consecutive patients having colectomy. Ann Intern Med. 1970;72:475.
61. Wee A, Ludwig J. Pericholangitis in chronic ulcerative colitis: primary sclerosing cholangitis of the small bile ducts? Ann Intern Med. 1985;102:581.
62. Stauffer MN, Sauer WG, Dearing WH *et al.* The spectrum of cholestatic hepatic disease. J Am Med Assoc. 1965;191:125–9
63. Porayko MK, Wiesner RH, LaRusso NF. The association of primary sclerosing cholangitis (PSC) and sarcoidosis. Hepatology. 1989;10:689[abstract].

31
Liver abnormalities in coeliac disease

M. B. JACOBSEN

Most review articles on coeliac disease contain information on associated manifestations. Changes in joints, muscle, skin, kidney and lungs, have been described, as well as liver diseases. New studies implicating genetic, immunological, and environmental factors in the pathogenesis of coeliac disease may contribute to the understanding of its diverse clinical features. The definition of the central intestinal manifestation may be summarized as: a chronic disease in which there is a characteristic, though not specific, mucosal lesion of the small intestine that impairs nutrient absorption. Extraintestinal, and in particular hepatic, involvement is less clearly defined. Green and Wollaeger[1] described liver pathology in coeliac disease, but Hagander et al.[2] were the first to firmly establish the connection between coeliac disease and liver involvement. They examined case records from 74 consecutive patients. Raised sGOT and/or sGPT were found in 29 of 53 patients, and abnormal liver histology in 12 of 13 patients. Of these 12 patients seven had chronic active hepatitis (CAH) or established cirrhosis. The cirrhotic patients with coeliac disease all displayed normal IgA levels. One patients developed hepatocellular carcinoma.

In our own series[3] we reviewed 171 patient records with the diagnosis of villous atrophy. The diagnostic criteria were marked reduction of villous height or flat mucosa on small intestinal biopsies. In 15 patients other causes of villous atrophy, e.g. pancreatic insufficiency, primary hypogammaglobulinaemia, or radiation injury were found. Twenty-four patients were omitted due to incomplete records; thus 132 patients fulfilled the criteria and had at some time responded favourably to a gluten-free diet. In our population, patients were thought to have liver pathology if ASAT, ALAT or both were elevated. ALP elevation alone was not considered diagnostic for liver disease. Other causes of liver involvement were ruled out by estimation of hepatitis B (HBV) serology, seFe TIBC, ferritin, α_1 antitrypsin and autoantibodies against smooth muscle and mitochondria. Hepatitis C (HCV) testing was not available for these patients. Liver involvement judged by ASAT ALAT and/or ALP was found in 62/132 patients (46%); ALP elevation alone was seen in 14; thus, according to

Table 1 Liver involvement in coeliac disease

Reference	Abnormal ASAT/ALAT/ALP	Abnormal histology
2	39%	12/13 patients
3	47%	32/37 patients
4	42%	

our definition, 48/132 (36%) patients had liver involvement. Liver biopsies were performed in 37/132 patients. Normal histology was seen in five patients, 25 had unspecified changes and seven fulfilled criteria for a specific diagnosis. The main histopathological changes were unspecified with increased number of Kupffer cells, expanded portal fields and increased mononuclear infiltration. The specific diseases were CAH in five patients, one of whom had established cirrhosis; primary sclerosing cholangitis (PSC) in one, and one patient had a toxic hepatitis induced by alcohol. Interestingly, the raised liver transaminases decreased towards normal values on a gluten-free diet in 32 of the 62 patients with liver involvement, and completely normalized in 24 (75%). In our series 16 of the 132 patients had a malignant disease. When these patients were grouped according to whether liver involvement was present or not, significantly more patients with liver involvement had malignant disease.

In 1995 Bardella et al.[4] published a series of studies involving 158 adult coeliac disease patients where 67(42%) had elevated ASAT; ALAT and or ALP values. In this population 89.5% of the 67 patients with liver injury improved their transaminases on a gluten-free diet. No association of liver injury with body mass index (BMI), gender, age or small intestinal histology was found. They found HBV and CAH in three, HBC and CAH in one, fatty liver in two and CAH in one patient. PSC or primary biliary cirrhosis was not found.

Interestingly, 73% of the patients reported by the Milano group had neither overt malabsorption, diarrhoea, or reduced BMI. This confirms previous observations that liver involvement may be the only presentation of coeliac disease. Mitchison et al.[5] reported in 1989 on three patients in whom the predominant clinical and laboratory features suggested liver disease, bowel symptoms were a minor part of the presentation and the diagnosis of coeliac disease was reached with a delay of 6 months. Prompted by this and other similar observations, Lindgren et al.[6] examined 327 patients referred for evaluation of liver disease to a university hospital. Their patients covered the whole spectrum of liver diseases from subtle biochemical abnormalities to end-stage diseases. Sera from these patients were examined for gluten antibodies, and 19 patients (6%) tested positive – a six-fold increase in prevalence compared to blood donors. Ten of the 19 patients had a specified diagnosis of liver disease; in the others it was classified as 'crypogenic'. This work confirms the need for small intestinal biopsies in the diagnostic work-up of undefined liver diseases. This is in line with the work of Lindberg et al.[7], who found villous atrophy in three of 16 patients with a diagnosis of CAH. Interestingly, no patient with CAH and coeliac disease displayed elevated IgM.

Logan *et al.*[8] described four patients with PBC and coeliac disease who responded to a gluten-free diet by normalization or amelioration of the small intestinal biopsies. The liver diseases, however, remained unchanged. In 1982 Olsson *et al.*[9] reported a series of 26 patients with PBC and small intestinal biopsies. Five patients showed villous atrophy. All had elevated titres of antimitochondrial antibodies and four had elevated smooth-muscle antibodies. The liver histology in these patients showed features of both PBC and CAH, with destruction of interlobular bile ducts, ductular proliferation and piecemeal necrosis. None of the patients showed any improvement in liver tests, autoantibody titres or serum globulins during 6–22 months follow-up.

Liver involvement is seen more often in coeliac disease than can be explained by coincidence. Most common are the unspecified changes which improve, or even disappear, on a gluten-free diet. However, an increased incidence of specific liver disease such as PBC, CAH and PSC is repeatedly documented in coeliac disease. The histological findings in liver biopsies often represent a mixture of changes compatible both with PBC and CAH. They may represent a common response to an underlying autoimmune mechanism, responsible both for the intestinal and hepatic lesions.

References

1. Green PA, Wollaeger EE. Gastroenterology. The clinical behaviour of spruce in the United States. 1960;38:399–40
2. Hagander B, Berg NO, Brandt L, Norden A, Sjolund K, Stenstam M. Hepatic injury in adult coeliac disease. Lancet 1977;2:270–2
3. Jacobsen MB, Fausa O, Elgjo K, Schrumpf E. Hepatic lesions in adult coeliac disease. Scand J Gastroenterol 1990;25:656–662
4. Bardella MT, Fraquelli M, Quatrini M, Molteni N, Bianchi P, Conte D. Prevalence of hypertransaminasemia in adult celiac patients and effect of gluten-free diet. Hepatology. 1995;22:833–6
5. Mitchison HC, Record CO, Bateson MC, Cobden I. Hepatic abnormalities in coeliac disease: three cases of delayed diagnosis. Postgrad Med J. 1989;65:920–2.
6. Lindgren S, Sjöberg K, Eriksson S. Unsuspected coeliac disease in chronic 'cryptogenic' liver disease. Scand J Gastroenterol. 1994;29:661–4.
7. Lindberg J, Åhren C, Iwarson S. Intestinal villous atrophy in chronic active hepatitis. Scand J Gastroenterol. 1979;14:1015–18.
8. Logan RFA, Ferguson A, Finlayson NDC, Weir DG. Primary biliary cirrhosis and coeliac disease: an association? Lancet. 1978; 1:230–3.
9. Olsson R, Kagevi I, Rydberg L. On the concurrence of primary biliary cirrhosis and intestinal villous atrophy. Scand J Gastroenterol 1982;17:625–8

32
Primary sclerosing cholangitis: new therapeutic strategies

A. STIEHL, C. BENZ, P. SAUER and L. THEILMANN

CLINICS OF PRIMARY SCLEROSING CHOLANGITIS (PSC)

PSC is a chronic inflammatory liver disease characterized by progressive fibrosis and obstruction of bile ducts leading to increasing cholestasis and finally to cirrhosis. In early stages the patients have elevated levels of serum alkaline phosphatase and gamma-glutamyl transpetidase (GGT), and only in later stages do serum bilirubin and serum cholesterol increase. In early stages the patients may be free of symptoms, and with progressive disease jaundice, pruritus and fatigue appear.

The disease in general is diagnosed by endoscopic retrograde cholangiography, which shows multiple intrahepatic and/or extrahepatic stenoses with prestenotic dilatations which give the biliary system its typical appearance. Approximately 90% of patients with PSC have inflammatory bowel disease and, on the contrary, 5–10% of patients with ulcerative colitis have PSC. As a consequence, in all patients with inflammatory bowel disease with an elevated serum alkaline phosphatase, an endoscopic retrograde cholangiopancreatography (ERCP) should be performed, and this will allow detection of the majority of patients with PSC.

TREATMENT WITH IMMUNOSUPPRESSIVE AGENTS

Treatment of PSC patients with immunosuppressive, anti-inflammatory or antifibrotic agents has not proved very successful. Reports on a beneficial effect of methotrexate need confirmation in controlled trials. Since repeated episodes of bacterial cholangitis are typical for the disease, immunosuppressive treatment may even be harmful.

The major breakthrough came with the observation that ursodeoxycholic acid (UDCA) has a beneficial effect in patients with primary biliary cirrhosis (PBC). Subsequently patients with various forms of cholestatic liver diseases, including PSC, have been treated with UDCA[1-5]. Stenoses of the major bile ducts represent a problem, as they cannot be treated with UDCA and need endoscopic treatment[6–14].

EFFECT OF UDCA ON LABORATORY PARAMETERS

Stimulated by the report of a beneficial effect of UDCA in PBC, in 1987 we started a trial in patients with PSC[1]. After a 1-year treatment period with UDCA, which showed similar beneficial effects as in PBC and good tolerance in patients with additional ulcerative colitis, a double-blind placebo-controlled study was initiated. UDCA administration led to significant improvement of acid phosphatase, GGT, alanine aminotransferase, and aspartate transaminase. Serum cholesterol decreased in patients with elevated levels before treatment, and was unchanged in the others[1]. Changes in immunoglobulins IgA, IgM, and IgG were not significant. The changes are similar to those in three other controlled studies (Table 1) in which, in contrast to our study, serum bilirubin also improved significantly[2,4,5]. In a further controlled study, in which a relatively low dose of UDCA (600 mg/day) was used, no improvement of laboratory parameters was observed[3], indicating that such a low dose is ineffective and that 10–15 mg/day of UDCA should be given.

SYMPTOMS

Only approximately one-third of our patients with PSC suffered from pruritus and one-half from fatigue[1]. During treatment with UDCA both symptoms improved in some patients but, in comparison to placebo, the effect was not significant.

EFFECT OF UDCA ON LIVER HISTOLOGY

In all three studies in which changes in liver histology were evaluated after UDCA treatment cellular infiltrates in the portal triads decreased significantly, whereas all other changes were not significant[1,2,6]. In the Mayo study the effect of UDCA treatment on liver histology was not reported[4]. A decrease in portal

Table 1 Ursodeoxycholic acid in primary sclerosing cholangitis: results of placebo-controlled studies[a]

Reference	n	AP, GGT, ALT or AST	Bilirubin	Histology
1	20	Improved	Unchanged	Favourable[b]
2	14	Improved	Improved	Favourable
4	105	Improved	Improved	–
5	24	Improved	Improved	Favourable

[a] Studies with UDCA doses > 10 mg/kg.
[b] Favourable effect in comparison to pretreatment histology.

inflammation after UDCA has also been observed in patients with PBC. It is unclear at present whether a decrease of the inflammation around the bile ducts in PSC will have an effect on the development of bile duct carcinomas in this disease.

STENOSES OF MAJOR BILE DUCTS

After the end of a controlled study period all our patients were enrolled in a prospective trial on the effect of UDCA on bile duct disease, in which repeat cholangiographies were performed[6]. During treatment with UDCA, of 65 patients treated for up to 8 years (mean 45 months) 10 developed progressive stenosis of major bile ducts. Endoscopic dilatation of these stenoses is highly effective[6-14]. Repeat cholangiography in patients with narrowing of major bile ducts seems essential for early detection of stenoses of major bile ducts[6]. It is evident that mechanical obstruction of major bile ducts cannot be effectively treated by UDCA, and that endoscopic measures are essential if conservative treatment is to be effective.

BILE DUCT CARCINOMA

An unresolved problem in the treatment of patients with PSC is the development of bile duct carcinomas. In a large multicentre study from Sweden, in which 305 PSC patients were followed over a median follow-up time of 63 months, a bile duct carcinoma was observed in 8% of patients, and 44% of these were asymptomatic at the time of diagnosis of PSC[15]. In 37% of the patients with bile duct carcinoma this diagnosis was made within 1 year after detection of PSC and, as a consequence, it seems possible that the patients already had a bile duct carcinoma when the PSC was recognized. This study at present represents the largest series available, and no factors were found which would allow the identification of patients who will later develop a bile duct carcinoma.

The 8% cacrcinomas in the Swedish multicentre study is similar to the figure reported by others[16-20], and appears much lower than that observed at the Mayo[21]. Very high rates of bile duct carcinomas have repeatedly been reported in studies coming from transplantation centres, and it appears that they reflect very selected patient groups. In patients treated with UDCA, 3% developed a bile duct carcinoma[6]. It is unclear at present whether UDCA treatment can reduce the incidence of bile duct carcinomas.

SURVIVAL

In a recent controlled 2-year study[4], in which endoscopic treatment of major duct stenoses was not used, UDCA treatment did not improve survival free of liver transplantation. This is in contrast to a prospective non-randomized study[6], in which (from May 1987 to December 1995) 65 patients were treated with UDCA and, whenever necessary, by additional endoscopic dilatations: the actuarial Kaplan–Meier estimate of survival after treatment with UDCA and dilatation of major duct stenoses was significantly improved compared to the predicted survival, with a p value of 0.001[6].

CONCLUSION

We conclude that PSC may be treated conservatively by UDCA with good treatment results and prolongation of survival free of liver transplantation only when patients who develop major duct stenoses are recognized early and are additionally treated by endoscopic means. In end-stage disease liver transplantation is indicated.

References

1. Stiehl A, Walker S, Stiehl L et al. Effects of ursodeoxycholic acid on liver and bile duct disease in primary sclerosing cholangitis. A 3 year pilot study with a placebo-controlled study period. J Hepatol. 1994;20:57–64.
2. Beuers U, Spengler U, Kruis W et al. Ursodeoxycholic acid for treatment of primary sclerosing cholangitis: a placebo controlled trial. Hepatology. 1992;16:707–14.
3. De Maria N, Colantoni A, Rosenblom E, Van Thiel DH. Ursodeoxycholic acid does not improve the clinical course of primary sclerosing cholangitis over a 2-year period. Hepato-Gastroenterology. 1996;43:1472–9.
4. Lindor KD and the Mayo PSC/UDCA study group. Ursodiol for the treatment of primary sclerosing cholangitis. N Engl J Med. 1997;336:691–5.
5. Mitchell SA, Bansi D, Hunt N et al. High dose ursodeoxycholic acid (UDCA) in primary sclerosing cholangitis (PSC): results after two years of a randomized double-blind, placebo-controlled trial. Gut. 1997;40(Suppl. 1):TH 115 (abstract).
6. Stiehl A, Rudolph G, Sauer P et al. Efficacy of ursodeoxycholic acid and endoscopic dilation of major duct stenoses in primary sclerosing cholangitis. An 8-year prospective study. J Hepatol. 1997;26:560–6.
7. Grijm R, Huibregtse K, Bartelsman J et al. Therapeutic investigations in primary sclerosing cholangitis. Dig Dis Sci. 1986;31:792–8.
8. Johnson GK, Geenen JE, Venu RP, Hogan WJ. Endoscopic treatment of biliary duct strictures in sclerosing cholangitis: Follow up assessment of a new therapeutic approach. Gastrointest Endosc. 1987;33:9–12.
9. Huitbregtse K. Therapeutic investigations in primary sclerosing cholangitis. In: Huitbregtse K, editor. Endoscopic biliary and pancreatic drainage. Stuttgart: Georg Thieme; 1988:78–85.
10. Cotton PB, Nickl N. Endoscopic and radiologic approaches to therapy in primary sclerosing cholangitis. Sem Liver Dis. 1991;11:40–8.
11. Craig PI, Hatfield RW. Endoscopic therapy in primary sclerosing cholangitis. Eur J Gastroentrol Hepatol. 1992;4:284–7.
12. Gaing AA, Geders JM, Cohen SA, Siegel JH. Endoscopic management of primary sclerosing cholangitis: review, and report of an open series. Am J Gastroenterol. 1993;88:2000–8.
13. Lee JG, Schutz SM, England RE, Leung JW, Cotton PB. Endoscopic therapy of sclerosing cholangitis. Hepatology. 1995;21:661–7.
14. van Milligen AWM, van Bracht J et al. Endoscopic stent therapy for dominant extrahepatic bile duct strictures in primary sclerosing cholangitis. Gastrointest Endosc. 1996;44:293–9.
15. Broome U, Olson R, Lööf L et al. Natural history and prognostic factors in 305 Swedish patients with primary sclerosing cholangitis. Gut. 1996;38:610–615.
16. Aadland E, Schrumpf E, Fausa O et al. Primary sclerosing cholangitis: long-term follow up study. Scand J Gastroenterol. 1987;22:655–64.
17. Helzberg JH, Petersen JM, Boyer JL. Improved survival with primary sclerosing cholangitis; a review of clinicopathologic features and comparison of symtomatic and asymptomatic patients. Gastroenterology. 1987;92:1869–75.
18. Lebovics E, Palmer M, Woo J et al. Outcome of primary sclerosing cholangitis. Arch Intern Med. 1987;147:729–31.

19. Herrmann R, Dooley J, Sherlock S, McIntyre N. Progression of asymptomatic primary sclerosing cholangitis. J Hepatol. 1988;7:S39(abstract).
20. Farrant MJ, Hayllar KM, Wilkinson ML *et al.* Natural history and prognostic variables in primary sclerosing cholangitis. Gastroenterology. 1991;100:1710–17.
21. Wiesner RH, Grambsch PM, Dickson ER *et al.* Natural history, prognostic factors, and survival analysis. Hepatology. 1989;10:430–6.

33
Jejunoileal bypass: an unintended model of steatohepatitis (NASH syndrome) in humans

D. L. KAMINSKI

INTRODUCTION

The liver has been recognized for many years to be abnormal in obese patients. Patients significantly overweight were found to have biopsy evidence of hepatic steatosis, inflammation and fibrosis compared to liver biopsy results from normal-weight patients. Exclusion of other potential factors which could produce the hepatic abnormality led the investigators to conclude that the problem was due to the obese state[1,2]. When patients lost weight by dietary methods, and interval liver biopsy and liver function tests were performed, the hepatic abnormality improved[3]. The disorder was categorized as non-alcoholic steatohepatitis, NASH syndrome[4] and further experience has demonstrated that it is not the mild self-limited disease process originally considered but a serious problem that can progress to extensive fibrosis and cirrhosis[5]. In addition to obesity, NASH syndrome has been associated with adult-onset type II diabetes and hypertriglyceri-daemia, and has been found to be more prevalent in women than in men with these associated disorders[6]. One of the most dramatic and reproducible forms of NASH syndrome is that produced by jejunoileal bypass operations.

It was obvious that patients who underwent resection of large amounts of small intestine for various reasons, for example mesenteric ischaemia and infarction of the small intestine, had significant weight loss and difficulty maintaining their weight due to limited absorptive surface[7]. It was not unexpected that the possibility of producing weight loss by reproducing the process in obese patients would be considered. Following a limited amount of experimentation[8], and even more limited, uncontrolled clinical experience, short-circuiting the gastrointestinal system began to be widely employed in large numbers of patients with various degrees of obesity[9,10]. The original operations bypassed large amounts of the small intestine and joined about 20 cm of proximal jejunum to the right colon[10]. This operative procedure was associated with profound, life-threatening metabolic problems, and jejunocolic bypass operations were quickly abandoned and replaced by jejunoileal bypass operations which were performed by joining approximately 14 cm of proximal jejunum to approximately 8 cm of distal ileum (Fig. 1). A variety of adaptations of this operation were performed, generally with the same overall results of weight loss, diarrhoea and a remarkable constellation of metabolic problems[11,12]. The frequency with which this operation was performed is unknown; however, estimates of the number of

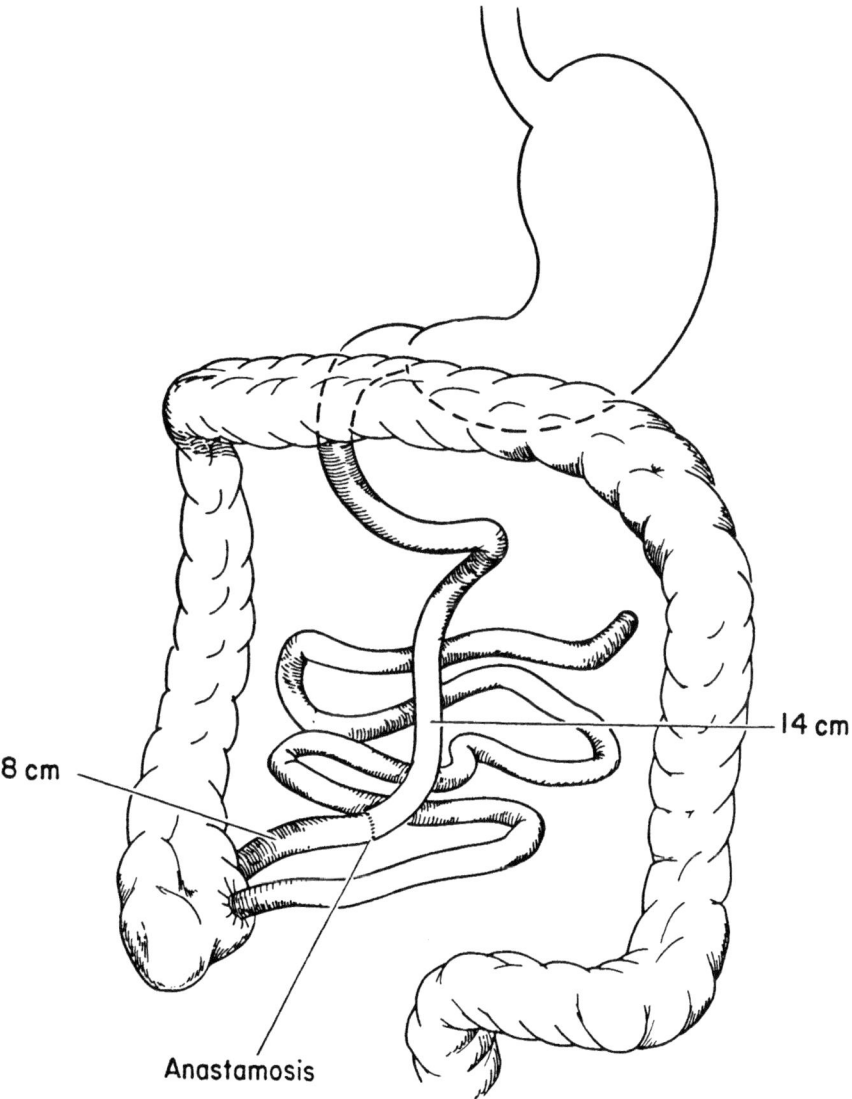

14 cm

8 cm

Anastamosis

Figure 1 Diagrammatic illustration of the general characteristics of jejunoileal bypass operations. The general characteristics of the operation resulted in malabsorption being produced by excluding approximately 90% of the small intestine from the incontinuity intestinal tract to produce weight loss

patients so treated in the United States, varying from 25 000 to 50 000[13], are likely to be a gross underestimation. The metabolic complications associated with the operation stimulated a National Institutes of Health Consensus Conference, during which time the consensus was that the operation should stop being performed, and a moratorium eliminating the performance of the operation appeared in 1978[14].

Following the brief initial experience with the operative procedure it quickly became apparent that the operation had adverse effects on the patients' livers[15]. Surgeons performing the operation began to biopsy the liver in order to ascertain the degree of steatohepatitis present when the operation was performed, to compare the biopsy to the histological appearance of the liver if the patient developed problems with the liver postoperatively. This resulted in a large amount of observational information being available, and for someone such as the author, involved in reconstructing these operations, every patient being reconstructed had an original liver biopsy specimen available to which the patient's current hepatic histology could be compared. This chapter represents a compilation of these data. Importantly, as we have observed this iatrogenic form of NASH syndrome over the past 20 years, all seven of the patients with jejunoileal bypass on whom we have reversed the operation during the past 2 years had clinical cirrhosis representing the end stage of this remarkable human experiment.

NASH SYNDROME

In order to understand the effect of jejunoileal bypass operations on the liver it is necessary to consider the effect of obesity on the liver. Operations on very obese individuals to perform gastric restrictive procedures provides the opportunity to evaluate the characteristics of the NASH syndrome. Our anecdotal experience is that males and females weighing over 350 lb generally always have gross evidence of NASH syndrome. Techniques have been developed that enable us, with informed consent and Institutional Review Board approval, to obtain flash-frozen liver specimens for lipid analysis and biopsies for histological analysis[16]. In collaboration with our pathologists a histological scoring system was developed (Table 1) that enables us to estimate the degree of steatosis present histo-

Table 1 Histological classification of the liver disease present in patients at the time of and following reconstruction of jejunoileal bypass

Inflammation			
A.	Focal inflammation		
B.	Portal inflammation	*Degree*	
C.	Focal necrosis	0 = None	
Lipid		1 = Mild	
D.	Steatosis	2 = Moderate	
Fibrosis		3 = Severe	
E.	Central fibrosis		
F.	Portal fibrosis		
G.	Lobular sinusoid fibrosis		
H.	Bridging fibrosis		

Table 2 Non-alcoholic steatohepatitis produced by morbid obesity (NASH syndrome)

	Normal	Obese
Mean body weight (lb)	162 ± 32	374 ± 18*
Total hepatic lipid (mg/g liver)	35 ± 3	84 ± 12*
Hepatic triglyceride (mg/g liver)	9 ± 1	57 ± 13*
Hepatic phospholipid (mg/g liver)	20 ± 3	21 ± 9
Hepatic cholesterol (mg/g liver)	3 ± 0.1	3 ± 0.3
Total hepatic protein (mg/g liver)	278 ± 19	238 ± 15
Hepatic steatosis (0–3)	0.2 ± 0.01	1.2 ± 0.1*
Hepatic inflammation (0–9)	0.2 ± 0.01	2.9 ± 0.3*
Hepatic fibrosis (0–12)	0.1 ± 0.01	1.0 ± 0.2*

Each value represents the mean ± SEM of six values obtained from liver specimens from six patients. Asterisks indicate that the obese patient's sample produced values significantly different from the values determined in the liver specimens from the normal-weight patients.

logically that has a significant correlation with the total hepatic lipid quantitated in the liver ($r = 0.73$). The data presented in Table 2 were determined from six consecutive patients between the ages of 30 and 47, including three males and three females in the normal weight group and in the obese patient group. The results indicate that patients with NASH syndrome have approximately six times more triglyceride in their liver than do normal-weight patients. This is associated with histological abnormalities including steatosis, hepatitis and early fibrosis. One can assume that a patient undergoing a jejunoileal bypass operation, at the time of the operation had the general liver abnormalities presented in Table 2.

EARLY HEPATIC EFFECTS OF JEJUNOILEAL BYPASS OPERATIONS

It was originally believed that patients undergoing jejunoileal bypass, during the period of rapid weight loss, experienced a severe insult to their livers with exacerbation of the steatohepatitis. This was associated with an approximately 7% incidence of liver failure treated with observation, nutritional support or reversal of the operation[17]. It was believed that, after weight stabilization following jejunoileal bypass operations, the steatohepatitis improved and the patient was no longer at risk for serious liver disease[18]. A large number of pre- and post-jejunoileal bypass liver specimens were available to the author[19], and the histological characteristics of the liver of patients 6 months following the operation is compared in Fig. 2 to the histological pattern of the liver when the operation was performed. Early following the operation there was primarily an exacerbation of steatosis and inflammation with no significant change in fibrosis.

LATE HEPATIC EFFECTS OF JEJUNOILEAL BYPASS OPERATIONS AND THE EFFECT OF RECONSTRUCTION ON THE LIVER

The hepatic histological information on 26 consecutive patients undergoing reconstruction of jejunoileal bypass operations for a wide variety of metabolic

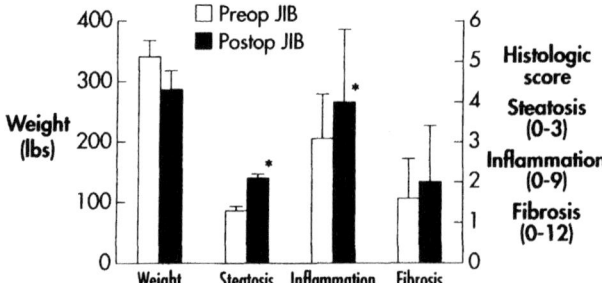

Figure 2 Early effects of jejunoileal bypass operations (JIB) on hepatic histology. Liver biopsy was performed on 24 consecutive patients at the time of JIB and at 6 months following the operation, and the slides evaluated by a blinded observer to assess the liver abnormality present utilizing the scoring system outlined in Table 1. Asterisks indicate that the value determined from the liver biopsy at the time of the postoperative biopsy was significantly different from the value from the biopsy specimen obtained at the time the JIB was performed

complications[12] is illustrated in Fig. 3. Patients having jejunoileal bypass operations for approximately 5 years had significant increases in the hepatic steatosis, inflammatory cell infiltrate and fibrosis. Nine of the 26 patients had gross cirrhosis. These patients underwent repeat liver biopsy 1–2 years following reconstruction of the jejunoileal bypass operation. As indicated in Fig. 3, significant improvement in hepatic steatosis and inflammation was evident, compared to the histological characteristics of the liver at the time the jejunoileal bypass operation was reversed. Hepatic fibrosis was not significantly decreased by reconstruction. While the appearance of the liver improves, fibrosis was decreased in 20 patients, unchanged in four patients and increased in two patients following reconstruction of the jejunoileal bypass. Following recon-

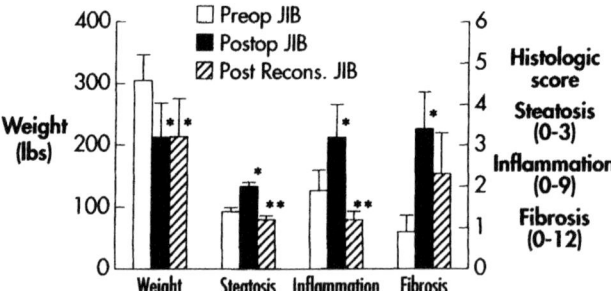

Figure 3 Late effects of jejunileal bypass operations (JIB) on hepatic histology and the effects of reconstruction on the histological appearance of the liver. Histological slides from liver specimens were evaluated in a blinded fashion by an experienced pathologist from 26 consecutive patients undergoing reconstruction of the JIB, 69 ± 19 months after the JIB, and compared to the histological appearance of the patients' livers at the time the JIB operation was performed. These patients underwent liver biopsies 14 ± 2 months following reconstruction of the JIB. Single asterisks indicate that the post-JIB value is significantly different from the pre-JIB value, and two asterisks indicate that the value obtained from the liver biopsy from the patients having the JIB reversed is significantly different from the value produced by the liver biopsy obtained at the time that the JIB was reversed

struction of the jejunoileal bypass operations, one patient died of liver failure and one patient has undergone liver transplantation.

The above information regarding changes in hepatic lipid content, as determined histologically, associated with reconstruction of jejunoileal bypass operations, was confirmed by quantitating the triglyceride content utilizing core needle biopsy specimens obtained at the time of reconstruction and 1–2 years following reconstruction[20]. Twenty-six patients 69 ± 19 months following jejunoileal bypass operations had 137 ± 7 mg triglyceride/100 mg protein in their liver, which was significantly decreased to 87 ± 5 at 1–2 years following reconstruction.

THE HEPATIC EFFECTS PRODUCED BY THE JEJUNOILEAL BYPASS COMPARED TO THOSE PRODUCED BY THE PATIENT'S OBESE STATE

It became apparent that patients who underwent reconstruction of the jejunoileal bypass operation and gained weight following reconstruction had a deterioration in their liver histology. We have been able to evaluate a group of eight patients who underwent reconstruction without a gastric restrictive procedure to control their weight, and a group of patients who did have a gastroplasty and who maintained their weight loss. As indicated in Table 3, weight gain was detrimental following reconstruction regarding triglyceride accumulation, while inflammation and fibrosis decreased regardless of whether the patients lost weight. This suggests that the bypassed intestine contributes to a great extent to the production of the inflammatory changes and subsequent fibrosis associated with jejunoileal bypass, while the steatosis may be more dependent on body weight.

AETIOLOGY OF JEJUNOILEAL BYPASS STEATOHEPATITIS

The mechanism of the production of the steatohepatitis associated with jejunoileal bypass is not known, similar to steatohepatitis related to other disease processes. Whether it has unique aetiological mechanisms, or whether all forms of steatohepatitis have a common aetiology, is unknown. The factors originally believed to contribute to jejunoileal bypass steatohepatitis are presented in Table 4. Clinical or experimental information was available to support various theoretical mechanisms, including protein deficiency[21], choline deficiency[22], bypass enterotoxins[23], and abnormal bile salt metabolism[24].

More recent information concerning the aetiology of steatohepatitis in general may provide the opportunity to better understand the steatohepatitis associated with jejunoileal bypass. The theoretical production of steatosis[25] associated with jejunoileal bypass is illustrated in Fig. 4. Obese and diabetic patients[25] and patients with jejunoileal bypass[26] have increased fatty acids delivered to the liver. This is associated with relative hyperinsulinaemia, which drives the lipid into triglyceride formation rather than ketone formation. Patients with jejunoileal bypass are hypoproteinaemic[21] and have decreased ability to form lipoproteins for transport of the triglyceride from the liver. The aetiology of the

Table 3 Comparison of the effect of weight gain on the results of reconstruction of jejunoileal bypass operations (JIB)

Change in body weight since Recon JIB[†]	Hepatic triglyceride (mg/100 mg protein)		Hepatic inflammation (0–9)		Hepatic fibrosis (0–12)	
	Pre-recon	Post-recon	Pre-recon	Post-recon	Pre-recon	Post-recon
+85 ± 23 lb	108 ± 33	205 ± 32[††]	3.0 ± 2.0	0.75 ± 0.3[††]	2.38 ± 1.2	1.62 ± 1.5
−33 ± 23 lb	142 ± 15	84 + 6[††]	3.3 ± 1.8	1.38 ± 1.2[††]	3.94 ± 2.0	2.44 ± 1.9

[†] Eight patients underwent reconstruction of the jejunoileal bypass without a gastric restrictive procedure, and 18 patients had a simultaneous gastric restrictive procedure. Liver specimens were obtained at the time of reconstruction of the jejunoileal bypass operations and > 1 year later. (Recon = reconstruction)
[††] indicates that the post-reconstruction value is significantly different from the pre-construction value.

Table 4 Original theoretical causes of liver disease associated with intestinal bypass operations for obesity

Early steatosis
Starvation
Protein deficiency
Choline deficiency
Late inflammation and cirrhosis
Bypass enterotoxins
Ruptured intracellular lipid droplets
Abnormal bile salt metabolism

Following Intestinal Bypass

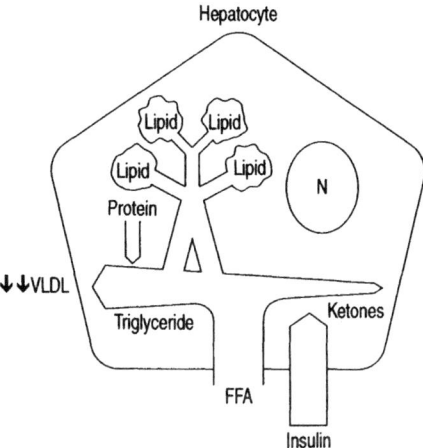

Figure 4 Diagrammatic illustration of the factors believed to contribute to steatosis in patients who have undergone jejunoileal bypass operations. Obese patients have increased fatty acid levels and relative hyperinsulinaemia. The increased insulin levels drive fatty acid metabolism from ketones towards triglycerides. Hypoprotinaemia decreases the hepatocyte's ability to export triglycerides as lipoproteins, resulting in triglycerides forming intracellular lipid droplets (steatosis)

inflammation in NASH syndrome has become focused on cytochrome P450IIE1[27]. As indicated in Fig. 5, the increased fatty acids associated with jejunoileal bypass may elevate cytochrome P450IIE1 levels which, along with enterotoxins from the small intestine, may increase reactive oxygen species[28], resulting in cell damage and inflammation. These theoretical considerations have produced avenues of research to follow in attempting to better understand NASH syndrome and find ways to prevent the disorder.

DISCUSSION

NASH syndrome occurring in association with various disorders such as severe obesity and in patients with jejunoileal bypass appears to be a chronic, indolent form of liver disease, the natural history of which may extend throughout a

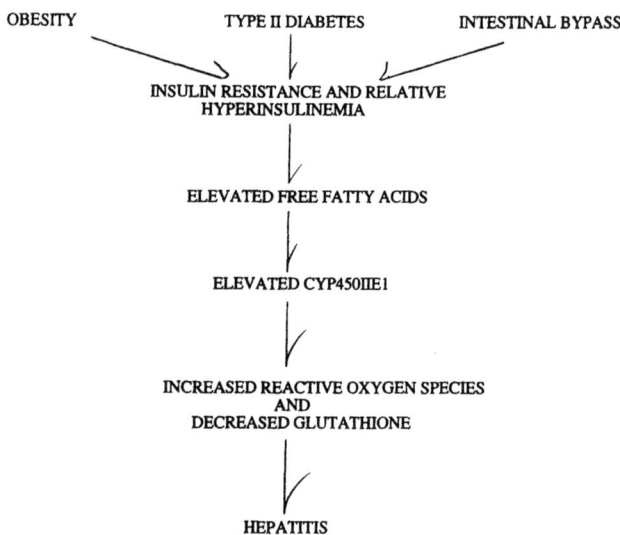

Figure 5 Schematic illustration of the theoretical mechanisms involved in producing inflammation in patients with steatohepatitis and steatonecrosis. Patients with intestinal bypass operations are proposed to have relative hyperinsulinaemia because they are encouraged to be hyperphagocytic. The known elevated free fatty acids are proposed to increase the amount of hepatocyte cytochrome P450IIE1, which as in alcoholic hepatitis induces the formation of reactive oxygen species and decreases glutathione formation resulting in inflammation (hepatitis)

lifetime. The frequency with which the disorder will compromise survival from liver failure is presently unknown. Our experience with NASH syndrome associated with jejunoileal bypass is that, following 20 years with what may represent the most severe form of NASH syndrome, these patients now all manifest clinical cirrhosis. While it was originally felt that some patients with jejunoileal bypass could be followed with interval liver biopsy[12], currently the information suggests that these patients will all have NASH syndrome and should undergo reversal of the jejunoileal bypass operation. The information presented above suggests that patients undergoing reversal of the operation may benefit by having their weight controlled by a gastric restrictive procedure, as resumption of the obese state will significantly exacerbate the steatotosis. This concept seems to be relevant in regard to patients with NASH syndrome, or patients with an intact jejunoileal bypass who have cirrhosis and have progressed to liver failure and undergo liver transplantation. Based on a small number of patients the information suggests that the transplanted liver will develop steatohepatitis unless the aetiological mechanism is controlled[29,30]. In patients with obesity, unless their obesity can be controlled with a gastric restrictive procedure their anticipated benefit from a liver transplant may be brief. Patients with jejunoileal bypass and clinical cirrhosis may benefit from reversal of the jejunoileal bypass and a gastric restrictive procedure prior to any consideration for liver transplantation. Our results indicate that approximately 65% of the patients undergoing this approach will have significant improvement in hepatic histology and liver function, and the patients may avoid transplantation[12]. If the patients continue to deteriorate, and do require liver transplantation, their liver will be protected from reoccurrence of the NASH syndrome produced by the jejunoileal bypass operation[30].

While NASH syndrome occurring in patients with jejunoileal bypass represents a small number of patients, NASH syndrome occurring in obesity does not[31]. Steatohepatitis occurs frequently in morbidly obese patients weighing >350 lb and frequently these patients have adult-onset, type II diabetes. There is evidence that weight loss produces improvement in the steatohepatitis associated with obesity[32], and patients with obesity-related steatohepatitis should be encouraged to permanently reduce their body weight by dietary, or dietary and pharmacological, means. If this approach fails to control their weight the patients may be well served by having a gastric restrictive procedure. Weight loss associated with gastric restrictive operative procedures may reverse the patient's NASH syndrome[33] and, if present, may also cure the patient's diabetes[34].

Acknowledgement

This work was supported in part by USPHS Grant DK27695.

References

1. Westwater JO, Fainer D. Liver impairment in the obese. Gastroenterology. 1958;34:686–93.
2. Zelman S. The liver in obesity. Arch Intern Med. 1952;90:141–8.
3. Rozental P, Biava C, Spencer H, Zimmerman HJ. Liver morphology and function tests in obesity and during total starvation. Am J Dig Dis. 1967;12:198–208.
4. Ludwig J, Viggiano TR, McGill DB, Ott BJ. Non-alcoholic steatohepatitis. Mayo Clinic experience with a hitherto unnamed disease. Mayo Clin Proc. 1980;55:424–38.
5. Bacon BR, Farahvash MJ, Janney CG, Neuschwander-Tetri BA. Nonalcoholic steatohepatitis: an expanded clinical entity. Gastroenterology. 1994;107:1103–9.
6. Weltman MD, Farrell GC, Liddle C. Increased hepatocyte CYP2E1 expression in a rat nutritional model of hepatic steatosis with inflammation. Gastroenterology. 1996;111:1645–53.
7. Joffe SN. Surgical management of morbid obesity. Gut. 1981;22:242–54.
8. Nachlas MM, Crawford DT, Pearl JM. Current status of jejunoileal bypass in the treatment of morbid obesity. Surg Gynecol Obstet. 1980;150:256–70.
9. Wood LC, Chremos AN. Treating obesity by 'short circuiting' the small intestine. J Am Med Asssoc. 1963;186:63–72.
10. Payne JH, DeWind LT, Commons RR. Metabolic observations in patients with jejunocolic shunts. Am J Surg. 1963;106:273–87.
11. Kaminski DL, Herrmann VM, Martin S. Late effects of jejunoileal bypass operations on hepatic inflammation, fibrosis, and lipid content. Hepatogastroenterology. 1985;32:185–9.
12. Dean P, Joshi S, Kaminski DL. Long-term outcome of reversal of small intestinal bypass operations. Am J Surg. 1990;159:118–23.
13. Requarth JA, Burchard KW, Colacchio TA et al. Long-term morbidity following jejunoileal bypass. Arch Surg. 1995;130:318–25.
14. Gastrointestinal surgery for severe obesity: consensus development conference panel. Ann Intern Med. 1991;115:956–61.
15. Maxwell JG, Richards RC, Albo D. Fatty degeneration of the liver after intestinal bypass for obesity. Am J Surg. 1968;116:648–52.
16. Styblo T, Martin S, Kaminski DL. The effects of reversal of jejunoileal bypass operations on hepatic triglyceride content and hepatic morphology. Surgery. 1984;96:632–41.
17. Haines NW, Baker AL, Boyer JL et al. Prognostic indicators of hepatic injury following jejunoileal bypass performed for refractory obesity: a prospective study. Hepatology. 1981;1:161–7.
18. Kern WH, Payne JH, Dewind LT. Hepatic changes after small-intestinal bypass for morbid obesity. Am J Clin Pathol. 1974;61:763–8.

19. Manes JL, Taylor HB, Starkloff GB. Relationship between hepatic morphology and clinical and biochemical findings in morbidly obese patients. J Clin Pathol. 1973;26:776–83.
20. Kaminski DL, Adams A, Jellinek M. The effects of hyperalimentation on hepatic lipid content and lipogenic enzyme activity in rats and man. Surgery. 1980;88:93–100.
21. Kaminski DL, Mueller E, Jellinek M. The effect of dietary manipulation on hepatic lipid accumulation in rats undergoing small intestinal bypass. Int J Obes. 1985;9:59–68.
22. Kaminski DL, Jellinek M, Ruwart MJ. Small intestinal bypass in nutritionally obese rats receiving choline supplementation. Surg Forum. 1976;27:449–51.
23. Kaminski DL, Jellinek M, Mueller EJ. The effect of antibiotics on hepatic lipid metabolism following small intestinal bypass. J Surg Res. 1980;28:97–102.
24. Sherr HP, Nair PP, White JJ, Banwell JG, Lockwood DH. Bile acid metabolism and hepatic disease following small-bowel bypass for obesity. Am J Clin Nutr. 1974;27:1369–79.
25. Wanless IR, Bargman JM, Oreopoulos DG, Vas SI. Subcapsular steatonecrosis in response to peritoneal insulin deliver: a clue to the pathogenesis of steatonecrosis in obesity. Mod Pathol. 1989;2:69–74.
26. Kallner A, Hallberg D, Backman L. Fatty acid patterns of serum triglycerides and subcutaneous adipose tissues after ileal bypass in obesity. Scand J Gastroenterol. 1975;10:763–7.
27. Weltman MD, Liddle C, Farrell GC. Hepatic CYP2E1 is increased in patients with nonalcoholic steatohepatitis. Hepatolology. 1996;24:202A.
28. Weltman MD, Liddle C, Farrell GC. Evidence that oxidative stress plays a role in steatohepatitis produced in a rat nutritional model. Hepatology. 1996;24:304A.
29. Carson K, Washington MK, Treem WR, Clavien PA, Hunt CM. Recurrence of nonalcoholic steatohepatitis in a liver transplant recipient. Liver Transplant Surg. 1997;3:174–6.
30. D'Souza-Grurek SM, Batts KP, Nikias GA, Wiesner RH, Krom RAF. Liver transplantation for jejunoileal bypass-associated cirrhosis: allograft histology in the setting of an intact bypassed limb. Liver Transplant Surg. 1997;3:23–7.
31. Wanless IR, Lentz JS. Fatty liver hepatitis (steatohepatitis) and obesity: an autopsy study with analysis of risk factors. Hepatology. 1990;12:1106–10.
32. Eriksson S, Eriksson KF, Bondesson L. Nonalcoholic steatohepatitis in obesity: a reversible condition. Acta Med Scand. 1986;220:83–8.
33. Ranlev I, Hardt F. Regression of liver steatosis following gastroplasty or gastric bypass for morbid obesity. Digestion. 1990;47:208–14.
34. Pories WJ, MacDonald KG, Flickinger EG et al. Is type II diabetes mellitus (NIDDM) a surgical disease? Ann Surg. 1992;215:633–43.

Index

acetaldehyde 130
  production, large intestine by colonic
    bacteria 125
acetamide 179
achlorhydria 334(table), 335
actin-ADP-ribosylating toxins 186,
  187(fig.)
adherence 6
adhesins 3
agglutinins 68
alanine 141, 142(fig.), 154(fig.), 156(fig.)
alcohol 36, 38(table), 39
  blood concentration 105, 108
  chronic consumption
    effect of 106
    rectal carcinogenesis 130
  effect on concentration 106–7
  effect on motility 310–12
    colon 312
    gastric emptying 311
    oesophagus 310–11
    small bowel motility 311–12
  endotoxaemia 129–30
  fermentation by intestinal microbes
    125
  first-pass metabolism *see* first-pass
    metabolism, alcohol
  functional implications 108
  gastric first-pass metabolism 104–18
  gastritis *see* gastritis, alcoholic
  gender/ethnicity differences 106
  induced mucosal injury in the upper
    GIT 282–8
  interaction with other drugs 106–7
  legal limits of intoxication 108
  misuse (chronic), intestinal
    permeability 38
  oral–coecal transit time 129
  oxidation, bacteriocolonic pathway
    127–8, 129(table)

alcohol dehydrogenase (ADH) 104, 125,
  126(fig.)
  gastric first-pass metabolism, role
    104–6
  human colonic flora 126–7
  sigma 106
alcohol-induced liver injury 222–36
  cytokine release and other mediators
    289–93
  endotoxin 223(fig.)
  free radicals 223(fig.)
    involvement 233–5
  hypoxia 223(fig.)
  Kupffer cells 223(fig.)
allopurinol 52
α-antiplasmin 263
α-macroglobulin 263
α-glucosidase inhibitors 33
amino acid(s)
  metabolism, gut 153–9
    metabolic cooperation of intestine
      and liver in vitro 157–8
  transport and cell function 139(fig.)
5-aminosalicylic acid 34
aminosugar-D-galactosamine (Gal N),
  hepatitis 206
ammonium 109, 154(fig.)
  role in chronic alcoholic gastritis
    110–13
ampicillin 7, 357
amyloidosis 394–5
antibiotics 66
  long-term prophylaxis, yeast
    overgrowth 7
  oral 49
    risk to bacterial translocation 49
antithrombin (AT) III 263
apoptotic cell death 206
apoptotic necrosis 207
arginine 154(fig.), 156(fig.)

ascites, culture-negative neutrocytic 341–2, 356
aspirin 107
asymptomatic bacteriascites 356
autoimmune chronic hepatitis 390–4
  clinical manifestations 391
  pathogenesis 390–1
  pathology 391–2
azathioprine 69
aztreonam 358

B cell(s)
  development 18(fig.)
  differentiation 17–19
  function 18(fig.)
Bacillus Calmette-Guerin 206
Bacillus megaterium 47(table)
bacterial drug metabolism
  effect of antibiotics 179–80
  principles 177–8
  small intestinal bacterial overgrowth, role 180
  under physiological conditions, role 178–9
bacterial overgrowth in alcoholics 283–4
bacterial peritonitis, spontaneous 341–51
  clinical course 348–50
  death, causes 350(table)
  definition 342(table)
  diagnosis 346–8
  epidemiology 341–3
  factors, predisposing 345–6
  features 342(table)
  microbia 343–5
  paracentesis 346–8
  pathophysiology 343
  prognostic factors 348–50
  risk factors 345(table)
  symptoms 346
  treatment and prophylaxis 354–60
    data 355–6
    diagnosis 356–7
    pathogenesis 354–5
    prophylaxis 358–60
    treatment 357–8
bacterial translocation 47–57
  animal models lacking T-cell-mediated immunity 53(table)
  host immune defence deficiency 54
  induced by a combination of promoting mechanisms 54–5
  pathogenesis, stages 56, 57(fig.)

promoted by:
  compromised host immune defences 52–4
  increased intestinal permeability 51–2
  physical damage to the intestinal mucosa 51–2
  promoted by intestinal bacterial overgrowth 48–51
bacteriocins 3
Bacteriodes fragilis 56
Bacteriodes spp 5, 177, 179, 299
Bacteroides vulgatus 9, 56, 245
β7 integrin 15
β-blockers 264
β-lactoglobulin A and B 65
Bifidobacterium spp 179
bile acids 141
  deconjugation 93–5
  7-deoxy, toxicity *see* 7-deoxy bile acids
  dehydroxylation 94–5
  intestinal bacteria 85–99
  metabolism 93–4
  modulation of small intestinal flora 99–100
  unconjugated
    absorption from the intestine 92–3
    metabolism in the liver 93
bile duct carcinoma 403
bile salt 87
bovine serum albumin 62, 65
bowel rest 66
Budd–Chiari syndrome 343

Campylobacter 113
canalicular multiple-drug resistance protein 22
Candida albicans 50, 125
Candida spp 359
carbon tetrachloride 225–6
cardiopulmonary bypass, small intestine injury 39
casein 65
CD11b/c expression 200–2
CD1d 15
CD25 20, 16
CD2 16
CD4+T helper cells type-1 17
CD40 16
CD45RA 20
CD45RO 20, 16
CD4 cells 16
CD71 16

CD80/86   16
CD8 cells   15
CD95 (fas/APO-1) system, apoptosis
      210–11
CD95/CD95L, ramifications   211
CD-71   20
cefonicid   358
cefotaxime   357–8
ceftizoxime   358
ceftriaxone   358
cell-mediated immunity   54
cellobiose   63
chemotherapeutic agents   36
chenodeoxycholic acid   86
Chlamydia trachomatis   347
cholangiocarcinoma   389
cholanoids
   primary
      chemistry   87–8
      modification by bacterial enzymes
         88–91
      unconjugated, physicochemical
         properties   91
cholelithiasis   388–9
cholera toxin   186(fig.), 17
cholestasis, endotoxaemia   299–302
   clinical features   300–1
   diagnosis   300–1
      differential   301–2
   incidence   299–300
   pathogenesis   300
   prognosis   300–1
cholestasis, sepsis-induced   299–302
cholesterol   87
   gallstones, deoxycholic acid input
      98–9
cimetidine   107, 109(fig.)
ciprofloxacin   188, 360
cirrhosis
   endotoxaemia and disseminated
      intravascular coagulation
      263–77
   portal hypertension   39
citrulline   154(fig.), 156(fig.)
clindamycin   49, 7
clonal anergy   23
Clostridium botulinum C2 toxin   186–7
Clostridium difficile
   associated colitis or diarrhoea   7
   toxins, effect on intestinal mucosa
      185–91
Clostridium perfringens   185–7
Clostridium spp   177

clotting activation, portal vein,
      endotoxaemia role   274–7
clotting, liver cirrhosis   263(table)
co-vitamin B_{12} 35(fig.), 34
cobra venom factor   199
coeliac disease   174, 398–400
   agglutinin   68
cofactors   3
colchicine   179
colitis
   antibiotic-associated   7
   dextran-sulphate sodium   68
   trinitrochlorobenzene   23
collagen arthritis   23
colonic flora   124
colonic permeability   33–4
colonization resistance, antibiotic-induced
      48–9
colony forming units   4
common mucosal immune system   15
Corynebacterium parvum   52
corrinoids   180
corticosteroids   69
   hepatic encephalopathy   117
Councilman bodies   206
Crohn's disease   9, 34, 64–5, 174,
      381(table)
   bowel rest   66
cryptogenic cirrhosis   392–3
   clinical manifestations   392
   fatty infiltration   392
   treatment   392
cyclophosphamide   54
cyclosporin   169(table) 174, 387
   A   81
CYP-1A1   172–3
CYP-3A4   164, 168(fig.), 170
CYP-3A   169–7
CYP-3AP   172
CYP-P450   163, 165, 166–8
   mediated intestinal drug metabolism,
      inhibition   169–70
cystic fibrosis   38(table)
cystic fibrosis transmembrane regulator
      185, 186(fig.)
cytokine
   burst syndrome   203
   factors influencing the effects
      290(table)
   induced neutrophil chemoattractant
      199
   mediated suppression of immune
      reaction   22

cytokine (*contd.*)
  release of peripheral blood monocytes
    292–9
  serum/plasma levels 291
cytosolic protein concentration 145
cytotoxic drugs 38(table)

deamidation 88
deconjugation 88
  intestinal site 89–91
deferoxamine 52
dehydroxylation at C-7 89
  intestinal site 89–91
7-deoxy bile acids
  endogenous
    adaptation preventing toxicity 96–8
    patients with cholesterol gallstones
      98–9
  exogenous, toxicity 95–6
detergents 36
dextrans 36
diabetes in the non-obese 23
diaphragm disease 36
diet, elemental 66
digestion
  endolytic 86
  xenolytic 86
digoxin 179
D-dimer 264
dimethyl-β-cyclodextrin 81
dimethylsulphoxide 52
drug metabolism, intestinal wall 163–75
drug-metabolising enzymes, assessment
  163–5
dysfibrinogenaemia 263(table)
dyspeptic symptoms 114

eicosanoids 204
endotoxaemia 39
  acute-phase response 286
  acute/chronic 195–202
    hepatic polymorphonuclear leukocyte
      influx 196–7
  alcohol-induced 129–30
  alcoholic liver disease 284–7
  changes induced by alcohol abuse in the
    intestine 294(fig.)
  cholestasis 299–302
  cirrhosis 251–61
  clotting activation in the portal vein
    274–7
  disseminated intravascular coagulation
    in cirrhosis 263–77

factors influencing activity of LPS
  288–9
hepatitis, chronic 251–61
hyperfibrinolysis and clotting activation
  267–274
portal 64
systemic 64
endotoxin 39, 52
  binding capacity of:
    albumin 253–4
    high density lipoprotein 253–4
    transferrin 253–4
  binding of plasma proteins 256–7
  clearance by reticuloendothelial system
    62
  core 65
  effect of ethanol 226–7, 232(fig.)
  effect on Kupffer and parenchymal cells
    225–6
  gut permeability 224
  gut-derived, experimental alcohol-
    induced liver injury 287
  inactivating rate of plasma,
    measurement 253
  plasma concentration 254–5
  relationship to liver function test
    255–6
  translocating 68
  uptake, Limulus assay 62
enteric bacteria, translocation 68
Enterobacter spp 345
Enterobacteriaceae 56–7
Enterococcus faecalis 56
erythromycin 169–70
Escherichia coli 9, 47(table), 299, 345
  C25, antagonism by indigenous
    anaerobes 49(table)
  heat-labile toxins 185
ethanol *see* alcohol
ethinyloestradiol 179
Eubacterium 5
experimental autoimmune
  encephalomyelitis 23
experimental autoimmune uveitis 23

ferritin expression 370–1
fibrin(ogen) degradation products 264
fibrinopeptide A 269
fibrosis
  mediastinal 382, 383(table)
  retroperitoneal 382, 383(table)
first-pass metabolism, alcohol 104–8
  after gastrectomy 106

during fasting 106
quantification 107–8
FITC-dextran 63
food allergies 24
free radicals
alcohol-induced liver injury 233–5
Fusobacterium 5
Fusobacterium russii 56

gadolinium chloride 225, 228(table)
D-galactosamine 226
GALT (gut-associated lymphoid tissues) 13
gastric antral vascular ectasia 308, 318
gastric permeability 33
gastritis
chronic, symptomatology 113
epidemic 113
histological scores 114(fig.)
effect of antibiotic treatment 115(fig.)
pathogenesis, role of ammonia, alcohol 114–8
gastritis, alcoholic
chronic 110–18
alcohol, role 110
ammonium, role 110–13
Helicobacter pylori, role 110–13
clinical observation 108–18
gastroduodenal ulcer, aetiological agent 109
gastroesophageal reflux disease 310
gastrointestinal bleeding 345
gastrointestinal immune system, structure 13–16
diffused mucosal lymphoid tissue 15–16
organised lymphoid tissues 13–15
gastrointestinal motility, altered 307–13
bacterial overgrowth 310
gastric emptying 307–9
motility, effect of ethanol 310–12
oesophageal motility, effect of sclerotherapy 312
small intestinal transit 309–10
gene expression 139(fig.)
germ-free paradox 158
giardiasis 34
Gilbert's syndrome 165–6
gliadin 65
glucagon 141–2
glutamate 139(fig.)

glutamine 141–2
intestinal
metabolism in humans 155
pathophysiological conditions 155–7
metabolism, rat intestine 153–4
glutathione 375
gluten 65
gluten-sensitive enteropathies 24, 174
glycine 141–2
glycogen synthesis 139(fig.)
glycogenolysis 139(fig.)
glycolysis 139(fig.)
glycoprotein Ib/IIb/IIIa 266
glycuronidation 93
gp180 15
guanine nucleotide dissociation stimulators/inhibitors 189
gut bacteria in drug metabolism, role 177–80
gut design 86–7
gut flora, alterations induced by diet of alcohol 224
gut mucosal barrier 61(fig.)
dysfunction 62–3
inflammatory bowel disease, experimental 63
function 62
inflammatory bowel disease 63–9
gut permeability
increased to macromolecules 283
to endotoxin, alcohol induced 224
gut-derived bacterial toxins 281–2

H2 blockers 107
action on blood alcohol level 107–8
haemochromatosis 365–77
genetic defect 365
incidence 365
iron metabolism 368–75
liver transplantation 375–7
protein, model 366(fig.)
Haemophilus influenzae 299
Hafnia alvei 130
Helicobacter pylori 282, 308, 317, 328
alcohol interaction 104
chronic alcoholic gastritis, role 110–13
gastroduodenal ulcer 109
hepatic encephalopathy, role 115–17
heparin cofactor II 263
hepatic abscess 395

hepatic apoptosis   206–14
  elicited by cytokines   208–11
  endotoxin-induced   207
  modulation   211–14
hepatic encephalopathy   345–6
  Helicobacter pylori, role   115–17
hepatic granulomas   394
hepatitis
  A, intestinal permeability   38
  chronic, with primary sclerosing
      cholangitis   385(table)
hepatobiliary inflammation   241–9
  genetically susceptible rats   242–5
  immune mechanisms   247–8
  luminal anaerobic bacteria, influence
      245–7
hepatocyte, cell volume signalling
      147(fig.)
HIV-AIDS   38(table)
HML-1 activation antigen   15, 19
homing   19
host defence, overactivation   203
humoral immunity   54
hydrogen sulphide   6
hydroxylation   93, 94(fig.)
hyodeoxycholic acid   96
hyperammonaemic coma   158
hyperfibrinolysis
  cirrhosis, bleeding complication   264–7
  clotting activation, role of
      endotoxaemia   267–74
hyperfibrinolytic syndrome   263(table)
hypochlorhydria   113
hypogammaglobulinaemia   38(table)

ileal pouch disease   8–9
immunoglobulin A   20–1, 54, 61(fig.)
  secretory   20–1, 12–13
indomethacin   328
inflammatory bowel disease
  agglutinins to enteric bacteria   68
  as an aggravating factor   67–8
  as an epiphenomenon   68
  clinical, gut mucosal barrier function
      63–9
    antibody response to dietary antigens
        65
    antibody response to enteric bacteria
        65
    bacterial translocation   64
    bowel rest   66
    circulating immune complexes
        65–6

endotoxaemia   64
intestinal permeability   64
intestinal protein loss   64–5
gut barrier dysfunction, clinical
    significance   66–9
primary event   66–7
insulin   141–2
insulin-like growth factor   141
interferon-γ 17, 23
interleukin-10   22
interleukin-1   204, 289
interleukin-2   17
interleukin-4   22
interleukin-8   291–2
International Agency for Research on
    Cancer   130
intestinal absorption, small particles
    75–81
intestinal bacteria, biochemical reactions
    178(table)
intestinal immune system   12–24
intestinal microflora   3
  (normal), factors influencing   5(table)
intestinal permeability
  barrier   31–9
  changes, localization   35(fig.)
  increased
    burn patient   39
    consequences, systemic/local
        37–8
    critically ill   39
    inflammatory bowel diesase   61–9
    liver disease   38–9
    luminal aggressors   38(table)
    mucosal defence, impaired   38(table)
    permeability breakers   38(table)
  tests, uses   34–7
    diagnostic screening/monitoring of
        therapeutic responses   34–6
    effect of drugs/toxins on intestinal
        integrity   36
    intestinal physiology   36–7
    pathogenesis of disease   36
intestinal proteolysis   21–2
intra-epithelial cells   15
iron
  induced cellular toxicity   374–5
  metabolism, physiology   366–8
  sulphur switch   370
ischaemia/reperfusion, following shock
    52
isoenzyme of nitric oxide (iNOS)   325
  gastrointestinal disease, role of   327–8

jaundice
  resulting from sepsis   301–2
  total parenteral nutrition-associated
    299
jejunoileal bypass   406–15
  steatohepatitis, aetiology   411–13
Jun-kinases   145, 148

6-keto-PGF1$_\alpha$ 318
ketoconazole   169(table)
Klebsiella   345
Klebsiella pneumoniae   50, 299
Kupffer cells
  activated by ethanol treatment, liver
    injury   230–2
  alcohol-induced liver injury
    223(fig.)
    in vivo   229–30
  endotoxin clearance   285

Lactobacillus acidophilus   52
Lactobacillus brevis   56
Lactobacillus spp   177, 224
lactose   36
lamina propria T cells   20(table)
large intestine, normal microbiota   4–5
leukotriene D$_4$ 204
Limulus
  enzyme   251
  gelation test   284
lipid A   65
lipid peroxidation   375
lipogenesis   139(fig.)
lipopolysaccharide   203–4
  effect on mediator release from
    monocytes/macrophages
    290(fig.)
lithocholic acid   86, 89
liver, apoptosis *see* hepatic apoptosis
liver cell hydration   134–49
  bile formation   144
  cell volume sensing and signalling
    145–8
  gene expression   145
  liver cell function   139–40
    effect of hypo-osmotic cell swelling
      140(table)
    physiological modulators   135–8
    cumulative substrate uptake
      135–6
    ethanol   136–8
    glucagon   137(table), 138
    insulin   137(table), 138

oxidative stress   138
  urea   138
  proteolysis   141–3
liver injury (experimental)
  role of lipopolysaccharide and
    cytokines   203
  sensitizers   206
liver transplantation
  end-stage primary sclerosing
    cholangitis   388
  genetic haemochromatosis   375–6
long-chain fatty acids   86
Lophophorus ihllysii   89, 90(fig.)
lower oesophageal sphincter, following
  sclerotherapy   312
LPAM-1   19
lymphoid tissues
  diffused   15–16
  organised   13–15

M (membranous) cells   13, 77,
  78–80(figs.)
macrophages, MHC class II   15
maize   65
major bile duct, stenosis   403
malnutrition   335
MALT (mucosa-associated lymphoid
  tissues)   13
mannitol   36, 63
melibiose   36
methotrexate   387
metronidazole   49, 179
MHC class I-like molecules   15
Michaelis–Menten formula, alcohol   107
microbial control mechanisms, basic
  5–6
microflora-associated characteristics
  177, 178(table)
midazolam   168(table), 169, 174
migrating motor complex (MMC) activity
  310, 311
mitogen-activated protein (MAP) kinase
  144–146
molybdenum-free diet   52
monoalide   19
morphine   179
mucosal homing   15
mucosal immune system
  inductive and effector sites   13,
    14(fig.)
  functional features   16–21
    B cell differentiation   17–19
    homing   19

mucosal immune system
 functional features contd.
  immunoglobulin A 20–1
  lamina propria T cells 20
  uptake of antigen, events following
   16–18
mucosal immunity 54
multiorgan failure 39, 52
mutanolysin 246–7

NASH syndrome 406–15
necrosis, secondary 207
New Italian Endoscopic Club Consensus
 Conference (1992) 316–17
Nippostrongylus brasiliensis 37
nitric oxide 204–5, 290(fig.)
 constitutive 324–5
 inducible 325
 synthase inhibitors 325, 327
non-steroidal anti-inflammatory drugs
 (NSAIDs) 32, 38(table), 66
 mucosal ulceration 62
norfloxacin 359
nutrient 5

3-*O*-methyl-D-glucose 34
oesophageal varices 264
ofloxacin 358, 360
omeprazole 107, 173
oral contraception, administration of
 antibiotics 180
oral tolerance 21–4
 characteristics 21
 features 22(table)
 humans 24
 mechanisms 21–3
 suppressions of disease in animal
  models 23
oxidation–reduction potential 4–6
oxytetracycline
 cirrhosis with encephalopathy 116–17
 effect on gastric ammonia 113(fig.)

P-glycoprotein (PgP) 19, 172
paracentesis, diagnostic 346–8
paradoxical mucosal iron deficiency 370
D-penicillamine 387
penicillin 49, 55(table), 179–80
pentoxifylline 248
peptoglycans 65
persorption 47(table)
Peyer's patches 13, 16, 19
phase II enzymes 165–6

phosphoenolpyruvate carboxykinase 145
phospholipase A2 198(fig.)
plasminogen 263
platelet abnormalities, liver cirrhosis
 263(table)
platelet-activating factor 225
poly-1g receptor 21
polyethylene glycol (PEG-400) 32–3,
 63–4
polymorphonuclear leukocyte
 function, gender differences 200–2
 hepatic accumulation, cytokine-induced
  neutrophil chemoattractant
  199
 liver recruited, differences between
  blood circulating (rats) 198–9
polysucrose-15000 37
portal hypertension 309
 colopathy 319–20
 enteropathy 318–19
 gastropathy 308, 316–18
 hepatic injury 328–9
portal hypertensive intestinal vasculopathy
 316–20
portal vein thrombosis 395
post-feeding hyperammonaemia, model
 for disturbed gut-liver cooperation
 158–9
pouchitis 8–9
prednisolone 54, 55(table)
primary biliary cirrhosis 384, 389
primary sclerosing cholangitis 382–8
 aetiopathological factors 384(table)
 clinical past manifestations 384–5
 clinics 401
 diagnosis, criteria 383(table)
 diseases associated 383(table)
 natural history 385–7
 pathogenesis 383–4
 survival 403–4
 symptoms 402
 treatment 387–8, 401–2
proctocolectomy 388
Propionibacterium acnes 52, 204
propranolol 318
prostacyclin 204, 318
prostaglandin E$_2$ 318
proteases 290(fig.)
protein C 263
protein phosphatase 2A 139(fig.)
protein S 263
protein synthesis 185–6
proteolysis 139(fig.)

Proteus mirabilis 50–1
Proteus spp 299
Pseudomonas aeruginosa 78, 80(fig.), 299

Rac proteins 189
radiation 38(table)
raffinose 36
ranitidine 106
reactive oxygen species 209, 290(fig.)
renal failure, chronic 38(table)
renal-hepatic syndrome 116
reticuloendothelial system 61(fig.)
L-rhamnose 32, 36–7
Rho proteins
  glucosylation
    Clostridium difficile toxins 188(fig.)
    functional consequences 190
  modifying toxins 187–8
  as targets for *Clostridium difficile* toxins 189–90
Riddle's thyroiditis 382
rifampicin 179
rifampin 171(fig.)
Rotavirus infection 34

Saccharomyces cerevisiae 65
salicylates 69
Salmonella 6, 38(table)
Salmonella enteridis 54
Salmonella typhimurium 50
sarcoidosis 395
sclerotherapy, oesophageal motility 312
secondary iron overload syndrome 368–9
secretory immunoglobulin A, cirrhosis 335
selective antibiotic decontamination 57
self-filling/emptying blind loops 241–9
sepsis 39
  cholestasis induced 299–302
Serratia marcescens 47(table)
Shiga toxin 186
Shigella 6, 38(table)
shock
  intestinal permeability 52
  models 51
short-chain fatty acids 86–7
small intestinal bacterial overgrowth 180
  chronic liver disease 332–6
    achlorhydria 335
    consequences in the setting 335–6

intestinal motility disturbances 334
local immunodeficiencies 335
malnutrition 335
possible causes involved 334
prevalence in patients 332–4
small intestinal permeability 32–3, 33–4
soluble tumour necrosis factor receptor type I 291
solvent drag 37
stachyose 36
Staphylococcus aureus 299–300
Staphylococcus epidermidis 51, 56
steatohepatitis 406–15
Streptococcus faecalis 47(table)
Streptococcus spp 177
Streptomyces globisporus 246
sucrose 33, 36
sulphapyridine 34
sulphasalazine 35(fig.), 178
swift increase in alcohol metabolism
  hypoxia in parenchymal cells 228–9
  interaction between Kupffer cells 227–8
systemic inflammatory response syndrome (SIRS) 203

T cell cytokine 17
T cells
  development 18(fig.)
  function 18(fig.)
taurocholate, effect on cellular hydration 144
Teprenone 318
terfenadine 170
Th2 cytokines 22
thrombin 269
thrombocytopenia 263(table)
thromboxane A2 204
thymectomy 52
tissue plasminogen activator 263–4, 268
TNF-R/TNF system 211
tobramycin 357
total dyspepsia score 114
total parenteral nutrition 66
  liver disease associated 301
transferrin 20, 370
  receptor 371(fig.)
transforming growth factor α 22–3
transjugular portosystemic shunt (TIPS) 274–6, 318
transmural migration 47(table)

trihydroxy bile acid 96
trimethoprim–sulphamethoxazol 360
tumour necrosis factor 204, 225
    β 199, 241, 289
    induced hepatic apoptosis 208–10
    β, growth inhibition, hepatic
        apoptosis 208
    particular role 205–6

UDP-glucurosyl transferase (UGT)
    izoenzymes 163
ulcerative colitis 9, 174
  Crohn's disease 381(table)
ursodeoxycholic acid 387, 401
  effect on:
    laboratory parameters 402
    liver histology 402–3

vasopressin 318
Veilonella spp 179
verapamil 171(fig.), 172(table), 174
vesicular transcellular bile acid transport
    144
Vibrio cholerae 6, 54
vitamin B_{12} 34
vitamin D 179
von Willebrand factor 266

watermelon stomach syndrome 318
xenobiotic metabolism, intestinal diseases
    173–4
xenolytic digestion 86–7

yeast cell wall mannan 65
Yersinia 38(table)

Falk Symposium Series

43. Reutter W, Popper H, Arias IM, Heinrich PC, Keppler D, Landmann L, eds.: *Modulation of Liver Cell Expression*. Falk Symposium No. 43. 1987 ISBN: 0-85200-677-2*
44. Boyer JL, Bianchi L, eds.: *Liver Cirrhosis*. Falk Symposium No. 44. 1987
ISBN: 0-85200-993-3*
45. Paumgartner G, Stiehl A, Gerok W, eds.: *Bile Acids and the Liver*. Falk Symposium No. 45. 1987 ISBN: 0-85200-675-6*
46. Goebell H, Peskar BM, Malchow H, eds.: *Inflammatory Bowel Diseases – Basic Research & Clinical Implications*. Falk Symposium No. 46. 1988 ISBN: 0-7462-0067-6*
47. Bianchi L, Holt P, James OFW, Butler RN, eds.: *Aging in Liver and Gastrointestinal Tract*. Falk Symposium No. 47. 1988 ISBN: 0-7462-0066-8*
48. Heilmann C, ed.: *Calcium-Dependent Processes in the Liver*. Falk Symposium No. 48. 1988 ISBN: 0-7462-0075-7*
50. Singer MV, Goebell H, eds.: *Nerves and the Gastrointestinal Tract*. Falk Symposium No. 50. 1989 ISBN: 0-7462-0114-1
51. Bannasch P, Keppler D, Weber G, eds.: *Liver Cell Carcinoma*. Falk Symposium No. 51. 1989 ISBN: 0-7462-0111-7
52. Paumgartner G, Stiehl A, Gerok W, eds.: *Trends in Bile Acid Research*. Falk Symposium No. 52. 1989 ISBN: 0-7462-0112-5
53. Paumgartner G, Stiehl A, Barbara L, Roda E, eds.: *Strategies for the Treatment of Hepatobiliary Diseases*. Falk Symposium No. 53. 1990 ISBN: 0-7923-8903-4
54. Bianchi L, Gerok W, Maier K-P, Deinhardt F, eds.: *Infectious Diseases of the Liver*. Falk Symposium No. 54. 1990 ISBN: 0-7923-8902-6
55. Falk Symposium No. 55 not published
55B. Hadziselimovic F, Herzog B, Bürgin-Wolff A, eds.: *Inflammatory Bowel Disease and Coeliac Disease in Children*. International Falk Symposium. 1990 ISBN 0-7462-0125-7
56. Williams CN, eds.: *Trends in Inflammatory Bowel Disease Therapy*. Falk Symposium No. 56. 1990 ISBN: 0-7923-8952-2
57. Bock KW, Gerok W, Matern S, Schmid R, eds.: *Hepatic Metabolism and Disposition of Endo- and Xenobiotics*. Falk Symposium No. 57. 1991 ISBN: 0-7923-8953-0
58. Paumgartner G, Stiehl A, Gerok W, eds.: *Bile Acids as Therapeutic Agents: From Basic Science to Clinical Practice*. Falk Symposium No. 58. 1991 ISBN: 0-7923-8954-9
59. Halter F, Garner A, Tytgat GNJ, eds.: *Mechanisms of Peptic Ulcer Healing*. Falk Symposium No. 59. 1991 ISBN: 0-7923-8955-7
60. Goebell H, Ewe K, Malchow H, Koelbel Ch, eds.: *Inflammatory Bowel Diseases – Progress in Basic Research and Clinical Implications*. Falk Symposium No. 60. 1991
ISBN: 0-7923-8956-5
61. Falk Symposium No. 61 not published
62. Dowling RH, Folsch UR, Löser Ch, eds.: *Polyamines in the Gastrointestinal Tract*. Falk Symposium No. 62. 1992 ISBN: 0-7923-8976-X
63. Lentze MJ, Reichen J, eds.: *Paediatric Cholestasis: Novel Approaches to Treatment*. Falk Symposium No. 63. 1992 ISBN: 0-7923-8977-8
64. Demling L, Frühmorgen P, eds.: *Non-Neoplastic Diseases of the Anorectum*. Falk Symposium No. 64. 1992 ISBN: 0-7923-8979-4
64B. Gressner AM, Ramadori G, eds.: *Molecular and Cell Biology of Liver Fibrogenesis*. International Falk Symposium. 1992 ISBN: 0-7923-8980-8

*These titles were published under the MTP Press imprint.

Falk Symposium Series

65. Hadziselimovic F, Herzog B, eds.: *Inflammatory Bowel Diseases and Morbus Hirschprung.* Falk Symposium No. 65. 1992   ISBN: 0-7923-8995-6
66. Martin F, McLeod RS, Sutherland LR, Williams CN, eds.: *Trends in Inflammatory Bowel Disease Therapy.* Falk Symposium No. 66. 1993   ISBN: 0-7923-8827-5
67. Schölmerich J, Kruis W, Goebell H, Hohenberger W, Gross V, eds.: *Inflammatory Bowel Diseases – Pathophysiology as Basis of Treatment.* Falk Symposium No. 67. 1993
ISBN: 0-7923-8996-4
68. Paumgartner G, Stiehl A, Gerok W, eds.: *Bile Acids and The Hepatobiliary System: From Basic Science to Clinical Practice.* Falk Symposium No. 68. 1993
ISBN: 0-7923-8829-1
69. Schmid R, Bianchi L, Gerok W, Maier K-P, eds.: *Extrahepatic Manifestations in Liver Diseases.* Falk Symposium No. 69. 1993   ISBN: 0-7923-8821-6
70. Meyer zum Büschenfelde K-H, Hoofnagle J, Manns M, eds.: *Immunology and Liver.* Falk Symposium No. 70. 1993   ISBN: 0-7923-8830-5
71. Surrenti C, Casini A, Milani S, Pinzani M , eds.: *Fat-Storing Cells and Liver Fibrosis.* Falk Symposium No. 71. 1994   ISBN: 0-7923-8842-9
72. Rachmilewitz D, ed.: *Inflammatory Bowel Diseases – 1994.* Falk Symposium No. 72. 1994   ISBN: 0-7923-8845-3
73. Binder HJ, Cummings J, Soergel KH, eds.: *Short Chain Fatty Acids.* Falk Symposium No. 73. 1994   ISBN: 0-7923-8849-6
73B. Möllmann HW, May B, eds.: *Glucocorticoid Therapy in Chronic Inflammatory Bowel Disease: from basic principles to rational therapy.* International Falk Workshop. 1996
ISBN 0-7923-8708-2
74. Keppler D, Jungermann K, eds.: *Transport in the Liver.* Falk Symposium No. 74. 1994
ISBN: 0-7923-8858-5
74B. Stange EF, ed.: *Chronic Inflammatory Bowel Disease.* Falk Symposium. 1995
ISBN: 0-7923-8876-3
75. van Berge Henegouwen GP, van Hoek B, De Groote J, Matern S, Stockbrügger RW, eds.: *Cholestatic Liver Diseases: New Strategies for Prevention and Treatment of Hepatobiliary and Cholestatic Liver Diseases.* Falk Symposium 75. 1994.
ISBN: 0-7923-8867-4
76. Monteiro E, Tavarela Veloso F, eds.: *Inflammatory Bowel Diseases: New Insights into Mechanisms of Inflammation and Challenges in Diagnosis and Treatment.* Falk Symposium 76. 1995.   ISBN 0-7923-8884-4
77. Singer MV, Ziegler R, Rohr G, eds.: *Gastrointestinal Tract and Endocrine System.* Falk Symposium 77. 1995.   ISBN 0-7923-8877-1
78. Decker K, Gerok W, Andus T, Gross V, eds.: *Cytokines and the Liver.* Falk Symposium 78. 1995.   ISBN 0-7923-8878-X
79. Holstege A, Schölmerich J, Hahn EG, eds.: *Portal Hypertension.* Falk Symposium 79. 1995.   ISBN 0-7923-8879-8
80. Hofmann AF, Paumgartner G, Stiehl A, eds.: *Bile Acids in Gastroenterology: Basic and Clinical Aspects.* Falk Symposium 80. 1995   ISBN 0-7923-8880-1
81. Riecken EO, Stallmach A, Zeitz M, Heise W, eds.: *Malignancy and Chronic Inflammation in the Gastrointestinal Tract – New Concepts.* Falk Symposium 81. 1995
ISBN 0-7923-8889-5
82. Fleig WE, ed.: *Inflammatory Bowel Diseases: New Developments and Standards.* Falk Symposium 82. 1995   ISBN 0-7923-8890-6

Falk Symposium Series

82B.Paumgartner G, Beuers U, eds.: *Bile Acids in Liver Diseases*. International Falk Workshop. 1995   ISBN 0-7923-8891-7

83. Dobrilla G, Felder M, de Pretis G, eds.: *Advances in Hepatobiliary and Pancreatic Diseases: Special Clinical Topics*. Falk Symposium 83. 1995.   ISBN 0-7923-8892-5

84. Fromm H, Leuschner U, eds.: *Bile Acids – Cholestasis – Gallstones: Advances in Basic and Clinical Bile Acid Research*. Falk Symposium 84. 1995   ISBN 0-7923-8893-3

85. Tytgat GNJ, Bartelsman JFWM, van Deventer SJH, eds.: *Inflammatory Bowel Diseases*. Falk Symposium 85. 1995   ISBN 0-7923-8894-1

86. Berg PA, Leuschner U, eds.: *Bile Acids and Immunology*. Falk Symposium 86. 1996
ISBN 0-7923-8700-7

87. Schmid R, Bianchi L, Blum HE, Gerok W, Maier KP, Stalder GA, eds.: *Acute and Chronic Liver Diseases: Molecular Biology and Clinics*. Falk Symposium 87. 1996
ISBN 0-7923-8701-5

88. Blum HE, Wu GY, Wu CH, eds.: *Molecular Diagnosis and Gene Therapy*. Falk Symposium 88. 1996   ISBN 0-7923-8702-3

88B.Poupon RE, Reichen J, eds.: *Surrogate Markers to Assess Efficacy of TReatment in Chronic Liver Diseases*. International Falk Workshop. 1996   ISBN 0-7923-8705-8

89. Reyes HB, Leuschner U, Arias IM, eds.: *Pregnancy, Sex Hormones and the Liver*. Falk Symposium 89. 1996   ISBN 0-7923-8704-X

89B.Broelsch CE, Burdelski M, Rogiers X, eds.: *Cholestatic Liver Diseases in Children and Adults*. International Falk Workshop. 1996   ISBN 0-7923-8710-4

90. Lam S-K, Paumgartner P, Wang B, eds.: *Update on Hepatobiliary Diseases 1996*. Falk Symposium 90. 1996   ISBN 0-7923-8715-5

91. Hadziselimovic F, Herzog B, eds.: *Inflammatory Bowel Diseases and Chronic Recurrent Abdominal Pain*. Falk Symposium 91. 1996   ISBN 0-7923-8722-8

91B.Alvaro D, Benedetti A, Strazzabosco M, eds.: *Vanishing Bile Duct Syndrome – Pathophysiology and Treatment*. International Falk Workshop. 1996
ISBN 0-7923-8721-X

92. Gerok W, Loginov AS, Pokrowskij VI, eds.: *New Trends in Hepatology 1996*. Falk Symposium 92. 1997   ISBN 0-7923-8723-6

93. Paumgartner G, Stiehl A, Gerok W, eds.: *Bile Acids in Hepatobiliary Diseases – Basic Research and Clinical Application*. Falk Symposium 93. 1997   ISBN 0-7923-8725-2

94. Halter F, Winton D, Wright NA, eds.: *The Gut as a Model in Cell and Molecular Biology*. Falk Symposium 94. 1997   ISBN 0-7923-8726-0

94B.Kruse-Jarres JD, Schölmerich J, eds.: *Zinc and Diseases of the Digestive Tract*. International Falk Workshop. 1997   ISBN 0-7923-8724-4

95. Ewe K, Eckardt VF, Enck P, eds.: *Constipation and Anorectal Insufficiency*. Falk Symposium 95. 1997   ISBN 0-7923-8727-9

96. Andus T, Goebell H, Layer P, Schölmerich J, eds.: *Inflammatory Bowel Disease – from Bench to Bedside*. Falk Symposium 96. 1997   ISBN 0-7923-8728-7

97. Campieri M, Bianchi-Porro G, Fiocchi C, Schölmerich J, eds. *Clinical Challenges in Inflammatory Bowel Diseases: Diagnosis, Prognosis and Treatment*. Falk Symposium 97. 1998   ISBN 0-7923-8733-3

98. Lembcke B, Kruis W, Sartor RB, eds. *Systemic Manifestations of IBD: The Pending Challenge for Subtle Diagnosis and Treatment*. Falk Symposium 98. 1998
ISBN 0-7923-8734-1

Falk Symposium Series

99. Goebell H, Holtmann G, Talley NJ, eds. *Functional Dyspepsia and Irritable Bowel Syndrome: Concepts and Controversies.* Falk Symposium 99. 1998

ISBN 0-7923-8735-X

100. Blum HE, Bode Ch, Bode JCh, Sartor RB, eds. *Gut and the Liver.* Falk Symposium 100. 1998   ISBN 0-7923-8736-8

Printed by Printforce, the Netherlands